Handbook of Medical Statistics

Handbook of Medical Statistics

editor

Ji-Qian Fang
Sun Yat-Sen University, China

World Scientific

NEW JERSEY • LONDON • SINGAPORE • BEIJING • SHANGHAI • HONG KONG • TAIPEI • CHENNAI • TOKYO

Published by

World Scientific Publishing Co. Pte. Ltd.
5 Toh Tuck Link, Singapore 596224
USA office: 27 Warren Street, Suite 401-402, Hackensack, NJ 07601
UK office: 57 Shelton Street, Covent Garden, London WC2H 9HE

Library of Congress Cataloging-in-Publication Data
Names: Fang, Ji-Qian, 1939– editor.
Title: Handbook of medical statistics / edited by Ji-Qian Fang.
Description: Hackensack, NJ : World Scientific, [2017] | Includes bibliographical references and index.
Identifiers: LCCN 2016059285 | ISBN 9789813148956 (hardcover : alk. paper)
Subjects: | MESH: Statistics as Topic--methods | Biomedical Research--methods | Handbooks
Classification: LCC R853.S7 | NLM WA 39 | DDC 610.72/7--dc23
LC record available at https://lccn.loc.gov/2016059285

British Library Cataloguing-in-Publication Data
A catalogue record for this book is available from the British Library.

Typeset by Stallion Press
Email: enquiries@stallionpress.com

Printed in Singapore

PREFACE

One day in May 2010, I received a letter from Dr. Don Mak, World Scientific Co., Singapore. It said, "You published a book on Medical Statistics and Computer Experiments for us in 2005. It is a quite good book and has garnered good reviews. Would you be able to update it to a new edition? Furthermore, we are currently looking for someone to do a handbook on medical statistics, and wondering whether you would have the time to do so ...". In response, I started to update the book of *Medical Statistics and Computer Experiments* and kept the issues of the handbook in mind.

On June 18, 2013, Don wrote to me again, "We discussed back in May 2010 the Medical statistics handbook, which we hope that you can work on after you finished the manuscript for the second edition of *Medical Statistics and Computer Experiments*. Can you please let me know the title of the Handbook, the approx. number of pages, the number of color pages (if any), and the approx. date that you can finish the manuscript? I will arrange to send you an agreement after."

After a brainstorming session, both Don and I agreed to the following: It would be a "handbook" with 500–600 pages, which does not try to "teach" systematically the basic concepts and methods widely used in daily work of medical professionals, but rather a "guidebook" or a "summary book" for learning medical statistics or in other words, a "cyclopedia" for searching for knowledge around medical statistics. In order to make the handbook useful across various fields of readers, it should touch on a wide array of content (even more than a number of textbooks or monographs). The format is much like a dictionary on medical statistics with several items packaged chapterwise by themes; and each item might consist of a few sub-items. The readers are assumed to not be naïve in statistics and medical statistics so that at the end of each chapter, they might be led to some references accordingly, if necessary.

In October 2014, during a national meeting on teaching material of statistics I proposed to publish a Chinese version of the aforementioned handbook first by the China Statistics Publishing Co. and then an English version by the World Scientific Co. Just as we expected, the two companies quickly agreed in a few days.

In January 2015, four leading statisticians in China, Yongyong Xu, Feng Chen, Zhi Geng and Songlin Yu, accepted my invitation to be the co-editors; along with the cohesiveness amongst us, a team of well-known experts were formed and responsible for the 26 pre-designed themes, respectively; among them were senior scholars and young elites, professors and practitioners, at home and abroad. We frequently communicated by internet to reach a group consensus on issues such as content and format. Based on an individual strengths and group harmonization the Chinese version was successfully completed in a year and was immediately followed with work on the English version.

Now that the English version has finally been completed, I would sincerely thank Dr. Don Mak and his colleagues at the World Scientific Co. for their persistency in organizing this handbook and great trust in our team of authors. I hope the readers will really benefit from this handbook, and would welcome any feedback they may have (handbookmedistat@126.com).

Jiqian Fang
June 2016 in Guangzhou, China

ABOUT THE EDITORS

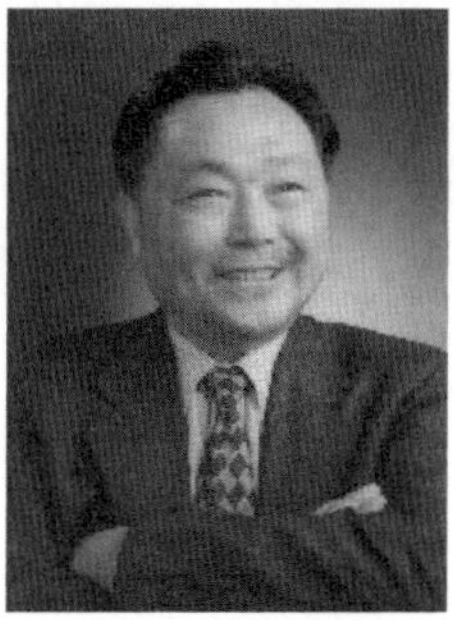

Ji-Qian Fang was honorably awarded as a National Teaching Master of China by the Central Government of China in 2009 due to his outstanding achievements in university education. Professor Fang received his BS in Mathematics from Fu-Dan University, China in 1961, and his PhD in Biostatistics from the University of California at Berkeley, U.S. in 1985. He served as Professor and Director of the Department of Biomathematics and Biostatistics at Beijing Medical University from 1985 to 1991 and since 1991, has been the Professor and Director of the Department of Medical Statistics at Sun Yat-Sen Medical University (now Sun Yat- Sen University). He also was an Adjunct Professor at Chinese University of Hong Kong from 1993 to 2009.

Professor Fang has completed 19 national and international research projects, and has received 14 awards for progression in research from the Provincial and Central Government. He is the Chief Editor of national textbooks of *Advanced Mathematics*, *Mathematical Statistics for Medicine* (1st and 2nd editions), *Health Statistics* (5–7th editions) for undergraduate program, and of *Statistical Methods for Bio-medical Research*, *Medical Statistics and Computer Experiments* (1st–4th editions, in Chinese and 1st and 2nd editions in English) for postgraduate program. The course of *Medical Statistics* led by Professor Fang has been recognized as the National Recommended Course in 2008 and National Demonstration Bi-lingual Course in 2010.

Professor Fang is the founder of Group China of the International Biometric Society, and also the founder of Committee of Medical Statistics Education of the Chinese Association of Health Informatics.

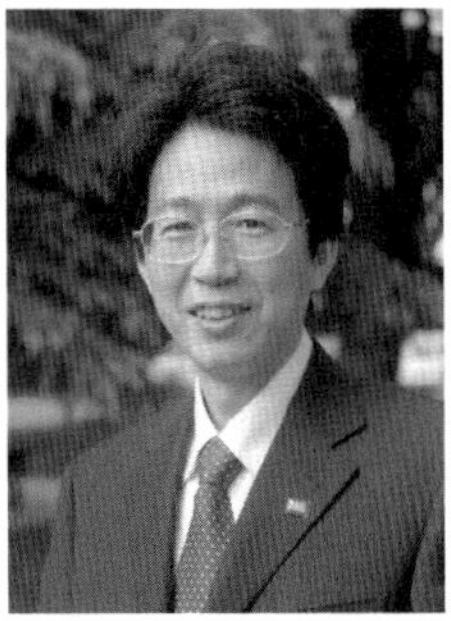

Feng Chen is Professor of Biostatistics in Nanjing Medical University. He earned his BSc in Mathematics from Sun Yat-Sen University in 1983, and continued on to receive an MSc in Biostatistics from Shanghai Second Medical University, and PhD in Biostatistics from West China University of Medical Sciences, 1994.

Dr. Feng Chen dedicated himself in statistical theory and methods in medical research, especially in the analysis of non-independent data, high-dimensional data and clinical trials. He studied multilevel models in London University in 1996. As a Visiting Scholar, he was engaged in the Genome-wide Association Study (GWAS) in Harvard University from April 2008 to March 2010. As a statistician, he was involved in writing dozens of grant, in charge of design, data management and statistical analysis. He has more than 180 papers and 18 textbooks and monographs published.

He is now the Chairperson of the China Association of Biostatistics, the Chairperson of China Clinical Trial Statistics (CCTS) working group, Vice Chair of IBS-China, member of the Drafting Committee of China Statistical Principles for Clinical Trials. He has been appointed Dean of the School of Public Health, Nanjing Medical University from 2012 and has been awarded as Excellent Teacher and Youth Specialist with Outstanding contribution in Jiangsu.

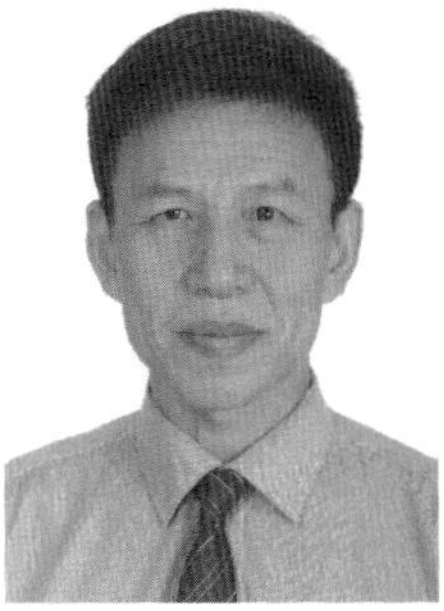

Zhi Geng is a Professor at the School of Mathematical Sciences in Peking University. He graduated from Shanghai Jiaotong University in 1982 and got his PhD degree from Kyushu University in Japan in 1989. He became an ISI elected member in 1996 and obtained the National Excellent youth fund of China in 1998. His research interests are causal inference, multivariate analysis, missing data analysis, biostatistics and epidemiological methods. The research works are published in journals of statistics, biostatistics, artificial intelligence and machine learning and so on.

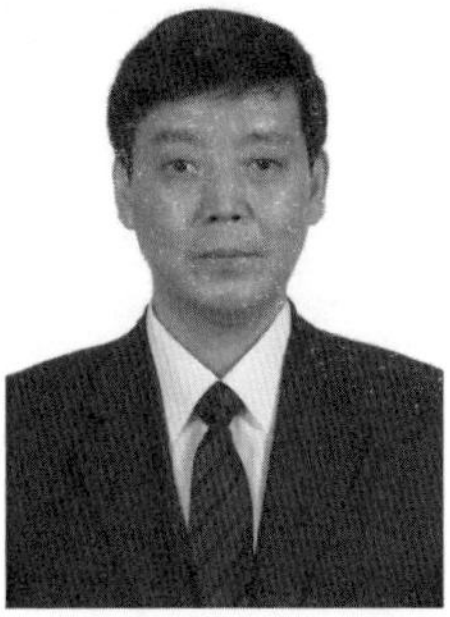

Yongyong Xu is Professor of Health Statistics and Head of the Institute of Health Informatics in Fourth Military Medical University. He is the Vice President of the Chinese Society of Statistics Education, Vice Director of the Committee of Sixth National Statistics Textbook Compilation Committee, the Chair of the Committee of Health Information Standardization of Chinese Health Information Society. For more than 30 years his research has mainly involved medical statistics and statistical methods in health administration. He takes a deep interest in the relationship between health statistics and health informatics in recent years. He is now responsible for the project of national profiling framework of health information and is also involved in other national projects on health information standardization.

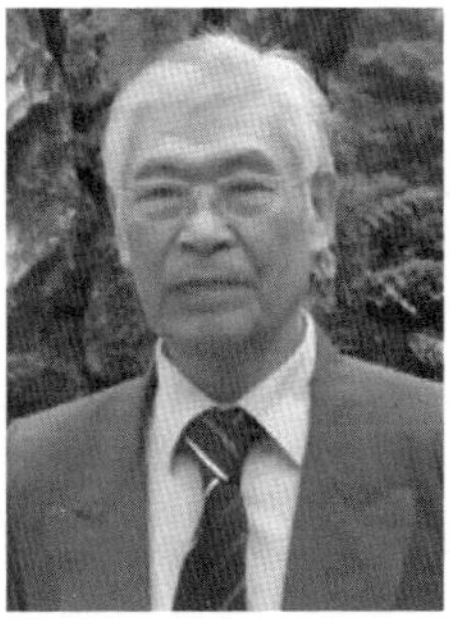

Songlin Yu is Professor of Medical Statistics of Tongji Medical College (TJMU), Huazhong University of Science and Technology in Wuhan, China. He graduated from Wuhan Medical College in 1960, and studied in NCI, NIH, the USA in 1982–1983. He was Vice-Chairman of the Department of Health Statistics, TJMU, from 1985 to 1994.

He has written several monographs: *Statistical Methods for Field Studies in Medicine* (1985), *Survival Analysis in Clinical Researches* (1993), *Analysis of Repeated Measures Data* (2001), *R Software and its Use in Environmental Epidemiology* (2014). He was the Editor-in-Chief of *Medical Statistics for Medical Graduates*, Vice Chief Editor of the book *Medical Statistics and Computer Experiments*, Editor of *Health Statistics*, *Medical Statistics* for medical students.

He served as one of the principal investigators of several programs: Multivariate Analytical Methods for Discrete Data (NSFC), Comparative Cost-Benefit Analysis between Two Strategies for Controlling Schistosomiasis in Two Areas in Hubei Province (TDR, WHO), Effects of Economic System Reformation on Schistosomiasis Control in Lake Areas of China (TDR, WHO), Research on Effects of Smoking Control in a Medical University (Sino Health Project organization, the USA). He suggested a method for calculating average age of menarche. He discovered the remote side effect of vacuum cephalo-extractor on intelligence development of chidren, etc.

CONTENTS

CHAPTER 1

PROBABILITY AND PROBABILITY DISTRIBUTIONS

Jian Shi*

1.1. The Axiomatic Definition of Probability[1,2]

There had been various definitions and methods of calculating probability at the early stage of the development of probability theory, such as those of classical probability, geometric probability, the frequency and so on. In 1933, Kolmogorov established the axiomatic system of probability theory based on the measure theory, which laid the foundation of modern probability theory.

The axiomatic system of probability theory: Let Ω be the set of point ω, and $\mathcal{F}$ be the set of subset A of Ω. $\mathcal{F}$ is called an σ-algebra of Ω if it satisfies the conditions:

(i) $\Omega \in \mathcal{F}$;
(ii) if $A \in \mathcal{F}$, then its complement set $A^c \in \mathcal{F}$;
(iii) if $A_n \in \mathcal{F}$ for $n = 1, 2, \ldots$, then $\cup_{n=1}^{\infty} A_n \in \mathcal{F}$.

Let $P(A)(A \in \mathcal{F})$ be a real-valued function on the σ-algebra $\mathcal{F}$. Suppose $P(\,)$ satisfies:

(1) $0 \leq P(A) \leq 1$ for every $A \in \mathcal{F}$;
(2) $P(\Omega) = 1$;
(3) $P(\cup_{n=1}^{\infty} A_n) = \sum_{n=1}^{\infty} P(A_n)$ holds for $A_n \in \mathcal{F}, n = 1, 2, \ldots$, where $A_i \cap A_j = \emptyset$ for $i \neq j$, and $\emptyset$ is the empty set.

Then, P is a probability measure on $\mathcal{F}$, or probability in short. In addition, a set in $\mathcal{F}$ is called an event, and $(\Omega, \mathcal{F}, P)$ is called a probability space.

Some basic properties of probability are as follows:

*Corresponding author: jshi@iss.ac.cn

1. $P(\emptyset) = 0$;
2. For events A and B, if $B \subseteq A$, then $P(A - B) = P(A) - P(B)$, $P(A) \geq P(B)$, and particularly, $P(A^c) = 1 - P(A)$;
3. For any events $A_1, \ldots, A_n$ and $n \geq 1$, there holds

$$P(\cup_{i=1}^{n} A_i) \leq \sum_{i=1}^{n} P(A_i);$$

4. For any events A and B, there holds

$$P(A \cup B) = P(A) + P(B) - P(A \cap B)$$

Suppose a variable X may represent different values under different conditions due to accidental, uncontrolled factors of uncertainty and randomness, but the probability that the value of X falls in a certain range is fixed, then X is a random variable.

The random variable X is called a discrete random variable if it represents only a finite or countable number of values with fixed probabilities. Suppose X takes values $x_1, x_2, \ldots$ with probability $p_i = P\{X = x_i\}$ for $i = 1, 2, \ldots$, respectively. Then, it holds that:

(1) $p_i \geq 0, i = 1, 2, \ldots$; and
(2) $\sum_{i=1}^{\infty} p_i = 1$.

The random variable X is called a continuous random variable if it can represent values from the entire range of an interval and the probability for X falling into any sub-interval is fixed.

For a continuous random variable X, if there exists a non-negative integrable function $f(x)$, such that

$$P\{a \leq X \leq b\} = \int_a^b f(x)dx,$$

holds for any $-\infty < a < b < \infty$, and

$$\int_{-\infty}^{\infty} f(x)dx = 1,$$

then $f(x)$ is called the density function of X.

For a random variable X, if $F(x) = P\{X \leq x\}$ for $-\infty < x < \infty$, then $F(x)$ is called the distribution function of X. When X is a discrete random variable, its distribution function is $F(x) = \sum_{i:x_i \leq x} p_i$ and similarly, when X is a continuous random variable, its distribution function is $F(x) = \int_{-\infty}^{x} f(t)dt$.

1.2. Uniform Distribution[2,3,4]

If the random variable X can take values from the interval [a, b] and the probabilities for X taking each value in [a, b] are equal, then we say X follows the uniform distribution over $[a,b]$ and denote it as $X \stackrel{d}{=} U(a,b)$. In particular, when $a = 0$ and $b = 1$, we say X follows the standard uniform distribution $U(0,1)$. The uniform distribution is the simplest continuous distribution.

If $X \stackrel{d}{=} U(a,b)$, then the density function of X is

$$f(x;a,b) = \begin{cases} \frac{1}{b-a}, & \text{if } a \le x \le b, \\ 0, & \text{otherwise}, \end{cases}$$

and the distribution function of X is

$$F(x;a,b) = \begin{cases} 0, & x < a, \\ \frac{x-a}{b-a}, & a \le x \le b, \\ 1, & x > b. \end{cases}$$

A uniform distribution has the following properties:

1. If $X \stackrel{d}{=} U(a,b)$, then the k-th moment of X is

$$E(X^k) = \frac{b^{k+1} - a^{k+1}}{(k+1)(b-a)}, \quad k = 1, 2, \ldots$$

2. If $X \stackrel{d}{=} U(a,b)$, then the k-th central moment of X is

$$E((X - E(X))^k) = \begin{cases} 0, & \text{when } k \text{ is odd}, \\ \frac{(b-a)^k}{2^k(k+1)}, & \text{when } k \text{ is even}. \end{cases}$$

3. If $X \stackrel{d}{=} U(a,b)$, then the skewness of X is $s = 0$ and the kurtosis of X is $\kappa = -6/5$.
4. If $X \stackrel{d}{=} U(a,b)$, then its moment-generating function and characteristic function are

$$M(t) = E(e^{tX}) = \frac{e^{bt} - e^{at}}{(b-a)t}, \quad \text{and}$$

$$\psi(t) = E(e^{itX}) = \frac{e^{ibt} - e^{iat}}{i(b-a)t},$$

respectively.

5. If X_1 and X_2 are independent and identically distributed random variables both with the distribution $U(-\frac{1}{2},\frac{1}{2})$, then the density function of $X = X_1 + X_2$, is

$$f(x) = \begin{cases} 1+x, & -1 \le x \le 0, \\ 1-x, & 0 \le x \le 1. \end{cases}$$

This is the so-called "Triangular distribution".

6. If X_1, X_2, and X_3 are independent and identically distributed random variables with common distribution $U(-\frac{1}{2},\frac{1}{2})$, then the density function of $X = X_1 + X_2 + X_3$ is

$$f(x) = \begin{cases} \frac{1}{2}(x+\frac{3}{2})^2, & -\frac{3}{2} \le x \le -\frac{1}{2}, \\ \frac{3}{4} - x^2, & -\frac{1}{2} < x \le \frac{1}{2}, \\ \frac{1}{2}(x-\frac{3}{2})^2, & \frac{1}{2} < x \le \frac{3}{2}, \\ 0, & \text{otherwise}. \end{cases}$$

The shape of the above density function resembles that of a normal density function, which we will discuss next.

7. If $X \stackrel{d}{=} U(0,1)$, then $1 - X \stackrel{d}{=} U(0,1)$.
8. Assume that a distribution function F is strictly increasing and continuous, F^{-1} is the inverse function of F, and $X \stackrel{d}{=} U(0,1)$. In this case, the distribution function of the random variable $Y = F^{-1}(X)$ is F.

In stochastic simulations, since it is easy to generate pseudo random numbers of the standard uniform distribution (e.g. the congruential method), pseudo random numbers of many common distributions can therefore be generated using property 8, especially for cases when inverse functions of distributions have explicit forms.

1.3. Normal Distribution[2,3,4]

If the density function of the random variable X is

$$\phi\left(\frac{x-\mu}{\sigma}\right) = \frac{1}{\sqrt{2\pi}\sigma}\exp\left\{-\frac{(x-\mu)^2}{2\sigma^2}\right\},$$

where $-\infty < x, \mu < \infty$ and $\sigma > 0$, then we say X follows the normal distribution and denote it as $X \stackrel{d}{=} N(\mu,\sigma^2)$. In particular, when $\mu = 0$ and $\sigma = 1$, we say that X follows the standard normal distribution $N(0,1)$.

If $X \stackrel{d}{=} N(\mu, \sigma^2)$, then the distribution function of X is

$$\Phi\left(\frac{x-\mu}{\sigma}\right) = \int_{-\infty}^{x} \phi\left(\frac{t-\mu}{\sigma}\right) dt.$$

If X follows the standard normal distribution, $N(0,1)$, then the density and distribution functions of X are $\phi(x)$ and $\Phi(x)$, respectively.

The Normal distribution is the most common continuous distribution and has the following properties:

1. If $X \stackrel{d}{=} N(\mu, \sigma^2)$, then $Y = \frac{X-\mu}{\sigma} \stackrel{d}{=} N(0,1)$, and if $X \stackrel{d}{=} N(0,1)$, then $Y = a + \sigma X \stackrel{d}{=} N(a, \sigma^2)$.
   Hence, a general normal distribution can be converted to the standard normal distribution by a linear transformation.
2. If $X \stackrel{d}{=} N(\mu, \sigma^2)$, then the expectation of X is $E(X) = \mu$ and the variance of X is $\mathrm{Var}(X) = \sigma^2$.
3. If $X \stackrel{d}{=} N(\mu, \sigma^2)$, then the k-th central moment of X is
$$E((X-\mu)^k) = \begin{cases} 0, & k \text{ is odd}, \\ \frac{k!}{2^{k/2}(k/2)!}\sigma^k, & k \text{ is even}. \end{cases}$$
4. If $X \stackrel{d}{=} N(\mu, \sigma^2)$, then the moments of X are
$$E(X^{2k-1}) = \sigma^{2k-1} \sum_{i=1}^{k} \frac{(2k-1)!!\mu^{2i-1}}{(2i-1)!(k-i)!2^{k-i}},$$
   and
$$E(X^{2k}) = \sigma^{2k} \sum_{i=0}^{k} \frac{(2k)!\mu^{2i}}{(2i)!(k-i)!2^{k-i}}$$
   for $k = 1, 2, \ldots$.
5. If $X \stackrel{d}{=} N(\mu, \sigma^2)$, then the skewness and the kurtosis of X are both 0, i.e. $s = \kappa = 0$. This property can be used to check whether a distribution is normal.
6. If $X \stackrel{d}{=} N(\mu, \sigma^2)$, then the moment-generating function and the characteristic function of X are $M(t) = \exp\{t\mu + \frac{1}{2}t^2\sigma^2\}$ and $\psi(t) = \exp\{it\mu - \frac{1}{2}t^2\sigma^2\}$, respectively.
7. If $X \stackrel{d}{=} N(\mu, \sigma^2)$, then
$$a + bX \stackrel{d}{=} N(a + b\mu, b^2\sigma^2).$$

8. If $X_i \overset{d}{=} N(\mu_i, \sigma_i^2)$ for $1 \leq i \leq n$, and $X_1, X_2, \ldots, X_n$ are mutually independent, then

$$\sum_{i=1}^{n} X_i \overset{d}{=} N\left(\sum_{i=1}^{n} \mu_i, \sum_{i=1}^{n} \sigma_i^2\right).$$

9. If $X_1, X_2, \ldots, X_n$ represent a random sample of the population $N(\mu, \sigma^2)$, then the sample mean $\bar{X}_n = \frac{1}{n}\sum_{i=1}^{n} X_i$ satisfies $\bar{X}_n \overset{d}{=} N(\mu, \frac{\sigma^2}{n})$.

The central limit theorem: Suppose that $X_1, \ldots, X_n$ are independent and identically distributed random variables, and that $\mu = E(X_1)$ and $0 < \sigma^2 = \mathrm{Var}(X_1) < \infty$, then the distribution of $T_n = \sqrt{n}(\bar{X}_n - \mu)/\sigma$ is asymptotically standard normal when n is large enough.

The central limit theorem reveals that limit distributions of statistics in many cases are (asymptotically) normal. Therefore, the normal distribution is the most widely used distribution in statistics.

The value of the normal distribution is the whole real axis, i.e. from negative infinity to positive infinity. However, many variables in real problems take positive values, for example, height, voltage and so on. In these cases, the logarithm of these variables can be regarded as being normally distributed.

Log-normal distribution: Suppose $X > 0$. If $\ln X \overset{d}{\sim} N(\mu, \sigma^2)$, then we say X follows the log-normal distribution and denote it as $X \overset{d}{\sim} LN(\mu, \sigma^2)$.

1.4. Exponential Distribution[2,3,4]

If the density function of the random variable X is

$$f(x) = \begin{cases} \lambda e^{-\lambda x}, & x \geq 0, \\ 0, & x < 0, \end{cases}$$

where $\lambda > 0$, then we say X follows the exponential distribution and denote it as $X \overset{d}{=} E(\lambda)$. Particularly, when $\lambda = 1$, we say X follows the standard exponential distribution $E(1)$.

If $X \overset{d}{=} E(\lambda)$, then its distribution function is

$$F(x; \lambda) = \begin{cases} 1 - e^{-\lambda x}, & x \geq 0, \\ 0, & x < 0. \end{cases}$$

Exponential distribution is an important distribution in reliability. The life of an electronic product generally follows an exponential distribution. When the life of a product follows the exponential distribution $E(\lambda)$, λ is called the failure rate of the product.

Exponential distribution has the following properties:

1. If $X \stackrel{d}{=} E(\lambda)$, then the k-th moment of X is $E(X^k) = k\lambda^{-k}, k = 1, 2, \ldots$.
2. If $X \stackrel{d}{=} E(\lambda)$, then $E(X) = \lambda^{-1}$ and $\mathrm{Var}(X) = \lambda^{-2}$.
3. If $X \stackrel{d}{=} E(\lambda)$, then its skewness is $s = 2$ and its kurtosis is $\kappa = 6$.
4. If $X \stackrel{d}{=} E(\lambda)$, then the moment-generating function and the characteristic function of X are $M(t) = \frac{\lambda}{\lambda - t}$ for $t < \lambda$ and $\psi(t) = \frac{\lambda}{\lambda - it}$, respectively.
5. If $X \stackrel{d}{=} E(1)$, then $\lambda^{-1}X \stackrel{d}{=} E(\lambda)$ for $\lambda > 0$.
6. If $X \stackrel{d}{=} E(\lambda)$, then for any $x > 0$ and $y > 0$, there holds
$$P\{X > x + y | X > y\} = P\{X > x\}.$$
This is the so-called "memoryless property" of exponential distribution. If the life distribution of a product is exponential, no matter how long it has been used, the remaining life of the product follows the same distribution as that of a new product if it does not fail at the present time.
7. If $X \stackrel{d}{=} E(\lambda)$, then for any $x > 0$, there hold $E(X|X > a) = a + \lambda^{-1}$ and $\mathrm{Var}(X|X > a) = \lambda^{-2}$.
8. If x and y are independent and identically distributed as $E(\lambda)$, then $\min(X, Y)$ is independent of $X - Y$ and
$$\{X|X + Y = z\} \stackrel{d}{\sim} U(0, z).$$
9. If $X_1, X_2, \ldots, X_n$ are random samples of the population $E(\lambda)$, let $X_{(1,n)} \le X_{(2,n)} \le \cdots \le X_{(n,n)}$ be the order statistics of $X_1, X_2, \ldots, X_n$. Write $Y_k = (n - k + 1)(X_{(k,n)} - X_{(k-1,n)}), 1 \le k \le n$, where $X_{(0,n)} = 0$. Then, $Y_1, Y_2, \ldots, Y_n$ are independent and identically distributed as $E(\lambda)$.
10. If $X_1, X_2, \ldots, X_n$ are random samples of the population of $E(\lambda)$, then $\sum_{i=1}^{n} X_i \stackrel{d}{\sim} \Gamma(n, \lambda)$, where $\Gamma(n, \lambda)$ is the Gamma distribution in Sec. 1.12.
11. If then $Y \stackrel{d}{\sim} U(0, 1)$, then $X = -\ln(Y) \stackrel{d}{\sim} E(1)$. Therefore, it is easy to generate random numbers with exponential distribution through uniform random numbers.

1.5. Weibull Distribution[2,3,4]

If the density function of the random variable X is

$$f(x; \alpha, \beta, \delta) = \begin{cases} \frac{\alpha}{\beta}(x - \delta)^{\alpha - 1} \exp\{-\frac{(x-\delta)^\alpha}{\beta}\}, & x \ge \delta, \\ 0, & x < \delta, \end{cases}$$

then we say X follows the Weibull distribution and denote it as $X \overset{d}{\sim} W(\alpha, \beta, \delta)$. Where δ is location parameter, $\alpha > 0$ is shape parameter, $\beta > 0$, is scale parameter. For simplicity, we denote $W(\alpha, \beta, 0)$ as $W(\alpha, \beta)$.

Particularly, when $\delta = 0, \alpha = 1$, Weibull distribution $W(1, \beta)$ is transformed into Exponential distribution $E(1/\beta)$.

If $X \overset{d}{\sim} W(\alpha, \beta, \delta)$, then its distribution function is

$$F(x; \alpha, \beta, \delta) = \begin{cases} 1 - \exp\{-\frac{(x-\delta)^\alpha}{\beta}\}, & x \geq \delta, \\ 0, & x < \delta, \end{cases}$$

Weibull distribution is an important distribution in reliability theory. It is often used to describe the life distribution of a product , such as electronic product and wear product.

Weibull distribution has the following properties:

1. If $X \overset{d}{\sim} E(1)$, then

$$Y = (X\beta)^{1/\alpha} + \delta \overset{d}{\sim} W(\alpha, \beta, \delta)$$

Hence, Weibull distribution and exponential distribution can be converted to each other by transformation.

2. If $X \overset{d}{\sim} W(\alpha, \beta)$, then the k-th moment of X is

$$E(X^k) = \Gamma\left(1 + \frac{k}{\alpha}\right)\beta^{k/\alpha},$$

where $\Gamma(\cdot)$ is the Gamma function.

3. If $X \overset{d}{\sim} W(\alpha, \beta, \delta)$, then

$$E(X) = \Gamma\left(1 + \frac{1}{\alpha}\right)\beta^{1/\alpha} + \delta,$$

$$\mathrm{Var}(X) = \left(\Gamma\left(1 + \frac{2}{\alpha}\right) - \Gamma^2\left(1 + \frac{1}{\alpha}\right)\right)\beta^{2/\alpha}.$$

4. Suppose $X_1, X_2, \ldots, X_n$ are mutually independent and identically distributed random variables with common distribution $W(\alpha, \beta, \delta)$, then

$$X_{1,n} = \min(X_1, X_2, \ldots, X_n) \overset{d}{\sim} W(\alpha, \beta/n, \delta),$$

whereas, if $X_{1,n} \overset{d}{\sim} W(\alpha, \beta/n, \delta)$, then $X_1 \overset{d}{\sim} W(\alpha, \beta, \delta)$.

1.5.1. *The application of Weibull distribution in reliability*

The shape parameter α usually describes the failure mechanism of a product. Weibull distributions with $\alpha < 1$ are called "early failure" life distributions, Weibull distributions with $\alpha = 1$ are called "occasional failure" life distributions, and Weibull distributions with $\alpha > 1$ are called "wear-out (aging) failure" life distributions.

If $X \overset{d}{\sim} W(\alpha, \beta, \delta)$ then its reliability function is

$$R(x) = 1 - F(x; \alpha, \beta, \delta) = \begin{cases} \exp\{-\frac{(x-\delta)^\alpha}{\beta}\}, & x \geq \delta, \\ 1, & x < \delta. \end{cases}$$

When the reliability R of a product is known, then

$$x_R = \delta + \beta^{1/\alpha}(-\ln R)^{1/\alpha}$$

is the Q-percentile life of the product.

If $R = 0.5$, then $x_{0.5} = \delta + \beta^{1/\alpha}(\ln 2)^{1/\alpha}$ is the median life; if $R = e^{-1}$, then $x_{e^{-1}}\delta + \beta^{1/\alpha}$ is the characteristic life; $R = \exp\{-\Gamma^\alpha(1 + \alpha^{-1})\}$, then $x_R = E(X)$, that is mean life.

The failure rate of Weibull distribution $W(\alpha, \beta, \delta)$ is

$$\lambda(x) = \frac{f(x; \alpha, \beta, \delta)}{R(x)} = \begin{cases} \frac{\alpha}{\beta}(x - \delta)^{\alpha - 1}, & x \geq \delta, \\ 0, & x < \delta. \end{cases}$$

The mean rate of failure is

$$\bar{\lambda}(x) = \frac{1}{x - \delta}\int_\delta^x \lambda(t)dt = \begin{cases} \frac{(x-\delta)^{\alpha-1}}{\beta}, & x \geq \delta, \\ 0, & x < \delta. \end{cases}$$

Particularly, the failure rate of Exponential distribution $E(\lambda) = W(1, 1/\lambda)$ is constant λ.

1.6. Binomial Distribution[2,3,4]

We say random variable follows the binomial distribution, if it takes discrete values and

$$P\{X = k\} = C_n^k p^k (1 - p)^{n-k}, \quad k = 0, 1, \ldots, n,$$

where n is positive integer, C_n^k is combinatorial number, $0 \leq p \leq 1$. We denote it as $X \overset{d}{\sim} B(n, p)$.

Consider n times independent trials, each with two possible outcomes "success" and "failure". Each trial can only have one of the two outcomes. The probability of success is p. Let X be the total number of successes in this

n trials, then $X \overset{d}{\sim} B(n,p)$. Particularly, if $n = 1, B(1,p)$ is called Bernoulli distribution or two-point distribution. It is the simplest discrete distribution.

Binomial distribution is a common discrete distribution.

If $X \overset{d}{\sim} B(n,p)$, then its density function is

$$B(x;n,p) = \begin{cases} \sum_{k=0}^{\min([x],n)} C_n^k p^k q^{n-k}, & x \geq 0, \\ 0, & x < 0, \end{cases}$$

where $[x]$ is integer part of $x, q = 1 - p$.

Let $B_x(a,b) = \int_0^x t^{a-1}(1-t)^{b-1}dt$ be the incomplete Beta function, where $0 < x < 1, a > 0, b > 0$, then $B(a,b) = B_1(a,b)$ is the Beta function. Let $I_x(a,b) = B_x(a,b)/B(a,b)$ be the ratio of incomplete Beta function. Then the binomial distribution function can be represented as follows:

$$B(x;n,p) = 1 - I_p(x+1, n-[x]), \quad 0 \leq x \leq n.$$

Binomial distribution has the following properties:

1. Let $b(k;n,p) = C_n^k p^k q^{n-k}$ for $0 \leq k \leq n$. If $k \leq [(n+1)p]$, then $b(k;n,p) \geq b(k-1;n,p)$; if $k > [(n+1)p]$, then $b(k;n,p) < b(k-1;n,p)$.
2. When $p = 0.5$, Binomial distribution $B(n, 0.5)$ is a symmetric distribution; when $p \neq 0.5$, Binomial distribution $B(n,p)$ is asymmetric.
3. Suppose $X_1, X_2, \ldots, X_n$ are mutually independent and identically distributed Bernoulli random variables with parameter p, then
$$Y = \sum_{i=1}^{n} X_i \overset{d}{\sim} B(n,p).$$
4. If $X \overset{d}{\sim} B(n,p)$, then
$$E(X) = np, \quad \mathrm{Var}(X) = npq.$$
5. If $X \overset{d}{\sim} B(n,p)$, then the k-th moment of X is
$$E(X^k) = \sum_{i=1}^{k} S_2(k,i) P_n^i p^i,$$
where $S_2(k,i)$ is the second order Stirling number, P_n^k is number of permutations.
6. If $X \overset{d}{\sim} B(n,p)$, then its skewness is $s = (1-2p)/(npq)^{1/2}$ and kurtosis is $\kappa = (1-6pq)/(npq)$.
7. If $X \overset{d}{\sim} B(n,p)$, then the moment-generating function and the characteristic function of X are $M(t) = (q + pe^t)^n$ and $\psi(t) = (q + pe^{it})^n$, respectively.

8. When n and x are fixed, the Binomial distribution function $b(x; n, p)$ is a monotonically decreasing function with respect to $p(0 < p < 1)$.
9. If $X_i \overset{d}{\sim} B(n_i, p)$ for $1 \le i \le k$, and $X_1, X_2, \ldots, X_k$ are mutually independent, then $X = \sum_{i=1}^k X_i \overset{d}{\sim} B(\sum_{i=1}^k n_i, p)$.

1.7. Multinomial Distribution[2,3,4]

If an $n(n \ge 2)$-dimensional random vector $\boldsymbol{X} = (X_1, \ldots, X_n)$ satisfies the following conditions:

(1) $X_i \ge 0$, $1 \le n$, and $\sum_{i=1}^n X_i = N$;
(2) Suppose $m_1, m_2, \ldots, m_n$ are any non-negative integers with $\sum_{i=1}^n m_i = N$ and the probability of the following event is $P\{X_1 = m_1, \ldots, X_n = m_n\} = \frac{N!}{m_1! \cdots m_n!} \Pi_{i=1}^n p_i^{m_i}$,

where $p_i \ge 0, 1 \le i \le n, \sum_{i=1}^n p_i = 1$, then we say X follows the multinomial distribution and denote it as $\boldsymbol{X} \overset{d}{\sim} PN(N; p_1, \ldots, p_n)$.

Particularly, when $n = 2$, multinomial distribution degenerates to binomial distribution.

Suppose a jar has balls with n kinds of colors. Every time, a ball is drawn randomly from the jar and then put back to the jar. The probability for the ith color ball being drawn is $p_i, 1 \le i \le n, \sum_{i=1}^n p_i = 1$. Assume that balls are drawn and put back for N times and X_i is denoted as the number of drawings of the ith color ball, then the random vector $\boldsymbol{X} = (X_1, \ldots, X_n)$ follows the Multinomial distribution $PN(N; p_1, \ldots, p_n)$.

Multinomial distribution is a common multivariate discrete distribution.

Multinomial distribution has the following properties:

1. If $(X_1, \ldots, X_n) \overset{d}{\sim} PN(N; p_1, \ldots, p_n)$, let $X_{i+1}^* = \sum_{j=i+1}^n X_i, p_{i+1}^* = \sum_{j=i+1}^n p_i$, $1 \le i < n$, then

   (i) $(X_1, \ldots, X_i, X_{i+1}^*) \overset{d}{\sim} PN(N; p_1, \ldots, p_i, p_{i+1}^*)$,
   (ii) $X_i \overset{d}{\sim} B(N, p_i), 1 \le i \le n$.

   More generally, let $1 = j_0 < j_1 < \cdots < j_m = n$, and $\tilde{X}_k = \sum_{i=j_{k-1}+1}^{j_k} X_i, \tilde{p}_k = \sum_{i=j_{k-1}+1}^{j_k} p_i, 1 \le k \le m$, then $(\tilde{X}_1, \ldots, \tilde{X}_m) \overset{d}{\sim} PN(N; \tilde{p}_1, \ldots, \tilde{p}_m)$.

2. If $(X_1, \ldots, X_n) \overset{d}{\sim} PN(N; p_1, \ldots, p_n)$, then its moment-generating function and the characteristic function of are

$$M(t_1, \ldots, t_n) = \left(\sum_{j=1}^{n} p_j e^{t_j}\right)^N \quad \text{and} \quad \psi(t_1, \ldots, t_n) = \left(\sum_{j=1}^{n} p_j e^{it_j}\right)^N,$$

respectively.

3. If $(X_1, \ldots, X_n) \overset{d}{\sim} PN(N; p_1, \ldots, p_n)$, then for $n > 1, 1 \leq k < n$,

$$(X_1, \ldots, X_k | X_{k+1} = m_{k+1}, \ldots, X_n = m_n) \overset{d}{\sim} PN(N - M; p_1^*, \ldots, p_k^*),$$

where

$$M = \sum_{i=k+1}^{n} m_i, \quad 0 < M < N,$$

$$p_j^* = \frac{p_j}{\sum_{i=1}^{k} p_i}, \quad 1 \leq j \leq k.$$

4. If X_i follows Poisson distribution $P(\lambda_i), 1 \leq i \leq n$, and $X_1, \ldots, X_n$ are mutually independent, then for any given positive integer N, there holds

$$\left(X_1, \ldots, X_n \middle| \sum_{i=1}^{n} X_i = N\right) \overset{d}{\sim} PN(N; p_1, \ldots, p_n),$$

where $p_i = \lambda_i / \sum_{j=1}^{n} \lambda_j, 1 \leq i \leq n$.

1.8. Poisson Distribution[2,3,4]

If random variable X takes non-negative integer values, and the probability is

$$P\{X = k\} = \frac{\lambda^k}{k!} e^{-\lambda}, \quad \lambda > 0, \quad k = 0, 1, \ldots,$$

then we say X follows the Poisson distribution and denote it as $X \overset{d}{\sim} P(\lambda)$.

If $X \overset{d}{\sim} P(\lambda)$, then its distribution function is

$$P\{X \leq x\} = P(x; \lambda) = \sum_{k=0}^{[x]} p(k; \lambda),$$

where $p(k; \lambda) = e^{-\lambda} \lambda^k / k!$, $k = 0, 1, \ldots$.

Poisson distribution is an important distribution in queuing theory. For example, the number of the purchase of the ticket arriving in ticket window in a fixed interval of time approximately follows Poisson distribution. Poisson distribution have a wide range of applications in physics, finance, insurance and other fields.

Poisson distribution has the following properties:

1. If $k < \lambda$, then $p(k;\lambda) > p(k-1;\lambda)$; if $k > \lambda$, then $p(k;\lambda) < p(k-1;\lambda)$. If λ is not an integer, then $p(k;\lambda)$ has a maximum value at $k = [\lambda]$; if λ is an integer, then $p(k,\lambda)$ has a maximum value at $k = \lambda$ and $\lambda - 1$.
2. When x is fixed, $P(x;\lambda)$ is a non-increasing function with respect to λ, that is

$$P(x;\lambda_1) \geq P(x;\lambda_2) \quad \text{if } \lambda_1 < \lambda_2.$$

When λ and x change at the same time, then

$$\begin{aligned} P(x;\lambda) &\geq P(x-1;\lambda-1) \quad \text{if } x \leq \lambda - 1, \\ P(x;\lambda) &\leq P(x-1;\lambda-1) \quad \text{if } x \geq \lambda. \end{aligned}$$

3. If $X \overset{d}{\sim} P(\lambda)$, then the k-th moment of X is $E(X^k) = \sum_{i=1}^{k} S_2(k,i)\lambda^i$, where $S_2(k,i)$ is the second order Stirling number.
4. If $X \overset{d}{\sim} P(\lambda)$, then $E(X) = \lambda$ and $\text{Var}(X) = \lambda$. The expectation and variance being equal is an important feature of Poisson distribution.
5. If $X \overset{d}{\sim} P(\lambda)$, then its skewness is $s = \lambda^{-1/2}$ and its kurtosis is $\kappa = \lambda^{-1}$.
6. If $X \overset{d}{\sim} P(\lambda)$, then the moment-generating function and the characteristic function of X are $M(t) = \exp\{\lambda(e^t - 1)\}$ and $\psi(t) = \exp\{\lambda(e^{\mathrm{i}t} - 1)\}$, respectively.
7. If $X_1, X_2, \ldots, X_n$ are mutually independent and identically distributed, then $X_1 \overset{d}{\sim} P(\lambda)$ is equivalent to $\sum_{i=1}^{n} X_i \overset{d}{\sim} P(n\lambda)$.
8. If $X_i \overset{d}{\sim} P(\lambda_i)$ for $1 \leq i \leq n$, and $X_1, X_2, \ldots, X_n$ are mutually independent, then

$$\sum_{i=1}^{n} X_i \overset{d}{\sim} P\left(\sum_{i=1}^{n} \lambda_i\right).$$

9. If $X_1 \overset{d}{\sim} P(\lambda_1)$ and $X_2 \overset{d}{\sim} P(\lambda_2)$ are mutually independent, then conditional distribution of X_1 given $X_1 + X_2$ is binomial distribution, that is

$$(X_1 | X_1 + X_2 = x) \overset{d}{\sim} B(x, p),$$

where $p = \lambda_1/(\lambda_1 + \lambda_2)$.

1.9. Negative Binomial Distribution[2,3,4]

For positive integer m, if random variable X takes non-negative integer values, and the probability is

$$P\{X = k\} = C_{k+m-1}^{k} p^m q^k, \quad k = 0, 1, \ldots,$$

where $0 < p < 1, q = 1 - p$, then we say X follows the negative binomial distribution and denotes it as $X \overset{d}{\sim} NB(m, p)$.

If $X \overset{d}{\sim} NB(m, p)$, then its distribution function is

$$NB(x; m, p) = \begin{cases} \sum_{k=0}^{[x]} C_{k+m-1}^{k} p^m q^k, & x \geq 0, \\ 0, & x < 0, \end{cases}$$

Negative binomial distribution is also called Pascal distribution. It is the direct generalization of binomial distribution.

Consider a success and failure type trial (Bernoulli distribution), the probability of success is p. Let X be the total number of trial until it has m times of "success", then $X - m$ follows the negative binomial distribution $NB(m, p)$, that is, the total number of "failure" follows the negative binomial distribution $NB(m, p)$.

Negative binomial distribution has the following properties:

1. Let $nb(k; m, p) = C_{k+m-1}^{k} p^m q^k$, where $0 < p < 1, k = 0, 1, \ldots,$ then

   $$nb(k + 1; m, p) = \frac{m + k}{k + 1} \cdot nb(k; m, p).$$

   Therefore, if $k < \frac{m-1}{p} - m, nb(k; m, p)$ increases monotonically; if $k > \frac{m-1}{p} - m, nb(k; m, p)$ decreases monotonically with respect to k.
2. Binomial distribution $B(m, p)$ and negative binomial distribution $NB(r, p)$ has the following relationship:

   $$NB(x; r, p) = 1 - B(r - 1; r + [x], p).$$

3. $NB(x; m, p) = I_p(m, [x] + 1)$, where $I_p(\cdot, \cdot)$ is the ratio of incomplete Beta function.
4. If $X \overset{d}{\sim} NB(m, p)$, then the k-th moment of X is

   $$E(X^k) = \sum_{i=1}^{k} S_2(k, i) m^{[i]} (q/p)^i,$$

   where $m^{[i]} = m(m + 1) \cdots (m + i - 1)$, $1 \leq i \leq k, S_2(k, i)$ is the second order Stirling number.

5. If $X \overset{d}{\sim} NB(m,p)$, then $E(X) = mq/p, \mathrm{Var}(X) = mq/p^2$.
6. If $X \overset{d}{\sim} NB(m,p)$, then its skewness and kurtosis are $s = (1+q)/(mq)^{1/2}$ and $\kappa = (6q+p^2)/(mq)$, respectively.
7. If $X \overset{d}{\sim} NB(m,p)$, then the moment-generating function and the characteristic function of X are $M(t) = p^m(1-qe^t)^{-m}$ and $\psi(t) = p^m(1-qe^{it})^{-m}$, respectively.
8. If $X_i \overset{d}{\sim} NB(m_i,p)$ for $1 \le i \le n$, and $X_1, X_2, \ldots, X_n$ are mutually independent, then

$$\sum_{i=1}^{n} X_i \overset{d}{\sim} NB\left(\sum_{i=1}^{n} m_i, p\right).$$

9. If $X \overset{d}{\sim} NB(m_i,p)$, then there exists a sequence random variables $X_1, \ldots, X_m$ which are independent and identically distributed as $G(p)$, such that

$$X \overset{d}{=} X_1 + \cdots + X_m - m,$$

where $G(p)$ is the Geometric distribution in Sec. 1.11.

1.10. Hypergeometric Distribution[2,3,4]

Let N, M, n be positive integers and satisfy $M \le N, n \le N$. If the random variable X takes integer values from the interval $[\max(0, M+n-N), \min(M,n)]$, and the probability for $X = k$ is

$$P\{X = k\} = \frac{C_M^k C_{N-M}^{n-k}}{C_N^n},$$

where $\max(0, M+n-N) \le k \le \min(M,n)$, then we say X follows the hypergeometric distribution and denote it as $X \overset{d}{\sim} H(M,N,n)$.

If $X \overset{d}{\sim} H(M,N,n)$, then the distribution function of X is

$$H(x;n,N,M) = \begin{cases} \sum_{k=K_1}^{\min([x],K_2)} \frac{C_M^k C_{N-M}^{n-k}}{C_N^n}, & x \ge K_1, \\ 0, & x < K_1, \end{cases}$$

where $K_1 = \max(0, M_n - N), K_2 = \min(M,n)$.

The hypergeometric distribution is often used in the sampling inspection of products, which has an important position in the theory of sampling inspection.

Assume that there are N products with M non-conforming ones. We randomly draw n products from the N products without replacement. Let

X be the number of non-conforming products out of this n products, then it follows the hypergeometric distribution $H(M, N, n)$.

Some properties of hypergeometric distribution are as follows:

1. Denote $h(k; n, N, M) = C_M^k C_{n-M}^{n-k} / C_N^n$, then

$$h(k; n, N, M) = h(k; M, N, n),$$
$$h(k; n, N, M) = h(N - n - M + k; N - n, N, M),$$

where $K_1 \le k \le K_2$.

2. The distribution function of the hypergeometric distribution has the following expressions

$$\begin{aligned} H(x; n, N, M) &= H(N - n - M + x; N - n, N, N - M) \\ &= 1 - H(n - x - 1; n, N, N - M) \\ &= 1 - H(M - x - 1; N - n, N, M) \end{aligned}$$

and

$$1 - H(n - 1; x + n, N, N - m) = H(x; n + x, N, M),$$

where $x \ge K_1$.

3. If $X \overset{d}{\sim} H(M, N, n)$, then its expectation and variance are

$$E(X) = \frac{nM}{N}, \quad \mathrm{Var}(X) = \frac{nM(N - n)(N - M)}{N^2(N - 1)}.$$

For integers n and k, denote

$$n^{(k)} = \begin{cases} n(n-1)\cdots(n-k+1), & k < n, \\ n! & k \ge n. \end{cases}$$

4. If $X \overset{d}{\sim} H(M, N, n)$, the k-th moment of X is

$$E(X^k) = \sum_{i=1}^{k} S_2(k, i) \frac{n^{(i)} M^{(i)}}{N^{(i)}}.$$

5. If $X \overset{d}{\sim} H(M, N, n)$, the skewness of X is

$$s = \frac{(N - 2M)(N - 1)^{1/2}(N - 2n)}{(NM(N - M)(N - n))^{1/2}(N - 2)}.$$

6. If $X \overset{d}{\sim} H(M, N, n)$, the moment-generating function and the characteristic function of X are

$$M(t) = \frac{(N-n)!(N-M)!}{N!(N-M-n)!}F(-n, -M; N-M-n+1; e^t)$$

and

$$\psi(t) = \frac{(N-n)!(N-M)!}{N!(N-M-n)!}F(-n, -M; N-M-n+1; e^{it}),$$

respectively, where $F(a, b; c; x)$ is the hypergeometric function and its definition is

$$F(a, b; c, x) = 1 + \frac{ab}{c}\frac{x}{1!} + \frac{a(a+1)b(b+1)}{c(c+1)}\frac{x^2}{2!} + \cdots$$

with $c > 0$.

A typical application of hypergeometric distribution is to estimate the number of fish. To estimate how many fish in a lake, one can catch M fish, and then put them back into the lake with tags. After a period of time, one re-catches $n(n > M)$ fish from the lake among which there are s fish with the mark. M and n are given in advance. Let X be the number of fish with the mark among the n re-caught fish. If the total amount of fish in the lake is assumed to be N, then X follows the hypergeometric distribution $H(M, N, n)$. According to the above property 3, $E(X) = nM/N$, which can be estimated by the number of fish re-caught with the mark, i.e., $s \approx E(X) = nM/N$. Therefore, the estimated total number of fish in the lake is $\hat{N} = \mathrm{nM}/s$.

1.11. Geometric Distribution[2,3,4]

If values of the random variable X are positive integers, and the probabilities are

$$P\{X = k\} = q^{k-1}p, \quad k = 1, 2, \ldots,$$

where $0 < p \leq 1, q = 1-p$, then we say X follows the geometric distribution and denote it as $X \overset{d}{\sim} G(p)$. If $X \overset{d}{\sim} G(p)$, then the distribution function of X is

$$G(x; p) = \begin{cases} 1 - q^{[x]}, & x \geq 0, \\ 0, & x < 0. \end{cases}$$

Geometric distribution is named according to what the sum of distribution probabilities is a geometric series.

In a trial (Bernoulli distribution), whose outcome can be classified as either a "success" or a "failure", and p is the probability that the trial is a "success". Suppose that the trials can be performed repeatedly and independently. Let X be the number of trials required until the first success occurs, then X follows the geometric distribution $G(p)$.

Some properties of geometric distribution are as follows:

1. Denote $g(k;p) = pq^{k-1}, k = 1, 2, \ldots, 0 < p < 1$, then $g(k;p)$ is a monotonically decreasing function of k, that is,
$$g(1;p) > g(2;p) > g(3;p) > \cdots.$$
2. If $X \overset{d}{\sim} G(p)$, then the expectation and variance of X are $E(X) = 1/p$ and $\mathrm{Var}(X) = q/p^2$, respectively.
3. If $X \overset{d}{\sim} G(p)$, then the k-th moment of X is
$$E(X^K) = \sum_{i=1}^{k} S_2(k,i)i!q^{i-1}/p^i,$$
where $S_2(k,i)$ is the second order Stirling number.
4. If $X \overset{d}{\sim} G(p)$, the skewness of X is $s = q^{1/2} + q^{-1/2}$.
5. If $X \overset{d}{\sim} G(p)$, the moment-generating function and the characteristic function of X are $M(t) = pe^t(1 - e^t q)^{-1}$ and $\psi(t) = pe^{it}(1 - e^{it}q)^{-1}$, respectively.
6. If $X \overset{d}{\sim} G(p)$, then
$$P\{X > n + m|X > n\} = P\{X > m\},$$
for any nature number n and m.

Property 6 is also known as "memoryless property" of geometric distribution. This indicates that, in a success-failure test, when we have done n trials with no "success" outcome, the probability of the even that we continue to perform m trials still with no "success" outcome has nothing to do with the information of the first n trials.

The "memoryless property" is a feature of geometric distribution. It can be proved that a discrete random variable taking natural numbers must follow geometric distribution if it satisfies the "memoryless property".

7. If $X \overset{d}{\sim} G(p)$, then
$$E(X|X > n) = n + E(X).$$
8. Suppose X and Y are independent discrete random variables, then $\min(X, Y)$ is independent of $X - Y$ if and only if both X and Y follow the same geometric distribution.

1.12. Gamma Distribution[2,3,4]

If the density function of the random variable X is

$$g(x;\alpha,\beta)=\begin{cases}\frac{\beta^{\alpha}x^{\alpha-1}e^{-\beta x}}{\Gamma(\alpha)}, & x\geq 0,\\ 0, & x<0,\end{cases}$$

where $\alpha>0,\beta>0,\Gamma(\cdot)$ is the Gamma function, then we say X follows the Gamma distribution with shape parameter α and scale parameter β, and denote it as $X\overset{d}{\sim}\Gamma(\alpha,\beta)$.

If $X\overset{d}{\sim}\Gamma(\alpha,\beta)$, then the distribution function of X is

$$\Gamma(x;\alpha,\beta)=\begin{cases}\frac{\beta^{\alpha}t^{\alpha-1}e^{-\beta x}}{\Gamma(\alpha)}dt, & x\geq 0,\\ 0, & x<0.\end{cases}$$

Gamma distribution is named because the form of its density is similar to Gamma function. Gamma distribution is commonly used in reliability theory to describe the life of a product.

When $\beta=1,\Gamma(\alpha,1)$, is called the standard Gamma distribution and its density function is

$$g(x;\alpha,1)=\begin{cases}\frac{x^{\alpha-1}e^{-x}}{\Gamma(\alpha)}, & x\geq 0,\\ 0, & x<0.\end{cases}$$

When $\alpha=1(1,\beta)$ is called the single parameter Gamma distribution, and it is also the exponential distribution $E(\beta)$ with density function

$$g(x;1,\beta)=\begin{cases}\beta e^{-\beta x}, & x\geq 0,\\ 0, & x<0.\end{cases}$$

More generally, the gamma distribution with three parameters can be obtained by means of translation transformation, and the corresponding density function is

$$g(x;\alpha,\beta,\delta)=\begin{cases}\frac{\beta^{\alpha}(x-\delta)^{\alpha-1}e^{-\beta(x-\delta)}}{\Gamma(\alpha)}, & x\geq 0,\\ 0, & x<\delta.\end{cases}$$

Some properties of gamma distribution are as follows:

1. If $X\overset{d}{\sim}\Gamma(\alpha,\beta)$, then $\beta X\overset{d}{\sim}\Gamma(\alpha,1)$. That is, the general gamma distribution can be transformed into the standard gamma distribution by scale transformation.

2. For $x \geq 0$, denote

$$I_\alpha(x) = \frac{1}{\Gamma(\alpha)} \int_0^x t^{\alpha-1} e^{-t} dt$$

to be the incomplete Gamma function, then $\Gamma(x; \alpha, \beta) = I_\alpha(\beta x)$. Particularly, $\Gamma(x; 1, \beta) = 1 - e^{-\beta x}$.

3. Several relationships between gamma distributions are as follows:

   (1) $\Gamma(x; \alpha, 1) - \Gamma(x; \alpha+1, 1) = g(x; \alpha, 1)$.
   (2) $\Gamma(x; \frac{1}{2}, 1) = 2\Phi(\sqrt{2x}) - 1$,

   where $\Phi(x)$ is the standard normal distribution function.

4. If $X \overset{d}{\sim} \Gamma(\alpha, \beta)$, then the expectation of X is $E(X) = \alpha/\beta$ and the variance of X is $\text{Var}(X) = \alpha/\beta^2$.
5. If $X \overset{d}{\sim} \Gamma(\alpha, \beta)$, then the k-th moment of X is $E(X^k) = \beta^{-k}\Gamma(k+\alpha)/\Gamma(\alpha)$.
6. If $X \overset{d}{\sim} \Gamma(\alpha, \beta)$, the skewness of X is $s = 2\alpha^{-1/2}$ and the kurtosis of X is $\kappa = 6/\alpha$.
7. If $X \overset{d}{\sim} \Gamma(\alpha, \beta)$, the moment-generating function of X is $M(t) = (\frac{\beta}{\beta-t})^\alpha$, and the characteristic function of X is $\psi(t) = (\frac{\beta}{\beta-it})^\alpha$ for $t < \beta$.
8. If $X_i \overset{d}{\sim} \Gamma(\alpha_i, \beta)$, for $1 \leq i \leq n$, and $X_1, X_2, \ldots, X_n$ and are independent, then

$$\sum_{i=1}^n X_i \overset{d}{\sim} \Gamma\left(\sum_{i=1}^n \alpha_i, \beta\right).$$

9. If $X \overset{d}{\sim} \Gamma(\alpha_1, 1), Y \overset{d}{\sim} \Gamma(\alpha_2, 1)$, and X is independent of Y, then $X+Y$ is independent of X/Y. Conversely, if X and Y are mutually independent, non-negative and non-degenerate random variables, and moreover $X+Y$ is independent of X/Y, then both X and Y follow the standard Gamma distribution.

1.13. Beta Distribution[2,3,4]

If the density function of the random variable X is

$$f(x; a, b) = \begin{cases} \frac{x^{a-1}(1-x)^{b-1}}{B(a,b)}, & 0 \leq x \leq 1, \\ 0, & \text{otherwise}, \end{cases}$$

where $a > 0, b > 0, B(\cdot, \cdot)$ is the Beta function, then we say X follows the Beta distribution with parameters a and b, and denote it as $X \overset{d}{\sim} BE(a, b)$.

If $X \overset{d}{\sim} BE(a,b)$, then the distribution function of X is

$$BE(x;a,b) = \begin{cases} 1, & x > 1, \\ I_x(a,b), & 0 < x \le 1, \\ 0, & x \le 0, \end{cases}$$

where $I_x(a,b)$ is the ratio of incomplete Beta function.

Similar to Gamma distribution, Beta distribution is named because the form of its density function is similar to Beta function.

Particularly, when $a = b = 1, BE(1,1)$ is the standard uniform distribution $U(0,1)$.

Some properties of the Beta distribution are as follows:

1. If $X \overset{d}{\sim} BE(a,b)$, then $1 - X \overset{d}{\sim} BE(b,a)$.
2. The density function of Beta distribution has the following properties:

   (1) when $a < 1, b \ge 1$, the density function is monotonically decreasing;
   (2) when $a \ge 1, b < 1$, the density function is monotonically increasing;
   (3) when $a < 1, b < 1$, the density function curve is U type;
   (4) when $a > 1, b > 1$, the density function curve has a single peak;
   (5) when $a = b$, the density function curve is symmetric about $x = 1/2$.

3. If $X \overset{d}{\sim} BE(a,b)$, then the k-th moment of X is $E(X^k) = \frac{B(a+k,b)}{B(a,b)}$.
4. If $X \overset{d}{\sim} BE(a,b)$, then the expectation and variance of X are $E(X) = a/(a+b)$ and $\text{Var}(X) = ab/((a+b+1)(a+b)^2)$, respectively.
5. If $X \overset{d}{\sim} BE(a,b)$, the skewness of X is $s = \frac{2(b-a)(a+b+1)^{1/2}}{(a+b+2)(ab)^2}$ and the kurtosis of X is $\kappa = \frac{3(a+b)(a+b+1)(a+1)(2b-a)}{ab(a+b+2)(a+b+3)} + \frac{a(a-b)}{a+b} - 3$.
6. If $X \overset{d}{\sim} BE(a,b)$, the moment-generating function and the characteristic function of X are $M(t) = \frac{\Gamma(a+b)}{\Gamma(a)} \sum_{k=0}^{\infty} \frac{\Gamma(a+k)}{\Gamma(a+b+k)} \frac{t^k}{\Gamma(k+1)}$ and $\psi(t) = \frac{\Gamma(a+b)}{\Gamma(a)} \sum_{k=0}^{\infty} \frac{\Gamma(a+k)}{\Gamma(a+b+k)} \frac{(it)^k}{\Gamma(k+1)}$, respectively.
7. Suppose $X_1, X_2, \ldots, X_n$ are mutually independent, $X_i \overset{d}{\sim} BE(a_i, b_i), 1 \le i \le n$, and $a_{i+1} = a_i + b_i, 1 \le i \le n-1$, then

$$\prod_{i=1}^{n} X_i \overset{d}{\sim} BE\left(a_1, \sum_{i=1}^{n} b_i\right).$$

8. Suppose $X_1, X_2, \ldots, X_n$ are independent and identically distributed random variables with common distribution $U(0,1)$, then $\min(X_1, \ldots, X_n)$

$\overset{d}{\sim} BE(1,n)$. Conversely, if $X_1, X_2, \ldots, X_n$ are independent and identically distributed random variables, and

$$\min(X_1,\ldots,X_n) \overset{d}{\sim} U(0,1),$$

then $X_1 \overset{d}{\sim} BE(1,1/n)$.

9. Suppose $X_1, X_2, \ldots, X_n$ are independent and identically distributed random variables with common distribution $U(0,1)$, denote

$$X_{(1,n)} \le X_{(2,n)} \le \cdots \le X_{(n,n)}$$

as the corresponding order statistics, then

$$X_{(k,n)} \overset{d}{\sim} BE(k, n-k+1), \quad 1 \le k \le n,$$

$$X_{(k,n)} - X_{(i,n)} \overset{d}{\sim} BE(k-i, n-k+i+1), \quad 1 \le i < k \le n.$$

10. Suppose $X_1, X_2, \ldots, X_n$ are independent and identically distributed random variables with common distribution $BE(a,1)$.
Let

$$Y = \min(X_1,\ldots,X_n),$$

then $Y^a \overset{d}{\sim} BE(1,n)$.

11. If $X \overset{d}{\sim} BE(a,b)$, where a and b are positive integers, then

$$BE(x;a,b) = \sum_{i=a}^{a+b-1} C_{a+b-1}^{i} x^i (1-x)^{a+b-1-i}.$$

1.14. Chi-square Distribution[2,3,4]

If $Y_1, Y_2, \ldots, Y_n$ are mutually independent and identically distributed random variables with common distribution $N(0,1)$, then we say the random variable $X = \sum_{i=1}^{n} Y_i^2$ change position with the previous math formula follows the Chi-square distribution (χ^2 distribution) with n degree of freedom, and denote it as $X \overset{d}{\sim} \chi_n^2$.

If $X \overset{d}{\sim} \chi_n^2$, then the density function of X is

$$f(x;n) = \begin{cases} \dfrac{e^{-x/2} x^{n/2-1}}{2^{n/2}\Gamma(n/2)}, & x > 0, \\ 0, & x \le 0, \end{cases}$$

where $\Gamma(n/2)$ is the Gamma function.

Chi-square distribution is derived from normal distribution, which plays an important role in statistical inference for normal distribution. When the degree of freedom n is quite large, Chi-square distribution χ_n^2 approximately becomes normal distribution.

Some properties of Chi-square distribution are as follows:

1. If $X_1 \overset{d}{\sim} \chi^2_n, X_2 \overset{d}{\sim} \chi^2_m, X_1$ and X_2 are independent, then $X_1+X_2 \overset{d}{\sim} \chi^2_{n+m}$. This is the "additive property" of Chi-square distribution.
2. Let $f(x;n)$ be the density function of Chi-square distribution χ^2_n. Then, $f(x;n)$ is monotonically decreasing when $n \le 2$, and $f(x;n)$ is a single peak function with the maximum point $n-2$ when $n \ge 3$.
3. If $X \overset{d}{\sim} \chi^2_n$, then the k-th moment of X is
$$E(X^k) = 2^k \frac{\Gamma(n/2+k)}{\Gamma(n/2)} = 2^k \Pi_{i=0}^{k-1} \Gamma\left(i+\frac{n}{2}\right).$$
4. If $X \overset{d}{\sim} \chi^2_n$, then
$$E(X) = n, \quad \mathrm{Var}(X) = 2n.$$
5. If $X \overset{d}{\sim} \chi^2_n$, then the skewness of X is $s = 2\sqrt{2}n^{-1/2}$, and the kurtosis of X is $\kappa = 12/n$.
6. If $X \overset{d}{\sim} \chi^2_n$, the moment-generating function of X is $M(t) = (1-2t)^{-n/2}$ and the characteristic function of X is $\psi(t) = (1-2it)^{-n/2}$ for $0 < t < 1/2$.
7. Let $K(x;n)$ be the distribution function of Chi-square distribution χ^2_n, then we have
   (1) $K(x;2n) = 1 - 2\sum_{i=1}^n f(x;2i)$;
   (2) $K(x;2n+1) = 2\Phi(x) - 1 - 2\sum_{i=1}^n f(x;2i+1)$;
   (3) $K(x;n) - K(x;n+2) = (\frac{x}{2})^{n/2} e^{-x/2}/\Gamma(\frac{n+2}{2})$, where $\Phi(x)$ is the standard normal distribution function.
8. If $X \overset{d}{\sim} \chi^2_m, Y \overset{d}{\sim} \chi^2_n, X$ and Y are independent, then $X/(X+Y) \overset{d}{\sim} BE(m/2, n/2)$, and $X/(X+Y)$ is independent of $X+Y$.
   Let $X_1, X_2, \ldots, X_n$ be the random sample of the normal population $N(\mu, \sigma^2)$. Denote
$$\bar{X} = \frac{1}{n}\sum_{i=1}^n X_i, \quad S^2 = \sum_{i=1}^n (X_i - \bar{X})^2,$$
   then $S^2/\sigma^2 \overset{d}{\sim} \chi^2_{n-1}$ and is independent of $\bar{X}$.

1.14.1. *Non-central Chi-square distribution*

Suppose random variables $Y_1, \ldots, Y_n$ are mutually independent, $Y_i \overset{d}{\sim} N(\mu_i, 1), 1 \le i \le n$, then the distribution function of the random variable $X = \sum_{i=1}^n Y_i^2$ is the non-central Chi-square distribution with the degree of freedom n and the non-central parameter $\delta = \sum_{i=1}^n \mu_i^2$, and is denoted as $\chi^2_{n,\delta}$. Particularly, $\chi^2_{n,0} = \chi^2_n$.

9. Suppose $Y_1, \ldots, Y_m$ are mutually independent, and $Y_i \overset{d}{\sim} \chi^2_{n_i,\delta_i}$ for $1 \leq i \leq m$, then $\sum_{i=1}^m Y_i \overset{d}{\sim} \chi^2_{n,\delta}$ where, $n = \sum_{i=1}^m n_i, \delta = \sum_{i=1}^m \delta_i$.
10. If $X \overset{d}{\sim} \chi^2_{n,\delta}$ then $E(X) = n + \delta, \mathrm{Var}(X) = 2(n + 2\delta)$, the skewness of X is $s = \sqrt{8}\frac{n+3\delta}{(n+2\delta)^{3/2}}$, and the kurtosis of X is $\kappa = 12\frac{n+4\delta}{(n+2\delta)^2}$.
11. If $X \overset{d}{\sim} \chi^2_{n,\delta}$, then the moment-generating function and the characteristic function of X are $M(t) = (1 - 2t)^{-n/2}\exp\{t\delta/(1 - 2t)\}$ and $\psi(t) = (1 - 2it)^{-n/2}\exp\{it\delta/(1 - 2it)\}$, respectively.

1.15. *t* Distribution[2,3,4]

Assume $X \overset{d}{\sim} N(0,1), Y \overset{d}{\sim} \chi^2_n$, and X is independent of Y. We say the random variable $T = \sqrt{n}X/\sqrt{Y}$ follows the t distribution with n degree of freedom and denotes it as $T \overset{d}{\sim} t_n$.

If $X \overset{d}{\sim} t_n$, then the density function of X is

$$t(x;n) = \frac{\Gamma(\frac{n+1}{2})}{(n\pi)^{1/2}\Gamma(\frac{n}{2})}\left(1 + \frac{x^2}{n}\right)^{-(n+1)/2},$$

for $-\infty < x < \infty$.

Define $T(x;n)$ as the distribution function of t distribution, t_n, then

$$T(x;n) = \begin{cases} \frac{1}{2}I_{n/(n+x^2)}(\frac{1}{2}, \frac{n}{2}), & x \leq 0, \\ \frac{1}{2} + \frac{1}{2}I_{n/(n+x^2)}(\frac{1}{2}, \frac{n}{2}), & x < 0, \end{cases}$$

where $I_{n/(n+x^2)}(\frac{1}{2}, \frac{n}{2})$ is the ratio of incomplete beta function.

Similar to Chi-square distribution, t distribution can also be derived from normal distribution and Chi-square distribution. It has a wide range of applications in statistical inference on normal distribution. When n is large, the t distribution t_n with n degree of freedom can be approximated by the standard normal distribution.

t distribution has the following properties:

1. The density function of t distribution, $t(x;n)$, is symmetric about $x = 0$, and reaches the maximum at $x = 0$.
2. $\lim_{n\to\infty} t(x;n) = \frac{1}{\sqrt{2\pi}}e^{-x^2/2} = \phi(x)$, the limiting distribution for t distribution is the standard normal distribution as the degree of freedom n goes to infinity.

3. Assume $X \overset{d}{\sim} t_n$. If $k < n$, then $E(X^k)$ exists, otherwise, $E(X^k)$ does not exist. The k-th moment of X is

$$E(X^k) = \begin{cases} 0 & \text{if } 0 < k < n, & \text{and } k \text{ is odd}, \\ \frac{\Gamma(\frac{k+1}{2})\Gamma(\frac{n-k}{2})\frac{k}{2}}{\sqrt{\pi}\Gamma(\frac{n}{2})} & \text{if } 0 < k < n, & \text{and } k \text{ is even}, \\ \text{doesn't exist} & \text{if } k \geq n, & \text{and } k \text{ is odd}, \\ \infty & \text{if } k \geq n, & \text{and } k \text{ is even}. \end{cases}$$

4. If $X \overset{d}{\sim} t_n$, then $E(X) = 0$. When $n > 3, \mathrm{Var}(X) = n/(n-2)$.
5. If $X \overset{d}{\sim} t_n$, then the skewness of X is 0. If $n \geq 5$, the kurtosis of X is $\kappa = 6/(n-4)$.
6. Assume that X_1 and X_2 are independent and identically distributed random variables with common distribution χ^2_n, then the random variable

$$Y = \frac{1}{2}\frac{n^{1/2}(X_2 - X_1)}{(X_1 X_2)^{1/2}} \overset{d}{\sim} t_n.$$

Suppose that $X_1, X_2, \ldots, X_n$ are random samples of the normal population $N(\mu, \sigma^2)$, define $\bar{X} = \frac{1}{n}\sum_{i=1}^n X_i$, $S^2 = \sum_{i=1}^n (X_i - \bar{X})^2$, then

$$T = \sqrt{n(n-1)}\frac{\bar{X} - \mu}{S} \overset{d}{\sim} t_{n-1}.$$

1.15.1. *Non-central t distribution*

Suppose that $X \overset{d}{\sim} N(\delta, 1), Y \overset{d}{\sim} \chi^2_n$, X and Y are independent, then $T = \sqrt{n}X/\sqrt{Y}$ is a non-central t distributed random variable with n degree of freedom and non-centrality parameter δ, and is denoted as $T \overset{d}{\sim} t_{n,\delta}$. Particularly, $t_{n,0} = t_n$.

7. Let $T(x; n, \delta)$ be the distribution function of the non-central t distribution $t_{n,\delta}$, then we have

$$T(x; n, \delta) = 1 - T(-x; n, -\delta), \quad T(0; n, \delta) = \Phi(-\delta),$$
$$T(1; 1, \delta) = 1 - \Phi^2(\delta/\sqrt{2}).$$

8. If $X \overset{d}{\sim} t_{n,\delta}$, then $E(X) = \sqrt{\frac{n}{2}}\frac{\Gamma(\frac{n-1}{2})}{\Gamma(\frac{n}{2})}\delta$ for $n > 1$ and $\mathrm{Var}(X) = \frac{n}{n-2}(1 + \delta^2) - (E(X))^2$ for $n > 2$.

1.16. F Distribution[2,3,4]

Let X and Y be independent random variables such that $X \overset{d}{\sim} \chi^2_m, Y \overset{d}{\sim} \chi^2_n$. Define a new random variable F as $F = \frac{X}{m} / \frac{Y}{n}$. Then the distribution of F is called the F distribution with the degrees of freedom m and n, denoted as $F \overset{d}{\sim} F_{m,n}$.

If $X \overset{d}{\sim} F_{m,n}$, then the density function of X is

$$f(x; m, n) = \begin{cases} \frac{(\frac{m}{n})^{\frac{m}{2}}}{B(\frac{m}{2}, \frac{n}{2})} x^{\frac{m-2}{2}} \left(1 + \frac{mx}{n}\right)^{-\frac{m+n}{2}}, & x > 0, \\ 0, & x \leq 0. \end{cases}$$

Let $F(x; m, n)$ be the distribution function of F distribution, $F_{m,n}$, then $F(x; m, n) = I_a(n/2, m/2)$, where $a = xm/(n + mx), I_a(\cdot, \cdot)$ is the ratio of incomplete beta function.

F distribution is often used in hypothesis testing problems on two or more normal populations. It can also be used to approximate complicated distributions. F distribution plays an important role in statistical inference.

F distribution has the following properties:

1. F distributions are generally skewed, the smaller of n, the more it skews.
2. When $m = 1$ or $2, f(x; m, n)$ decreases monotonically; when $m > 2, f(x; m, n)$ is unimodal, the mode is $\frac{n(m-2)}{(n+2)m}$.
3. If $X \overset{d}{\sim} F_{m,n}$, then $Y = 1/X \overset{d}{\sim} F_{n,m}$.
4. If $X \overset{d}{\sim} t_n$, then $X^2 \overset{d}{\sim} F_{1,n}$.
5. If $X \overset{d}{\sim} F_{m,n}$, then the k-th moment of X is

$$E(X^k) = \begin{cases} (\frac{n}{m})^k \frac{\Gamma(\frac{m}{2}+k)\Gamma(\frac{n}{2}-k)}{\Gamma(\frac{m}{2})\Gamma(\frac{n}{2})}, & 0 < k < n/2, \\ \infty, & k \geq n/2. \end{cases}$$

6. Assume that $X \overset{d}{\sim} F_{m,n}$. If $n > 2$, then $E(X) = \frac{n}{n-2}$; if $n > 4$, then $\text{Var}(X) = \frac{2n^2(m+n-2)}{m(n-2)^2(n-4)}$.
7. Assume that $X \overset{d}{\sim} F_{m,n}$. If $n > 6$, then the skewness of X is $s = \frac{(2m+n-2)(8(n-4))^{1/2}}{(n-6)(m(m_n-2))^{1/2}}$; if $n > 8$, then the kurtosis of X is $\kappa = \frac{12((n-2)^2(n-4)+m(m+n-2)(5n-22))}{m(n-6)(n-8)(m+n-2)}$.

8. When m is large enough and $n > 4$, the normal distribution function $\Phi(y)$ can be used to approximate the F distribution function $F(x; m, n)$, where $y = \frac{\frac{x-n}{n-2}}{\frac{n}{n-2}(\frac{2(n+m-2)}{m(n-4)})^{1/2}}$, that is, $F(x; m, n) \approx \Phi(y)$.

Suppose $X \overset{d}{\sim} F_{m,n}$. Let $Z_{m,n} = \ln X$, when both m and n are large enough, the distribution of $Z_{m,n}$ can be approximated by the normal distribution $N(\frac{1}{2}(\frac{1}{n} - \frac{1}{m}), \frac{1}{2}(\frac{1}{m} + \frac{1}{n}))$, that is,

$$Z_{m,n} \overset{d}{\approx} N\left(\frac{1}{2}\left(\frac{1}{n} - \frac{1}{m}\right), \quad \frac{1}{2}\left(\frac{1}{m} + \frac{1}{n}\right)\right).$$

Assume that $X_1, \ldots, X_m$ are random samples of the normal population $N(\mu_1, \sigma_1^2)$ and $Y_1, \ldots, Y_n$ are random samples of the normal population $N(\mu_2, \sigma_2^2)$. The testing problem we are interested in is whether σ_1 and σ_2 are equal.

Define $\hat{\sigma}_1^2 = (m-1)^{-1}\sum_{i=1}^m (X_i - \bar{X})^2$ and $\hat{\sigma}_2^2 = (n-1)^{-1}\sum_{i=1}^n (Y_i - \bar{Y})^2$ as the estimators of σ_1^2 and σ_2^2, respectively. Then we have

$$\hat{\sigma}_1^2/\sigma_1^2 \overset{d}{\sim} \chi_{m-1}^2, \quad \hat{\sigma}_2^2/\sigma_2^2 \overset{d}{\sim} \chi_{n-1}^2,$$

where $\hat{\sigma}_1^2$ and $\hat{\sigma}_2^2$ are independent. If $\sigma_1^2 = \sigma_2^2$, by the definition of F distribution, the test statistics

$$F = \frac{(n-1)^{-1}\sum_{i=1}^m (X_i - \bar{X})^2}{(m-1)^{-1}\sum_{i=1}^n (Y_i - \bar{Y})^2} = \frac{\hat{\sigma}_1^2/\sigma_1^2}{\hat{\sigma}_2^2/\sigma_2^2} \overset{d}{\sim} F_{m-1,n-1}.$$

1.16.1. *Non-central F distribution*

If $X \overset{d}{\sim} \chi_{m,\delta}^2, Y \overset{d}{\sim} \chi_n^2, X$ and Y are independent, then $F = \frac{X}{m}/\frac{Y}{n}$ follows a non-central F distribution with the degrees of freedom m and n and non-centrality parameter δ. Denote it as $F \overset{d}{\sim} F_{m,n,\delta}$. Particularly, $F_{m,n,0} = F_{m,n}$.

10. If $X \overset{d}{\sim} t_{n,\delta}$, then $X^2 \overset{d}{\sim} F_{1,n,\delta}$.
11. Assume that $X \overset{d}{\sim} F_{1,n,\delta}$. If $n > 2$ then $E(X) = \frac{(m+\delta)n}{(n-2)m}$; if $n > 4$, then $\mathrm{Var}(X) = 2(\frac{n}{m})^2 \frac{(m+\delta)^2 + (m+2\delta)(n-2)}{(n-2)^2(n-4)}$.

1.17. Multivariate Hypergeometric Distribution[2,3,4]

Suppose $\boldsymbol{X} = (X_1, \ldots, X_n)$ is an n-dimensional random vector with $n \geq 2$, which satisfies:

(1) $0 \leq X_i \leq N_i, 1 \leq i \leq n, \sum_{i=1}^{n} N_i = N$;
(2) let $m_1, \ldots, m_n$ be positive integers with $\sum_{i=1}^{n} m_i = m$, the probability of the event $\{X_1 = m_1, \ldots, X_n = m_n\}$ is

$$P\{X_1 = m_1, \ldots, X_n = m_n\} = \frac{\prod_{i=1}^{n} C_{N_i}^{m_i}}{C_N^m},$$

then we say X follows the multivariate hypergeometric distribution, and denote it as $\boldsymbol{X} \stackrel{d}{\sim} MH(N_1, \ldots, N_n; m)$.

Suppose a jar contains balls with n kinds of colors. The number of balls of the ith color is $N_i, 1 \leq i \leq n$. We draw m balls randomly from the jar without replacement, and denote X_i as the number of balls of the ith color for $1 \leq i \leq n$. Then the random vector $(X_1, \ldots, X_n)$ follows the multivariate hypergeometric distribution $MH(N_1, \ldots, N_n; m)$.

Multivariate hypergeometric distribution has the following properties:

1. Suppose $(X_1, \ldots, X_n) \stackrel{d}{\sim} MH(N_1, \ldots, N_n; m)$.

For $0 = j_0 < j_1 < \cdots < j_s = n$, let $X_k^* = \sum_{i=j_{k-1}+1}^{j_k} X_i, N_k^* = \sum_{i=j_{k-1}+1}^{j_k} N_i$, $1 \leq k \leq s$, then $(X_1^*, \ldots, X_s^*) \stackrel{d}{\sim} MH(N_1^*, \ldots, N_s^*; m)$.

Combine the components of the random vector which follows multivariate hypergeometric distribution into a new random vector, the new random vector still follows multivariate hypergeometric distribution.

2. Suppose $(X_1, \ldots, X_n) \stackrel{d}{\sim} MH(N_1, \ldots, N_n; m)$, then for any $1 \leq k < n$,, we have

$$P\{X_1 = m_1, \ldots, X_k = m_k\} = \frac{C_{N_1}^{m_1} C_{N_2}^{m_2} \cdots C_{N_k}^{m_k} C_{N_{k+1}^*}^{m_{k+1}^*}}{C_N^m},$$

where $N = \sum_{i=1}^{n} N_i, N_{k+1}^* = \sum_{i=k+1}^{n} N_i, m_{k+1}^* = m - \sum_{i=1}^{k} m_i$.

Especially, when $k = 1$, we have $P\{X_1 = m_1\} = \frac{C_{N_1}^{m_1} C_{N_2^*}^{m_2^*}}{C_N^m}$, that is $X_1 \stackrel{d}{\sim} H(N_1, N, m)$.

Multivariate hypergeometric distribution is the extension of hypergeometric distribution.

3. Suppose $(X_1,\ldots,X_n) \stackrel{d}{\sim} MH(N_1,\ldots,N_n;m), 0<k<n$, then

$$\begin{aligned}&P\{X_1=m_1,\ldots,X_k=m_k|X_{k+1}=m_{k+1},\ldots,X_n=m_n\}\\&=\frac{C_{N_1}^{m_1}\cdots C_{N_k}^{m_k}}{C_{N^*}^{m^*}},\end{aligned}$$

where, $N^*=\sum_{i=1}^k N_i, m_{k+1}^*=m-\sum_{i=k+1}^n m_i$. This indicates that, under the condition of $X_{k+1}=m_{k+1},\ldots,X_n=m_n$, the conditional distribution of $(X_1,\ldots,X_k)$ is $MH(N_1,\ldots,N_k;m^*)$.

4. Suppose $X_i \stackrel{d}{\sim} B(N_i,p), 1\le i\le n, 0<p<1$, and $X_1,\ldots,X_n$ are mutually independent, then

$$\left(X_1,\ldots,X_n\,\middle|\,\sum_{i=1}^n X_i=m\right)\stackrel{d}{\sim} MH(N_1,\ldots,N_n;m).$$

This indicates that, when the sum of independent binomial random variables is given, the conditional joint distribution of these random variables is a multivariate hypergeometric distribution.

5. Suppose $(X_1,\ldots,X_n) \stackrel{d}{\sim} MH(N_1,\ldots,N_n;m)$. If $N_i/N \to p_i$ when $N\to\infty$ for $1\le i\le n$, then the distribution of $(X_1,\ldots,X_n)$ converges to the multinomial distribution $PN(N;p_1,\ldots,p_n)$.

In order to control the number of cars, the government decides to implement the random license-plate lottery policy, each participant has the same probability to get a new license plate, and 10 quotas are allowed each issue. Suppose 100 people participate in the license-plate lottery, among which 10 are civil servants, 50 are individual household, 30 are workers of state-owned enterprises, and the remaining 10 are university professors. Denote X_1,X_2,X_3,X_4 as the numbers of people who get the license as civil servants, individual household, workers of state-owned enterprises and university professors, respectively. Thus, the random vector (X_1,X_2,X_3,X_4) follows the multivariate hypergeometric distribution. $MH(10,50,30,10;10)$. Therefore, in the next issue, the probability of the outcome $X_1=7, X_2=1, X_3=1$, $X_4=1$ is

$$P\{X_1=7,X_2=1,X_3=1,X_4=1\}=\frac{C_{10}^7C_{50}^1C_{30}^1C_{10}^1}{C_{100}^{10}}.$$

1.18. Multivariate Negative Binomial Distribution[2,3,4]

Suppose $\boldsymbol{X} = (X_1, \ldots, X_n)$ is a random vector with dimension $n(n \geq 2)$ which satisfies:

(1) X_i takes non-negative integer values, $1 \leq i \leq n$;
(2) If the probability of the event $\{X_1 = x_1, \ldots, X_n = x_n\}$ is

$$P\{X_1 = x_1, \ldots, X_n = x_n\} = \frac{(x_1 + \cdots + x_n + k - 1)!}{x_1! \cdots x_n!(k-1)!} p_0^k p_1^{x_1} \cdots p_n^{x_n},$$

where $0 < p_i < 1, 0 \leq i \leq n, \sum_{i=0}^n p_i = 1, k$ is a positive integer, then we say $\boldsymbol{X}$ follows the multivariate negative binomial distribution, denoted as $\boldsymbol{X} \overset{d}{\sim} MNB(k; p_1, \ldots, p_n)$.

Suppose that some sort of test has $(n+1)$ kinds of different results, but only one of them occurs every test with the probability of $p_i, 1 \leq i \leq (n+1)$. The sequence of tests continues until the $(n+1)$-th result has occurred k times. At this moment, denote the total times of the i-th result occurred as X_i for $1 \leq i \leq n$, then the random vector $(X_1, \ldots, X_n)$ follows the multivariate negative binomial distribution $MNB(k; p_1, \ldots, p_n)$.

Multivariate negative binomial distribution has the following properties:

1. Suppose $(X_1, \ldots, X_n) \overset{d}{\sim} MNB(k; p_1 \ldots, p_n)$. For $0 = j_0 < j_1 < \cdots < j_s = n$, let $X_k^* = \sum_{i=j_{k-1}+1}^{j_k} X_i, p_k^* = \sum_{i=j_{k-1}+1}^{j_k} p_i$, $1 \leq k \leq s$, then $(X_1^*, \ldots, X_s^*) \overset{d}{\sim} MNB(k; p_1^* \ldots, p_s^*)$.
   Combine the components of the random vector which follows multivariate negative binomial distribution into a new random vector, the new random vector still follows multivariate negative binomial distribution.
2. If $(X_1, \ldots, X_n) \overset{d}{\sim} MNB(k; p_1 \ldots, p_n)$, then $E(X_1^{r_1} \cdots X_n^{r_n}) = (k + \sum_{i=1}^n r_i - 1)^{\sum_{i=1}^n r_i} \Pi_{i=1}^n (p_i/p_0)^{r_i}$, where $p_0 = 1 - \sum_{i=1}^n p_i$.
3. If $(X_1, \ldots, X_n) \overset{d}{\sim} MNB(k; p_1 \ldots, p_n), 1 \leq s < n$, then $(X_1, \ldots, X_s) \overset{d}{\sim} MNB(k; p_1^* \ldots, p_s^*)$, where $p_i^* = p_i/(p_0 + p_1 + \cdots + p_s), 1 \leq i \leq s, p_0 = 1 - \sum_{i=1}^n p_i$.

Especially, when $s = 1, X_1 \overset{d}{\sim} NB(k, \frac{p_0}{p_0+p_1})$.

1.19. Multivariate Normal Distribution[5,2]

A random vector $\boldsymbol{X} = (X_1, \ldots, X_p)'$ follows the multivariate normal distribution, denoted as $\mathbf{X} \overset{d}{\sim} N_p(\mu, \sum)$, if it has the following density function

$$f(\mathbf{x}) = (2\pi)^{-\frac{p}{2}} \left|\sum\right|^{-\frac{1}{2}} \exp\left\{-\frac{1}{2}(\mathbf{x} - \mu)' \sum^{-1} (\mathbf{x} - \mu)\right\},$$

where $\mathbf{x} = (x_1, \ldots, x_p)' \in R^p, \mu \in R^p, \sum$ is a $p \times p$ positive definite matrix, "$|\cdot|$" denotes the matrix determinant, and "$'$" denotes the transition matrix transposition.

Multivariate normal distribution is the extension of normal distribution. It is the foundation of multivariate statistical analysis and thus plays an important role in statistics.

Let $X_1, \ldots, X_p$ be independent and identically distributed standard normal random variables, then the random vector $\mathbf{X} = (X_1, \ldots, X_p)'$ follows the standard multivariate normal distribution, denoted as $X \overset{d}{\sim} N_p(0, \mathbf{I}_p)$, where $\mathbf{I}_p$ is a unit matrix of p-th order.

Some properties of multivariate normal distribution are as follows:

1. The necessary and sufficient conditions for $\mathbf{X} = (X_1, \ldots, X_p)'$ following multivariate normal distribution is that $\mathbf{a}'\mathbf{X}$ also follows normal distribution for any $\mathbf{a} = (a_1, \ldots, a_p)' \in R^p$.
2. If $\mathbf{X} \overset{d}{\sim} N_p(\mu, \sum)$, we have $E(\mathbf{X}) = \mu, \mathrm{Cov}(\mathbf{X}) = \sum$.
3. If $\mathbf{X} \overset{d}{\sim} N_p(\mu, \sum)$, its moment-generating function and characteristic function are $M(\mathbf{t}) = \exp\{\mu'\mathbf{t} + \frac{1}{2}\mathbf{t}' \sum \mathbf{t}\}$ and $\psi(\mathbf{t}) = \exp\{i\mu'\mathbf{t} - \frac{1}{2}\mathbf{t}' \sum \mathbf{t}\}$ for $\mathbf{t} \in R^p$, respectively.
4. Any marginal distribution of a multivariate normal distribution is still a multivariate normal distribution. Let $\mathbf{X} = (X_1, \ldots, X_p)' \overset{d}{\sim} N(\mu, \sum)$, where $\mu = (\mu_1, \ldots, \mu_p)', \sum = (\sigma_{ij})_{p \times p}$. For any $1 \leq q < p$, set $\mathbf{X}^{(1)} = (X_1, \ldots, X_q)', \mu^{(1)} = (\mu_1, \ldots, \mu_q)', \sum_{11} = (\sigma_{ij})_{1 \leq i,j \leq 1}$, then we have $\mathbf{X}^{(1)} \overset{d}{\sim} N_q(\mu^{(1)}, \sum_{11})$. Especially, $X_1 \overset{d}{\sim} N(\mu_i, \sigma_{ii}), 1 \leq i \leq p$.
5. If $\mathbf{X} \overset{d}{\sim} N_p(\mu, \sum)$, $\mathbf{B}$ denotes an $q \times p$ constant matrix and $\mathbf{a}$ denotes an $q \times 1$ constant vector, then we have

$$\mathbf{a} + \mathbf{B}\mathbf{X} \overset{d}{\sim} N_q\left(\mathbf{a} + \mathbf{B}\mu, \mathbf{B} \sum \mathbf{B}'\right),$$

which implies that the linear transformation of a multivariate normal random vector still follows normal distribution.
6. If $\mathbf{X}_i \overset{d}{\sim} N_p(\mu_i, \sum_i), 1 \leq i \leq n$, and $\mathbf{X}_1, \ldots, \mathbf{X}_n$ are mutually independent, then we have $\sum_{i=1}^n \mathbf{X}_i \overset{d}{\sim} N_p(\sum_{i=1}^n \mu_i, \sum_{i=1}^n \sum_i)$.
7. If $\mathbf{X} \overset{d}{\sim} N_p(\mu, \sum)$, then $(\mathbf{X} - \mu)' \sum^{-1} (\mathbf{X} - \mu) \overset{d}{\sim} \chi_p^2$.
8. Let $\mathbf{X} = (X_1, \ldots, X_p)' \overset{d}{\sim} N_p(\mu, \sum)$, and divide $\mathbf{X}, \mu$ and $\sum$ as follows:

$$\mathbf{X} = \begin{pmatrix} \mathbf{X}^{(1)} \\ \mathbf{X}^{(2)} \end{pmatrix}, \quad \mu = \begin{pmatrix} \mu^{(1)} \\ \mu^{(2)} \end{pmatrix}, \quad \sum = \begin{pmatrix} \sum_{11} & \sum_{12} \\ \sum_{21} & \sum_{22} \end{pmatrix},$$

where $\mathbf{X}^{(1)}$ and $\mu^{(1)}$ are $q \times 1$ vectors, and $\sum_{11}$ is an $q \times q$ matrix, $q < p$, then $\mathbf{X}^{(1)}$ and $\mathbf{X}^{(2)}$ are mutually independent if and only if $\sum_{12} = 0$.

9. Let $\mathbf{X} = (X_1, \ldots, X_p)' \overset{d}{\sim} N_p(\mu, \sum)$, and divide $\mathbf{X}, \mu$ and $\sum$ in the same manner as property 8, then the conditional distribution of $\mathbf{X}^{(1)}$ given $\mathbf{X}^{(2)}$ is $N_q(\mu^{(1)} + \sum_{12}\sum_{22}^{-1}(\mathbf{X}^{(2)} - \mu^{(2)}), \sum_{11} - \sum_{12}\sum_{22}^{-1}\sum_{21})$.
10. Let $\mathbf{X} = (X_1, \ldots, X_p)' \overset{d}{\sim} N_p(\mu, \sum)$, and divide $\mathbf{X}, \mu$ and in $\sum$ the same manner as property 8, then $\mathbf{X}^{(1)}$ and $\mathbf{X}^{(2)} - \sum_{21}\sum_{11}^{-1}\mathbf{X}^{(1)}$ are independent, and $\mathbf{X}^{(1)} \overset{d}{\sim} N_q(\mu^{(1)}, \sum_{11})$,

$$\mathbf{X}^{(2)} - \Sigma_{21}\Sigma_{11}^{-1}\mathbf{X}^{(1)} \overset{d}{\sim} N_{p-q}\left(\mu^{(2)} - \Sigma_{21}\Sigma_{11}^{-1}\mu^{(1)}, \Sigma_{22} - \Sigma_{21}\Sigma_{11}^{-1}\Sigma_{12}\right).$$

Similarly, $\mathbf{X}^{(2)}$ and $\mathbf{X}^{(1)} - \sum_{12}\sum_{22}^{-1}\mathbf{X}^{(2)}$ are independent, and $\mathbf{X}^{(2)} \overset{d}{\sim} N_{p-q}$ $(\mu^{(2)}, \sum_{22})$,

$$\mathbf{X}^{(1)} - \Sigma_{12}\Sigma_{22}^{-1}\mathbf{X}^{(2)} \overset{d}{\sim} N_q\left(\mu^{(1)} - \Sigma_{12}\Sigma_{22}^{-1}\mu^{(2)}, \Sigma_{11} - \Sigma_{12}\Sigma_{22}^{-1}\Sigma_{21}\right).$$

1.20. Wishart Distribution[5,6]

Let $X_1, \ldots, X_n$ be independent and identically distributed p-dimensional random vectors with common distribution $N_p(0, \sum)$, and $\mathbf{X} = (X_1, \ldots, X_n)$ be an $p \times n$ random matrix. Then, we say the p-th order random matrix $\mathbf{W} = \mathbf{XX}' = \sum_{i=1}^{n} X_i X_i'$ follows the p-th order (central) Wishart distribution with n degree of freedom, and denote it as $\mathbf{W} \overset{d}{\sim} W_p(n, \sum)$. Here the distribution of a random matrix indicates the distribution of the random vector generated by matrix vectorization.

Particularly, if $p = 1$, we have $\mathbf{W} = \sum_{i=1}^{n} X_i^2 \overset{d}{\sim} \sum \chi_n^2$, which implies that Wishart distribution is the extension of Chi-square distribution.

If $\mathbf{W} \overset{d}{\sim} W_p(n, \sum)$, and $\sum > 0, n \geq p$, then density function of W is

$$f_p(\mathbf{W}) = \frac{|\mathbf{W}|^{(n-p-1)/2} \exp\{-\frac{1}{2}tr(\sum^{-1}\mathbf{W})\}}{2^{(np/2)}|\sum|^{n/2}\pi^{(p(p-1)/4)}\prod_{i=1}^{p}\Gamma(\frac{(n-i+1)}{2})},$$

where $\mathbf{W} > 0$, and "*tr*" denotes the trace of a matrix.

Wishart distribution is a useful distribution in multivariate statistical analysis and plays an important role in statistical inference for multivariable normal distribution.

Some properties of Wishart distribution are as follows:

1. If $\mathbf{W} \overset{d}{\sim} W_p(n, \sum)$, then $E(\mathbf{W}) = n\sum$.

2. If $\mathbf{W} \overset{d}{\sim} W_p(n, \sum)$, and $\mathbf{C}$ denotes an $k \times p$ matrix, then $\mathbf{CWC}' \overset{d}{\sim} W_k(n, \mathbf{C} \sum \mathbf{C}')$.
3. If $\mathbf{W} \overset{d}{\sim} W_p(n, \sum)$, its characteristic function is $E(e^{\{itr(\mathbf{TW})\}}) = |\mathbf{I}_p - 2i \sum \mathbf{T}|^{-n/2}$, where $\mathbf{T}$ denotes a real symmetric matrix with order p.
4. If $\mathbf{W}_i \overset{d}{\sim} W_p(n_i, \sum), 1 \le i \le k$, and $\mathbf{W}_1, \dots, \mathbf{W}_k$ are mutually independent, then $\sum_{i=1}^k \mathbf{W}_i \overset{d}{\sim} W_p(\sum_{i=1}^k n_i, \sum)$.
5. Let $X_1, \dots, X_n$ be independent and identically distributed p-dimensional random vectors with common distribution $N_p(0, \sum), \sum > 0$, and $\mathbf{X} = (X_1, \dots, X_n)$.

   (1) If $\mathbf{A}$ is an n-th order idempotent matrix, then the quadratic form matrix $\mathbf{Q} = \mathbf{XAX}' \overset{d}{\sim} W_p(m, \sum)$, where $m = r(\mathbf{A}), r(\cdot)$ denotes the rank of a matrix.

   (2) Let $\mathbf{Q} = \mathbf{XAX}', \mathbf{Q}_1 = \mathbf{XBX}'$, where both $\mathbf{A}$ and $\mathbf{B}$ are idempotent matrices. If $\mathbf{Q}_2 = \mathbf{Q} - \mathbf{Q}_1 = \mathbf{X}(\mathbf{A} - \mathbf{B})\mathbf{X}' \ge 0$, then $\mathbf{Q}_2 \overset{d}{\sim} W_p(m - k, \sum)$, where $m = r(\mathbf{A}), k = r(\mathbf{B})$. Moreover, $\mathbf{Q}_1$ and $\mathbf{Q}_2$ are independent.

6. If $\mathbf{W} \overset{d}{\sim} W_p(n, \sum), \sum > 0, n \ge p$, and divide $\mathbf{W}$ and $\sum$ into q-th order and $(p - q)$-th order parts as follows:

$$\mathbf{W} = \begin{pmatrix} \mathbf{W}_{11} & \mathbf{W}_{12} \\ \mathbf{W}_{21} & \mathbf{W}_{22} \end{pmatrix}, \quad \sum = \begin{pmatrix} \sum_{11} & \sum_{12} \\ \sum_{21} & \sum_{22} \end{pmatrix},$$

   then

   (1) $\mathbf{W}_{11} \overset{d}{\sim} W_q(n, \sum_{11})$;

   (2) $\mathbf{W}_{22} - \mathbf{W}_{21}\mathbf{W}_{11}^{-1}\mathbf{W}_{12}$ and $(\mathbf{W}_{11}, \mathbf{W}_{21})$ are independent;

   (3) $\mathbf{W}_{22} - \mathbf{W}_{21}\mathbf{W}_{11}^{-1}\mathbf{W}_{12} \overset{d}{\sim} W_{p-q}(n - q, \sum_{2|1})$ where $\sum_{2|1} = \sum_{22} - \sum_{21} \sum_{11}^{-1} \sum_{12}$.

7. If $\mathbf{W} \overset{d}{\sim} W_p(n, \sum), \sum > 0, n > p + 1$, then $E(\mathbf{W}^{-1}) = \frac{1}{n-p-1} \sum^{-1}$.
8. If $\mathbf{W} \overset{d}{\sim} W_p(n, \sum), \sum > 0, n \ge p$, then $|\mathbf{W}| \overset{d}{=} |\sum| \prod_{i=1}^p \gamma_i$, where $\gamma_1, \dots, \gamma_p$ are mutually independent and $\gamma_i \overset{d}{\sim} \chi^2_{n-i+1}, 1 \le i \le p$.
9. If $\mathbf{W} \overset{d}{\sim} W_p(n, \sum), \sum > 0, n \ge p$, then for any p-dimensional non-zero vector $\mathbf{a}$, we have

$$\frac{\mathbf{a}' \sum^{-1} \mathbf{a}}{\mathbf{a}'\mathbf{W}^{-1}\mathbf{a}} \overset{d}{\sim} \chi^2_{n-p+1}.$$

1.20.1. *Non-central Wishart distribution*

Let $X_1, \ldots, X_n$ be independent and identically distributed p-dimensional random vectors with common distribution $N_p(\mu, \sum)$, and $\mathbf{X} = (X_1, \ldots, X_n)$ be an $p \times n$ random matrix. Then, we say the random matrix $\mathbf{W} = \mathbf{XX}'$ follows the non-central Wishart distribution with n degree of freedom. When $\mu = 0$, the non-central Wishart distribution becomes the (central) Wishart distribution $W_p(n, \sum)$.

1.21. Hotelling T^2 Distribution[5,6]

Suppose that $\mathbf{X} \overset{d}{\sim} N_p(0, \sum)\mathbf{W} \overset{d}{\sim} W_p(n, \sum), \mathbf{X}$ and $\mathbf{W}$ are independent. Let $\mathbf{T}^2 = n\mathbf{X}'\mathbf{W}^{-1}\mathbf{X}$, then we say the random variable $\mathbf{T}^2$ follows the (central) Hotelling T^2 distribution with n degree of freedom, and denote it as $\mathbf{T}^2 \overset{d}{\sim} T_p^2(n)$.

If $p = 1$, Hotelling T^2 distribution is the square of univariate t distribution. Thus, Hotelling $\mathbf{T}^2$ distribution is the extension of t distribution.

The density function of Hotelling $\mathbf{T}^2$ distribution is

$$f(t) = \frac{\Gamma((n+1)/2)}{\Gamma(p/2)\Gamma((n-p+1)/2)} \frac{(t/n)^{(p-2)/2}}{(1+t/n)^{(n+1)/2}}.$$

Some properties of Hotelling $\mathbf{T}^2$ distribution are as follows:

1. If $\mathbf{X}$ and $\mathbf{W}$ are independent, and $\mathbf{X} \overset{d}{\sim} N_p(0, \sum), \mathbf{W} \overset{d}{\sim} W_p(n, \sum)$, then $\mathbf{X}'\mathbf{W}^{-1}\mathbf{X} \overset{d}{=} \frac{\chi_p^2}{\chi_{n-p+1}^2}$, where the numerator and denominator are two independent Chi-square distributions.
2. If $\mathbf{T}^2 \overset{d}{\sim} T_p^2(n)$, then

$$\frac{n-p+1}{np}\mathbf{T}^2 \overset{d}{=} \frac{\frac{\chi_p^2}{p}}{\frac{\chi_{n-p+1}^2}{n-p+1}} \overset{d}{\sim} F_{p,n-p+1}.$$

Hence, Hotelling $\mathbf{T}^2$ distribution can be transformed to F distribution.

1.21.1. *Non-central* T^2 *distribution*

Assume $\mathbf{X}$ and $\mathbf{W}$ are independent, and $\mathbf{X} \overset{d}{\sim} N_p(\mu, \sum), \mathbf{W} \overset{d}{\sim} W_p(n, \sum)$, then the random variable $\mathbf{T}^2 = n\mathbf{X}'\mathbf{W}^{-1}\mathbf{X}$ follows the non-central Hotelling $\mathbf{T}^2$ distribution with n degree of freedom.

When $\mu = 0$, non-central Hotelling $\mathbf{T}^2$ distribution becomes central Hotelling $\mathbf{T}^2$ distribution.

3. Suppose that $\mathbf{X}$ and $\mathbf{W}$ are independent, $\mathbf{X} \overset{d}{\sim} N_p(\mu, \sum), \mathbf{W} \overset{d}{\sim} W_p(n, \sum)$. Let $\mathbf{T}^2 = n\mathbf{X}'\mathbf{W}^{-1}\mathbf{X}$, then

$$\frac{n-p+1}{np}\mathbf{T}^2 \overset{d}{=} \frac{\frac{\chi^2_{p,a}}{p}}{\frac{\chi^2_{n-p+1}}{n-p+1}} \overset{d}{\sim} F_{p,n-p+1,a},$$

where $a = \mu' \sum^{-1} \mu$.

Hotelling $\mathbf{T}^2$ distribution can be used in testing the mean of a multivariate normal distribution. Let $\mathbf{X}_1, \ldots, \mathbf{X}_n$ be random samples of the multivariate normal population $N_p(\mu, \sum)$, where $\sum > 0, \sum$ is unknown, $n > p$. We want to test the following hypothesis:

$$\mathbf{H}_0\colon \mu = \mu_0, \quad vs\ \mathbf{H}_1\colon \mu \neq \mu_0.$$

Let $\bar{\mathbf{X}}_n = n^{-1}\sum_{i=1}^n \mathbf{X}_i$ be the sample mean and $\mathbf{V}_n = \sum_{i=1}^n(\mathbf{X}_i - \bar{\mathbf{X}}_n)(\mathbf{X}_i - \bar{\mathbf{X}}_n)'$ be the sample dispersion matrix. The likelihood ratio test statistic is $\mathbf{T}^2 = n(n-1)(\bar{\mathbf{X}}_n - \mu_0)'\mathbf{V}_n^{-1}(\bar{\mathbf{X}}_n - \mu_0)$. Under the null hypothesis $\mathbf{H}_0$, we have $\mathbf{T}_2 \overset{d}{\sim} T_p^2(n-1)$. Moreover, from property 2, we have $\frac{n-p}{(n-1)p}\mathbf{T}^2 \overset{d}{\sim} F_{p,n-p}$. Hence, the p-value of this Hotelling $\mathbf{T}^2$ test is $p = P\{F_{p,n-p} \geq \frac{n-p}{(n-1)p}T^2\}$.

1.22. Wilks Distribution[5,6]

Assume that $\mathbf{W}_1$ and $\mathbf{W}_2$ are independent, $\mathbf{W}_1 \overset{d}{\sim} W_p(n, \sum), \mathbf{W}_2 \overset{d}{\sim} W_p(m, \sum)$, where $\sum > 0, n \geq p$. Let

$$\mathbf{A} = \frac{|\mathbf{W}_1|}{|\mathbf{W}_1 + \mathbf{W}_2|},$$

then the random variable $\mathbf{A}$ follows the Wilks distribution with the degrees of freedom n and m, and denoted as $\Lambda_{p,n,m}$.

Some properties of Wilks distribution are as follows:

1. $\Lambda_{p,n,m} \overset{d}{=} B_1 B_2 \cdots B_p$, where $B_i \overset{d}{\sim} BE((n-i+1)/2, m/2), 1 \leq i \leq p$, and $B_1, \ldots, B_p$ are mutually independent.
2. $\Lambda_{p,n,m} \overset{d}{=} \Lambda_{m,n+m-p,p}$.
3. Some relationships between Wilks distribution and F distribution are:
   (1) $\frac{n}{m}\frac{1-\Lambda_{1,n,m}}{\Lambda_{1,n,m}} \overset{d}{\sim} F_{m,n}$;
   (2) $\frac{n+1-p}{p}\frac{1-\Lambda_{p,n,1}}{\Lambda_{p,n,1}} \overset{d}{\sim} F_{p,(n+1-p)}$;
   (3) $\frac{n-1}{m}\frac{1-\sqrt{\Lambda_{2,n,m}}}{\sqrt{\Lambda_{2,n,m}}} \overset{d}{\sim} F_{2m,2(n-1)}$;

(4) $\frac{n+1-p}{p}\frac{1-\sqrt{\Lambda_{p,n,2}}}{\sqrt{\Lambda_{p,n,2}}} \overset{d}{\sim} F_{2p,2(n+1-p)}$.

Wilks distribution is often used to model the distribution of a multivariate covariance. Suppose we have k mutually independent populations $\mathbf{X}_j \overset{d}{\sim} N_p(\mu_j, \sum)$, where $\sum > 0$ and $\sum$ is unknown. Let $x_{j1}, \ldots, x_{jn_j}$ be the random samples of population $\mathbf{X}_j, 1 \leq j \leq k$. Set $n = \sum_{j=1}^k n_j$, and we have $n \geq p + k$. We want to test the following hypothesis:

$$\mathbf{H}_0\colon \mu_1 = \cdots = \mu_k, \textit{ vs } \mathbf{H}_1\colon \mu_1, \ldots, \mu_k \text{ are not identical.}$$

Set

$$\bar{x}_j = n_j^{-1}\sum_{i=1}^{n_j} x_{ji}, \quad 1 \leq j \leq k,$$

$$V_j = \sum_{i=1}^{n_j}(x_{ji} - \bar{x}_j)(x_{ji} - \bar{x}_j)', \quad 1 \leq j \leq k,$$

$$\bar{x} = \sum_{j=1}^{k} n_j\bar{x}_j/n,$$

$\mathbf{SSB} = \sum_{j=1}^k n_j(\bar{x}_j - \bar{x})(\bar{x}_j - \bar{x})'$ be the between-group variance, $\mathbf{SSB} = \sum_{j=1}^k V_j$ be the within-group variance.

The likelihood ratio test statistic is

$$\Lambda = \frac{|\mathbf{SSW}|}{|\mathbf{SSW} + \mathbf{SSB}|}.$$

Under the null hypothesis $\mathbf{H}_0$, we have $\Lambda \overset{d}{\sim} \Lambda_{p,n-k,k-1}$. Following the relationships between Wilks distribution and F distribution, we have following conclusions:

(1) If $k = 2$, let

$$\mathbf{F} = \frac{n-p-1}{p} \cdot \frac{1-\Lambda}{\Lambda} \overset{d}{\sim} F_{p,n-p-1},$$

then the p-value of the test is

$$p = P\{F_{p,n-p-1} \geq \mathbf{F}\}.$$

(2) If $p = 2$, let

$$\mathbf{F} = \frac{n-k-1}{k-1} \cdot \frac{1-\sqrt{\Lambda}}{\sqrt{\Lambda}} \overset{d}{\sim} F_{2(k-1),2(n-k-1)},$$

then the p-value of the test is

$$p = P\{F_{2(k-1),2(n-k-1)} \geq \mathbf{F}\}.$$

(3) If $k = 3$, let

$$\mathbf{F} = \frac{n-p-2}{p} \cdot \frac{1-\sqrt{\Lambda}}{\sqrt{\Lambda}} \overset{d}{\sim} F_{2p,2(n-p-2)},$$

then the p-value of the test is

$$p = P\{F_{2p,2(n-p-2)} \geq \mathbf{F}\}.$$

References

1. Chow, YS, Teicher, H. *Probability Theory: Independence, Interchangeability, Martingales.* New York: Springer, 1988.
2. Fang, K, Xu, J. *Statistical Distributions.* Beijing: Science Press, 1987.
3. Krishnamoorthy, K. *Handbook of Statistical Distributions with Applications.* Boca Raton: Chapman and Hall/CRC, 2006.
4. Patel, JK, Kapadia, CH, and Owen, DB. *Handbook of Statistical Distributions.* New York: Marcel Dekker, 1976.
5. Anderson, TW. *An Introduction to Multivariate Statistical Analysis.* New York: Wiley, 2003.
6. Wang, J. *Multivariate Statistical Analysis.* Beijing: Science Press, 2008.

About the Author

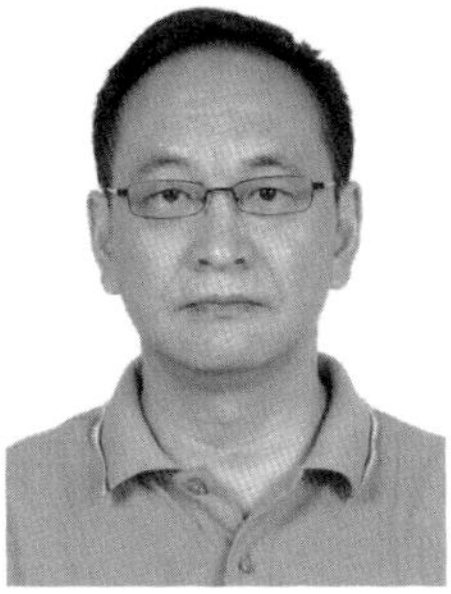

Dr. Jian Shi, graduated from Peking University, is Professor at the Academy of Mathematics and Systems Science in Chinese Academy of Sciences. His research interests include statistical inference, biomedical statistics, industrial statistics and statistics in sports. He has held and participated in several projects of the National Natural Science Foundation of China as well as applied projects.

CHAPTER 2

FUNDAMENTALS OF STATISTICS

Kang Li*, Yan Hou and Ying Wu

2.1. Descriptive Statistics[1]

Descriptive statistics is used to present, organize and summarize a set of data, and includes various methods of organizing and graphing the data as well as various indices that summarize the data with key numbers. An important distinction between descriptive statistics and inferential statistics is that while inferential statistics allows us to generalize from our sample data to a larger population, descriptive statistics allows us to get an idea of what characteristics the sample has. Descriptive statistics consists of numerical, tabular and graphical methods.

The numerical methods summarize the data by means of just a few numerical measures before any inference or generalization is drawn from the data. Two types of measures are used to numerically summarize the data, that is, measure of location and measure of variation (or dispersion or spread). One measure of location for the sample is arithmetic mean (or average, or mean or sample mean), usually denoted by $\bar{X}$, and is the sum of all observations divided by the number of observations, and can be written in statistical terms as $\bar{X} = n^{-1}\sum_{i=1}^{n} X_i$. The arithmetic mean is a very natural measure of location. One of the limitations, however, is that it is oversensitive to extreme values. An alternative measure of location is the median or sample median. Suppose there are n observations in a sample and all observations are ordered from smallest to largest, if n is odd, the median is the $(n+1)/2$th largest observation; if n is even, the median is the average of the $n/2$th and $(n/2+1)$th largest observations. Contrary to the arithmetic mean, the main

*Corresponding author: likang@ems.hrbmu.edu.cn

strength of the sample median is that it is insensitive to extreme values. The main weakness of the sample median is that it is determined mainly by the middle points in this sample and may take into less account the actual numeric values of the other data points. Another widely used measure of location is the mode. It is the most frequently occurring value among all the observations in a sample. Some distributions have more than one mode. The distribution with one mode is called unimodal; two modes, bimodal; three modes, trimodal, and so forth. Another popular measure of location is geometric mean and it is always used with skewed distributions. It is preferable to work in the original scale by taking the antilogarithm of $\log(X)$ to form the geometric mean, $G = \log^{-1}(n^{-1}\sum_{i=1}^{n}\log(X_i))$.

Measures of dispersion are used to describe the variability of a sample. The simplest measure of dispersion is the range. The range describes the difference between the largest and the smallest observations in a sample. One advantage of the range is that it is very easy to compute once the sample points are ordered. On the other hand, a disadvantage of the range is that it is affected by the sample size, i.e. the larger sample size, the larger the range tends to be. Another measure of dispersion is quantiles (or percentiles), which can address some of the shortcomings of the range in quantifying the spread in a sample. The xth percentile is the value P_x and is defined by the $(y+1)$th largest sample point if $nx/100$ is not an integer (where y is the largest integer less than $nx/100$) or the average of the $(nx/100)$th and $(nx/100+1)$th largest observations if $nx/100$ is an integer. Using percentiles is more advantageous over the range since it is less sensitive to outliers and less likely to be affected by the sample size. Another two measures of dispersion are sample variance and standard deviation, (SD) which are defined as $S^2 = (n-1)^{-1}\sum_{i=1}^{n}(X_i - \bar{X})^2$ and $S = \sqrt{S^2} = \sqrt{\text{sample variance}}$, where S is the sample SD. The SD is more often used than the variance as a measure of dispersion, since the SD and arithmetic mean use the same units whereas the variance and the arithmetic mean are not. Finally, the coefficient of variation, a measure of dispersion, is defined as $\text{CV} = S/\bar{X} \times 100\%$. This measure is most useful in comparing the variability of several different samples, each with different arithmetic means.

In continuation, tabular and graphical methods are the two other components of descriptive statistics. Although there are various ways of organizing and presenting data, the creation of simple tables for grouped data and graphs, however, still represents a very effective method. Tables are designed to help the readers obtain an overall feeling for the data at a glance. Several graphic techniques for summarizing data, including traditional methods, such as the bar graph, stem-and-leaf plot and box plot, are widely used. For more details, please refer to statistical graphs.

2.2. Statistical Graphs and Tables[2]

Statistical graphical and tabular methods are commonly used in descriptive statistics. The graphic methods convey the information and the general pattern of a set of data. Graphs are often an easy way to quickly display data and provide the maximum information indicating the principle trends in the data as well as suggesting which portions of the data should be examined in more detail using methods of inferential statistics. Graphs are simple, self-explanatory and often require little or no additional explanation. Tables always include clearly-labeled units of measurement and/or the magnitude of quantities.

We provide some important ways of graphically describing data including histograms, bar charts, linear graphs, and box plots. A histogram is a graphical representation of the frequency distribution of numerical data, in which the range of outcomes are stored in bins, or in other words, the range is divided into different intervals, and then the number of values that fall into each interval are counted. A bar chart is one of the most widely used methods for displaying grouped data, where each bar is associated with a different proportion. The difference between the histogram and the bar chart is whether there are spaces between the bars; the bars of histogram touch each other, while those of bar charts do not. A linear graph is similar to a bar graph, but in the case of a linear graph, the horizontal axis represents time. The most suitable application to use line graphs is a binary characteristic which is observed instances over time. The instances are observed in consecutive time periods such as years, so that a line graph is suitable to illustrate the outcomes over time. A box plot is used to describe the skewness of a distribution based on the relationships between the median, upper quartile, and lower quartile. Box plots may also have lines extending vertically from the boxes, known as whiskers, indicating the variability outside the upper and lower quartiles, hence the box plot's alternate names are box-and-whisker plot and box-and-whisker diagram. Box-and-whisker plots are uniform in their use of the box: The bottom and top of the box are always the first and third quartiles, and the band inside the box is always the second quartile (the median). However, the ends of the whiskers can represent several possible alternative values: either the minimum and maximum of the observed data or the lowest value within 1.5 times the interquartile range (IQR) of the lower quartile, and the highest value within 1.5 IQR of the upper quartile.

Box plots such as the latter are known as the Tukey box plot. In the case of a Tukey box plot, the outliers can be defined as the values outside 1.5 IQR, while the extreme values can be defined as the values outside 3 IQR. The main guideline for graphical representations of data sets is that the results should be understandable without reading the text. The captions, units and axes on graphs should be clearly labeled, and the statistical terms used in tables and graphs should be well defined.

Another way of summarizing and displaying features of a set of data is in the form of a statistical table. The structure and meaning of a statistical table is indicated by headings or labels and the statistical summary is provided by numbers in the body of the table. A statistical table is usually two-dimensional, in that the headings for the rows and columns define two different ways of categorizing the data. Each portion of the table defined by a combination of row and column is called a cell. The numerical information may be counts of individuals in different cells, mean values of some measurements or more complex indices.

2.3. Reference Range[3,4]

In health-related fields, the reference range or reference interval is the range of values for particular measurements in persons deemed as healthy, such as the amount of creatinine in the blood. In common practice, the reference range for a specific measurement is defined as the prediction interval between which 95% of the values of a reference group fall into, i.e. 2.5% of sample values would be less than the lower limit of this interval and 2.5% of values would be larger than the upper limit of this interval, regardless of the distribution of these values. Regarding the target population, if not otherwise specified, the reference range generally indicates the outcome measurement in healthy individuals, or individuals that are without any known condition that directly affects the ranges being established. Since the reference group is from the healthy population, sometimes the reference range is referred to as normal range or normal. However, using the term normal may not be appropriate since not everyone outside the interval is abnormal, and people who have a particular condition may still fall within this interval.

Methods for establishing the reference ranges are mainly based on the assumption of a normal distribution, or directly from the percentage of interest. If the population follows a normal distribution, the commonly used 95% reference range formula can be described as the mean $\pm$ 1.96 SDs. If the population distribution is skewed, parametric statistics are not valid and non-parametric statistics should be used. The non-parametric approach involves establishing the values falling at the 2.5 and 97.5 percentiles of the population as the lower and upper reference limits.

The following problems are noteworthy while establishing the reference range: (1) When it comes to classifying the homogeneous subjects, the influence to the indicators of the following factors shall be taken into consideration, e.g. regions, ethnical information, gender, age, pregnancy; (2) The measuring method, the sensitivity of the analytical technology, the purity of the reagents, the operation proficiency and so forth shall be standardized if possible; (3) The two-sided or one-sided reference range should be chosen correctly given the amount of professional knowledge at hand, e.g. it may be that it is abnormal when the numeration of leukocyte is too high or too low, but for the vital capacity, we say it is abnormal only if it is too low. In the practical application, it is preferable to take into account the characteristics of distribution, the false positive rate and false negative rate for an appropriate percentile range.

2.4. Sampling Errors[5]

In statistics, sampling error is incurred when the statistical characteristics of a population are estimated from a particular sample, in which the sampling error is mainly caused by the variation of the individuals. The statistics calculated from samples usually deviate from the true values of population parameters, since the samples are just a subset of population and sampling errors are mainly caused from sampling the population. In practice, it is hard to precisely measure the sampling error because the actual population parameters are unknown, but it can be accurately estimated from the probability model of the samples according to the law of large numbers. One of the major determinants of the accuracy of a sample statistic is whether the subjects in the sample are representative of the subjects in the population. The sampling error could reflect how representative the samples are relative to the population. The bigger the sampling error, the less representative the samples are to the population, and the less reliable the result; on the contrary, the smaller the sampling error, the more representative the samples are to the population, and the more reliable the sampling result.

It can be proved in theory that if the population is normally distributed with mean μ and SD σ, then the sample mean $\bar{X}$ is approximately a normal distribution with a mean equal to population mean μ and a SD $\sigma/\sqrt{n}$. According to the central limit theorem, in situations that the sample size n is arbitrarily large enough (e.g. $n \geq 50$), the distribution of the sample mean $\bar{X}$ is approximately normally distributed $N(\mu, \sigma^2/n)$ regardless of the underlying distribution of the population. The SD of a sample measures the variation of individual observations while the standard error of mean refers to the variations of the sample mean. Obviously, the standard error is smaller than the SD of the original measurements. The smaller the standard error, the more accurate the estimation, thus, the standard error of mean can be a good measure of the sampling error of the mean. In reality, for unlimited populations or under the condition of sampling with replacement, the sampling error of the sample mean can be estimated as follows:

$$S_{\bar{X}} = \frac{S}{\sqrt{n}},$$

where S is the sample SD, n is the sample size. For finite populations or situations of sampling without replacement, the formula to estimate the standard error is

$$S_{\bar{X}} = \sqrt{\frac{S^2}{n}\left(\frac{N-n}{N-1}\right)},$$

where N is the population size.

The standard error of the sample probability for binary data can be estimated according to the properties of a binomial distribution. Under the condition of sampling with replacement, the standard error formula of the frequency is

$$S_p = \sqrt{\frac{P(1-P)}{n}},$$

where P is the frequency of the "positive" response in the sample. Under the condition of sampling without replacement, the standard error of the frequency is

$$S_p = \sqrt{\frac{P(1-P)}{n}\left(\frac{N-n}{N-1}\right)},$$

where N is the population size and n is the sample size.

The factors that affect the sampling error are as follows: (1) The amount of variation within the individual measurements, such that the bigger the variation, the bigger the sampling error; (2) For a binomial distribution, the closer the population rate is to 0.5, the bigger the sampling error; (3) In terms of sample size, the larger the sample size, the less the corresponding sampling error; (4) Sampling error also depends on the sampling methods utilized.

2.5. Parameter Estimation[6,7]

Parameter estimation is the process of using the statistics of a random sample to estimate the unknown parameters of the population. In practice, researchers often need to analyze or infer the fundamental regularities of population data based on sample data, that is, they need to infer the distribution or numerical characteristics of the population from sample data.

Parameter estimation is an important part of statistical inference, and consists of point estimation and interval estimation. Point estimation is the use of sample information $X_1, \ldots, X_n$ to create the proper statistic $\hat{\theta}(X_1, \ldots, X_n)$, and to use this statistic directly as the estimated value of the unknown population parameter. Some common point estimation methods include moment estimation, maximum likelihood estimation (MLE), least square estimation, Bayesian estimation, and so on. The idea of moment estimation is to use the sample moment to estimate the population moment, e.g. to estimate the population mean using the sample mean directly. MLE is the idea of constructing the likelihood function using the distribution density of the sample, and then calculating the estimated value of the parameter by maximizing the likelihood function. The least square estimation mainly applies to the linear model where the parameter value is estimated by minimizing the residual sum of squares. Bayesian estimation makes use of one of the characteristic values of the posterior distribution to estimate the population parameter, such as the mean of the posterior distribution (posterior expected estimation), median (posterior median estimation) or the estimated value of the population parameter that maximizes the posterior density (posterior maximum estimation). In general, these point estimation methods are different, except for when the posterior density is symmetrically distributed. The reason for the existence of different estimators is that different loss functions in the posterior distribution lead to different estimated values. It is practical to select an appropriate estimator according to different needs.

Due to sampling error, it is almost impossible to get 100% accuracy when we estimate the population parameter using the sample statistic. Thus, it is necessary to take the magnitude of the sampling error into consideration. Interval estimation is the use of sample data to calculate an interval that can cover the unknown population parameters according to a predefined probability. The predefined probability $1 - \alpha$ is defined as the confidence level (usually 0.95 or 0.99), and this interval is known as the confidence interval (CI). The CI consists of two confidence limits defined by two values: the lower limit (the smaller value) and the upper limit (the bigger value). The formula for the confidence limit of the mean that is commonly used in practice is $\bar{X} \pm t_{\alpha/2,\nu} S_{\bar{X}}$, where $S_{\bar{X}} = S/\sqrt{n}$ is the standard error, $t_{\alpha/2,\nu}$ is the quartile of the t distribution located on the point of $1 - \alpha/2$ (two-sided critical value), and $\nu = n - 1$ is the degree of freedom. The CI of the probability is $p \pm z_{\alpha/2} S_p$, where $S_p = \sqrt{p(1-p)/n}$ is the standard error, p is the sample rate, and $z_{\alpha/2}$ is the quartile of the normal distribution located on the point $1-\alpha/2$ (two-sided critical value). The CI of the probability can be precisely calculated according to the principle of the binomial distribution when the sample size is small (e.g. $n < 50$). It is obvious that the precision of the interval estimation is reflected by the width of the interval, and the reliability is reflected in the confidence level $(1 - \alpha)$ of the range that covers the population parameter.

Many statistics are used to estimate the unknown parameters in practice. Since there are various methods to evaluate the performance of the statistic, we should make a choice according to the nature of the problems in practice and the methods of theoretical research. The common assessment criteria include the small-sample and the large-sample criterion. The most commonly used small-sample criteria mainly consist of the level of unbiasedness and effectiveness of the estimation (minimum variance unbiased estimation). On the other hand, the large-sample criteria includes the level of consistency (compatibility), optimal asymptotic normality as well as effectiveness.

2.6. The Method of Least Squares[8,9]

In statistics, the method of least squares is a typical technique for estimating a parameter or vector parameter in regression analysis. Consider a statistical model

$$Y = \xi(\theta) + e,$$

where ξ is a known parametric function of the unknown parameter θ and a random error e. The problem at hand is to estimate the unknown parameter θ. Suppose $Y_1, Y_2, \ldots, Y_n$ are n independent observations and $\hat{Y}_1, \hat{Y}_2, \ldots, \hat{Y}_n$ are the corresponding estimated values given by

$$\hat{Y} = \xi(\hat{\theta}),$$

where $\hat{\theta}$ is an estimator of θ, then the deviation of the sample point Y_i from the model is given by

$$e_i = Y_i - \hat{Y}_i = Y_i - \xi(\hat{\theta}).$$

A good-fitting model would make these deviations as small as possible. Because $e_i, i = 1, \ldots, n$ cannot all be zero in practice, the criterion $Q_1 =$ sum of absolute deviation $s = \sum_{i=1}^{n} |e_i|$ can be used and the estimator $\hat{\theta}$ that minimizes Q_1 can be found. However, for both theoretical reasons and ease of derivation, the criterion Q = sum of the squared deviations $= \sum_{i=1}^{n} e_i^2$ is commonly used. The principle of least squares minimizes Q instead and the resulting estimator of θ is called the least squares estimate. As a result, this method of estimating the parameters of a statistical model is known as the method of least squares. The least squares estimate is a solution of the least square equations that satisfy $dS/d\theta = 0$.

The method of least squares has a widespread application where ξ is a linear function of θ. The simplest case is that $\xi = \alpha + \beta X$, where X is a covariate or explanatory variable in a simple linear regression model

$$Y = \alpha + \beta X + e.$$

The corresponding least squares estimates are given by

$$\hat{\beta} = \frac{L_{xy}}{L_{xx}} \quad \text{and} \quad \hat{\alpha} = \bar{Y} - \hat{\beta}\bar{X} = \frac{\left(\sum_{i=1}^{n} Y_i - \hat{\beta}\sum_{i=1}^{n} X_i\right)}{n},$$

where L_{XX} and L_{XY} denote the corrected sum of squares for X and the corrected sum of cross products, respectively, and are defined as

$$L_{XX} = \sum_{i=1}^{n} (X_i - \bar{X})^2 \quad \text{and} \quad L_{XY} = \sum_{i=1}^{n} (X_i - \bar{X})(Y_i - \bar{Y}).$$

The least squares estimates of parameters in the model $Y = \xi(\theta) + e$ are unbiased and have the smallest variance among all unbiased estimators for a wide class of distributions where e is a $N(0, \sigma^2)$ error. When e is not normally distributed, a least squares estimation is no longer relevant, but rather the maximum likelihood estimation MLE (refer to 2.19) usually is applicable. However, the weighted least squares method, a special case of generalized least squares which takes observations with unequal care, has computational applications in the iterative procedures required to find the MLE. In particular, weighted least squares is useful in obtaining an initial value to start the iterations, using either the Fisher's scoring algorithm or Newton–Raphson methods.

2.7. Property of the Estimator[6,10,11]

The estimator is the function of estimation for observed data. The attractiveness of different estimators can be judged by looking at their properties, such as unbiasedness, consistency, efficiency, etc. Suppose there is a fixed parameter θ that needs to be estimated, the estimate is $\hat{\theta} = \hat{\theta}(X_1, X_2, \ldots, X_n)$. The estimator $\hat{\theta}$ is an unbiased estimator of θ if and only if $E(\hat{\theta}) = \theta$. If $E(\hat{\theta}) \neq \theta$ but $\lim_{n\to\infty} E(\hat{\theta}) = \theta, \hat{\theta}$ is called the asymptotically unbiased estimate of θ. $\hat{\theta}$ is interpreted as a random variable corresponding to the observed data. Unbiasedness does not indicate that the estimate of a sample from the population is equal to or approaching the true value or that the estimated value of any one sample from the population is equal to or approached to the true value, but rather it suggests that the mean of the estimates through data collection by sampling *ad infinitum* from the population is an unbiased value. For example, when sampling from an infinite population, the sample mean

$$\bar{X} = \frac{X_1 + X_2 + \cdots + X_n}{n} = \frac{\sum_{i=1}^{n} X_i}{n},$$

is an unbiased estimator of the population mean μ, that is, $E(\bar{X}) = \mu$. The sample variance is an unbiased estimator of the population variance σ^2, that is, $E(S^2) = \sigma^2$.

The consistency of the parameter estimation, also known as the compatibility, is that increasing the sample size increases the probability of the estimator being close to the population parameter. When the sample size $n \to \infty$, $\hat{\theta}$ converges to θ, and $\hat{\theta}$ is the consistent estimate of θ. For example, the consistency for a MLE is provable. If the estimation is consistent, the accuracy and reliability for the estimation can be improved by increasing the sample size. Consistency is the prerequisite for the estimator. Estimators without consistency should not be taken into consideration.

The efficiency of an estimator compares the different magnitudes of different estimators to the same population. Generally, a parameter value has multiple estimators. If all estimators of a parameter are unbiased, the one with the lowest variance is the efficient estimator. Suppose there are two estimators $\hat{\theta}_1$ and $\hat{\theta}_2$, the efficiency is defined as: under the condition that $E(\hat{\theta}_1) = \theta$ and $E(\hat{\theta}_2) = \theta$, if $\text{Var}(\hat{\theta}_1) < \text{Var}(\hat{\theta}_2)$, then $\hat{\theta}_1$ is deemed more efficiency than $\hat{\theta}_2$. In some cases, an unbiased efficient estimator exists, which, in addition to having the lowest variance among unbiased estimators, must satisfy the Cramér–Rao bound, which is an absolute lower bound on variance for statistics of a variable.

Beyond the properties of estimators as described above, in practice, the shape of the distribution is also a property evaluated for estimators as well.

2.8. Hypothesis Testing[12]

Hypothesis testing is an important component of inferential statistics, and it is a method for testing a hypothesis about a parameter in a population using data measured in a sample. The hypothesis is tested by determining the likelihood that a sample statistic could have been selected, given that the hypothesis regarding the population parameter were true. For example, we begin by stating that the value of population mean will be equal to sample mean. The larger the actual difference or discrepancy between the sample mean and population mean, the less likely it is that the sample mean is equal to the population mean as stated. The method of hypothesis testing can be summarized in four steps: stating the hypothesis, setting the criteria for a decision, computing the test statistic, and finally making a conclusion. In stating the hypothesis in this case, we first state the value of the population mean in a null hypothesis and alternative hypothesis. The null hypothesis, denoted as H_0, is a statement about a population parameter, such as the population mean in this case, that is assumed to be true. The alternative hypothesis, denoted as H_1, is a statement that directly contradicts the null hypothesis, stating that the actual value of a population parameter is less than, greater than, or not equal to the value stated in the null hypothesis. In the second step, where we set the criteria for a decision, we state the level of significance for a test. The significance level is based on the probability of obtaining a statistic measured in a sample if the value stated in the null hypothesis were true and is typically set at 5%. We use the value of the test statistic to make a decision about the null hypothesis. The decision is based on the probability of obtaining a sample mean, given that the value stated in the null hypothesis is true. If the probability of obtaining a sample mean is less than the 5% significance level when the null hypothesis is true, then the conclusion we make would be to reject the null hypothesis. Various methods of hypothesis testing can be used to calculate the test statistic, such as a t-test, ANOVA, chi-square test and Wilcoxon rank sum test.

On the other hand when we decide to retain the null hypothesis, we can either be correct or incorrect. One such incorrect decision is to retain a false null hypothesis, which represents an example of a Type II error, or β error. With each test we make, there is always some probability that the decision could result in a Type II error. In the cases where we decide to reject the null hypothesis, we can be correct or incorrect as well. The incorrect decision is to reject a true null hypothesis. This decision is an example of a Type I error, or the probability of rejecting a null hypothesis that is actually true. With each test we make, there is always some probability that our decision is a Type I error. Researchers directly try to control the probability of committing this type of error. Since we assume the null hypothesis is true, we control for Type I error by stating a significance level. As mentioned before, the criterion is usually set at 0.05 ($\alpha = 0.05$) and is compared to the p value. When the probability of a Type I error is less than 5% ($p < 0.05$), we decide to reject the null hypothesis; otherwise, we retain the null hypothesis. The correct decision is to reject a false null hypothesis. There is always a good probability that we decide that the null hypothesis is false when it is indeed false. The power of the decision-making process is defined specifically as the probability of rejecting a false null hypothesis. In other words, it is the probability that a randomly selected sample will show that the null hypothesis is false when the null hypothesis is indeed false.

2.9. *t*-test[13]

A t-test is a common hypothesis test for comparing two population means, and it includes the one sample t-test, paired t-test and two independent sample t-test.

The one sample t-test is suitable for comparing the sample mean $\bar{X}$ with the known population mean μ_0. In practice, the known population mean μ_0 is usually the standard value, theoretical value, or index value that is relatively stable based on a large amount of observations. The test statistic is

$$t = \frac{\bar{X} - \mu_0}{S/\sqrt{n}}, \quad \nu = n - 1,$$

where S is the sample SD, n is the sample size and ν is the degree of freedom.

The paired t-test is suitable for comparing two sample means of a paired design. There are two kinds of paired design: (1) homologous pairing, that is, the same subject or specimen is divided into two parts, which are randomly assigned one of two different kinds of treatments; (2) non-homologous pairing, in which two homogenous test subjects are assigned two kinds of treatments in order to get rid of the influence of the confounding factors. The test statistic is

$$t = \frac{\bar{d}}{S_d/\sqrt{n}}, \quad \nu = n - 1,$$

where $\bar{d}$ is the sample mean of paired measurement differences, S_d is the SD of the differences, n is the number of the pairs and ν is the degree of freedom.

The two independent sample t-test is suitable for comparing two sample means of a completely randomized design, and its purpose is to test whether two population means are the same. The testing conditions include the assumptions of normal distribution and equal variance, which can be confirmed by running the test of normality and test of equal variance, respectively. The test statistic is

$$t = \frac{|\bar{X}_1 - \bar{X}_2| - 0}{S_{\bar{X}_1 - \bar{X}_2}} = \frac{|\bar{X}_1 - \bar{X}_2|}{S_{\bar{X}_1 - \bar{X}_2}}, \quad \nu = n_1 + n_2 - 2,$$

where

$$S_{\bar{X}_1 - \bar{X}_2} = \sqrt{S_c^2 \left(\frac{1}{n_1} + \frac{1}{n_2} \right)},$$

n_1 and n_2 are the sample sizes of the two groups, respectively, and S_c^2 is the pooled variance of the two groups

$$S_c^2 = \frac{(n_1 - 1)S_1^2 + (n_2 - 1)S_2^2}{n_1 + n_2 - 2}.$$

If the variances of the two populations are not equal, Welch's t-test method is recommended. The test statistic is

$$t = \frac{X_1 - X_2}{S_{\bar{X}_1 - \bar{X}_2}}, \quad \nu = \frac{(S_1^2/n_1 + S_2^2/n_2)^2}{\frac{(S_1^2/n_1)^2}{n_1 - 1} + \frac{(S_2^2/n_2)^2}{n_2 - 1}},$$

where

$$S_{\bar{X}_1 - \bar{X}_2} = \sqrt{\frac{S_1^2}{n_1} + \frac{S_2^2}{n_2}}.$$

The actual distribution of the test statistic is dependent on the variances of two unknown populations (please refer to the Behrens–Fisher problem for details).

When the assumptions of normality or equal variance are not met, the permutation t-test can be taken into account (please refer to Chapter 13 for details). In the permutation t-test, the group labels of the samples are randomly permuted, and the corresponding t value is calculated. After repeating this process several times, the simulation distribution is obtained, which can be accepted as the distribution of the t statistic under the null hypothesis. At this stage, the t value from the original data can be compared with the simulation distribution to calculate the accumulated one-tailed probability or two-tailed probability, that is, the p-value of the one-sided or two-sided permutation t-test for comparing two independent sample means. Finally, the p-value can be compared with the significance level of α to make a decision on whether to retain or reject the null hypothesis.

2.10. Analysis of Variance (ANOVA)[14,15]

ANOVA, also known as F-test, is a kind of variance decomposition method, which decomposes, compares and tests the observed variation from different sources and can be used to analyze the differences among data sets as well as linear regression analysis. ANOVA can be used to analyze data from various experimental designs, such as completely randomized design, randomized block design, factorial design and so on. When ANOVA is used for comparing multiple sample means, the specific principle is to partition the total variation of all observations into components that each represent a different source of variation as such:

$$\mathrm{SS}_{\mathrm{Total}} = \mathrm{SS}_{\mathrm{Treatment}} + \mathrm{SS}_{\mathrm{Error}}.$$

The test statistic F can be calculated as:

$$F = \frac{\mathrm{SS}_{\mathrm{Treatment}}/\nu_{\mathrm{Treatment}}}{\mathrm{SS}_{\mathrm{Error}}/\nu_{\mathrm{Error}}},$$

where $\mathrm{SS}_{\mathrm{Treatment}}$ and $\mathrm{SS}_{\mathrm{Error}}$ are the variations caused by treatment and individual differences, respectively, and $\nu_{\mathrm{Treatment}}$ and ν_{Error} are the corresponding degrees of freedom. The test statistic F follows the F-distribution, so we can calculate the p-value according to the F-value and F-distribution. If two-sample t-test is used for multiple comparisons between means, the overall type I error will increase. The assumptions of ANOVA include the following: the observations are mutually independent, the residuals follow a normal distribution and the population variances are the same. The independence of observations can be judged by professional knowledge and research background. The normality of residuals can be tested by a residual plot or other diagnostic statistics. The homogeneity of variances can be tested by F-test, Levene test, Bartlett test or Brown–Forsythe test. The null hypothesis of ANOVA is that the population means are equal between two or more groups. The rejection of the null hypothesis only means that the population means of different groups are not equal, or not all the population means are equal. In this case, pairwise comparisons are needed to obtain more detailed information about group means. The commonly used pairwise comparison methods are Dunnett-t-test, LSD-t-test, SNK-q (Student–Newman–Keuls) test, Tukey test, Scheffé test, Bonferroni t-test, and Sidak t-test. In practice, the pairwise comparison method should be adopted according to the research purposes.

ANOVA can be divided into one-way ANOVA and multi-way ANOVA according to the research purposes and number of treatment factors. One-way ANOVA refers to that there is only one treatment factor and the purpose is to test whether the effects of different levels of this factor on the observed variable is statistically significant. The fundamental principle of one-way ANOVA is to compare the variations caused by treatment factor and uncontrolled factors. If the variation caused by the treatment factor makes up the major proportion of the total variation, it indicates that the variation of the observed variable is mainly caused by the treatment factor. Otherwise, the variation is mainly caused by the uncontrolled factors. Multi-way ANOVA indicates that two or more study factors affect the observed variable. It can not only analyze the independent effects of multiple treatment factors on the observed variable, but also identify the effects of interactions between or among treatment factors.

In addition, the ANOVA models also include the random-effect model and covariance analysis model. The random-effect model can include the fixed effect and random effect at the same time, and the covariance analysis model can adjust the effects of covariates.

2.11. Multiple Comparisons[16,17]

The term of multiple comparisons refers to carrying out multiple analyses on the basis of subgroups of subjects defined *a priori*. A typical case is to perform the comparisons of every possible pair of multiple groups after ANOVA; another case is to perform the comparisons of repeated measurement data. The multiple comparisons also occur when one is considering multiple endpoints within the same study. In these cases, several significance tests are carried out and the issue of multiple comparisons is raised. For example, in a clinical trial of a new drug for the treatment of hypertension, blood pressures need to be measured within eight weeks of treatment once a week. If the test group and control group are compared at each visit using the t-test procedure, then some significant differences are likely to be found just by chance. It can be proved that the total significance level is $\bar{\alpha} = 1-(1-\alpha)^m$ when m times of independent comparison are performed, from which we can see that $\bar{\alpha}$ will increase as the number of comparisons increases. In the above example, $\bar{\alpha}$ will be $\bar{\alpha} = 1 - (1 - 0.05)^8 = 0.3366$.

Several multiple comparison procedures can ensure that the overall probability of declaring any significant differences between all comparisons is maintained at some fixed significance level α. Multiple comparison procedures may be categorized as single-step or stepwise procedures. In single-step procedures, multiple tests are carried out using the same critical value for each component test. In stepwise procedures, multiple tests are carried out in sequence using unequal critical values. Single-step procedures mainly include Bonferroni adjustment, Tukey's test, Scheffé method, etc. Stepwise procedures mainly include SNK test, Duncan's multiple range test (MRT), Dunnett-t test, etc. The method of Bonferroni adjustment is one of the simplest and most widely used multiple comparison procedures. If there are k comparisons, each comparison is conducted at the level of significance $\alpha' = \alpha/k$. The Bonferroni procedure is conservative and may not be applicable if there are too many comparisons. In Tukey's testing, under the normality and homogeneous variance assumptions, we calculate the q test statistic for every pair of groups and compare it with a critical value determined by studentized range. Scheffé method is applicable for not only comparing pairs of means but also comparing pairs of linear contrasts. SNK test is similar to Tukey's test that both procedures use the studentized range statistics. They differ in the way that the significance level for every comparison is fixed. Duncan's MRT is a modification of the SNK test, which leads to an increasing of the statistical power. Dunnett-t test mainly applies to the comparisons of every test group with the same control group.

2.12. Chi-square Test[6,18]

Chi-square (χ^2) test is a hypothesis testing method based on the chi-square distribution. The common methods include Pearson χ^2 test, McNemar χ^2 test, test of goodness of fit and so on.

Pearson χ^2 test is a main statistical inference method used for contingency table data, of which the main purpose is to infer whether there is a significant difference between two or more population proportions, or to test whether the row and column factors are mutually independent. The form of $R \times C$ two-way contingency table is shown in Table 2.12.1, in which N_{ij} indicates the actual frequency in the i-th row and j-th column, and N_{i+} and N_{+j} indicate the sum of frequencies in the corresponding rows and columns, respectively.

The formula of the test statistic of Pearson χ^2 is as follows:

$$\chi^2 = \sum_{i=1}^{R}\sum_{j=1}^{C}\frac{(N_{ij} - T_{ij})^2}{T_{ij}}$$

and the degree of freedom is

$$\nu = (R-1)(C-1),$$

where T_{ij} is the theoretical frequency, and the formula is

$$T_{ij} = \frac{N_{i+}N_{+j}}{N}.$$

Table 2.12.1. The general form of two-way contingency table.

Row factor	Column factor (observed frequencies) $j = 1$	$j = 2$	$\ldots$	$j = C$	Row sum
$i = 1$	N_{11}	N_{12}	$\ldots$	N_{1C}	N_{1+}
$i = 2$	N_{21}	N_{22}	$\ldots$	N_{2C}	N_{2+}
$\vdots$	$\vdots$	$\vdots$		$\vdots$	$\vdots$
$i = R$	N_{R1}	N_{R2}	$\ldots$	N_{RC}	N_{R+}
Column sum	N_{+1}	N_{+2}	$\ldots$	N_{+C}	N

Table 2.12.2. An example of 2×2 contingency table of two independent groups.

Row factor	Column factor Positive	Negative	Row sum
Level 1	a	b	$a + b$
Level 2	c	d	$c + d$
Column sum	$a + c$	$b + d$	n

This indicates the theoretical frequency in the corresponding grid when the null hypothesis H_0 is true. The statistic χ^2 follows a chi-square distribution with degrees of freedom ν. The null hypothesis can be rejected when χ^2 is bigger than the critical value corresponding to a given significant level. The χ^2 statistic reflects how well the actual frequency matches the theoretical frequency, so it can be inferred whether there are any differences in the frequency distribution between or among different groups. In practice, if it is a 2×2 contingency table and the data form can be shown as in Table 2.12.2, the formula can be abbreviated as

$$\chi^2 = \frac{(ad - bc)^2 n}{(a + b)(c + d)(a + c)(b + d)}.$$

McNemar χ^2 test is suitable for the hypothesis testing of the 2×2 contingency table data of a paired design. For example, Table 2.12.3 shows the results of each individual detected by different methods at the same time, and it is required to compare the difference of the positive rates between the two methods.

This is the comparison of two sets of dependent data, and McNemar χ^2 test should be used. In this case, only the data related to different outcomes

Table 2.12.3. An example of 2×2 contingency table of paired data.

	Method 2		
Method 1	Positive	Negative	Row sum
Positive	a	b	$a+b$
Negative	c	d	$c+d$
Column sum	$a+c$	$b+d$	n

by the two methods will be considered, and the test statistic is

$$\chi^2 = \frac{(b-c)^2}{b+c},$$

where the degree of freedom is 1. When b or c is relatively small ($b+c < 40$), the adjusted statistics should be used:

$$\chi^2 = \frac{(|b-c|-1)^2}{b+c}.$$

2.13. Fisher's Exact Test[6,19]

Fisher's exact test is a hypothesis testing method for contingency table data. Both Fisher's exact test and Pearson χ^2 test can be used to compare the distribution proportions of two or more categorical variables in different categories. When the sample size is small, the Pearson χ^2 test statistic would result in an inferior goodness-of-fit for the χ^2 distribution. In this case, the analysis results of Pearson χ^2 test may be inaccurate, while Fisher's exact test could be an alternative. When comparing two probabilities, the 2×2 contingency table (Table 2.13.1) is usually used.

The null hypothesis of the test is that the treatment has no influence on the probability of the observation results. Under the null hypothesis, the

Table 2.13.1. The general form of 2×2 contingency table data of two independent groups.

	Results		
Row factor	Positive	Negative	Row sum
Level 1	a	b	n
Level 2	c	d	m
Column sum	S	F	N

Table 2.13.2. The calculating table of Fisher's exact probability test.

k	Combinations a	b	c	d	Occurrence probability
0	0	n	S	$F-n$	P_0
1	1	$n-1$	$S-1$	$F-n+1$	P_1
2	2	$n-2$	$S-2$	$F-n+2$	P_2
$\vdots$	$\vdots$	$\vdots$	$\vdots$	$\vdots$	$\vdots$
$\min(n,S)$	$\ldots$	$\ldots$	$\ldots$	$\ldots$	$\ldots$

occurrence probabilities of all possible combinations (see Table 2.12.2) with fixed margins S, F, n, m can be calculated based on the hyper geometric distribution, and the formula is

$$p_k = \frac{C_S^k C_F^{n-k}}{C_N^n}.$$

The one-sided or two-sided accumulated probabilities are then selected according to the alternative hypothesis, and the statistical inference can be made according to the significance level. If the alternative hypothesis is that the positive rate of level 1 is larger than that of level 2 in the one-sided test, the formula for p value is

$$p = \sum_{k=a}^{\min(n,S)} \frac{C_S^k C_F^{n-k}}{C_N^n}.$$

There is no unified formula for calculating the p value in a two-sided test. The specific method is to get the p value through summing all the two-sided accumulated probabilities which are lower than the occurrence probability for the current sample, and then compare it with the given significance level. To select whether a one-sided test or two-sided test for data analysis should be determined according to the study purposes at the design stage, Fisher's exact test can be implemented by various common statistical analysis software.

Although Fisher's exact test is applicable for a small sample size, its results are relatively conservative. The mid-p test improved on this basis can enhance the power to a certain extent, and the calculation principle of the mid-p value is

$$\begin{aligned}&\text{mid-}p\\&\quad=\Pr(\text{Situations that are more favorable to } H_1\\&\qquad\quad \text{than the current status } |H_0)\\&\qquad+\frac{1}{2}\Pr(\text{Situations that have the same favor for } H_1\\&\qquad\qquad \text{as the current status}|H_0),\end{aligned}$$

H_1 is the alternative hypothesis. For the standard Fisher's exact test, the calculation principle of p-value is

$$\begin{aligned}p=\Pr(&\text{Situations that have more or the same favor for } H_1\\&\text{than the current status } |H_0).\end{aligned}$$

Thus, the power of the mid-p test is higher than that of the standard Fisher's exact test. Statistical analysis software StatXact could be used to calculate the mid-p value.

Fisher's exact test can be extended to $R \times C$ contingency table data, and is applicable to multiple testing of $R \times 2$ contingency table as well. However, there is still the problem of type I error expansion.

2.14. Goodness-of-fit Test[6,20]

The goodness-of-fit test may compare the empirical distribution function (EDF) of the sample with the cumulative distribution function of the proposed distribution, or assess the goodness of fit of any statistical models. Two famous tests of goodness of fit are chi-squared test (χ^2) and Kolmogorov–Smirnov (K–S) test. The basic idea behind the chi-square test is to assess the agreement between an observed set of frequencies and the theoretical probabilities. Generally, the null hypothesis (H_0) is that, the observed sample data $X_1, X_2, \ldots, X_n$ follow a specified continuous distribution function: $F(x;\theta) = \Pr(X < x|\theta)$, where θ is an unknown parameter of the population. For example, to test the hypothesis that a sample has been drawn from a normal distribution, first of all, we should estimate the population mean μ and variance σ^2 using the sample data. Then we divided the sample into k non-overlapping intervals, denoted as $(a_0, a_1], (a_1, a_2], \cdots (a_{k-1}, a_k]$, according to the range of expected values. If the null hypothesis is true, the probability of any X that fell into ith interval can be calculated as

$$\pi_i(\theta) = Pr(a_{i-1} < X_i \leq a_i) = \int_{a_{i-1}}^{a_i} dF(x;\theta).$$

The theoretical numbers in the ith interval is given by $m_j = n\pi_j(\theta)$, and subsequently, the test statistic can be calculated by

$$\chi^2 = \sum_{i=1}^{k} \frac{(N_i - m_i)^2}{m_i}.$$

The test statistic asymptotically follows a chi-squared distribution with k-r-1 degrees of freedom, where k is the number of intervals and r is the number of estimated population parameters. Reject H_0 if this value exceeds the upper α critical value of the $\chi^2_{\nu,\alpha}$ distribution, where α is the desired level of significance.

Random interval goodness of fit is an alternative method to resolve the same issue. Firstly, we calculate the probabilities of the k intervals, which are denoted as $\pi_1, \pi_2, \ldots, \pi_k$, as well as the thresholds of each interval judged by the probabilities, and then calculate the observed frequencies and expected frequencies of each interval. Provided that $F(x;\theta)$ is the distribution function under null hypothesis, the thresholds can be calculated by

$$a_i(\theta) = F^{-1}(\pi_1 + \pi_2 + \cdots + \pi_i; \theta), \quad i = 1, 2, \ldots, k,$$

where $F^{-1}(c;\theta)\inf[x\colon F(x;\theta) \geq c]$ and θ and can be replaced by the sample estimated value $\hat{\theta}$. Once the thresholds of each random interval is determined, the theoretical frequency that fell into each interval, as well as the calculation of test statistics, is consistent with that of fixed intervals.

The K–S test is based on the EDF, which is used to investigate if a sample is drawn from a population of a specific distribution, or to compare two empirical distributions. To compare the cumulative frequency distribution of a sample with a specific distribution, if the difference is small, we can support the hypothesis that the sample is drawn from the reference distribution. The two-sample K–S test is one of the most useful non-parametric methods for comparing two samples, as it is sensitive to differences in both location and shape of the empirical cumulative distribution functions of the two samples.

For the single sample K–S test, the null hypothesis is that, the data follow a specified distribution defined as $F(X)$. In most cases, $F(X)$ is one-dimensional continuous distribution function, e.g. normal distribution, uniform distribution and exponential distribution. The test statistic is defined by

$$Z = \sqrt{n}\max(|F_n(X_{i-1}) - F(X_i)|, |F_n(X_i) - F(X_i)|),$$

where $F_n(x_i)$ is the cumulative probability function of the random sample. Z converges to the Kolmogorov distribution. Compared with chi-square test, the advantage of K–S test is that it can be carried out without dividing the sample into different groups.

For the two-samples K–S test, the null hypothesis is that the two data samples come from the same distribution, denoted as $F_1(X) = F_2(X)$. Given $D_i = F_1(X_i) = F_2(X_i)$, the test statistic is defined as

$$Z = \max |D_i| \sqrt{\frac{n_1 n_2}{n_1 + n_2}},$$

where n_1 and n_2 are the observations of two samples, respectively. Z asymptotically follows a standard normal distribution when the null hypothesis is true.

2.15. Test of Normality[21,22]

Many statistical procedures are based on the assumption of normally distributed population, like two-sample t-test, ANOVA, or decision of reference value. Test of normality is used to determine whether a data set is well modeled by a normal distribution and to compute how likely the underlying population is normally distributed. There are numerous methods for normality test. The most widely used methods include moment test, chi-square test and EDF.

Graphical methods: One of the usual graphical tools for assessing normality is the probability–probability plot (P–P plot). P–P plot is a scatter plot of the cumulative frequency of observed data against normal distribution. For normal population the points plotted in the P–P plot should fall approximately on a straight line from point (0,0) to point (1,1). The deviation of the points indicates the degree of non-normality. Quantile–quantile plot (Q–Q plot) is similar to P–P plot but uses quantiles instead.

Moment test: Deviations from normality could be described by the standardized third and fourth moments of a distribution, defined as

$$\sqrt{\beta_1} = \frac{\mu_2}{\sigma^2} \quad \text{and} \quad \beta_2 = \frac{\mu_4}{\sigma^4}.$$

Here $\mu_i = E(X - E(X))^i, i = 3, 4$ is the ith central moment for $i = 3, 4$, and $\sigma^2 = E(X - \mu)^2$ is the variance. If a distribution is symmetric about its mean, then $\sqrt{\beta_1} = 0$. Values different from zero indicate skewness and so non-normality. β_2 characterizes kurtosis (or peakedness and tail thickness) of a distribution. Since $\beta_2 = 3$ for normal distribution, other values indicate non-normality. Tests of normality following from this are based on $\sqrt{\beta_1}$ and

β_2, respectively, given as

$$\sqrt{b_1} = \frac{m_3}{m_2^{3/2}}, \quad b_2 = \frac{m_4}{m_2^2},$$

where

$$m_k = \sum \frac{(X - \bar{X})^k}{n}, \quad \bar{X} = \frac{\sum X}{n}.$$

Here n is the sample size. The moment statistics in combination with extensive tables of critical points and approximations can be applied separately to tests of non-normality due specifically to skewness or kurtosis. They can also be applied jointly for an omnibus test of non-normality by employing various suggestions given by D'Agostino and Pearson.

Chi-square Test: The chi-square test can also be used for testing for normality by using the goodness-of-fit. For this test the data are categorized into k non-overlapping categories. The observed values and expected values are calculated for each category. Under the null hypothesis of normality, the chi-square statistic is then computed as

$$\chi^2 = \sum_{i=1}^{k} \frac{(A_i - T_i)^2}{T_i}.$$

Here the statistic has an approximate chi-square distribution, with the degrees of freedom $k - r - 1$, where r is the number of parameters to be estimated. A nice feature of this test is that it can be employed for censored samples. The moment tests need complete samples.

EDF: Another general procedure applicable for testing normality is the class of tests called the EDF test. For these tests the theoretical cumulative distribution function of the normal distribution, $F(X; \mu, \sigma)$, is contrasted with the EDF of the data, defined as

$$F_n(x) = \frac{\#(X < x)}{n}.$$

A famous test in this class is the Kolmogorov test, defined by the test statistic

$$D = \sup_x |F_n(X) - F(X; \mu, \sigma)|.$$

Large values of D indicate non-normality. If μ and σ are known, then the original Kolmogorov test can be used. When they are not known they can be replaced by sample estimates, resulting an adjusted critical values for D developed by Stephens.

2.16. Test of Equal Variances[23,24]

To perform two-sample t-test or multi-sample ANOVA, it requires that the underlying population variances are the same (namely the assumption of equal variances is established), which may bias the testing results otherwise. There are several methods to test the equality of variances, and the commonly used are F-test, Levene test, Brown–Forsythe test and Bartlett test.

F-test is suitable for testing the equality of two variances. The null hypothesis H_0 denotes that the variances of two populations are the same, and the test statistic is

$$F = \frac{S_1^2}{S_2^2},$$

where $S_i^2 (i = 1, 2)$ indicate the sample variance of the ith population, respectively. The formula of S_i^2 is

$$S_i^2 = \frac{1}{n_i - 1} \sum_{k=1}^{n_i} (X_{ik} - \bar{X}_i)^2,$$

where n_i and $\bar{X}_i$ indicate the sample size and sample mean of the ith population.

When the null hypothesis is true, this statistic follows an F distribution with the degrees of freedom n_1 and n_2. If the F value is bigger than the upper critical value, or smaller than the lower critical value, the null hypothesis is rejected. For simplicity, F statistic can also be defined as: the numerator is the bigger sample variance and the denominator is the smaller sample variance, and then the one-sided test method is used for hypothesis testing. The F-test method for testing the equality of two population variances is quick and simple, but it assumes that both populations are normally distributed and is sensitive to this assumption. By contrast, Levene test and Bartlett test is relatively robust.

The null hypothesis of Levene test is that the population variances of k samples are the same. The test statistic is

$$W = \frac{(N - k) \sum_{i=1}^{k} N_i (Z_{i+} - Z_{++})^2}{(k - 1) \sum_{i=1}^{k} \sum_{j=1}^{N_i} (Z_{ij} - Z_{i+})^2}.$$

When the null hypothesis is true, W follows a F distribution with degrees of freedom $k - 1$ and $N - k$. Levene test is a one-sided test. When W is bigger than the critical value of $F_{\alpha,(k-1,N-k)}$, the null hypothesis is rejected, which means that not all the population variances are the same. In the formula, N_i is the sample size of the i-th group, N is the total sample size, $Z_{ij} = |X_{ij} - \bar{X}_i|, X_{ij}$ is the value of the j-th observation in the ith group, $\bar{X}_i$ is the sample mean of the ith group. Besides,

$$Z_{++} = \frac{1}{N}\sum_{i=1}^{k}\sum_{j=1}^{N_i} Z_{ij}, \quad Z_{i+} = \frac{1}{N_i}\sum_{j=1}^{N_i} Z_{ij}$$

To ensure the robustness and statistical power of the test method, if the data do not meet the assumption of symmetric distribution or normal distribution, two other definitions for Z_{ij} can be used, namely

$$Z_{ij} = |X_{ij} - \tilde{X}_i| \quad \text{or } Z_{ij} = |X_{ij} - \bar{X}_i^{\prime}|,$$

where $\tilde{X}_i$ is the median of the ith group, and it is suitable for skewed-distributed data. In this case, Levene test is Brown–Forsythe test. $\bar{X}_i^{\prime}$ is the 10% adjusted mean of the ith group, namely the sample mean within the scope of $[P_5, P_{95}]$, and it is suitable for the data with extreme values or outliers.

Bartlett test is an improved goodness-of-fit test and can be used to test the equality of multiple variances. This method assumes that the data are normally distributed, and the test statistic is

$$\chi^2 = \frac{Q_1}{Q_2}, \quad \nu = k - 1,$$

where

$$Q_1 = (N-k)\ln(S_c^2) - \sum_{i=1}^{k}(n_i - 1)\ln(S_i^2),$$

$$Q_2 = 1 + \frac{1}{3 \times (k-1)}\left(\sum_{i=1}^{k}\frac{1}{n_i - 1} - \frac{1}{N-k}\right),$$

where n_i and S_i^2 is the sample size and sample variance of the ith group, k is the number of groups, N is the total sample size, and S_c^2 is the pooled sample variance. The formula of S_c^2 is

$$S_c^2 = \frac{1}{N-k}\sum_{i=1}^{k}(n_i - 1)S_i^2.$$

When the null hypothesis is true, this χ^2 statistic approximately follow a χ^2 distribution with the degrees of freedom $k - 1$. When $\chi^2 > \chi^2_{\alpha,k-1}$, the null hypothesis is rejected, where $\chi^2_{\alpha,k-1}$ is the upper αth percentile of the χ^2 distribution with the degrees of freedom $k - 1$.

2.17. Transformation[6]

In statistics, data transformation is to apply a deterministic mathematical function to each observation in a dataset — that is, each data point Z_i is replaced with the transformed value Y_i where $Y_i = f(Z_i), f(\cdot)$ is the transforming function. Transforms are usually applied to make the data more closely meet the assumptions of a statistical inference procedure to be applied, or to improve the interpretability or appearance of graphs.

There are several methods of transformation available for data preprocessing, i.e. logarithmic transformation, power transformation, reciprocal transformation, square root transformation, arcsine transformation and standardization transformation. The choice takes account of statistical model and data characteristics. The logarithm and square root transformations are usually applied to data that are positive skew. However, when 0 or negative values observed, it is more common to begin by adding a constant to all values, producing a set of non-negative data to which the transformation can be applied. Power and reciprocal transformations can be meaningfully applied to data that include both positive and negative values. Arcsine transformation is for proportions. Standardization transformation, that is to reduce the dispersion within the datum includes

$$Z = (X - \bar{X})/S \quad \text{and} \quad Z = [X - \min(\boldsymbol{X})]/[\max(\boldsymbol{X}) - \min(\boldsymbol{X})],$$

where X is each data point, and S are the mean and SD of the sample, $\min(\boldsymbol{X})$ and $\max(\boldsymbol{X})$ are maximal and minimal values of the dataset, X is the vector of all data point.

Data transformation involves directly in statistical analyses. For example, to estimate the CI of population mean, if the population is substantially skewed and the sample size is at most moderate, the approximation provided by the central limit theorem can be poor. Thus, it is common to transform the data to a symmetric distribution before constructing a CI.

In linear regression, transformations can be applied to a response variable, an explanatory variable, or to a parameter of the model. For example, in simple regression, the normal distribution assumptions may not be satisfied for the response Y, but may be more reasonably supposed for some transformation of Y such as its logarithm or square root. As for logarithm transformation, the formula is presented as $\log(Y) = \alpha + \beta X$. Furthermore, transformations may be applied to both response variable and explanatory variable, as shown as $\log(Y) = \alpha + \beta \log(X)$, or the quadratic function $Y = \alpha + \beta X + \gamma X^2$ is used to provide a first test of the assumption of a linear relationship. Note that transformation is not recommended for least square estimation for parameters.

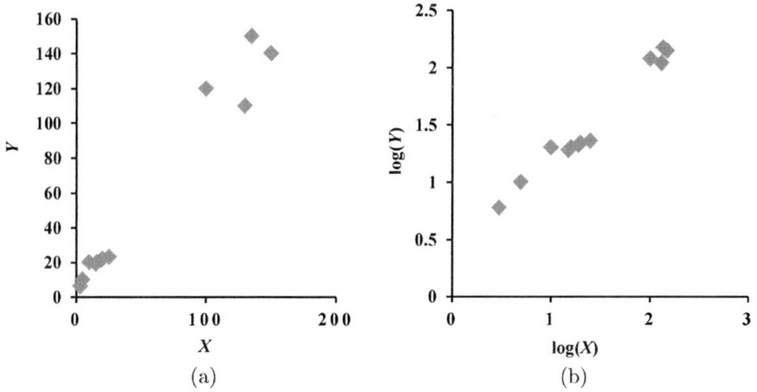

Fig. 2.17.1. Improve the visualization by data transformation.

Probability P is an basic concept in statistics though its application somewhat confined by the range of values, (0,1). Viewing at this, its transformations $Odds = P/(1-P)$ and $\ln Odds = \ln[P/(1-P)]$ provide much convenience for statistical inference so that they are widely used in epidemiologic studies; the former ranges in $(0, +\infty)$, and the latter ranges in $(-\infty, +\infty)$.

Transformations also play roles in data visualization. Taking Figure 2.17.1 as an example, in scatterplot, raw data points largely overlap in bottom left corner in the graph, while the rest points sparsely scattered (Figure 2.17.1a). However, following logarithmic transformations of both X and Y, the points will be spread more uniformly in the graph (Figure 2.17.1b).

2.18. Outlier[6,25]

An outlier is an observation so discordant from the majority of the data that it raises suspicion that it may not have plausibly come from the same statistical mechanism as the rest of the data. On the other hand, observations that did not come from the same mechanism as the rest of the data may also appear ordinary and not outlying. Naive interpretation of statistical results derived from data sets that include outliers may be misleading, thus these outliers should be identified and treated cautiously before making a statistical inference. There are various methods of outlier detection. Some are graphical such as normal probability plots, while others are model-based such as Mahalanobis distance. Finally, the nature of a box and whisker plot proves that it is a hybrid method.

Making a normal probability plot of residuals from a multiple regression and labeling any cases that appear too far from the line as outliers is an informal method of flagging questionable cases. The histogram and box plot are used to detect outliers of one-dimensional data. Here, it is only the largest and the smallest values of the data that reside at the two extreme ends of the histogram or are not included between the whiskers of the box plot. The way in which histograms depict the distribution of the data is somewhat arbitrary and depends heavily on the choice of bins and bin-widths.

More formal methods for identifying outliers remove the subjective element and are based on statistical models. The most commonly used methods are the pseudo-F test method, Mahalanobis distance and likelihood ratio method. The pseudo-F test method uses the variation analysis method to identify and test the outliers. It is suitable for the homoscedastic normal linear model (including the linear regression model and variance analysis model). Firstly, use part of the observations to fit the target model and denote the residual sum of squares as S_0 and the degrees of freedom as v. Next, delete one skeptical observation and refit the model while denoting the new residual sum of squares as S_1. The pseudo-F ratio is as such

$$F = \frac{(v-1)(S_0 - S_1)}{S_1}.$$

Compare the pseudo-F ratio to the quantiles of an F distribution with 1 and $v-1$ degrees of freedom. If the F-value is bigger, then the skeptical observation can be considered as an outlier. The method that the common statistic software utilizes to identify the outliers is using a t-statistic, whose square is equal to the F statistic. Next, the Mahalanobis distance is a common method to identify multivariate outliers, and the whole concept is based on the distance of each single data point from the mean. Let $\bar{X}$ and S represent the sample mean vector and covariance matrix, respectively, then the distance of any individual X_i from the mean can be measured by its squared Mahalanobis distance D_i, that is,

$$D_i = (X_i - \bar{X})' S^{-1} (X_i - \bar{X}).$$

If D_i is larger than $\chi^2_{\alpha,v}$, the individual value can be deemed as an outlier at the significance level α. Sequential deletion successively trims the observation with the largest D_i from the current sample.

Finally, the likelihood ratio method is appropriate for detecting outliers in generalized linear models, including the Poisson regression, logistic regression and log-linear model. Let S_0 represent the likelihood ratio statistic of the original fitted model and let S_1 represent the likelihood ratio statistic of the refitted model after deleting some skeptical observations. Then $S_0 - S_1$ is the deviance explained by deleting the suspect cases and can refer to its asymptotic χ^2 distribution to get an outlier identification and test. This frame work can also apply to the detection of outliers in contingency tables. For example, if the frequencies of all the cells are independent except for a select few, it is reasonable to delete a questionable cell, refit the model, and then calculate the change in deviance between the two fits. This gives an outlier test statistic for the particular cell.

Correct handling of an outlier depends on the cause. Outliers resulting from the testing or recording error may be deleted, corrected, or even transformed to minimize their influence on analysis results. It should be noted that no matter what statistical method is used to justifiably remove some data that appears as an outlier, there is a potential danger, that is, some important effects may come up as a result. It may be desirable to incorporate the effect of this unknown cause into the model structure, e.g. by using a mixture model or a hierarchical Bayes model.

2.19. MLE[26,27]

In statistics, the maximum likelihood method refers to a general yet useful method of estimating the parameters of a statistical model. To understand it we need to define a likelihood function. Consider a random variable Y with a probability-mass or probability-density function $f(y;\boldsymbol{\theta})$ and an unknown vector parameter $\boldsymbol{\theta}$. If $Y_1, Y_2, \ldots, Y_n$ are n independent observations of Y, then the likelihood function is defined as the probability of this sample given $\boldsymbol{\theta}$; thus,

$$L(\boldsymbol{\theta}) = \prod_{i=1}^{n} f(Y_i;\boldsymbol{\theta}).$$

The MLE of the vector parameter $\boldsymbol{\theta}$ is the value $\hat{\boldsymbol{\theta}}$ for which the expression $L(\boldsymbol{\theta})$ is maximized over the set of all possible values for $\boldsymbol{\theta}$. In practice, it is usually easier to maximize the logarithm of the likelihood, $\ln L(\boldsymbol{\theta})$, rather than the likelihood itself. To maximize $\ln L(\boldsymbol{\theta})$, we take the derivative of $\ln L(\boldsymbol{\theta})$ with respect to $\boldsymbol{\theta}$ and set the expression equal to 0. Hence,

$$\frac{\partial \ln L(\boldsymbol{\theta})}{\partial \boldsymbol{\theta}} = 0.$$

Heuristically, the MLE can be thought of as the values of the parameter $\boldsymbol{\theta}$ that make the observed data seem the most likely given $\boldsymbol{\theta}$.

The rationale for using the MLE is that the MLE is often unbiased and has the smallest variance among all consistent estimators for a wide class of distributions, particularly in large samples. Thus it is often the best estimate possible. The following are the three most important properties of the MLE in large samples:

(1) Consistency. The sequence of MLEs converges in probability to the true value of the parameter.
(2) Asymptotic normality. As the sample size gets large, the distribution of the MLE tends to a normal distribution with a mean of $\boldsymbol{\theta}$ and a covariance matrix that is the inverse of the Fisher information matrix, i.e. $\hat{\boldsymbol{\theta}} \sim N(\boldsymbol{\theta}, \boldsymbol{I}^{-1}/n)$.
(3) Efficiency. In terms of its variance, the MLE is the best asymptotically normal estimate when the sample size tends to infinity. This means that there is no consistent estimator with a lower asymptotic mean squared error than the MLE.

We now illustrate the MLE with an example. Suppose we have n observations of which k are successes and $n-k$ are failures, where Y_i is 1 if a certain event occurs and 0 otherwise. It can be assumed that each observation is a binary random variable and has the same probability of occurrence θ. Furthermore, $\Pr(Y=1)=\theta$ and $\Pr(Y=0)=1-\theta$. Thus, the likelihood of the sample can be written as

$$L(\theta) = \prod_{i=1}^{n} \theta^{Y_i}(1-\theta)^{1-Y_i} = \theta^k(1-\theta)^{n-k}.$$

In this example, $\boldsymbol{\theta}$ is a single parameter θ. The log likelihood is

$$\ln L(\theta) = k\ln(\theta) + (n-k)\ln(1-\theta).$$

To maximize this function we take the derivative of log L with respect to θ and set the expression equal to 0. Hence, we have the following score equation:

$$\frac{\partial \ln L(\theta)}{\partial\theta} = \frac{k}{\theta} - \frac{n-k}{1-\theta} = 0,$$

which has the unique solution $\hat{\theta} = k/n$. Thus, k/n is the MLE of θ.

The method of maximum likelihood can be used for a wide range of statistical models and is not always as easy as the above example shows. More often that not, the solution to the likelihood score equations must be posed as a nonlinear optimization problem. It involves solving a system of nonlinear equations that must be arrived at by numerical methods, such as the Newton–Raphson or *quasi*-Newton methods, the Fisher scoring algorithm, or the expectation–maximization (EM) algorithm.

2.20. Measures of Association[28]

Measures of association quantitatively show the degree of relationship between two or more variables. For example, if the measure of association between two variables is high, the awareness of one variable's value or magnitude could improve the power to accurately predict the other variable's value or magnitude. On the other hand, if the degree of association between two variables is rather low, the variables tend to be mutually independent.

For the continuous variables of a normal distribution, the most common measure of association is the Pearson product-moment correlation coefficient, or correlation coefficient in short, which is used to measure the degree and direction of the linear correlation between two variables. If $(X_1, Y_1), (X_2, Y_2), \ldots, (X_n, Y_n)$ are n pairs of observations, then the calculation formula of correlation coefficient r is

$$r = \frac{\sum_{i=1}^{n}(X_i - \bar{X})(Y_i - \bar{Y})}{[\sum_{i=1}^{n}(X_i - \bar{X})^2 \sum_{i=1}^{n}(Y_i - \bar{Y})^2]^{1/2}},$$

where $\bar{X}$ and $\bar{Y}$ indicate the sample mean of X_i and Y_i, respectively. The value of r ranges between -1 and 1. If the value of r is negative, it indicates a negative correlation; if the value of r is positive, it indicates a positive correlation. The bigger the absolute value of r, the closer the association. Thus, if it equals 0, it signifies a complete independence, and if it equals 1, it represents a perfect correlation, indicating that there is a linear functional relationship between X and Y. Therefore, if the functional relationship $Y = \alpha + \beta X$ is correct (for example, this is to describe the relationship between Fahrenheit Y and Celsius X), then $\beta > 0$ (as described in the case above) means $r = 1$ and $\beta < 0$ means $r = -1$.

In biology, the functional relationship between and among variables are usually nonlinear, thus the value of the correlation coefficient generally falls within the range of the critical values, but rarely is -1 or $+1$. There is a close relationship between correlation and linear regression. If $\beta_{Y,X}$ indicates the slope of the linear regression function of $Y \sim X$, and $\beta_{X,Y}$ indicates the slope of the linear regression function of $X \sim Y$, then

$$\beta_{Y,X} = \frac{\sum_{i=1}^{n}(X_i - \bar{X})(Y_i - \bar{Y})}{\sum_{i=1}^{n}(X_i - \bar{X})^2}, \quad \beta_{X,Y} = \frac{\sum_{i=1}^{n}(X_i - \bar{X})(Y_i - \bar{Y})}{\sum_{i=1}^{n}(Y_i - \bar{Y})^2}.$$

According to the definition of the correlation coefficient, $\beta_{Y,X}\beta_{X,Y} = r^2$ can be obtained. Because $r^2 \leq 1$ and $|\beta_{Y,X}| \leq |1/\beta_{X,Y}|$, the equal marks are justified only when there is a complete correlation. Therefore, the two regression curves usually intersect at a certain angle. Only when $r = 0$ and both $\beta_{Y,X}$ and $\beta_{X,Y}$ are 0 do the two regression curves intersect at a right angle.

For any value of X, if Y_0 indicates the predictive value obtained from the linear regression function, the variance of residuals from the regression $E[(Y - Y_0)^2]$ is equal to $\sigma_Y^2(1 - r^2)$. Thus, another interpretation of the correlation coefficient is that the square of the correlation coefficient indicates the percentage of the response variable variation that is explained by the linear regression from the total variation.

Under the assumption of a bivariate normal distribution, the null hypothesis of $\rho = 0$ can be set up, and the statistic below

$$t = \frac{(n-2)^{1/2}r}{(1-r^2)^{1/2}}$$

follows a t distribution with $n - 2$ degrees of freedom. ρ is the population correlation coefficient.

The measures of association for contingency table data are usually based on the Pearson χ^2 statistic (see chi-square test), while ϕ coefficient and Pearson contingency coefficient C are commonly used as well. Although the χ^2 statistic is also the measure of association between variables, it cannot be directly used to evaluate the degree of association due to its correlation with the sample size. With regard to the measures of association for ordered categorical variables, the Spearman rank correlation coefficient and Kendall's coefficient are used, which are referred to in Chapter 5.

2.21. Software for Biostatistics[6]

In statistics, there are many software packages designed for data manipulation and statistical analysis. To date, more than 1000 statistical software packages are available for various computer platforms. Among them, the most widely used ones are Statistical Analysis System (SAS), Statistical Package for the Social Sciences (SPSS), Stata, S-Plus and R.

The SAS is the most famous one available for Windows and UNIX/Linux operating systems. SAS was developed at North Carolina State University from 1966 to 1976, when SAS Institute was incorporated. SAS is designed in a style with modularized components that cover a wide range of functionalities like data access, management and visualization. The main approach to using SAS is through its programming interface, which provides users powerful abilities for data processing and multi-task data manipulation. Experienced users and statistical professionals will benefit greatly from the advanced features of SAS.

The SPSS released its first version in 1968 after being developed by Norman H. Nie, Dale H. Bent, and C. Hadlai Hull. The most prominent feature of SPSS is its user-friendly graphical interface. SPSS versions 16.0 and later run under Windows, Mac, and Linux. The graphical user interface is written in Java. SPSS uses windows and dialogs as an easy and intuitive way of guiding the user through their given task, thus requiring very limited statistical knowledge. Because of its rich, easy-to-use features and its appealing output, SPSS is widely utilized for statistical analysis in the social sciences, used by market researchers, health researchers, survey companies, government, education researchers, marketing organizations, data miners, and many others.

Stata is a general-purpose statistical software package created in 1985 by Stata Corp. Most of its users work in research, especially in the fields of economics, sociology, political science, biomedicine and epidemiology. Stata is available for Windows, Mac OS X, Unix, and Linux. Stata's capabilities include data management, statistical analysis, graphics, simulations, regression, and custom programming. Stata integrates an interactive command line interface so that the user can perform statistical analysis by invoking one or more commands. Comparing it with other software, Stata has a relatively small and compact package size.

S-PLUS is a commercial implementation of the S programming language sold by TIBCO Software Inc. It is available for Windows, Unix and Linux. It features object-oriented programming (OOP) capabilities and advanced analytical algorithms. S is a statistical programming language developed primarily by John Chambers and (in earlier versions) Rick Becker as well as Allan Wilks of Bell Laboratories. S-Plus provides menus, toolsets and dialogs for easy data input/output and data analysis. S-PLUS includes thousands of packages that implement traditional and modern statistical methods for users to install and use. Users can also take advantage of the S language to develop their own algorithms or employ OOP, which treats functions, data, model as objects, to experiment with new theories and methods. S-PLUS is well suited for statistical professionals with programming experience.

R is a programming language as well as a statistical package for data manipulation, analysis and visualization. The syntax and semantics of the R language is similar to that of the S language. To date, more than 7000 packages for R are available at the Comprehensive R Archive Network (CRAN), Bioconductor, Omegahat, GitHub and other repositories. Many cutting-edge algorithms are developed in R language. R functions are first class, which means functions, expressions, data and objects can be passed into functions as parameters. Furthermore, R is freely available under the GNU General Public License, and pre-compiled binary versions are provided for various operating systems.

Other than the general statistical analysis software, there are software for specialized domains as well. For example, BUGS is used for Bayesian analysis, while StatXact is a statistical software package for analyzing data using exact statistics, boasting the ability to calculate exact p-values and CIs for contingency tables and non-parametric procedures.

Acknowledgments

Special thanks to Fangru Jiang at Cornell University in the US, for his help in revising the English of this chapter.

References

1. Rosner, B. *Fundamentals of Biostatistics.* Boston: Taylor & Francis, Ltd., 2007.
2. Anscombe, FJ, Graphs in statistical analysis. *Am. Stat.*, 1973, 27: 17–21.
3. Harris, EK, Boyd, JC. *Statistical Bases of Reference Values in Laboratory Medicine.* New York: Marcel Dekker, 1995.
4. Altman, DG. Construction of age-related reference centiles using absolute residuals. *Stat. Med.*, 1993, 12: 917–924.
5. Everitt, BS. *The Cambridge Dictionary of Statistics.* Cambridge: CUP, 2003.
6. Armitage, P, Colton, T. *Encyclopedia of Biostatistics* (2nd edn.). John Wiley & Sons, 2005.
7. Bickel, PJ, Doksum, KA. *Mathematical Statistics: Basic Ideas and Selected Topics.* New Jersey: Prentice Hall, 1977.
8. York, D. Least-Square Fitting of a straight line. *Can. J. Phys.* 1966, 44: 1079–1086.
9. Whittaker, ET, Robinson, T. The method of least squares. Ch.9 in *The Calculus of Observations: A Treatise on Numerical Mathematics* (4th edn.). New York: Dover, 1967.
10. Cramer, H. *Mathematical Methods of Statistics.* Princeton: Princeton University Press, 1946.
11. Bickel, PJ, Doksum, KA. *Mathematical Statistics.* San Francisco: Holden-Day, 1977.
12. Armitage, P. Trials and errors: The emergence of clinical statistics. *J. R. Stat. Soc. Series A*, 1983, 146: 321–334.
13. Hogg, RW, Craig, AT. *Introduction to Mathematical Statistics.* New York: Macmillan, 1978.
14. Fisher, RA. *Statistical Methods for Research Workers.* Edinburgh: Oliver & Boyd, 1925.
15. Scheffé, H. *The Analysis of Variance.* New York: Wiley, 1961.
16. Bauer, P. Multiple testing in clinical trials. *Stat. Med.*, 1991, 10: 871–890.
17. Berger, RL, Multiparameter hypothesis testing and acceptance sampling. *Technometrics*, 1982, 24: 294–300.
18. Cressie, N, Read, TRC. Multinomial goodness-of-fit tests. *J. R. Stat. Soc. Series B*, 1984, 46: 440–464.

19. Lancaster, HO. The combination of probabilities arising from data in discrete distributions. *Biometrika*, 1949, 36: 370–382.
20. Rao, KC, Robson, DS. A chi-squared statistic for goodness-of-fit tests within the exponential family. *Communi. Stat. Theor.*, 1974, 3: 1139–1153.
21. D'Agostino, RB, Stephens, MA. *Goodness-of-Fit Techniques.* New York: Marcel Dekker, 1986.
22. Stephens, MA. EDF statistics for goodness-of-fit and some comparisons. *J. Amer. Stat. Assoc.*, 1974, 65: 1597–1600.
23. Levene, H. Robust tests for equality of variances. *Contributions to Probability and Statistics: Essays in Honor of Harold Hotelling* Stanford: Stanford University Press, 1960.
24. Bartlett, MS. Properties of sufficiency and statistical tests. *Proc. R. Soc. A.*, 1937, 160: 268–282.
25. Barnett, V, Lewis, T. *Outliers in Statistical Data.* New York: Wiley, 1994.
26. Rao, CR, Fisher, RA. The founder of modern statistics. *Stat. Sci.*, 1992, 7: 34–48.
27. Stigler, SM. *The History of Statistics: The Measurement of Uncertainty Before 1900.* Cambridge: Harvard University Press, 1986.
28. Fisher, RA. Frequency distribution of the values of the correlation coefficient in samples from an indefinitely large population. *Biometrika*, 1915, 10: 507–521.

About the Author

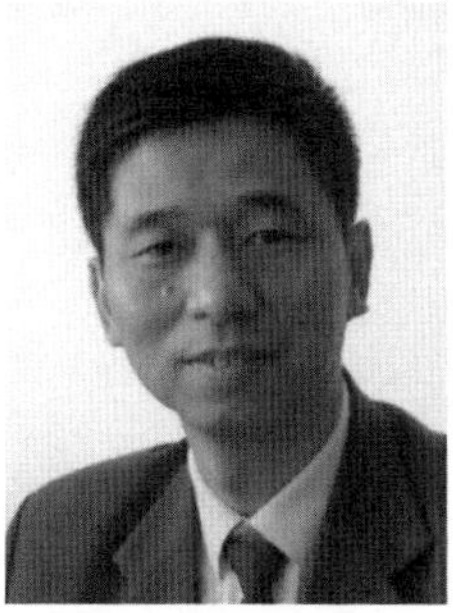

Kang Li, Professor, Ph.D. supervisor, Director of Medical Statistics, Editor of a planned Medical Statistics textbook (6th edn.) for national 5-year clinical medicine education, Associate Editor of "statistical methods and its application in medical research" (1st edn.) for postgraduates, Associate Editor of a planned textbook "health information management" (1st and 2nd edns.) for preventive medicine education. He is in charge of five grants from the National Natural Science Foundation of China and has published over 120 scientific papers. He is also Vice Chairman of Health Statistics Committee of Chinese Preventive Medicine Association, Vice Chairman of Statistical Theory and Methods Committee of Chinese Health Information Association Vice Chairman of System Theory Committee of Systems Engineering Society of China and Member of the Standing Committee of International Biometric Society China.

CHAPTER 3

LINEAR MODEL AND GENERALIZED LINEAR MODEL

Tong Wang*, Qian Gao, Caijiao Gu, Yanyan Li, Shuhong Xu, Ximei Que, Yan Cui and Yanan Shen

3.1. Linear Model[1]

Linear model is also called classic linear model or general linear model. If the dependent variable Y is continuously distributed, the linear model will be the first choice often in order to describe the relationship between dependent variable Y and independent variables Xs. If X is a categorical variable, the model is called analysis of variance (ANOVA); If X is a continuous variable, it is called regression model; if X contains both categorical variable and continuous variable, it is called covariance analysis model.

We can make Y as a function of other variables $x_1, x_2, \ldots, x_p$, or write the expectation of Y as $E(Y) = f(x)$, $f(x)$ is function of $x_1, x_2, \ldots, x_p$, which can be a vector X. If y is observed value of the random variable Y, then $y - f(x)$ is also random and it is called residual error or error:

$$e = y - E(Y) = y - f(x).$$

So, $y = f(x) + e$.

Theoretically, $f(x)$ can be any function about x. In linear model, it is a linear function $\beta_1 x_1 + \beta_2 x_2 + \cdots + \beta_k x_k$ about $\beta_1, \ldots, \beta_k$. If the model contains the parameter β_0 which means the first column of vector X always equals 1, then

$$y = \beta_0 + \beta_1 x_1 + \beta_2 x_2 + \cdots + \beta_k x_k + e,$$

*Corresponding author: wtstat@21cn.com

where β_0 is the intercept, $\beta_1, \ldots, \beta_k$ is the slope, and they are both called regression coefficient. Applying the above equation to all the observations, we get

$$y_i = \beta_0 + \beta_1 x_{i1} + \beta_2 x_{i2} + \cdots + \beta_k x_{ik} + e_i.$$

It can be written as $y = X\beta + e$.

This is the expression of general linear model. According to the definition $e_i = y_i - E(y_i)$, $E(e) = 0$, so the covariance of $y = X\beta + e$ can be written as

$$\text{var}(y) = \text{var}(e) = E[y - E(y)][y - E(y)]' = E(ee') = V.$$

We usually assume that each e_i equals a fixed variance σ^2, and the covariance of different e_i equals 0, so $V = \sigma^2 I$.

When we estimate the values of regression coefficients, there is no need to make a special assumption to the probability distribution of Y, but assumption for a conditional normal distribution is needed when we make statistical inference.

Generalized least squares estimation or the ordinary least squares estimation is always used to estimate the parameter β.

The estimation equation of the ordinary least squares is

$$X'X\hat{\beta} = X'y,$$

and that for generalized least squares is

$$X'V^{-1}X\hat{\beta} = X'V^{-1}y,$$

where V is non-singular; when it is singular matrix, the estimation equation is

$$X'V^{-}X\hat{\beta} = X'V^{-}y.$$

All these equations do not need to make special assumption to the distribution of e.

3.2. Generalized Linear Model[2]

Generalized linear model is an extension of the general linear model, it can establish linear relationship between μ, the expectation of the dependent variable Y, and independent variables through some kinds of transformations. This model was first introduced by Nelder and Wedderburn.

This model supposes that the expected value of Y is μ, and the distribution of y belongs to an exponential family. The probability density function (for continuous variable) or probability function (for discrete variable) has the form,

$$f_{y_i}(y_i; \theta_i, \phi) = \exp\left\{\frac{\theta_i y_i - b(\theta_i)}{a_i(\phi)} + c_i(y_i, \phi)\right\},$$

where θ_i is the natural parameter, and constant φ is the scale parameter. Many commonly used distributions belong to the exponential family, such as normal distribution, inverse normal distribution, Gamma distribution, Poisson distribution, Binomial distribution, negative binomial distribution and so on. The Poisson distribution, for instance, can be written as

$$f_y(y; \theta, \phi) = \exp[\theta y - e^{\theta} - \log(y!)],$$

$$y = 0, 1, 2 \ldots,$$

where $\theta = \log(\mu)$, $a(\phi) = 1$, $b(\theta) = e^{\theta}$, $c(y, \phi) = -\log(y!)$.

The Binomial distribution can be written as

$$f_y(y; \theta, \phi) = \exp\left[\frac{\theta y - \log(1 + e^{\theta})}{n^{-1}} + \log(C_n^{ny})\right], \quad y = 0, \frac{1}{n}, \frac{2}{n}, \ldots, 1,$$

where $\theta = \log[\pi/(1-\pi)]$, $a(\phi) = 1/n$, $b(\theta) = \log(1 + e^{\theta})$, $c(y, \phi) = \log(C_n^{ny})$.

The normal distribution can be written as

$$f_y(y; \theta, \phi) = \exp\left\{\left(\frac{\theta y - \theta^2}{2}\right) \Big/ \phi - \frac{1}{2}\left[\frac{y^2}{\phi + \log(2\pi\phi)}\right]\right\}, \quad -\infty < y < +\infty,$$

where $\theta = \mu$, $\varphi = \sigma^2$, $a(\phi) = \sigma^2$, $b(\theta) = \theta^2/2$, $c(y, \phi) = -\frac{1}{2}[\frac{y^2}{\phi + \log(2\pi\phi)}]$.

The linear combination of independent variables and their regression coefficients in a generalized linear model, written as $\eta = \beta_0 + \sum_{i=1}^{n} \beta_i x_i$, can link to the expectation of dependent variable through a link function $g(\mu)$, $g(\mu) = \eta = \beta_0 + \sum_{i=1}^{n} \beta_i x_i$.

The link function is very important in these models. The typical link functions of some distributions are shown in Table 3.2.1. When the link function is an identical equation $\mu = \eta = g(\mu)$, the generalized linear model is reduced to general linear model.

Table 3.2.1. The typical link of some commonly used distributions.

Distribution	Symbol	Mean	Typical link
Normal	$N(\mu, \sigma^2)$	μ	identity
Poisson	$P(\mu)$	μ	log
Binomial	$B(m, \pi)/m$	$m\pi$	logit

The parameters of these models can be obtained by maximum likelihood estimation.

3.3. Coefficient of Determination[3,4]

Coefficient of determination is a commonly used statistic in regression to evaluate the goodness-of-fit of the model. As is shown in Figure 3.3.1, y_i represents the observed value of the dependent variable of the ith observation, and $\hat{y}_i$ is the predicted value of the y_i based on regression equation, while $\bar{y}$ denotes the mean of n observations. The total sum of squared deviations $\sum_{i=1}^{n}(y_i - \bar{y})^2$ could be divided into the sum of squares for residuals and the sum of squares for regression which represent the contribution of the regression effects. The better the effect of the fit, the bigger the proportion of regression in the total variation, the smaller that of the residual in the total variation. The ratio of the sum of squared deviations for regression and the total sum of squared deviations is called determination coefficient, which reflects the proportion of the total variation of y explained by the model, denoted as

$$R^2 = \frac{\text{SSR}}{\text{SST}} = \frac{\sum_{i=1}^{n} (\hat{y}_i - \bar{y})^2}{\sum_{i=1}^{n} (y_i - \bar{y})^2},$$

where $0 \leq R^2 \leq 1$, and its value measures the contribution of the regression. The larger the R^2, the better the fit. So R^2 is an important statistic in regression model.

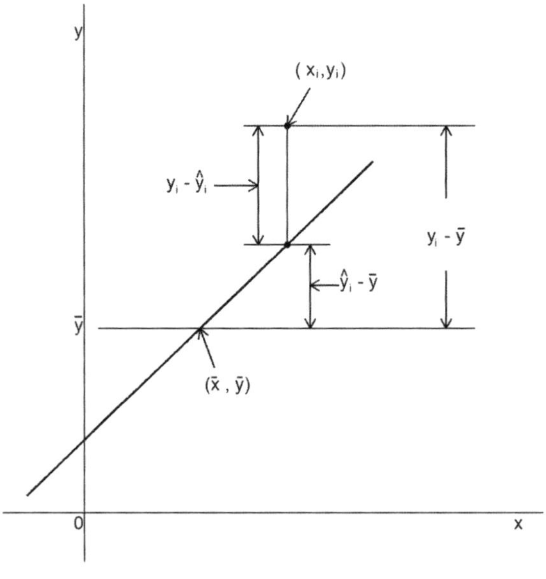

Fig. 3.3.1. Decomposing of variance in regression.

However, in multiple regression model, the value of R^2 always increases when more independent variables are added in. So, it is unreasonable to compare the goodness-of-fit between two models using R^2 directly without considering the number of independent variables in each model. The adjusted determination coefficient R_c^2, which has taken the number of the variables in models into consideration, can be written as

$$R_c^2 = 1 - (1 - R^2)\frac{n-1}{n-p-1},$$

where p is the number of the independent variables in the model. It is obvious that R_c^2 is decreased with the increase of p when R^2 is fixed.

In addition to describing the effect of the regression fit, R^2 can also be used to make statistical inference for the model. The test statistic is

$$F = \frac{R^2}{(1-R^2)/(n-2)}, \quad v_1 = 1, \ v_2 = n-2,$$

when R^2 is used to measure the association between two random variables in bivariate correlation analysis, the value of R^2 is equal to the squared Pearson's product-moment linear correlation coefficient r, that is, $R^2 = r^2$ or $r = \sqrt{R^2}$. Under this circumstance, the result of the hypothesis testing about R^2 and r is equivalent. $R = \sqrt{R^2}$, called multiple correlation coefficient, can be used to measure the association between dependent variable Y and multiple independent variables $X_1, X_2, \ldots, X_m$, which actually is the correlation between Y and $\hat{Y}$.

3.4. Regression Diagnostics[5]

Regression diagnostics are methods for detecting disagreement between a regression model and the data to which it is fitted. The data deviated far from the basic assumptions of the model are known as outliers, also called abnormal points, singular points or irregular points. Outliers usually refer to outlying points with respect to their Y values, such as points A and B in Figure 3.4.1. Observations B and C are called leverage points since their X values are far away from the sample space. It is easier to pull the regression line to itself and if works like a lever if one point is outlying with respect to both its X and Y spaces. But it is worth noting that not all outlying values have leverage effect on the fitted regression function. One point would not have such leverage effect if it is only outlying with regard to its X space while its Y value is consistent with the regression relation displayed in most observations. That is to say, the leverage effect depends on its position both in Y and X spaces. The observations which are outlying in both X and Y

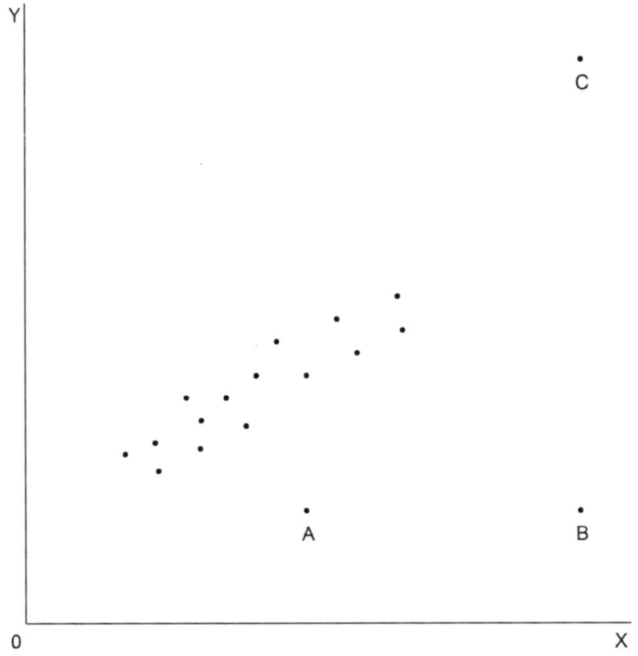

Fig. 3.4.1. Scatter plot for illustrating outliers, leverage points, and influential points.

axis are named influential points as it has a large effect on the parameter estimation and statistical inference of regression, such as observation B in the figure. Generally speaking, outliers include points that are only outlying with regard to its Y value; points that are only outlying with regard to its X value, and influential points that are outlying with respect to both its X and Y values.

The source of outliers in regression analysis is very complicated. It can mainly result from gross error, sampling error and the unreasonable assumption of the established model.

(1) The data used for regression analysis is based on unbalanced design. It is easier to produce outliers in the X space than in ANOVA, especially for data to which independent variable can be a random variable. The other reason is that one or several important independent variables may have been omitted from the model or incorrect observation scale has been used when fitting the regression function.
(2) The gross error is mostly derived from the data collection process, for example, wrong data entry or data grouping, which may result in outliers.

(3) In the data analysis stage, outliers mainly reflect the irrationality or even mistakes in the mode assumptions. For example, the real distribution of the data may be a heavy tailed one compared with the normal distribution; the data may be subject to a mixture of two kinds of distributions; the variances of the error term are not constant; the regression function is not linear.
(4) Even if the real distribution of data perfectly fits with the assumption of the established model, the occurrence of a small probability event in a certain position can also lead to the emergence of outliers.

The regression diagnostics are mostly based on residual, such as ordinary residual, standardized residual, and deleted residual.

In principle, we should study outliers with caution when they occur. And we should be alerted when outliers are present on certain characteristics as they may indicate an unexpected phenomenon or a better model. At this time, we should collect more data adjacent to outliers to affirm their structural features, or we can resort to transformation of the original variables before carrying out the regression analysis. Only when the best model has been confirmed and the study focus is placed on main body of data instead of outliers may we consider discarding outliers deliberately.

3.5. Influential Points[6]

What is more important than the identification of outliers is using diagnostic methods to identify influential observations. Outliers are not necessarily influential points. Influential points are those which will lead to significant changes of analysis results when they are deleted from the original data set. These points may be outliers with large residual corresponding to a certain model, or outliers away from the design space. Sometimes, it is hard to identify influential points as such observations may alone or jointly with other observations affect the analysis results.

We can use hat matrix, also known as projection matrix, to identify outlying X observation.

The hat matrix is defined as

$$H = X(X'X)^{-1}X'.$$

If $X'X$ is non-singular matrix, then

$$\hat{\beta} = (X'X)^{-1}X'y$$
$$\hat{y} = Hy = x\hat{\beta} = X(X'X)^{-1}X'y.$$

The hat matrix is a symmetric idempotent projection matrix, in which the element h_{ij} is used to measure the influence of observation data y_j to the fitted value $\hat{y}_i$. The diagonal element h_{ii} in the hat matrix is called leverage and has several useful properties:

$$0 \leq h_{ii} \leq 1 \qquad \sum_{i=1}^{n} h_{ii} = p = \text{rank of X}.$$

It indicates how remote, in the space of the carriers, the ith observation is from the other $n-1$ observations. A leverage value is usually considered to be large if $h_i > 2p/n$. That is to say, the observations are outlying with regard to its X value. Take simple linear regression as an example: $h_i = (1/n) + (x_i - \bar{x})/\sum(x_i - \bar{x})^2$. For a balanced experimental design, such as a D-optimum design, all $h_i = p/n$. For a point with high leverage, the larger h_i is, the more important the value of x_i, determining the fitted value $\hat{y}_{(i)}$ is. In extreme cases where $h_i = 1$, the fitted value $\hat{y}_{(i)}$ is forced to equal the observed value, this will lead to small variance of ordinary residual and observations with high leverage would be entered in to the model mistakenly.

Take general linear model for example, Cook's distance proposed by Cook and Weisberg is used to measure the impact of ith observation value on the estimated regression coefficients when it is deleted:

$$\begin{aligned} D_{\text{i}} &= (\hat{\beta}_{(i)} - \hat{\beta})^T X^T X (\hat{\beta}_{(i)} - \hat{\beta})/ps^2 \\ &= (1/p) r_i'^2 [h_i/(1-h_i)]. \end{aligned}$$

By comparing D_i with the percentile of corresponding F distribution (the degree of freedom is $(p, n-p)$), we can judge the influence of observed value on the fitted regression function. The square root of quantity is modified so as to make the obtained results multiples of residuals. One such quantity is called the modified Cook statistic as shown below:

$$C_{\text{i}} = \left(\frac{n-p}{p}\frac{h_i}{1-h_i}\right)^{1/2} |r_i^*|.$$

The leverage measures, residuals, and versions of Cook's statistics can be plotted against observation number to yield index plots, which can be used to conduct regression diagnostics.

The methods of identifying influential points can be extended from the multiple regression model to nonlinear model and to general inference based on the likelihood function, for example, generalized linear models. If interested in inference about the vector parameter θ, influence measures can be derived from the distance $\hat{\theta} - \hat{\theta}_{(i)}$.

3.6. Multicollinearity[7]

In regression analysis, sometimes the estimators of regression coefficients of some independent variables are extremely unstable. By adding or deleting an independent variable from the model, the regression coefficients and the sum of squares change dramatically. The main reason is that when independent variables are highly correlated, the regression coefficient of an independent variable depends on other independent variables which may or may not be included in the model. A regression coefficient does not reflect any inherent effect of the particular independent variable on the dependent variable but only a marginal or partial effect, given that other highly correlated independent variables are included in the model.

The term multicollinearity in statistics means that there are highly linear relationships among some independent variables. In addition to changing the regression coefficients and the sum of squares for regression, it can also lead to the situation that the estimated regression coefficients individually may not be statistically significant even though a definite statistical relation exists between the dependent variable and the set of independent variables.

Several methods of detecting the presence of multicollinearity in regression analysis can be used as follows:

1. As one of the indicators of multicollinearity, the high correlations among the independent variables can be identified by means of variance inflation factor (VIF) or the reciprocal of VIF as $1 - R_{ip}^2$ (i corresponds to the ith independent variable, p corresponds to the independent variables entered into the model before the ith independent variable). Tolerance limit for VIF is 10. The value of VIF greater than 10 indicates the presence of multicollinearity.
2. One or more regression coefficients or standardized coefficients of independent variables are very large.
3. Another indicator of multicollinearity is that one or more standard errors of regression coefficients of independent variables are very large. It may lead to the wide confidence intervals of regression coefficients.

When the serious multicollinearity is identified, some remedial measures are available to eliminate multicollinearity.

1. One or several independent variables may be dropped from the model in order to reduce the standard errors of the estimated regression coefficients of the independent variables remaining in the model.

2. Some computational methods such as orthogonalization can be used. In principal components (PC) regression, one finds the set of orthonormal eigenvectors of the correlation matrix of the independent variables. Then, the matrix of PC is calculated by the eigenmatrix with the matrix of independent variables. Finally, the regression model on the PC is fitted and then the regression model on the original variables can be obtained.
3. The method of ridge regression can be used when the multicollinearity exists. It is a statistic method that modifies the method of least squares in order to eliminate multicollinearity and allows biased estimators of the regression coefficients.

3.7. PC Regression[8]

As a combination of PC analysis and regression analysis, PC regression is often used to model data with problem of multicollinearity or relatively high-dimensional data.

The way PC regression works can be summarized as follows. Firstly, one finds the set of orthonormal eigenvectors of the correlation matrix of the independent variables. Secondly, the matrix of PCs is calculated by the eigenmatrix with the matrix of independent variables. The first PC in the matrix of PCs will exhibit the maximum variance. The second one will account for the maximum possible variance of the remaining variance which is uncorrelated with the first PC, and so on. As a set of new regressor variables, the score of PCs then is used to fit the regression model. Upon completion of this regression model, one transforms back to the original coordinate system.

To illustrate the procedure of PC regression, it is assumed that the m variables are observed on the n subjects.

1. To calculate the correlation matrix, it is useful to standardize the variables:

$$X'_{ij} = (X_{ij} - \bar{X}_j)/S_j, \quad j = 1, 2, \ldots, m.$$

2. The correlation matrix has eigenvectors and eigenvalues defined by

$$|X'X - \lambda_i I| = 0, \quad i = 1, 2, \ldots, m.$$

The m non-negative eigenvalues are obtained and then ranked by descending order as

$$\lambda_1 \geq \lambda_2 \geq \cdots \geq \lambda_m \geq 0.$$

Then, the corresponding eigenmatrix $\mathbf{a}_i = (\alpha_{i1}, \alpha_{i2}, \ldots, \alpha_{im})'$ of each eigenvalue λ_i is computed by $(X'X - \lambda'_i I)\mathbf{a}_i = 0$ $\mathbf{a}'_i\mathbf{a}_i = 1$. Finally, the

PC matrix is obtained by

$$Z_i = \mathbf{a}_i'\mathbf{X} = a_{i1}X_1 + a_{i2}X_2 + \cdots + a_{im}X_m, \quad i = 1, 2, \ldots, m.$$

3. The regression model is fitted as

$$Y = X\beta + \varepsilon = Z\mathbf{a}_i\beta + \varepsilon,$$
$$h = \mathbf{a}_i\beta \quad \text{or} \quad \beta = h\mathbf{a}_i,$$

where β is the coefficients vector obtained from the regression on the original variables, h is the coefficients vector obtained from the regression on the PCs. After the fitting of regression model, one needs to only interpret the linear relationships between the original variables and dependent variables namely β and does not need to be concerned with the interpretation of the PCs.

During the procedure of PC regression, there are several selection rules for picking PCs one needs to pay attention.

1. The estimation of coefficients in the PC regression is biased, since the PCs one picked do not account for all variation or information in the original set of variables. Only keep all PCs can yield the unbiased estimation.
2. Keeping those PCs with the largest eigenvalues tends to minimize the variances of the estimators of the coefficients.
3. Keeping those PCs which are highly correlated with the dependent variable can minimize the mean square errors of the estimators of the coefficients.

3.8. Ridge Regression[9]

In general linear regression model, β can be obtained by ordinary least squares:

$$\hat{\beta}_{LS} = (X'X)^{-1}XY,$$

which is the unbiased estimator of the true parameter. It requires that the determinant $|X'X|$ is not equal to zero, namely non-singular matrix. When there is a strong linear correlation between the independent variables or the variation in independent variable is small, the determinant $|X'X|$ will become smaller and even closer to 0. In this case, $X'X$ is often referred to as ill-conditioned matrix, regression coefficient which is obtained by the method of least squares will be very unstable and variance of estimator $\text{var}(\hat{\beta})$ will be very large.

Therefore, Hoerl and Kennard brought forward the ridge regression estimation to solve this problem in 1970. That is, adding a positive constant matrix λI to $X'X$ to make $(X'X)^{-1}$ limited, thus preventing the exaggerated variance of estimator and improving its stability. Because the offset was introduced into the estimation, so ridge regression is no longer an unbiased estimation.

If the residual sum of squares of the ordinary least squares estimator is expressed as

$$\mathrm{RSS}(\beta)_{LS} = \sum_{i=1}^{n}\left(Y_i - \beta_0 - \sum_{j=1}^{p} X_{ij}\beta_j\right)^2,$$

then the residual sum of squares defined by the ridge regression is referred to as L_2 penalized residual sum of squares:

$$\mathrm{PRSS}(\beta)_{L_2} = \sum_{i=1}^{n}\left(Y_i - \beta_0 - \sum_{j=1}^{p} X_{ij}\beta_j\right)^2 + \lambda\sum_{j=1}^{p}\beta_j^2$$

after derivation, we get

$$\frac{\partial \mathrm{PRSS}(\beta)_{L_2}}{\partial\beta} = -2X^T(Y - X\beta) + 2\lambda\beta.$$

Make it equal to 0 to obtain further solution

$$\hat{\beta}_{\mathrm{ridge}} = (X^TX + \lambda I)^{-1}X^TY.$$

It can be proved theoretically that there is a λ, which is greater than 0, and it makes the mean square error of $\hat{\beta}_{\mathrm{ridge}}(\lambda)$ less than the mean square error of $\hat{\beta}_{LS}$, but the value of λ, which makes the mean square error to achieve the minimum, depends on unknown parameters $\hat{\beta}_{\mathrm{ridge}}$ and variance σ^2, so the determination of λ value is the key of ridge regression analysis.

Commonly used methods of determining λ value in ridge regression estimation are ridge trace plot, the VIF, C_p criterion, the $H - K$ formula and $M - G$. Hoerl and Kennard pointed out that if the value of λ has nothing to do with the sample data y, then ridge regression estimator $\hat{\beta}_{(\lambda)}$ is a linear estimator. For different λ, there is only a group of solutions $\hat{\beta}_{(\lambda)}$, so different λ can depict the track of ridge regression solutions, namely the ridge trace plot. The ridge parameter λ of ridge trace plot generally starts from 0 with step size 0.01 or 0.1, calculate estimators of $\hat{\beta}_{(\lambda)}$ under different λ, then make $\hat{\beta}_{j(\lambda)}$ as a function of λ, respectively, and plot the changes of $\hat{\beta}_{j(\lambda)}$ with λ in the same plane coordinate system, namely the ridge trace. According to the characteristics of ridge trace plot, one can select the estimated value of $\hat{\beta}_{j(\lambda)}$ corresponding to λ, whose ridge estimators of each regression parameters are roughly stable, the signs of the regression coefficients are rational, and the residual sum of squares does not rise too much. When λ equals 0, the $\hat{\beta}_{(\lambda)}$ is equivalent to the least square estimator. When λ approaches infinity, $\hat{\beta}_{(\lambda)}$ tends to 0, so λ cannot be too large.

3.9. Robust Regression[10]

Robust regression is aimed to fit the structure reflected in most of the data, avoiding the influences from the potential outliers, influential points and identifying the deviation structure from the model assumptions. When the error is normally distributed, the estimation is almost as good as that of least squares estimation, while the least squares estimation conditions are violated, the robust estimation is superior to the least squares.

Robust regression includes M estimation based on Maximum likelihood, L estimation based on order statistic of certain linear transformation for residual, R estimation based on rank of residuals with its generalized estimation and some high breakdown point estimation such as LMS estimation, LTS estimation, S estimation, and τ estimation.

It is very significant that Huber has introduced the M estimation in robust regression theory because of its good mathematical property and basic theory about robustness that Huber and Hampel continuously explored. M estimations have become a classical method of robust regression and subsequently other estimation methods traced deeply from it. Its optimized principle is that when coming to the large sample cases, minimize the maximum possible variance. Given different definition to the weight function, we can get different estimations. Commonly used includes Huber, Hampel, Andrew, Tukey estimation function and others. The curves of these functions are different, but all of the large residuals are smoothly downweighted with a compromise between the ability of rejection of outliers and estimation efficiency. Although these estimations have some good properties, they are still sensitive to outliers occurring in x-axis. After reducing weight of outliers of x-axis, we can obtain a bounded influence regression, also called generalized (GM). M estimation Different weight functions lead to different estimations, such as Mallows estimation, Schweppe estimation, Krasker estimation, Welsch estimation and so on.

R estimation is a non-parametric regression method which was put forward by Jackel. This method will not square the residuals but make a certain function of the residual's rank as weight function to reduce the influences of outliers. R estimation is also sensitive to influential points in x-axis, Tableman and others put forward a Generalized R estimation which belongs to bound influence regression method too.

Considering the definition of classical LS estimation is minimizing the sum squares of residuals, which equals minimizing the arithmetic mean of squares, obviously arithmetic mean is not robust when the data are deviating from the normal distribution, while the median is quite robust in this case, so changing the estimation function of LS estimation to minimize the median squares in order to get the least median of squares regression. Similarly, as the trimmed mean is robust to outliers, if abandoning the larger residuals in regression, we can get the least trimmed sum of squares estimation with estimation function aimed to minimize the smaller residual squares after the larger residuals being trimmed. This kind of high breakdown point method could tolerate relative high proportion of outliers in the data, including S estimation, GS estimation, τ estimation.

3.10. Quantile Regression[11]

Conditional mean model, which is used to describe how the conditional mean of dependent variable varies with the changing of the independent variable, is the most common model in the analysis of regression. Using conditional mean to summarize the information of dependent variable will average the effect of the regression and hide the extreme impact of some independent variable to dependent variable. At the same time, the estimation of conditional mean model seems to lack robustness faced with potential outliers. Given the independent variable, the quantile regression describes the trend of dependent variable in the formation of varying quantile. The quantile regression can not only measure the impact of independent variable to the distribution center of dependent variable, but also characterize the influence to the lower and upper tails on its distribution, which highlight the association between local distributions. If the conditional variance of dependent has heterogeneity, the quantile regression can reveal local characters while the conditional mean model cannot.

The minimum mean absolute deviation regression, which has extended to the quantile regression by Hogg, Koenker and Bassett *et al.*, constructs model for conditional distribution function of dependent variable under linear assumption. The quantile regression can be written as

$$Q_{Y|X}(\tau; x) = x_i'\beta(\tau) + \varepsilon_i,$$

where $Q_{Y|X}(\tau; x)$ is ith population quantile of Y given x and satisfied $P\{Y \leq Q_{Y|X}|X = x\} = \tau$, that is,

$$Q_{Y|\underline{X}}(\tau; \underline{x}) = \overset{-1}{F_{Y|X}}(\tau; x) = \inf\{y : P\{Y \leq y|X = x\} = \tau\},$$

where $F_{Y|X}(\tau; x)$ is the conditional distribution of Y.

$\beta(\tau)$ is an unknown $(P \times 1)$ vector of regression coefficient. The error, $\varepsilon_i (i = 1, 2, \ldots, n)$, is an independent random variable whose distribution is

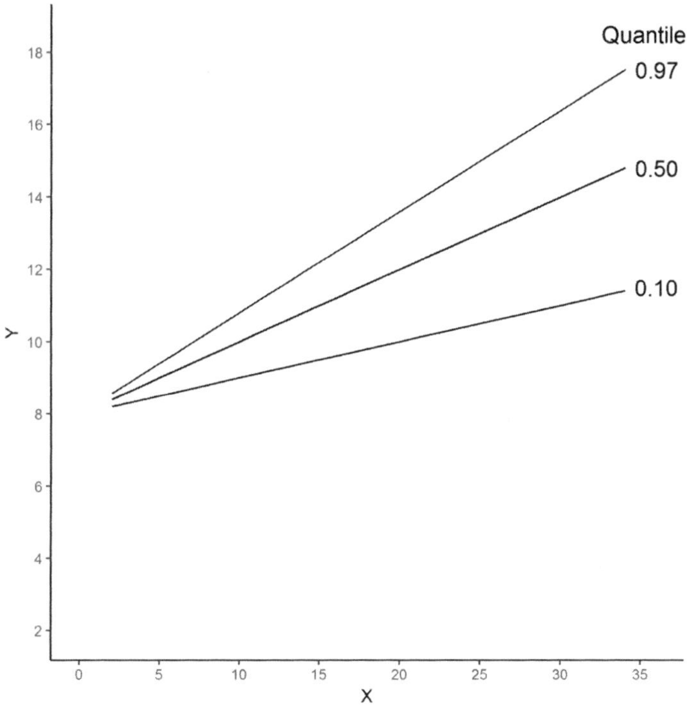

Fig. 3.10.1. The regression line for different quantiles.

free of specification. The population conditional median of ε_i is 0. $\beta(\tau)$ can vary with changes in τ and $0 < \tau < 1$.

Figure 3.10.1 shows the changing of different conditional quantiles of dependent variable with independent variable. While using a standard regression model (roughly corresponding to the regression line with $\tau = 0.5$), an obvious difference between distribution tails of dependent variable is not clear. When $\tau = 0.5$, the quantile regression can also be called median regression.

From the perspective of analytic geometry, τ is the percentage of the dependent variable under the regression line or regression plane. We can adjust the direction and position of the regression plane by taking any value of τ between 0 and 1. Quantile regression estimates the different quantile of dependent variable, which can represent all the information of the data to some extent, but more focused on a specific area of the corresponding quantile. The advantages of quantile regression are as follows:

1. Distribution of random error in the model is not specified, so this makes the model more robust than the classic one.

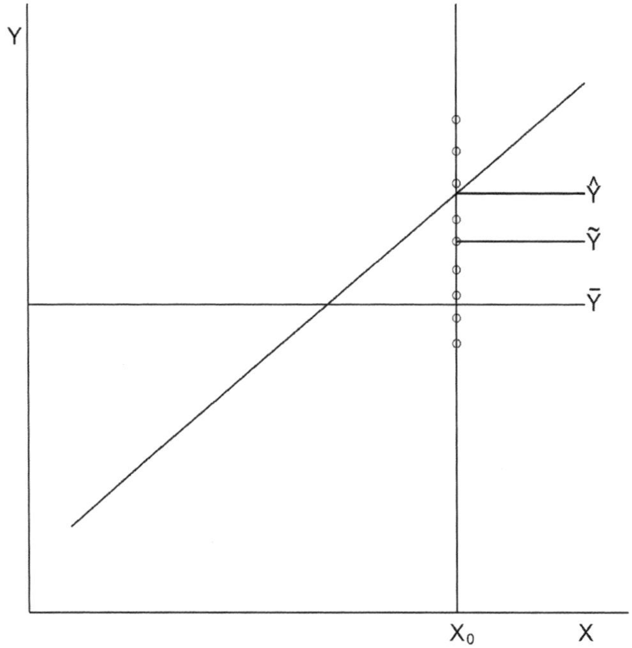

Fig. 3.11.1. Decomposing of random error and lack of fit.

2. Quantile regression is a regression for all quantiles, so it is resistant to outliers.
3. Quantile regression is monotonous invariant for dependent variable.
4. The parameters estimated by quantile regression are asymptotically optimal under the large sample theory.

3.11. Lack-of-Fit[12]

In general, there may be more than one candidate statistical model in the analysis of regression. For example, if both linear and quadratic models have statistical significance, which one is better for observed data? The simplest way to select an optimal model is to compare some statistics reflecting the goodness-of-fit. If there are many values of dependent variable observed for the fixed value of independent variable, we can evaluate the goodness-of-fit by testing lack-of-fit.

For fixed x, if there are many observations of Y (as illustrated in Figure 3.11.1), the conditional sample mean of Y is not always exactly equal to $\hat{Y}$. We denote this conditional sample mean as $\tilde{Y}$. If the model is specified correctly, the conditional sample mean of Y, that is $\tilde{Y}$, is close or equal to the model mean $\hat{Y}$, which is estimated by the model. According to this idea, we can construct corresponding F statistics by decomposing sum of squares and degrees of freedom for testing the difference between two conditional mean ($\tilde{Y}$ and $\hat{Y}$), which indicates whether the model is fitted insufficiently. In other words, we are testing whether the predicted model mean $\hat{Y}$ based on the model is far away from observed conditional mean $\tilde{Y}$.

Suppose that there are n different points on X, and k varying values of Y for each fixed point X_i ($i = 1, 2, \ldots, n$), which can be denoted as Y_{ij} ($i = 1, 2, \ldots, n$, $j = 1, 2, \ldots, k$). So, there is a total data of $nk = N$.

The sum squares of residuals of lack-of-fit test and degrees of freedom is as follows:

$$\mathrm{SS}_{\mathrm{Error}} = \sum_{i=1}^{n}\sum_{j=1}^{k}(\tilde{\mathrm{Y}}_{\mathrm{i}} - \hat{\mathrm{Y}}_{\mathrm{i}})^2 \quad df_{\mathrm{Error}} = k - 2,$$

$$\mathrm{SS}_{\mathrm{Lack}} = \sum_{i=1}^{n}\sum_{j=1}^{k}(\mathrm{Y}_{\mathrm{ij}} - \tilde{\mathrm{Y}}_{\mathrm{i}})^2 \quad df_{\mathrm{Lack}} = nk - k = N - k,$$

where $\mathrm{SS}_{\mathrm{sum}} = \mathrm{SS}_{\mathrm{Error}} + \mathrm{SS}_{\mathrm{Lack}}$, $df_{\mathrm{sum}} = df_{\mathrm{Error}} + df_{\mathrm{Lack}}$.

For a fixed x value, because $\tilde{Y}$ is the sample mean calculated by k numbers of corresponding Y value. $\mathrm{SS}_{\mathrm{Error}}/df_{\mathrm{Error}}$ represents pure random error, while $\mathrm{SS}_{\mathrm{Lack}}/df_{\mathrm{Lack}}$ represents the deviation of model fitting values $\hat{Y}$ and its conditional mean $\tilde{Y}$. If the model specification is correct, the error of lack of fitting will not be too large, when it is greater than the random error to a certain extent, the model fitting is not good.

When null hypothesis H_0 is correct, the ratio of the two parts will follow an F distribution:

$$F_{\mathrm{Lack}} = \frac{\mathrm{SS}_{\mathrm{Error}}/df_{\mathrm{Error}}}{\mathrm{SS}_{\mathrm{Lack}}/df_{\mathrm{Lack}}}, \quad df_{\mathrm{Error}} = k - 2,$$

$$df_{\mathrm{Lack}} = nk - k = N - k.$$

If F_{Lack} is greater than the corresponding threshold value, the model is recognized as not fitting well, it implies existence of a better model than the current one.

3.12. Analysis of Covariance[13]

Analysis of covariance is a special form of ANOVA, which is used to compare the differences between means from each group; the former can also control the confounding effects for quantitative variables but not for the latter.

Analysis of covariance is a combination of ANOVA and regression. Assumptions of the following conditions should be met: Firstly, the observed values are mutually independent and variance in populations is homogenous. Secondly, Y and X have a linear relationship and population regression coefficients are the same in each treatment group (the regression lines are parallel).

In a completely randomized trial, assume that there are three groups and each group has n_i subjects. The ith observation in group g can be expressed as a regression model $Y_{gi} = \mu + \alpha_g + \beta(X_{gi} + \bar{X}) + \varepsilon_{gi}$, it is clear that the formula is a combination of linear regression with ANOVA based on a completely random design. In this formula, u is the population mean of Y; the α_g is the effect of the treatment group; β is regression coefficient of Y_{gi} on X_{gi}, and ε_{gi} is the random error of Y_{gi}.

In order to understand it more easily, the model can be transformed into another form like this: $Y_{gi} = \beta X_{gi} + \beta\bar{X} = \mu + \alpha_g + \varepsilon_{gi}$. The left side of the equation is the residual of the ith subject in group g, in which the influence of X_{gi} has been removed, added with the regression effect assuming the value of independent variable for all the subjects in each group fixed in position of $\bar{X}$. The formula manifests the philosophy of covariance analysis After equalizing the covariant X that has linear correlation with dependent variable Y, and then testing the significant differences of the adjusted means of the Y between groups.

The basic idea of analysis of covariance is to get residual sum of squares using linear regression between covariant X and dependent variable Y, then carrying on ANOVA based on the decomposing of the residual sum of squares. The corresponding sum of squares is decomposed as follows:

$$\mathrm{SS}_{\mathrm{res}} = \sum_{g}^{k}\sum_{i}^{n_i}(Y_{gi} - Y_{\tau gi})^2,$$

this denotes the total residual sum of squares, namely, the sum of the squares between all the subjects and their population regression line, the associated degree of freedom is $v'_{res} = n - 2$.

$$\mathrm{SS}_E = \sum_{g}^{k}\sum_{i}^{n_i}(Y_{gi} - \hat{Y}_{gi})^2,$$

this denotes the residual deviations within groups, namely, it is the total sum of squares between subjects in each group and the paralleled regression line, the associated degree of freedom is $v'_E = n - k - 1$,

$$\mathrm{SS}_B = \sum_{g}^{k}\sum_{i}^{n_i}(\hat{Y}_{gi} - Y_{\tau gi})^2,$$

this denotes the residual deviations between groups, namely the sum of squared differences between the estimated values of the corresponding parallel regression lines of each group and the estimated values of the population regression line, the associated degree of freedom is $v'_B = K - 1$.

The following F statistic can be used to compare the adjusted means between groups:

$$F = \frac{\mathrm{SS}_E/v'_E}{\mathrm{SS}_B/v'_B} = \frac{\mathrm{MS}_E}{\mathrm{MS}_B}.$$

3.13. Dummy Variable[14]

The dummy variable encoding is a method to transform the independent variable to the nominal or ordered variable in the linear model. Supposing there is a study to explore influence factors on the average annual income, one of the independent variables is the educational status which involve the following three classes: (a) below high school (b) high school (c) college or above. If the educational status (a), (b), and (c) are assigned with 1, 2, and 3, respectively, as quantitative variables, the explanation of regression coefficients of this variable does not make sense because equidistance cannot be ensured in the differences between the three categories cannot. Assigning continuous numbers to nominal variable will lead to an absurd result under this circumstance.

Dummy variable encoding is commonly used to deal with this problem. If the original variable has k categories, it will be redefined as $k - 1$ dummy variables. For example, the educational status has three categories, which can be broken down into two dummy variables. One of the categories is set to be the reference level, and the others can be compared with it.

According to the encoding scheme in Table 3.13.1, if the education level is below high school, the dummy variables of college or above and high school are both encoded as 0; if the education level is college or above, the dummy variable of college or above is 1 and that of high school is 0; if the

Table 3.13.1. The dummy variable encoding of educational status.

	Dummy variables	
Educational status	College or above	High school
College or above	1	0
High school	0	1
Below high school	0	0

education level is high school, the dummy variable of college or above is 0 and that of high school is 1. It does not matter which category is chosen as reference mathematically. If there is no clear reason to decide which one is the reference, we can choose the one with the largest sample size to get a smaller standard error. Hardy put forward three suggestions on how to choose reference on dummy variable encoding:

1. If there is an ordered variable, it is better to choose the maximum or minimum category as reference.
2. Using a well-defined category variable rather than using an unclear defined one like "others" as reference.
3. Choose the one with maximum sample size.

In particular, if there is a category variable as independent variable in linear model, it is not recommended to use dummy variable to perform stepwise regression directly. Under this situation, we can take it as nominal variable with degree of freedom as $k-1$ and first perform an ANOVA, based on a statistically significant testing result, then we can define each category with a suitable dummy variable encoding scheme, and calculate respective regression coefficients compared with the reference level. This procedure can keep each level of the dummy variables as a whole when faced with variable selection in regression model.

3.14. Mixed Effects Model[15]

The linear model $y = X\beta + e$ can be divided into three kinds of models based on whether the parameters of covariates were random, which includes fixed, random and mixed effects models.

For example, we measured the content of some compounds in serum of six mice by four methods. The linear model was

$$Y_{ij} = u + \delta_i + e_{ij},$$

$i = 1, \ldots, 4$ was the different methods, and $\delta_1, \delta_2, \delta_3, \delta_4$ were the effects. $j = 1, \ldots, 6$ represents the different mice, and e_{ij} was error, where $E(e) = 0$, $\mathrm{var}(e) = \sigma_e^2$.

If the aim of this analysis was just comparing the differences in the four methods, and the results will not be extrapolated, the effects should be considered as the fixed effects; otherwise, if the results will be expanded to the sampling population, that is, each measurement represents a population, which was randomly sampled from various measurements, the effects should be considered as random effects. Random effects were more focused on interpretations of dependent variable variation caused by the variation of the treatment effect. In general, if all the treatment effects were fixed, the model was fixed effects model; if all the treatment effects were random, the model was random effects model. The mixed model contains both fixed effects and random effects. The form of mixed effects model was

$$y = X\beta + Z\gamma + e.$$

X and Z were known design matrixes of $n \times p$ and $n \times q$, respectively. β was unknown fixed effected vector of $p \times 1$, γ was unknown random effected vector of $q \times 1$, e was error term, where $E(\gamma) = 0$, $\mathrm{cov}(y) = D$, $\mathrm{cov}(\gamma, e) = 0$, $\mathrm{cov}(e) = R$. D and R were positive defined matrix. Then,

$$E(Y) = X\beta, \quad \mathrm{cov}(y) = ZDZ' + R = V.$$

If the random component was $u = Z\gamma + e$, then:

$$y = X\beta + u, \quad E(u) = 0, \quad \mathrm{cov}(u) = V.$$

For solving the variance components in random effects model, commonly used methods include maximum likelihood estimation, Restricted Maximum Likelihood Estimation, Minimum Norm Quadratic Unbiased Estimation, variance analysis and so on. As the estimations need iterative calculation, some variance component may be less than 0, and we can use Wald test to decide whether the component of variance was 0. If the result did not reject the null hypothesis, then we made it to 0.

3.15. Generalized Estimating Equation[16]

In analysis of longitudinal data, repeated measurement data or clustering data, an important feature is that observations are not independent, so it does not meet the applicable conditions of the traditional general linear regression model. The generalized estimating equation, developed on the basis of the generalized linear model, is dedicated to handling longitudinal data and achieving the robust parameter estimation.

Assuming Y_{ij} is the j measurement of the i object, $(i = 1, \ldots, k;\ j = 1, \ldots, t)$, $x_{ij} = (x_{ij1}, \ldots, x_{ijp})$, is $p \times 1$ vector corresponding to Y_{ij}. Define the marginal mean of Y_{ij} as known function of the linear combination of x_{ij}, the marginal variance of Y_{ij} as known function of the marginal mean, the covariance of Y_{ij} as the function of the marginal mean and the parameter α, namely:

$$E(y_{ij}) = \mu_{ij}, \quad g(\mu_{ij}) = X\beta,$$
$$\mathrm{Var}(Y_{ij}) = V(\mu_{ij}) \bullet \phi,$$
$$\mathrm{Cov}(Y_{is}, Y_{it}) = c(\mu_{is}, \mu_{it}; \alpha).$$

$g(\mu_{ij})$ is a link function, $\beta = (\beta_1, \beta_2, \ldots, \beta_p)'$ is the parameter vector the model needs to estimate, $V(\mu_{ij})$ is the known function; ϕ is the scale parameter indicating that part of the variance of Y cannot be explained by $V(\mu_{ij})$. This parameter ϕ also needs to estimate, but for both the binomial and Poisson distribution, $\phi = 1$; $c(\mu_{is}, \mu_{it}; \alpha)$ is the known function, α is the correlation parameter, s and t respectively refer to the s and the t measurement.

Make $R(\alpha)$ as $n \times n$ symmetric matrix, and $R(\alpha)$ is the working correlation matrix. Defining $V_i = A_i^{1/2} R_i(\alpha) A_i^{1/2} / \phi$, A_i is a t-dimensional diagonal matrix with $V(\mu_{ij})$ as the ith element, V_i indicates the working covariance matrix, $R_i(\alpha)$ is the working correlation matrix of Y_{ij}. Devote the magnitude of the correlation between each repeated measurements of dependent variable, namely the mean correlation between objects. If $R(\alpha)$ is the correlation matrix of Y_i, V_i is equal to $\mathrm{Cov}(Y_i)$. Then we can define the generalized estimating equations as

$$\sum_{i}^{n} \left(\frac{\partial \mu_1}{\partial \beta} \right) V_i^{-1}(\alpha)(Y_i - \mu_i) = 0.$$

Given the values of the ϕ and α, we can estimate the value of the β. Iterative algorithm is needed to get the parameter estimation by generalized estimating equations. When the link function is correct and the total number of observations is big enough, even though the structure of $R_i(\alpha)$ is not correctly defined, the confidence intervals of β and other statistics of the model are asymptotically right, so the estimation is robust to selection of the working correlation matrix.

3.16. Independent Variable Selection[17,18]

The variable selection in regression model is aimed to identify significant influential factors on dependent variable or to include only effective variables for reducing the error of prediction, or simply to reduce the number of variables for enhancing the robustness of regression equation. If any prior knowledge is available in the process of selecting independent variables, it is a good strategy to reduce the number of variables as much as possible by making use of such prior knowledge. Such a reduction not only helps to select a stable model, but also saves computation time.

1. Testing Procedures: Commonly used methods of variable selection include forward inclusion, backward elimination, and a mixed stepwise inclusion and elimination. In the backward elimination, for example, starting from the full model, eliminate one variable at a time. At any step of backward elimination, where the current model is p, if $\min_j F(p - \{j\}, p)$ is not statistically significant, then the variable j is eliminated from p, otherwise, the elimination process is terminated. The most widely used level of the test is 10% or 5%. Only when the order of variables entering into model is specified explicitly before applying the procedure can we estimate overall power as well as the type I error. Obviously, the order of entry differs with observation. To overcome such difficulties, the simultaneous testing procedure is proposed by Aitkin or McKay.
2. Criterion Procedure: In order to predict or control, many criteria have been proposed. The first group of criteria is based on RSS(p), each of which can be represented by the final prediction error FEP_α:

$$\text{FEP}_\alpha(p) = \text{RSS}(p) + \alpha \text{kRSS}(\bar{p})/(n - K).$$

General information criterion proposed by Atkinson is an extension of Akaike's information criterion (AIC):

$$C(\alpha, p) = \alpha k \text{RSS}(p) + \alpha k.$$

The selected model is obtained by minimizing these criteria.

Mallows propose the C_p criterion:

$$C_p = \text{RSS}(p)/\hat{\sigma}^2 + 2k - n,$$

which is equivalent to FEP_2 when $\text{RSS}(\bar{p})/(n - K)$ is regarded as an estimation of σ^2.

Hannan and Quinn showed that if α is a function of n, the necessary and sufficient condition of strong consistency of procedure is that $\alpha < 2c \log \log n$ for some $c > 1$.

The criterion with $\alpha = 2c \log \log n$ is called HQ criterion, which is the most conservative one among all criteria with the above form. What is more, this criterion has a tendency to overestimate in the case of small sample. From the perspective of Bayesian theory, Schwarz proposed $\alpha = \log n$, which is known as Bayesian information criterion (BIC).

The mean squared error of prediction criterion (MSEP), which is proposed by Allen, is similar to FEP_2. However, MSEP is based on the prediction error at a specified point x. Another group of criteria includes cross-validation. Allen also proposed the prediction sum-squares criterion: $\text{PRESS}(p) = \sum_1^n (y_i - \hat{y}_i(-i))^2$, where $\hat{y}_i(-i)$ is a prediction of y_i under the model P which is based on all observations except the i-th one. This criteria can also be represented as $\sum_1^n[(y_i - \hat{y}_i)/\ (1-\alpha_i)]^2$, where $\hat{y} = X\hat{\beta}(p)$ is an ordinary least-squares predictor and $\alpha_i = x_i'(X'X)^{-1}x_i$. It is obvious that this criterion is a special case of cross-validation. Cross-validation is asymptotically equivalent to AIC or general information criterion with $\alpha = 2$, that is, $C(2, p)$.

In recent years, along with the development of bioinformation technology, the method of variable selection in the case of high-dimensional data (such as gene number) is making some progress. For instance, inspired by Bridge Regression and Non-negative Garrote Tibshirani[17] proposed a method of variable selection, which is called Least Absolute Shrinkage and Selection Operator (LASSO). This method uses the absolute function of model coefficients as penalty strategy to compress the model confidents, that is, the coefficient, which is weakly correlated with the effect of y, will decrease even to zero. So LASSO can provide a sparse solution. Before the Least Angle Regression (LARS) algorithm appeared, LASSO lacked statistical support and the advantage of sparseness had not been widely recognized. What is more, high-dimensional data at that time is uncommon. In recent years, with the rapid development of computer technology, along with production of a large number of high-throughput omics data, much attention has been paid to LASSO, which results in LASSO's optimizing, for example, LARS algorithm and Co-ordinate Descent algorithm among others. Based on classical LASSO theory, the Elastic Net, Smoothly Clipped Absolute Deviation (SCAD), Sure Independence Screening (SIS), Minimax Concave Penalty (MCP) and other penalty methods are developed.

3.17. Least Absolute Shrinkage and Selection Operator

It is also known as "Lasso estimation", which is a "penalized least square" estimation proposed by Tibshirani.[17] That is, under the condition of L1-norm penalty, making the residual squares sum to the minimum so as to obtain the shrinkage estimation of regression coefficients.

Generally, a linear regression model is expressed as $Y_i = X_i\beta + \varepsilon_i = \sum_{j=0}^p X_{ij}\beta_j + \varepsilon_i$.

Among them, X_i is the independent variable, Y_i is the dependent variable, $i = 1, 2, \ldots, n$, and p is the number of independent variables. If the observed values are independent, X_{ij} is the standardized variable (the mean is 0, the variance is 1), then the Lasso estimator of the regression coefficient is $\hat{\beta}_{\text{Lasso}} = \sum_{i=1}^n (Y_i - \sum_{j=0}^p X_{ij}\beta_j)^2$, under the condition that $\sum_{j=1}^p |\beta_j| \leq t$, where t is the tuning parameter or the penalty parameter. When t is small enough, the partial regression coefficient can be compressed to 0.

1. LAR: Lasso regression is essentially a solution of constrained quadratic programming problems. Because of the limited computation resources of that time and the less demand of high-dimensional data for model sparsity, when LASSO was first put forward, the academic society does not pay much attention to it, so that its application is restricted. Efron[18] proposed the LAR algorithm to solve the calculation problem of Lasso regression. The algorithm is similar to forward stepwise regression, but instead of including variables at each step, the estimated parameters are increased in a direction equiangular to each one's correlations with the residual. The computational complexity is comparable to that of the least squares estimation. One can usually choose tuning parameters through k-fold cross-validation or generalized cross-validation method.

The main advantages of the lasso regression are as follows: First, the choice of the independent variable is realized and the explanation of the model is improved at the same time of parameter estimation. Second, the estimated variance is reduced, and the prediction accuracy of the model is improved by a small sacrifice of the unbiasedness of the regression coefficient estimator. Third, the problem of multicollinearity of the independent variables in the regression analysis can be solved by the shrinkage estimation of partial regression coefficients. Its main disadvantages are: First, the estimation of regression coefficient is always biased, especially for the shrinkages of the larger coefficients of the absolute value. Second, for all regression coefficients, the degrees of shrinkage are the same and the relative importance of the independent variables is ignored. Third, it does not have the consistency of parameters and the asymptotic properties of parameter estimation (Oracle property). Fourth, it failed to deal with the situation with large p and small n, and cannot select more than n independent variables and opt for a too sparse model. Fifth, when there is a high degree of correlation between independent variables (such as >0.95), it cannot get relative importance of the independent variables.

Dealing with the limitations of lasso regression, a lot of improved estimators have emerged, such as adaptive Lasso and elastic net. The former is the weighted Lasso estimation; the latter is a convex combination of Lasso regression and ridge regression. Both methods have the Oracle property and generally do not shrink parameters excessively; elastic net can handle the problem of a large p and a small n.

3.18. Linear Model Selection[22]

1. The Model Selection Criteria and Model Selection Tests:

Suppose there are n observed values $y(n \times 1)$ with design matrix $X(n \times p)$, $(n \geq p)$ when X is of full rank $[rank(x) = p]$, we can consider fitting a linear model:

$$y = X\beta + \varepsilon\varepsilon \sim N(0, \sigma^2 I).$$

Assume further that both $C_n = n^{-1}X'X$ and $\lim_{n\to\infty} C_n = C$ are positive definite.

Use $r_j - R_j\beta = 0$ $(j = 1, 2, \ldots)$ nested so that $r_j = G_j r_{j+1}$ and $R_j = G_j R_{J+1}$ is $m_j \times p$ with $m_1 < m_2 < \cdots m_h = p$ $\text{rank}(R_j) = m_j$, denote a series of h linear constraints on β. If the linear model satisfied $r_j - R_j\beta = 0$ for $j \leq j_0$ but not for $j > j_0$, we can denote M_{j_0} with the unrestricted model $(m_0 = 0)M_0$.

Obviously, M_{j_0} have $p - m_{j_0}$ free parameters. Because these are nested, we have $M_0 \supset M_1 \supset M_2 \supset \cdots \supset M_h$.

Model selection criteria (MSC) can be used to decide which of the models $M_0, M_1, M_2, \ldots, M_h$ is appropriate. Three, types of MSC are commonly used:

$$\begin{aligned} MSC1(M_j) &= \ln\hat{\sigma}^2 + (p - m_j)n^{-1}f(n, 0), \\ MSC2(M_j) &= \hat{\sigma}_j^2 + (p - m_j)\sigma^2 n^{-1}f(n, 0), \\ MSC3(M_j) &= \hat{\sigma}^2 + (p - m_j)\hat{\sigma}_j^2 n^{-1}f(n, p - m_j), \end{aligned}$$

where $f(\ldots) > 0$, $\lim_{n\to\infty} f(n, z) = 0$ for all z, and $\hat{\sigma}_j^2 = n^{-1}$.

The customary decision rule in using the MSC is that we can choose the model M_g if $MSC(M_g) = \min_{j=0,1,\ldots,h} MSC(M_j)$. Another strategy is to perform formal tests of significance sequentially. The test which is called MST started by testing M_0 against M_1, then M_1 against M_2, and so on, until the first rejection. For example, if the first rejection occurs on testing M_g against M_{g+1}, then the model M_g is chosen.

2. Sequential Testing:

That is, choosing a nested model from $M_0 \supset M_1 \supset M_2 \supset \cdots \supset M_h$ by using common MST. Assume that $m_j = j$, $j = 1, \ldots, h$. As mentioned above, the conditional testing starts from assuming that M_0, which is the least restrictive model, is true. The individual statistics follow $F_{1,n-k_j}$ distributions and is independent of each other.

The difference between MSC and MST is that the former compare all possible models simultaneously while the latter is the comparison of the two in sequence. Ostensibly, using MSC instead of MST seems to make us from choosing significance levels. Many criteria with varying small sample properties are available, and the selection between these criteria is equivalent to choosing the significance level of MSC rule.

References

1. Wang Songgui. *The Theory and Application of Linear Model.* Anhui Education Press, 1987.
2. McCullagh, P, Nelder, JA. *Generalized Linear Models* (2nd edn). London: Chapman & Hall, 1989.
3. Draper, N, Smith, H. *Applied Regression Analysis*, (3rd edn.). New York: Wiley, 1998.
4. Glantz, SA, Slinker, BK. *Primer of Applied Regression and Analysis of Variance*, (2nd edn.). McGraw-Hill, 2001.
5. Cook, RD, Weisberg, S. *Residuals and Influence in Regression.* London: Chapman & Hall, 1982.
6. Belsley, DA, Kuh, E, Welsch, R. *Regression Diagnostics: Identifying Influential Data and Sources of Collinearity.* New York: Wiley, 1980.
7. Gunst, RF, Mason, RL. *Regression Analysis and Its Application.* New York: Marcel Dekker, 1980.
8. Hoerl, AE, Kennard, RW, Baldwin, KF. Ridge regression: Some simulations. *Comm. Stat. Theor*, 1975, 4: 105–123.
9. Rousseeuw, PJ, Leroy, AM. *Robust Regression and Outlier Detection.* New York: John Wiley & Sons, 1987.
10. Roger K. *Quantile Regression* (2nd edn.). New York: Cambridge University Press, 2005.
11. Su, JQ, Wei, LJ. A lack-of-fit test for the mean function in a generalized linear model. *J. Amer. Statist. Assoc.* 1991, 86: 420–426.
12. Bliss, CI. Statistics in Biology. (Vol. 2), New York: McGraw-Hill, 1967.
13. Goeffrey, R, Norman, DL, Streiner, BC. *Biostatistics, The bare essentials* (3rd edn.). London: Decker, 1998.
14. Searle, SR, Casella, G, MuCullo, C. *Variance Components.* New York: John Wiley, 1992.
15. Liang, KY, Zeger, ST. Longitudinal data analysis using generalized linear models. *Biometrics*, 1986, 73(1): 13.
16. Bühlmann, P, Sara, G. *Statistics for High-Dimensional Data Methods, Theory and Applications.* New York: Springer, 2011.
17. Tibshirani, R. Regression shrinkage and selection via the lasso. *J. R. Stat. Soc. S. B*, 1996, 58(1): 267–288.
18. Efron, B, Hastie, T, Johnstone, I *et al.* Least angle regression. *Annal Stat.*, 2004, 32(2): 407–499.
19. Hastie, T, Tibshirani, R, Wainwright, M. *Statistical Learning with Sparsity: The Lasso and Generalizations.* Boca Raton: CRC Press, 2015.
20. Anderson, TW. The *Statistical Analysis of Time Series.* New York: Wiley, 1971.

About the Author

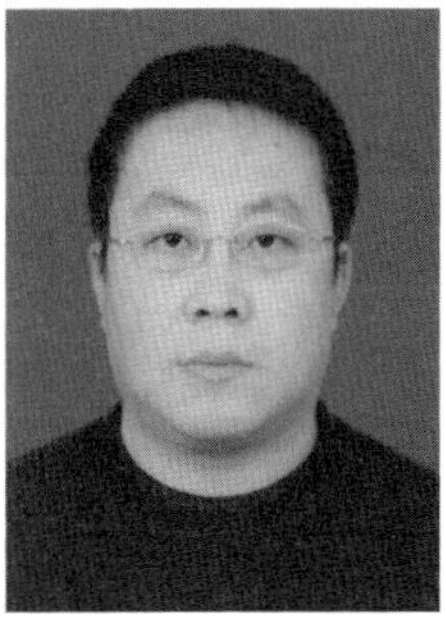

Tong Wang is a Professor at the Department of Health Statistics, School of Public Health, Shanxi Medical University. He is the Deputy Chair of the Biostatistics Division of the Chinese Preventive Medicine Association, Standing Director of IBS-CHINA, Standing Director of the Chinese Health Information Association, Standing Director of the Chinese Statistic Education Association, Deputy Chair of the Medical Statistics Education Division and Standing Director of Statistical Theory and Method Division of the Chinese Health Information Association. Dr. Wang was the PI of National Natural Science Foundations a key project of National Statistic Science Research and the Ministry of Education of China.

CHAPTER 4

MULTIVARIATE ANALYSIS

Pengcheng Xun* and Qianchuan He

4.1. Multivariate Descriptive Statistics[1,2]

Descriptive statistics is of particular importance not only because it enables us to present data in a meaningful way, but also because it is a preliminary step of making any further statistical inference. Multivariate descriptive statistics mainly includes mean vector, variance–covariance matrix, deviation of sum of squares and cross-products matrix (DSSCP), and correlation matrix.

Mean vector, a column vector, consists of mean of each variable, denoted as $\bar{\boldsymbol{X}}$. For simplicity, it can be expressed as the transpose of a row vector

$$\bar{X} = (\bar{x}_1, \bar{x}_2, \ldots, \bar{x}_m)'. \quad (4.1.1)$$

Variance–covariance matrix consists of the variances of the variables along the main diagonal and the covariance between each pair of variables in the other matrix positions. Denoted by $\boldsymbol{V}$, the variance–covariance matrix is often just called "covariance matrix". The formula for computing the covariance of the variables x_i and x_j is

$$v_{ij} = \frac{\sum_{k=1}^{n}(x_{ik} - \bar{x}_i)(x_{jk} - \bar{x}_j)}{n-1}, \quad 1 \le i, j \le m, \quad (4.1.2)$$

where n denotes sample size, m is the number of variables, and $\bar{x}_i$ and $\bar{x}_j$ denote the means of the variables x_i and x_j, respectively.

DSSCP is denoted as $\boldsymbol{SS}$, and consists of the sum of squares of the variables along the main diagonal and the cross products off diagonals. It is

*Corresponding author: pxun@indiana.edu; xunpc@163.com

also known as corrected SSCP. The formula for computing the cross-product between the variables x_i and x_j is

$$\mathrm{ss}_{ij} = \sum_{k=1}^{n}(x_{ik} - \bar{x}_i)(x_{jk} - \bar{x}_j), \quad 1 \leq i, j \leq m. \tag{4.1.3}$$

It is created by multiplying the scalar $n - 1$ with $\boldsymbol{V}$, i.e. $\boldsymbol{SS} = (n - 1)V$.

Correlation matrix is denoted as $\boldsymbol{R}$, and consists of 1s in the main diagonal and the correlation coefficients between each pair of variables in off-diagonal positions. The correlation between x_i and x_j is defined by

$$r_{ij} = \frac{v_{ij}}{\sqrt{v_{ii}v_{jj}}}, \quad 1 \leq i, j \leq m, \tag{4.1.4}$$

where v_{ij} is the covariance between x_i and x_j as defined in Eq. (4.1.2), and v_{ii} and v_{jj} are variance of x_i and x_j, respectively.

Since the correlation of x_i and x_j is the same as the correlation between x_j and x_i, $\boldsymbol{R}$ is a symmetric matrix. As such we often write it as a lower triangular matrix

$$\boldsymbol{R} = \begin{bmatrix} 1 & & & \\ r_{21} & 1 & & \\ \cdots & \cdots & & \\ r_{m1} & r_{m2} & \cdots & 1 \end{bmatrix} \tag{4.1.5}$$

by leaving off the upper triangular part. Similarly, we can also re-write $\boldsymbol{SS}$ and $\boldsymbol{V}$ as lower triangular matrices.

Of note, the above-mentioned statistics are all based on the multivariate normal (MVN) assumption, which is violated in most of the "real" data. Thus, to develop descriptive statistics for non-MVN data is sorely needed. Depth statistics, a pioneer in the non-parametric multivariate statistics based on data depth (DD), is such an alternative.

DD is a scale to provide a center-outward ordering or ranking of multivariate data in the high dimensional space, which is a generalization of order statistics in univariate situation (see Sec. 5.3). High depth corresponds to "centrality", and low depth to "outlyingness". The center consists of the point(s) that globally maximize depth. Therefore, the deepest point with maximized depth can be called "*depth median*". Based on depth, dispersion, skewness and kurtosis can also be defined for multivariate data.

Subtypes of DDs mainly include Mahalanobis depth, half-space depth, simplicial depth, project depth, and L^p depth. And desirable depth functions should at least have the following properties: affine invariance, the maximality at center, decreasing along rays, and vanishing at infinity.

DD extends to the multivariate setting in a unified way the univariate methods of sign and rank, order statistics, quantile, and outlyingness measure. In particular, the introduction of its concept substantially advances the development of non-parametric multivariate statistics, and provides a useful exploration of describing high-dimensional data including its visualization.

In addition, distance, a prime concept of descriptive statistics, plays an important role in multivariate statistics area. For example, Mahalanobis distance is widely used in multivariate analysis of variance (MANOVA) (see Sec. 4.3) and discriminant analysis (see Sec. 4.15). It is also closely related to Hotelling's T-squared distribution (see Sec. 4.2) and Fisher's linear discriminant function.

4.2. Hotelling's T-squared Test[1,3,4]

It was named after Harold Hotelling, a famous statistician who developed Hotelling's T-squared distribution as a generalization of Student's t-distribution in 1931. Also called multivariate T-squared test, it can be used to test whether a set of means is zero, or two set of means are equal. It commonly takes into account three scenarios:

(1) One sample T-squared test, testing whether the mean vector of the population, from which the current sample is drawn, is equal to the known population mean vector, i.e. $H_0\colon \boldsymbol{\mu} = \boldsymbol{\mu}_0$ with setting the significance level at 0.05. Then, we define the test statistic as

$$T^2 = n[\bar{\boldsymbol{X}} - \boldsymbol{\mu}_0]'\boldsymbol{V}^{-1}[\bar{\boldsymbol{X}} - \boldsymbol{\mu}_0], \tag{4.2.1}$$

where n is the sample size, $\bar{\boldsymbol{X}}$ and $\boldsymbol{\mu}_0$ stand for sample and population mean vector, respectively, $\boldsymbol{V}$ is the sample covariance matrix.

H_0 is rejected if and only if

$$\frac{n-m}{(n-1)m}T^2 \geq F_{m,n-m,(\alpha)}.$$

Or simply, if and only if

$$T^2 \geq \frac{(n-1)m}{n-m}F_{m,n-m,(\alpha)},$$

where m is the number of variables and α is the significance level.

In fact, T^2 in Eq. (4.2.1) is a multivariate generalization of the square of the univariate t-ratio for testing $H_0\colon \mu = \mu_0$, that is

$$t = \frac{\bar{X} - \mu_0}{s/\sqrt{n}}. \tag{4.2.2}$$

Squaring both sides of Eq. (4.2.2) leads to

$$t^2 = n(\bar{X} - \mu_0)(s^2)^{-1}(\bar{X} - \mu_0),$$

which is exactly equivalent to T^2 in case of $m = 1$.

(2) Two matched-sample T-squared test, which is the multivariate analog of paired t-test for two dependent samples in univariate statistics. It can also be considered as a special case of one sample T-squared test, which tests whether the sample mean vector of difference equals the population mean vector of difference (i.e., zero vector), in other words, tests whether a set of differences is zero jointly.

(3) Two independent-sample T-squared test, an extension of t-test for two independent samples in univariate statistics, tests H_0: $\boldsymbol{\mu}_A = \boldsymbol{\mu}_B$

T^2can be defined as

$$T^2 = \frac{n_A n_B}{n_A + n_B}[\bar{\boldsymbol{X}}_A - \bar{\boldsymbol{X}}_B]'\boldsymbol{V}^{-1}[\bar{\boldsymbol{X}}_A - \bar{\boldsymbol{X}}_B], \qquad (4.2.3)$$

where n_A and n_B are sample size for group A and B, respectively, and $\bar{\boldsymbol{X}}_A$ and $\bar{\boldsymbol{X}}_B$ stand for two sample mean vectors and $\boldsymbol{V}$ is the sample covariance matrix.

We reject the null hypothesis H_0 under the consideration if and only if

$$\frac{n_A + n_B - m - 1}{(n_A + n_B - 2)m}T^2 \geq F_{m,n_A+n_B-m-1,(\alpha)}.$$

Compared to t-test in univariate statistics, Hotelling T-squared test has several advantages/properties that should be highlighted: (1) it controls the overall type I error well; (2) it takes into account multiple variables' interrelationships; (3) It can make an overall conclusion when the significances from multiple t-tests are inconsistent.

In real data analysis, Hotelling T-squared test and standard t-test are complementary. Taking two independent-sample comparison as an example, Hotelling T-squared test summarizes between-group difference from all the involved variables; while standard t-test answers specifically which variable(s) are different between two groups. When Hotelling T-squared test rejects H_0, then we can resort to standard t-test to identify where the difference comes from. Therefore, to use them jointly is of particular interest in practice, which helps to interpret the data more systematically and thoroughly.

Independency among observations and MVN are generally assumed for Hotelling T-squared test. Homogeneity of covariance matrix is also assumed for two independent-sample comparison, which can be tested by likelihood ratio test under the assumption of MVN.

4.3. MANOVA[1,5–7]

MANOVA is a procedure using the variance–covariance between variables to test the statistical significance of the mean vectors among multiple groups. It is a generalization of ANOVA allowing multiple dependent variables and tests

H_0: $\boldsymbol{\mu}_1 = \boldsymbol{\mu}_2 = \cdots = \boldsymbol{\mu}_g$;

H_1: at least two mean vectors are unequal;

$$\alpha = 0.05.$$

Wilks' lambda (Λ, capital Greek letter lambda), a likelihood ratio test statistic, can be used to address this question:

$$\Lambda = \frac{|\boldsymbol{W}|}{|\boldsymbol{W} + \boldsymbol{B}|}, \tag{4.3.1}$$

which represents a ratio of the determinants of the within-group and total SSCP matrices.

From the well-known sum of squares partitioning point of view, Wilks' lambda stands for the proportion of variance in the combination of m dependent variables that is unaccounted for by the grouping variable g.

When the m is not too big, Wilks' lambda can be transformed (mathematically adjusted) to a statistic which has approximately an F distribution, as shown in Table 4.3.1.

Outside the tabulated range, the large sample approximation under null hypothesis allows Wilks's lambda to be approximated by a chi-squared distribution

$$-\left(\frac{n - 1 - (m + g)}{2}\right) \ln \Lambda \sim \chi^2_{m(g-1)}. \tag{4.3.2}$$

Table 4.3.1. The exact distributions of Wilks' Λ.

m	g	Λ's exact distribution
$m = 1$	$g \geq 2$	$\left(\frac{n-g}{g-1}\right)\left(\frac{1-\Lambda}{\Lambda}\right) \sim F_{g-1,n-g}$
$m = 2$	$g \geq 2$	$\left(\frac{n-g-1}{g-1}\right)\left(\frac{1-\sqrt{\Lambda}}{\sqrt{\Lambda}}\right) \sim F_{2(g-1),2(n-g-1)}$
$m \geq 1$	$g = 2$	$\left(\frac{n-m-1}{m}\right)\left(\frac{1-\Lambda}{\Lambda}\right) \sim F_{m,n-m-1}$
$m \geq 1$	$g = 3$	$\left(\frac{n-m-2}{m}\right)\left(\frac{1-\sqrt{\Lambda}}{\sqrt{\Lambda}}\right) \sim F_{2m,2(n-m-2)}$

*m, g, and n stand for the number of dependent variables, the number of groups, and sample size, respectively.

Rao C. R found the relation between Wilks' lambda and F

$$\frac{1-\Lambda^{1/s}}{\Lambda^{1/s}}\frac{\nu_2'}{\nu_1'} \sim F_{(\nu_1',\nu_2')}, \tag{4.3.3}$$

where

$$v_1' = m\nu_T, \qquad s = \sqrt{\frac{m^2 v_T^2-4}{m^2+v_T^2-5}}.$$

$$v_2' = \left(v_T + \nu_E - \frac{m+\nu_T+1}{2}\right)\sqrt{\frac{m^2\nu_T^2-4}{m^2+\nu_T^2-5}} - \frac{m\nu_T-2}{2},$$

Here, v_T and v_E denote the degree of freedom for treatment and error.

There are a number of alternative statistics that can be calculated to perform a similar task to that of Wilks' lambda, such as Pillai's trace, Lawley–Hotelling's trace, and Roy's greatest eigenvalue; however, Wilks' lambda is the most-widely used.

When MANOVA rejects the null hypothesis, we conclude that at least two mean vectors are unequal. Then we can use descriptive discriminant analysis (DDA) as a post hoc procedure to conduct multiple comparisons, which can determine why the overall hypothesis was rejected. First, we can calculate Mahalanobis distance between group i and j as

$$D_{ij}^2 = [\bar{\boldsymbol{X}}_i - \bar{\boldsymbol{X}}_j]'\boldsymbol{V}^{-1}[\bar{\boldsymbol{X}}_i - \bar{\boldsymbol{X}}_j], \tag{4.3.4}$$

where $\boldsymbol{V}$ denotes pooled covariance matrix, which equals pooled SSCP divided by $(n-g)$.

Then, we can make inference based on the relation of D_{ij}^2 with F distribution

$$\frac{(n-g-m+1)n_i n_j}{(n-g)m(n_i+n_j)} D_{ij}^2 \sim F_{m,n-m-g+1}.$$

In addition to comparing multiple mean vectors, MANOVA can also be used to rank the relative "importance" of m variables in distinguishing among g groups in the discriminant analysis. We can conduct m MANOVAs, each with $m-1$ variables, by leaving one (the target variable itself) out each time. The variable that is associated with the largest decrement in overall group separation (i.e. increase in Wilk's lambda) when deleted is considered the most important.

MANOVA test, technically similar to ANOVA, should be done only if n observations are independent from each other, m outcome variables approximate an m-variate normal probability distribution, and g covariance matrices are approximately equal. It has been reported that MANOVA test is robust to relatively minor distortions from m-variate normality, provided that the sample sizes are big enough. Box's M-test is preferred for testing the equality of multiple variance–covariance matrices. If the equality of multiple variance–covariance matrices is rejected, James' test can be used to compare multiple mean vectors directly, or the original variables may be transformed to meet the homogenous covariance matrices assumption.

If we also need to control other covariates while comparing multiple mean vectors, then we need to extend MANOVA to multivariate analysis of variance and covariance (MANCOVA).

4.4. Multivariate Linear Regression (MVLR)[8–10]

MVLR, also called multivariate multiple linear regression (MLR), extends one response variable in MLR to multiple response variables with the same set of independent or explanatory variables. It can be expressed as

$$\boldsymbol{Y} = \boldsymbol{X}\boldsymbol{B} + \boldsymbol{E}, \tag{4.4.1}$$

where $\boldsymbol{Y}$ is $n \times q$ response matrix, and $\boldsymbol{X}$ is $n \times (p+1)$ input matrix.

From the theory of the *least squares* (LS) in univariate regression, we can get the estimator of $\boldsymbol{B}$ by minimizing $\boldsymbol{E'E}$, where $\hat{\boldsymbol{E}} = \boldsymbol{Y} - \boldsymbol{X}\hat{B}$ is $n \times q$ error matrix.

We can minimize $\boldsymbol{E'E}$ by giving constraints to non-negative matrix, the trace, the determinant, and the largest eigenvalue, i.e. estimating $\hat{\boldsymbol{B}}$ to meet the following inequalities for all the possible matrices of $\boldsymbol{B}$, respectively:

$$(\boldsymbol{Y} - \boldsymbol{X}\hat{\boldsymbol{B}})'(\boldsymbol{Y} - \boldsymbol{X}\hat{\boldsymbol{B}}) \leq (\boldsymbol{Y} - \boldsymbol{X}\boldsymbol{B})'(\boldsymbol{Y} - \boldsymbol{X}\boldsymbol{B}), \tag{4.4.2}$$

$$\mathrm{trac}(\boldsymbol{Y} - \boldsymbol{X}\hat{\boldsymbol{B}})'(\boldsymbol{Y} - \boldsymbol{X}\hat{\boldsymbol{B}}) \leq \mathrm{trac}(\boldsymbol{Y} - \boldsymbol{X}\boldsymbol{B})'(\boldsymbol{Y} - \boldsymbol{X}\boldsymbol{B}), \tag{4.4.3}$$

$$|(\boldsymbol{Y} - \boldsymbol{X}\hat{\boldsymbol{B}})'(\boldsymbol{Y} - \boldsymbol{X}\hat{\boldsymbol{B}})| \leq |(\boldsymbol{Y} - \boldsymbol{X}\boldsymbol{B})'(\boldsymbol{Y} - \boldsymbol{X}\boldsymbol{B})|, \tag{4.4.4}$$

$$\max \mathrm{eig}\{(\boldsymbol{Y} - \boldsymbol{X}\hat{\boldsymbol{B}})'(\boldsymbol{Y} - \boldsymbol{X}\hat{\boldsymbol{B}})\} \tag{4.4.5}$$
$$\leq \max \mathrm{eig}\{(\boldsymbol{Y} - \boldsymbol{X}\boldsymbol{B})'(\boldsymbol{Y} - \boldsymbol{X}\boldsymbol{B})\}.$$

In fact, the above four criteria are equivalent to each other.[10] Under any criterion of the four, we can get the same LS estimator of $\boldsymbol{B}$, given by

$$\hat{\boldsymbol{B}} = (\boldsymbol{X'X})^{-1}\boldsymbol{X'Y}, \tag{4.4.6}$$

which is best linear unbiased estimation (BLUE).

We can also use penalization technique to get shrinkage estimates of $\boldsymbol{B}$ by assigning different penalty functions to minimize the sum of square errors

$$\boldsymbol{E}'\boldsymbol{E} = \text{trac}(\boldsymbol{Y} - \boldsymbol{XB})'(\boldsymbol{Y} - \boldsymbol{XB}) = (\boldsymbol{Y} - \boldsymbol{XB})'(\boldsymbol{Y} - \boldsymbol{XB}).$$

If the optimization is subject to $\sum_i \sum_j |\beta_{ij}| \leq t$, which can be written more compactly as the "*L_1-norm constraint*" $\|\beta\|_1 \leq t$, then we get a similar estimator to the Lasso estimator (see Sec. 3.17). If the optimization is subject to $|\boldsymbol{B}'\boldsymbol{B}| \leq t$, then we get the "*determinant constraint*" estimator, which benefits for digging the interrelationship between parameters by making use of the nice property of the determinant of the matrix. If the optimization is subject to $\text{trac}\{\boldsymbol{B}'\boldsymbol{B}\} \leq t$, then we get the "*trace constraint*" estimator, which not only has the same advantages as the "determinant constraint" estimator, but also it simplifies the computation. If the optimization is subject to $\max \text{eig}\{\boldsymbol{B}'\boldsymbol{B}\} \leq t$, it is called "*maximum eigenvalue constraint*" estimator, which mainly considers the role of maximum eigenvalue as in principal component analysis (PCA). Here, the bound t is kind of "budget": it gives a certain limit to the parameter estimates.

The individual coefficients and standard errors produced by MVLR are identical to those that would be produced by regressing each response variable against the set of independent variables separately. The difference lies in that the MVLR, as a joint estimator, also estimates the between-equation covariance, so we can test the interrelationship between coefficients across equations.

As to variable selection strategy, we have procedures such as forward section, backward elimination, stepwise forward, and stepwise backward as in univariate regression analysis. We can also use statistics such as *Cp*, and the AIC (Akaike, H., 1973),[8] to evaluate the goodness-of-fit of the model.

In addition, multivariate regression is related to Zellner's seemingly unrelated regression (SUR); however, SUR does not require each response variable to have the same set of independent variables.

4.5. Structural Equation Model (SEM)[11–13]

SEM is a multivariate statistical technique designed to model the intrinsic structure of a certain phenomenon, which can be expressed by a covariance matrix of original variables or sometimes a mean vector as well with a relatively few parameters. Subsequently, SEM will estimate the parameters, and test the related hypotheses. From a statistical point of view, SEM is a unifying technique using both confirmatory factor analysis (CFA) (see Sec. 4.10) and path analysis (PA).

4.5.1. *Model structure*

Basically, SEM mainly includes two models as follows:

(1) Measurement model characterizes the interrelationship between the latent variables and the observed variables

$$\begin{aligned} \boldsymbol{Y} &= \boldsymbol{\Lambda_Y}\boldsymbol{\eta} + \boldsymbol{\varepsilon} \\ \boldsymbol{X} &= \boldsymbol{\Lambda_X}\boldsymbol{\xi} + \boldsymbol{\delta}' \end{aligned} \tag{4.5.1}$$

where $\boldsymbol{Y}$ and $\boldsymbol{\eta}$ are endogenous vectors for observed variables (measurable) and latent variables, respectively. $\boldsymbol{X}$ and $\boldsymbol{\xi}$ denote exogenous vectors for observed variables (measurable) and latent variables, respectively. $\boldsymbol{\Lambda_Y}$ and $\boldsymbol{\Lambda_X}$ are respective matrices for regression coefficients; $\boldsymbol{\varepsilon}$ and $\boldsymbol{\delta}$ are the related error vectors.

From Eq. (4.5.1), it can be seen that measurement model is a CFA model because all the observed variables are indictors of the related latent variables. It also can be considered as a description of the reliability of the measurements of vector $\boldsymbol{Y}$ and vector $\boldsymbol{X}$.

(2) Structural model is a PA model that describes the relation among latent vectors including both endogenous and exogenous

$$\boldsymbol{\eta} = \boldsymbol{B}\boldsymbol{\eta} + \boldsymbol{I}\boldsymbol{\xi} + \boldsymbol{\zeta}, \tag{4.5.2}$$

where $\boldsymbol{\eta}$ is an endogenous latent vector, $\boldsymbol{\xi}$ is an exogenous latent vector, $\boldsymbol{B}$ is effect matrix among endogenous latent variables, $\boldsymbol{I}$ is effect matrix of exogenous variables on endogenous variables, and $\boldsymbol{\zeta}$ is the vector for error.

SEM assumes: (1) The expectations of all the error vectors in two models are zero vectors; (2) In the measurement model, error vector is independent of latent vector, and two error vectors are independent from each other; (3) In the structural model, error vector is also independent of latent vector; (4) Error vectors in two models are independent from each other.

4.5.2. *Model estimation*

Based on the constructed models (equations) between the observed variables in the real dataset and the hypothesized factors, we can estimate all the parameters including coefficient matrix and error matrix. Currently, there are several major estimation methods in SEM, including maximum likelihood (ML), LS, weighted least squares (WLS), generalized least squares (GLS), and Bayes.

4.5.3. *Model evaluation*

If the SEM model is correct, there should be no difference between covariance matrix re-generated from the model and the matrix from the original dataset, i.e.

$$\sum = \sum(\boldsymbol{\theta}), \tag{4.5.3}$$

where Σ is the population covariance matrix of the observed variables, which can be estimated by sample covariance matrix $\boldsymbol{S}$; $\boldsymbol{\theta}$ is parameter vector from the model, and $\sum(\theta)$ is the population covariance matrix described by model parameters.

A full model evaluation should include the evaluation of measurement model, structural model and the full model as a whole. The evaluation indexes mainly include two groups: (1) fitness index, e.g. chi-squared statistic, and goodness-of-fit index (GFI); (2) error index, e.g. root mean square error of approximation (RMSEA).

The main advantages of SEM lie in: (1) It can effectively explore latent variables, which discloses the essential factors or dominators behind a phenomenon, and meanwhile solves the collinearity concern between the observed variables; (2) It isolates the measurement error ("noise") from latent variables ("signal"), which is likely to give stronger results if the latent variables are subsequently used as an independent or dependent variable in a structural model; (3) It can estimate measurement error and its variance; (4) It can not only explore the relation between latent variables, but also explore the potential link between latent variables and observed variables.

In practice, we may meet some problems during the model fitting. Examples are: (1) Covariance matrix is not positive definite; (2) The model cannot converge; (3) Get unreasonable estimation of variance; or even (4) The lack of fit of the whole model. Then we need to reconsider the model structure and the plausibility of the parameter setting, and modify the model accordingly to get a final model with good explanations.

4.6. Logistic Regression[1,14,15]

In linear model (LM), the dependent variable or outcome (denoted as Y) is continuous, and the conditional value of Y given a fixed x should be normally distributed. When Y is a binary response coded as 0 or 1, we can model the log-likelihood ratio (i.e. the log odds of the positive response) as the linear combination of a set of independent variables ($x_1, x_2, \ldots, x_m$), i.e.

$$\log \frac{\pi}{1-\pi} = \beta_0 + \beta_1 x_1 + \beta_2 x_2 + \cdots + \beta_m x_m, \tag{4.6.1}$$

where π denotes probability of $Y = 1$ conditionally on a certain combination of the predictors. β_0 is the intercept term, and $\beta_1, \beta_2, \ldots, \beta_m$ are the regression coefficients. The model is called ordinary (binary-outcome) logistic regression model, and is part of a broader class of models called generalized linear models (GLMs) (see Sec. 3.2). The word "logit" was coined by Berkson.[14]

4.6.1. *Parameter estimation*

The estimation of a logistic regression is achieved through the principle of ML, which can be considered as a generalization of the LS principle of ordinary linear regression. Occasionally, ML estimation may not converge or may yield unrealistic estimates, then one can resort to exact logistic regression.

4.6.2. *Coefficient interpretation*

The regression coefficient β_i in the logistic regression model stands for the average change in logit P with 1 unit change in the explanatory variable x_i regardless of the values of the covariate combination. Due to the particular role of logit P in risk assessment of disease state, the interpretation of β_i can be immediately linked to the familiar epidemiologic measure odds ratio (OR) and adjusted OR, which depends on the form of the independent variable x_i (also called the exposure in epidemiological area): (1) If x_i is dichotomous with 1 and 0 denoting the exposure and the non-exposure group, respectively, then β_i is the change in log odds comparing the exposed to the unexposed group, the exponentiated $\beta_i (= e^{\beta_i})$ is the OR, namely, the ratio of two odds of the disease; (2) If x_i is ordinal $(0, 1, 2, \ldots)$ or continuous, then β_i is the average change in log odds associated with every 1 unit increment in exposure level; (3) If x_i is polychotomous $(0, 1, 2, \ldots, k)$, then x_i must enter the model with $k - 1$ dummy variables, and β_i is the change in log odds comparing on specific level to the reference level of the exposure.

4.6.3. *Hypothesis test*

In risk assessment of disease, it is meaningful to test whether there is association between exposure and risk of disease, which is testing OR $= 1$ or beta $= 0$. Three well-known tests including the likelihood test, the Wald test and the Score test are commonly used. The likelihood test is a test based on the difference in deviances: the deviance without the exposure in the model minus the deviance with the exposure in the model. The Wald statistic is constructed from the ratio of the estimated beta coefficient over its standard error. In general, the likelihood test is believed to be more powerful than the Wald test, whereas the Score test is a normal approximation to the likelihood test.

4.6.4. *Logistic regression family*

In matched pairs studies (e.g. in a matched case-control study), matching is used as a special technique intended to control the potential confounders from the very beginning of the study, i.e. the design stage. Under matching, the likelihood of the data depends on the "conditional probability" — the probability of the observed pattern of positive and negative responses within strata conditional on the number of positive outcome being observed. Therefore, logistic regression under this situation is also called "conditional logistic regression", which differs from ordinary logistic regression (also known as "unconditional logistic regression") under unmatched design or modeling the strata as dummy variables in an ordinary logistic regression.

If Y is multinomial, to construct multiple ordinary logistic regression models will definitely increase the overall type I error. Thus, multinomial logistic regression, a simple extension of binary logistic regression, is the solution to evaluate the probability of categorical membership by using ML estimation. Ordinal logistic regression is used when Y is ordinal, which mainly includes cumulative odds logit model and adjacent odds logit model.

4.6.5. *Some notes*

(1) Logistic regression is mainly used to explore risk factors of a disease, to predict the probability of a disease, and to predict group membership in logistic discriminant analysis. (2) It assumes independence and linearity (i.e. logit P is linearly associated with independent variables) (3) In cumulative odds model, if we consider the odds, $\text{odds}(k) = P(Y \leq k)/P(Y > k)$, then $\text{odds}(k_1)$ and $\text{odds}(k_2)$ have the same ratio for all independent variable combinations, which means that the OR is independent of the cutoff point. This proportional-odds assumption could be evaluated by modeling multiple binary logistic regression models. (4) In adjacent odds model, we have the same OR comparing any adjacent two categories of outcome for all independent variable combinations. (5) For cohort studies, unconditional logistic regression is typically used only when every patient is followed for the same length of time. When the follow-up time is unequal for each patient, using logistic regression is improper, and models such as Poisson regression (see Sec. 4.7) and Cox model that can accommodate follow-up time are preferred.

4.7. Poisson Regression[1,16]

In regression analysis, if the dependent variable or outcome (denoted as Y) is a non-negative count of events or occurrences that could occur at any time during a fixed unit of time (or anywhere within a spatial region), then Y can be modeled as a Poisson-distributed variable with probability mass function

$$P(y) = \frac{\exp(-\lambda)\lambda^y}{y!}, \quad y = 0, 1, 2, \ldots; \quad \lambda > 0, \tag{4.7.1}$$

where λ is the only parameter, i.e. the *intensity*. If λ is influenced by $x_1, x_2, \ldots, x_m$, then we can link λ to a set of independent variables by a log function, i.e.

$$\log(\lambda) = \beta_0 + \beta_1 x_1 + \beta_2 x_2 + \cdots + \beta_m x_m, \tag{4.7.2}$$

which is called Poisson regression model. Since the additivity holds on the log scale of measurement, it is called multiplicative Poisson model on the original scale of measurement.

If the additivity holds on the original scale, i.e.

$$\lambda = \beta_0 + \beta_1 x_1 + \beta_2 x_2 + \cdots + \beta_m x_m, \tag{4.7.3}$$

then it is called additive Poisson model.

In the multiplicative Poisson model, the log transformation guarantees that the predictions for average counts of the event will never be negative. In contrast, there is no such property in the additive model, especially when the event rate is small. This problem limits its wide use in practice.

Obviously, the regression coefficient β_i in Poisson regression model stands for the average change in λ (additive model) or $\log(\lambda)$ (multiplicative model) with 1 unit change in the explanatory variable x_i regardless of the values of the covariate combination.

As to modeling incidence rate, if the observation unit is n_i and the event number is y_i, then the corresponding multiplicative model is

$$\log\left(\frac{y_i}{n_i}\right) = \beta_0 + \sum_{i=1}^{m} \beta_i x_i. \tag{4.7.4}$$

In other words,

$$\log(y_i) = \beta_0 + \sum_{i=1}^{m} \beta_i x_i + \log(n_i), \tag{4.7.5}$$

where $\log(n_i)$ is called the offset.

Similar to the case of Logistic regression, the ML estimation is the most common choice for Poisson model. Since there are no closed-form solutions, the estimators can be obtained by using iterative algorithms such as Newton–Raphson, iteratively re-weighted LS, etc. The standard trinity of likelihood-based tests including likelihood ratio, Wald, and Lagrange multiplier (LM) are commonly used for basic inference about coefficients in the model.

Goodness-of-fit of the model can be evaluated by using Pearson chi-squared statistic or the deviance (D). If a model fits, its Pearson χ^2 or D will be lower than the degrees of freedom $(n - p)$. The closer the ratio of the statistics to its degree of freedom approaches 1, the better the model is. If the ratio is far from 1, then it indicates a huge variation of data, which means a poor goodness-of-fit. A residual analysis is often used for further exploration.

Poisson regression is constructed to modeling the average number of events per interval against a set of potential influential factors based on Poisson distribution. Therefore, it can only be used for Poisson-distributed data, such as the number of bacterial colonies in a Petri dish, the number of drug or alcohol abuse in a time interval, the number of certain events in unit space, and the incidence of rare diseases in specific populations.

Of note, Poisson distribution theoretically assumes that its conditional variance equals its conditional mean. However, practical issues in the "real" data have compelled researchers to extend Poisson regression in several directions. One example is the "overdispersion" case, which means the variance is greater than the mean. In this situation, naïve use of Poisson model will result in an underestimated variance and will therefore inflate the overall type I error in hypothesis testing. Models such as negative binomial regression (NBR) (see Sec. 4.8) are designed to model the overdispersion in the data. Another important example is the "excess zeros" case, which could be modeled by zero-inflated Poisson (ZIP) regression. Moreover, if the data has features of both over-dispersed and zero-inflated, then zero-inflated negative binomial regression (ZINB) is a potential solution.

4.8. NBR[17–19]

The equidispersion assumption in the Poisson regression model is a quite serious limitation because overdispersion is often found in the real data of event count. The overdispersion is probably caused by non-independence among the individuals in most situations. In medical research, a lot of events occur non-independently such as infectious disease, genetic disease, seasonally-variated disease or endemic disease. NBR has become the standard method for accommodating overdispersion in count data since its implementation into commercial software.

In fact, negative binomial distribution is an extension to Poisson distribution in that the intensity parameter λ is a gamma-distributed random variable; therefore it is also called Gamma–Poisson mixture distribution, which can be written as

$$P(y) = \int_0^{\infty} \frac{\exp(-\lambda)\lambda^y}{y!} \frac{\beta^\alpha \lambda^{\alpha-1} e^{-\beta\lambda}}{\Gamma(\alpha)} \quad (y = 0, 1, \ldots; \lambda > 0), \qquad (4.8.1)$$

where α is the shape parameter (constant), and λ is the intensity parameter; λ is not fixed as that in Poisson distribution, but a random variable related to independent variables.

Both NBR and Poisson regression can handle event count data by modeling the intensity of an event (λ)

$$\log(\hat{\lambda}) = \beta_0 + \beta_1 x_1 + \beta_2 x_2 + \cdots + \beta_m x_m. \qquad (4.8.2)$$

One important feature of the NBR model is that the conditional mean function is the same as that in the Poisson model. The difference lies in that the variance in NBR model equals $\hat{\lambda}(1 + \kappa\hat{\lambda})$, which is greater than that in the Poisson model by including an additional parameter κ. Here, "$1 + \kappa\hat{\lambda}$" is called variance inflation factor or overdispersion parameter. When $\kappa = 0$, NBR is Poisson model. $\kappa \neq 0$ indicates the event is not random, and clustered; in other words, some important factors may have been neglected in the research. To test whether κ equals 0 is one way of testing the assumption of equidispersion.

The parameter estimation, hypothesis testing and model evaluation can be referred to Sec. 4.7.

NBR model overcomes the severe limitation of Poisson model — the equidispersion assumption, and therefore is more widely used, especially when the intensity of an event is not fixed in a specific population (e.g. the incidence of a rare disease). However, it is of note that NBR model, similar to Poisson model, allows the prediction of event to be infinity, which means that the unit time or unit space should be infinite. Thus, it is improper to use either NBR or Poisson model to explore the influential factors of the intensity of an event when the possible event numbers are limited, or even small, in a fixed unit of time or spatial region. Likewise, when NBR is used to explore the potential risk and/or protective factors of the incidence of a disease within one unit population, the numbers of the individuals in this population should be theoretically infinite and the incidence rate should be differential.

If we extend the shape parameter α in NBR model from a constant to a random variable related to independent variables, then NBR model is extended to generalized NBR model.

Though NBR model might be the most important extension of Poisson model by accommodating the overdispersion in the count data, other issues are still commonly encountered in "real" data practice. Zero-inflation and truncation are considered as two major ones. ZINB is an ideal solution to zero-inflated over-dispersion count data. Truncated negative binomial regression (TNB) and negative Logit-Hurdle model (NBLH) are commonly used to handle truncated overdispersed count data.

4.9. PCA[1,20–23]

PCA is commonly considered as a multivariate data reduction technique by transforming p correlated variables into $m(m \le p)$ uncorrelated linear combinations of the variables that contain most of the variance. It originated with the work of Pearson K. (1901)[23] and then developed by Hotelling H. (1933)[21] and others.

4.9.1. *Definition*

Suppose, the original p variables are $X_1, X_2, \ldots, X_p$, and the corresponding standardized variables are $Z_1, Z_2, \ldots, Z_p$, then the first principal component C_1 is a unit-length linear combination of $Z_1, Z_2, \ldots, Z_p$ with the largest variance. The second principal component C_2 has maximal variance among all unit-length linear combinations that are uncorrelated to C_1. And C_3 has maximal variance among all unit-length linear combinations that are uncorrelated to C_1 and C_2, etc. The last principal component has the smallest variance among all unit-length linear combinations that are uncorrelated to all the earlier components.

It can be proved that: (1) The coefficient vector for each principal component is the unit eigenvector of the correlation matrix; (2) The variance of C_i is the corresponding eigenvalue λ_i; (3) The sum of all the eigenvalues equals p, i.e. $\sum_{i=1}^{p} \lambda_i = p$.

4.9.2. *Solution*

Steps for extracting principal components:

(1) Calculate the correlation matrix $\boldsymbol{R}$ of the standardized data $\boldsymbol{Z}$.
(2) Compute the eigenvalues $\lambda_1, \lambda_2, \ldots, \lambda_p, (\lambda_1 \ge \lambda_2 \ge \cdots \ge \lambda_p \ge 0)$ and the corresponding eigenvectors $\boldsymbol{a}_1, \boldsymbol{a}_2, \ldots, \boldsymbol{a}_p$, each of them having

length 1, that is $a_i^{'}a_i = 1$ for $i = 1, 2, \ldots, p$. Then, $y_1 = a_1^{'}Z, y_2 = a_2^{'}Z, \ldots, y_p = a_p^{'}Z$ are the first, second, $\ldots$, pth principal components of Z. Furthermore, we can calculate the contribution of each eigenvalue to the total variance as $\lambda_i / \sum_{i=1}^{p} \lambda_i = \lambda_i / p$, and the cumulative contribution of the first m components as $\sum_{i=1}^{m} \lambda_i / p$.

(3) Determine m, the maximum number of meaningful components to retain. The first few components are assumed to explain as much as possible of the variation present in the original dataset. Several methods are commonly used to determine m: (a) to keep the first m components that account for a particular percentage (e.g. 60%, or 75%, or even 80%) of the total variation in the original variables; (b) to choose m to be equal to the number of eigenvalues over their mean (i.e. 1 if based on $\boldsymbol{R}$); (c) to determine m via hypothesis test (e.g. Bartlett chi-squared test). Other methods include Cattell scree test, which uses the visual exploration of the scree plot of eigenvalues to find an obvious cut-off between large and small eigenvalues, and derivative eigenvalue method.

4.9.3. *Interpretation*

As a linear transformation of the original data, the complete set of all principal components contains the same information as the original variables. However, PCs contain more meaningful or "active" contents than the original variables do. Thus, it is of particular importance of interpreting the meaningfulness of PCs, which is a crucial step in comprehensive evaluation. In general, there are several experience-based rules in interpreting PCs: (1) First, the coefficients in a PC stand for the information extracted from each variable by the PC. The variables with coefficients of larger magnitude in a PC have larger contribution to that component. If the coefficients in a PC are similar to each other in the magnitude, then this PC can be considered as a comprehensive index of all the variables. (2) Second, the sign of one coefficient in a PC denotes the direction of the effect of the variable on the PC. (3) Third, if the coefficients in a PC are well stratified by one factor, e.g. the coefficients are all positive when the factor takes one value, and are all negative when it takes the other value, then this PC is strongly influenced by this specific factor.

4.9.4. *Application*

PCA is useful in several ways: (1) Reduction in the dimensionality of the input data set by extracting the first m components that keep most variation;

(2) Re-ordering or ranking of the original sample (or individual) by using the first PC or a weighted score of the first m PCs; (3) Identification and elimination of multicollinearity in the data. It is often used for reducing the dimensionality of the highly correlated independent variables in regression models, which is known as principal component regression (see Sec. 3.7).

Principal curve analysis and principal surface analysis are two of the extensions of PCA. Principal curves are smooth one-dimensional curves that pass through the middle of high-dimensional data. Similarly, principal surfaces are two-dimensional surfaces that pass through the middle of the data. More details can be found in Hastie.[20]

4.10. Factor Analysis (FA)[24–27]

FA, in the sense of exploratory factor analysis (EFA), is a statistical technique for data reduction based on PCA. It aims to extract m latent, unmeasurable, independent and determinative factors from p original variables. These m factors are abstract extractions of the commonality of p original variables. FA originated with the work of Charles Spearman, an English psychologist, in 1904, and has since witnessed an explosive growth, especially in the social science. EFA can be conducted in two ways: when factors are commonly calculated based on the correlation matrix between the variables, then it is called R-type FA; when factors are calculated from the correlation matrix between samples, then it is called Q-type FA.

4.10.1. *Definition*

First, denote a vector of p observed variables by $\boldsymbol{x} = (\boldsymbol{x}_1, \boldsymbol{x}_2, \ldots, \boldsymbol{x}_p)'$, and m unobservable factors as $(f_1, f_2, \ldots, f_m)$. Then x_i can be represented as a linear function of these m latent factors:

$$x_i = \mu_i + l_{i1}f_1 + l_{i2}f_2 + \cdots + l_{im}f_m + e_i, \quad i = 1, 2, \ldots, p, \qquad (4.10.1)$$

where $\mu_i = E(x_i)$; $f_1, f_2, \ldots, f_m$ are called common factors; $l_{i1}, l_{i2}, \ldots, l_{im}$ are called factor loadings; and e_i is the residual term or alternatively uniqueness term or specific factor.

4.10.2. *Steps of extracting factors*

The key step in FA is to calculate the factor loadings (pattern matrix). There are several methods that can be used to analyze correlation matrix such as principal component method, ML method, principal-factor method, and method of iterated principal-factor. Taking principal component method as an example, the steps for extracting factors are:

(1) Calculate the correlation matrix $\boldsymbol{R}$ of the standardized data.
(2) Compute the eigenvalues $\lambda_1, \lambda_2, \ldots, \lambda_p$ and the corresponding eigenvectors $a_1, a_2, \ldots, a_p$, calculate the contribution of each eigenvalue to the total variance and the cumulative contribution of the first m components.
(3) Determine m, the maximum number of common factors. The details of the first three steps can be referred to those in PCA.
(4) Estimate the initial factor loading matrix L.
(5) Rotate factors. When initial factors extracted are not evidently meaningful, they could be rotated. Rotations come in two forms — orthogonal and oblique. The most common orthogonal method is called varimax rotation.

4.10.3. *Interpretation*

Once the factors and their loadings have been estimated, they are interpreted albeit in a subjective process. Interpretation typically means examining the l_{ij}'s and assigning names to each factor. The basic rules are the same as in interpreting principal components in PCA (see Sec. 4.9).

4.10.4. *Factor scores*

Once the common factors have been identified, to estimate their values for each of the individuals is of particular interest to subsequent analyses. The estimated values are called *factor scores* for a particular observation on these unobservable dimensions. Factor scores are estimates of abstract, random, latent variables, which is quite different from traditional parametric estimation. Theoretically, factor scores cannot be exactly predicted by linear combination of the original variables because the factor loading matrix $\boldsymbol{L}$ is not invertible. There are two commonly-used methods for obtaining factor score estimates. One is WLS method (Bartllett, M. S., 1937),[24] and the other one is regression method (Thomson, G. H., 1951)[27]; neither of them can be viewed as uniformly better than the other.

4.10.5. *Some notes*

(1) Similar to PCA, FA is also a decomposition of covariance structure of the data; therefore, homogeneity of the population is a basic assumption. (2) The ML method assumes normality for the variable, while other methods

do not. (3) Since the original variables are expressed as linear combination of factors, the original variables should contain information of latent factors, the effect of factors on variables should be additive, and there should be no interaction between factors. (4) The main functions of FA are to identify basic covariance structure in the data, to solve collinearity issue among variables and reduce dimensionality, and to explore and develop questionnaires. (5) The researchers' rational thinking process is part and parcel of interpreting factors reasonably and meaningfully. (6) EFA explores the possible underlying factor structure (the existence and quantity) of a set of observed variables without imposing a preconceived structure on the outcome. In contrast, CFA aims to verify the factor structure of a set of observed variables, and allows researchers to test the association between observed variables and their underlying latent factors, which is postulated based on knowledge of the theory, empirical research (e.g. a previous EFA) or both.

4.11. Canonical Correlation Analysis (CCA)[28–30]

CCA is basically a descriptive statistical technique to identify and measure the association between two sets of random variables. It borrows the idea from PCA by finding linear combinations of the original two sets of variables so that the correlation between the linear combinations is maximized. It originated with the work of Hotelling H.,[29] and has been extensively used in a wide variety of disciplines such as psychology, sociology and medicine.

4.11.1. *Definition*

Given two correlated sets of variables,

$$\begin{aligned} \boldsymbol{X} &= (X_1, X_2, \ldots, X_p) \\ \boldsymbol{Y} &= (Y_1, Y_2, \ldots, Y_q) \end{aligned}, \tag{4.11.1}$$

and considering the linear combinations U_i and V_i,

$$\begin{aligned} U_i &= a_{i1}X_1 + a_{i2}X_2 + \cdots + a_{ip}X_p \equiv a'x \\ V_i &= b_{i1}Y_1 + b_{i2}Y_2 + \cdots + b_{iq}Y_q \equiv b'y \end{aligned}, \tag{4.11.2}$$

one aims to identify vectors $a_1'x$ and $b_2'y$ so that:

$$\rho(a_1'x, b_1'y) = \max \rho(a'x, b'y),$$

$$\mathrm{var}(a_1'x) = \mathrm{var}(b_2'y) = 1.$$

The idea is in vein with the PCA.

Then $a_1'x, b_2'y$ is called the first pair of canonical variables, and their correlation is called the first canonical correlation coefficient. Similarly, we can get the second, third, ..., and m pair of canonical variables to make them uncorrelated with each other, and then get the corresponding canonical correlation coefficients. The number of canonical variable pairs is equal to the smaller one of p and q, i.e. $\min(p, q)$.

4.11.2. *Solution*

(1) Calculate the total correlation matrix $\boldsymbol{R}$:

$$\boldsymbol{R} = \begin{pmatrix} \boldsymbol{R}_{XX} & \boldsymbol{R}_{XY} \\ \boldsymbol{R}_{YX} & \boldsymbol{R}_{YY} \end{pmatrix}, \tag{4.11.3}$$

where $\boldsymbol{R}_{XX}$ and $\boldsymbol{R}_{YY}$ are within-sets correlation matrices of X and Y, respectively, and $\boldsymbol{R}_{XY} = \boldsymbol{R}'_{YX}$ is the between-sets correlation matrix.

(2) Compute matrix $\boldsymbol{A}$ and $\boldsymbol{B}$:

$$\begin{aligned} \boldsymbol{A} &= (\boldsymbol{R}_{XX})^{-1}\boldsymbol{R}_{XY}(\boldsymbol{R}_{YY})^{-1}\boldsymbol{R}_{YX} \\ \boldsymbol{B} &= (\boldsymbol{R}_{YY})^{-1}\boldsymbol{R}_{YX}(\boldsymbol{R}_{XX})^{-1}\boldsymbol{R}_{XY} \end{aligned}. \tag{4.11.4}$$

(3) Calculate the eigenvalues of the matrix $\boldsymbol{A}$ and $\boldsymbol{B}$:

$$|\boldsymbol{A} - \lambda \boldsymbol{I}| = |\boldsymbol{B} - \lambda I| = 0. \tag{4.11.5}$$

Computationally, matrix $\boldsymbol{A}$ and $\boldsymbol{B}$ have same eigenvalues. The sample canonical correlations are the positive square roots of the non-zero eigenvalues among them:

$$r_{ci} = \sqrt{\lambda_i}. \tag{4.11.6}$$

Canonical correlation is best suited for describing the association between two sets of random variables. The first canonical correlation coefficient is greater than any simple correlation coefficient between any pair of variables selected from these two sets of variables in magnitude. Thus, the first canonical correlation coefficient is often of the most interest.

(4) Estimate the eigenvectors of the matrix $\boldsymbol{A}$ and $\boldsymbol{B}$:
The vectors corresponding to each pair of canonical variables and each eigenvalue can be obtained as the solution of

$$\begin{aligned} (\boldsymbol{R}_{XX})^{-1}\boldsymbol{R}_{XY}(\boldsymbol{R}_{YY})^{-1}\boldsymbol{R}_{YX}a_i &= r_i^2 a_i \\ (\boldsymbol{R}_{YY})^{-1}\boldsymbol{R}_{YX}(\boldsymbol{R}_{XX})^{-1}\boldsymbol{R}_{XY}b_i &= r_i^2 b_i \end{aligned}, \tag{4.11.7}$$

with the constraint $\mathrm{var}(a'x) = \mathrm{var}(b'y) = 1$.

4.11.3. *Hypothesis test*

Assume that both sets of variables have MVN distribution and sample size n is greater than the sum of variable numbers $(p+q)$. Consider the hypothesis testing problem

$$H_0\colon \rho_{s+1} = \ldots = \rho_p = 0, \tag{4.11.8}$$

which means that only the first s canonical correlation coefficients are non-zero. This hypothesis can be tested by using methods (e.g. chi-squared approximation, F approximation) based on Wilk's Λ (a likelihood ratio statistic)

$$\Lambda = \sum_{i=1}^{m} (1 - r_i^2), \tag{4.11.9}$$

which has Wilk's Λ distribution (see Sec. 4.3).

Other statistics such as Pillai's trace, Lawley–Hotelling's trace, and Roy's greatest root can be also used for testing the above H_0.

Of note, conceptually, while "*canonical correlation*" is used to describe the linear association between two sets of random variables, the correlation between one variable and another set of random variable can be characterized by "*multiple correlation*". Similarly, the simple correlation between two random variables with controlling for other covariates can be expressed by "*partial correlation*".

Canonical correlation can be considered as a very general multivariate statistical framework that unifies many of methods including multiple linear regression, discriminate analysis, and MANOVA. However, the roles of canonical correlations in hypothesis testing should not be overstated, especially when the original variables are qualitative. Under such situations, their p values should be interpreted with caution before drawing any formal statistical conclusions. It should also be mentioned that the canonical correlation analysis of two-way categorical data is essentially equivalent to correspondence analysis (CA), a topic discussed in 4.12.

4.12. CA[31–33]

CA is a statistical multivariate technique based on FA, and is used for exploratory analysis of contingency table or data with contingency-like structure. It originated from 1930s to 1940s, with its concept formally put forward by J. P. Benzécri, a great French mathematician, in 1973. It basically seeks to offer a low-dimensional representation for describing how the row and column variables contribute to the inertia (i.e. Pearson's phi-squared, a measure of dependence between row and column variables) in a contingency table. It can be used on both qualitative and quantitative data.

4.12.1. *Solution*

(1) Calculate normalized probability matrix: suppose we have n samples with m variables with data matrix $\boldsymbol{X}_{n\times m}$. Without loss of generality, assume $x_{ij} \geq 0$ (otherwise a constant number can be added to each entry), and define the correspondence table as the *correspondence matrix* $\boldsymbol{P}$:

$$\boldsymbol{P}_{n\times m} = \frac{1}{x_{..}}\boldsymbol{X}\hat{=}(p_{ij})_{n\times m}, \tag{4.12.1}$$

where $x_{..} = \sum_{i=1}^{n}\sum_{j=1}^{m} x_{ij}$, such that the overall sum meets $\sum_{i=1}^{n}\sum_{j=1}^{m} p_{ij} = 1$ with $0 < p_{ij} < 1$.

(2) Implement correspondence transformation: based on the matrix P, calculate the standardized residual matrix $\boldsymbol{Z} \hat{=} (z_{ij})_{n\times m}$ with elements:

$$z_{ij} = \frac{p_{ij} - p_{i.}p_{.j}}{\sqrt{p_{i.}p_{.j}}} = \frac{x_{ij} - x_{i.}x_{.j}/x_{..}}{\sqrt{x_{i.}x_{.j}}}. \tag{4.12.2}$$

Here, z_{ij} is a kind of the decomposition of chi-squared statistic. $\sum z_{ij}^2$ is Pearson's phi-squared, also known as the "inertia", and equals Pearson's chi-squared statistic divided by sample size n.

(3) Conduct a type-R FA: Calculate r non-zero eigenvalues ($\lambda_1 \geq \lambda_2 \geq \cdots \geq \lambda_r$) of the matrix $\boldsymbol{R} = \boldsymbol{Z}'\boldsymbol{Z}$ and the corresponding eigenvectors $u_1, u_2, \ldots, u_r$; normalize them, and determine k, the maximum number of common factors (usually $k = 2$, which is selected on similar criteria as in PCA, e.g. depending on the cumulative percentage of contribution of the first k dimension to inertia of a table); and then get the factor loading matrix $\boldsymbol{F}$. For example, when $k = 2$, the loading matrix is:

$$F = \begin{pmatrix} u_{11}\sqrt{\lambda_1} & u_{11}\sqrt{\lambda_2} \\ u_{21}\sqrt{\lambda_1} & u_{22}\sqrt{\lambda_2} \\ \vdots & \vdots \\ u_{m1}\sqrt{\lambda_1} & u_{m2}\sqrt{\lambda_2} \end{pmatrix}. \tag{4.12.3}$$

(4) Conduct a type-Q FA: similarly, we can get the factor loading matrix $\boldsymbol{G}$ from the matrix $Q = \boldsymbol{Z}\boldsymbol{Z}'$.

(5) Make a correspondence biplot: First, make a single scatter plot of variables ("column categories") using F_1 and F_2 in type-R FA; then make a similar plot of sample points ("row categories") using G_1 and G_2 extracted in type-Q FA; finally overlap the plane $F_1 - F_2$ and the plane $G_1 - G_2$. Subsequently, we will get the presentation of relation within variables, the relation within samples, and the relation between variables and samples all together in one two-dimensional plot.
However, when the cumulative percentage of the total inertia accounted by the first two or even three leading dimensions is low, then making a plot in a high-dimensional space becomes very difficult.
(6) Explain biplot: here are some rules of thumb when explaining biplot: Firstly, clustered variable points often indicate relatively high correlation of the variable; Secondly, clustered sample points suggest that these samples may potentially come from one cluster; Thirdly, if a set of variables is close to a group of samples, then it often indicates that the features of these samples are primarily characterized by these variables.

4.12.2. *Application*

CA can be used: (1) To analyze contingency table by describing the basic features of the rows and columns, disclosing the nature of the association between the rows and the columns, and offering the best intuitive graphical display of this association; (2) To explore whether a disease is clustered in some regions or a certain population, such as studying the endemic of cancers.

To extend the simple CA of a cross-tabulation of two variables, we can perform multiple correspondence analysis (MCA) or joint correspondence analysis (JCA) on a series of categorical variables.

In certain aspects, CA can be thought of as an analogue to PCA for nominal variables. It is also possible to interpret CA in canonical correlation analysis and other graphic techniques such as optimal scaling.

4.13. Cluster Analysis[34–36]

Cluster analysis, also called unsupervised classification or class discovery, is a statistical method to determine the natural groups (clusters) in the data. It aims to group objects into clusters such that objects within one cluster are more similar than objects from different clusters. There are four key issues in cluster analysis: (1) How to measure the similarity between the objects; (2) How to choose the cluster algorithm; (3) How to identify the number of clusters; (4) How to evaluate the performance of the clustering results.

The clustering of objects is generally based on their distance from or similarity to each other. The distance measures are commonly used to emphasize the difference between samples, and large values in a distance matrix indicate dissimilarity. Several commonly-used distance functions are the absolute distance, the Euclidean distance and the Chebychev distance. Actually, all the three distances are special cases of the Minkowski distance (also called Lq-norm metric, $q \geq 1$) when $q = 1, q = 2$, and $q \to \infty$

$$d_{ij}(q) = \left(\sum_{k=1}^{p} |x_{ik} - x_{jk}|^q \right)^{1/q}, \tag{4.13.1}$$

where x_{ik} denotes the values of the kth variable for sample i.

However, the Minkowski distance is related to the measurement units or scales, and does not take the possible correlation between variables into consideration. Thus, we can instead use standardized/weighted statistical distance functions to overcome these limitations. Note that, the Mahalanobis distance can also take into account the correlations of the covariates and is scale-invariant under the linear transformations. However, this distance is not suggested for cluster analysis in general, but rather widely used in the discriminant analysis.

We can also investigate the relationship of the variables by similarity measures, where the most commonly used ones are the cosine, the Pearson correlation coefficient, etc. In addition to the distance measures and the similarity measures, some other measures such as the entropy can be used to measure the similarity between the objects as well.

4.13.1. *Hierarchical cluster analysis*

First, we consider n samples as n clusters where each cluster contains exactly one sample. Then we merge the closest pair of clusters into one cluster so that we have $n - 1$ clusters. We can repeat the step until all the samples are merged into a single cluster of size n. Dendrogram, a graphic display of the hierarchical sequence of the clustering assignment, can be used to illustrate the process, and to further determine the number of the clusters.

Depending on different definitions of between-cluster distance, or the linkage criteria, the hierarchical clustering can be classified into single linkage (i.e. nearest-neighbor linkage) clustering, complete-linkage (i.e. furthest-neighbor linkage) clustering, median-linkage clustering, centroid-linkage clustering, average-linkage clustering, weighted average-linkage clustering, and minimum variance linkage clustering (i.e. Wald's method). We can have different clustering results using different linkage criteria, and different linkages tend to yield clusters with different characteristics. For example, the single-linkage tends to find "stingy" elongated or S-shaped clusters, while the complete-, average-, centroid-, and Wald's linkage tend to find ellipsoid clusters.

4.13.2. *Cluster analysis by partitioning*

In contrast to the hierarchical clustering, the cluster analysis by partitioning starts with all the samples in one cluster, and then splits into two, three until n clusters by some optimal criterion. A similar dendrogram can be used to display the cluster arrangements for this method.

These two clustering methods share some common drawbacks. First, the later stage clustering depends solely on the earlier stage clustering, which can never break the earlier stage clusters. Second, the two algorithms require the data with a nested structure. Finally, the computational costs of these two algorithms are relatively heavy. To overcome these drawbacks, we can use the dynamic clustering algorithms such as k-means and k-medians or clustering methods based on models, networks and graph theories.

To evaluate the effectiveness of the clustering, we need to consider: (1) Given the number of clusters, how to determine the best clustering algorithm by both internal and external validity indicators; (2) As the number of the clusters is unknown, how to identify the optimal number. In general, we can determine the number of clusters by using some visualization approaches or by optimizing some objective functions such as $CH(k)$ statistic, $H(k)$ statistic, Gap statistic, etc.

The cluster analysis has several limitations. Firstly, it is hard to define clusters in the data set; in some situations, "cluster" is a vague concept, and the cluster results differ with different definitions of cluster itself as well as the between cluster distance. Secondly, the cluster analysis does not work well for poorly-separated clusters such as clusters with diffusion and interpenetration structures. Thirdly, the cluster results highly depend on the subjective choices of the clustering algorithms and the parameters in the analysis.

4.14. Biclustering[37–40]

Biclustering, also called block clustering, co-clustering, is a multivariate data mining technique for the clustering of both samples and variables. The method is a kind of the subspace clustering. B. Mirkin was the first to use the term "bi-clustering" in 1996,[40] but the idea can be seen earlier in J. A.

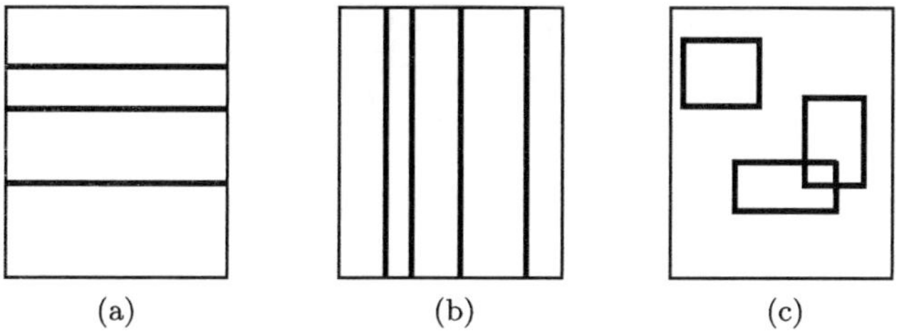

Fig. 4.14.1. Traditional clustering (*a* and *b*) and bi-clustering (*c*).

Hartingan *et al.* (1972).[38] Since Y. Z. Cheng and G. M. Church proposed a biclustering algorithm in 2000 and applied it to gene expression data,[37] a number of algorithms have been proposed in the gene expression biclustering field, which substantially promote the application of this method.

Taking the genetic data as an example, the traditional clustering is a one-way clustering, which can discover the genes with similar expressions by clustering on genes, or discover the structures of samples (such as pathological features or experimental conditions) by clustering on samples.

However, in practice, the researchers are more interested in finding the associated information between the genes and the samples, e.g. a subset of genes that show similar activity patterns (either up-regulated or down-regulated) under certain experimental conditions, as shown in Figure 4.14.1.

Figure 4.14.1 displays the genetic data as a matrix, where by the one-way clustering, Figures 4.14.1(*a*) and (*b*) group the row clusters and the column clusters (one-way clusters) after rearranging the rows and the columns, respectively. As seen in Figure (*c*), biclustering aims to find the block clusters (biclusters) after the rearrangement of both the rows and the columns. Furthermore, the bi-clustering is a "local" clustering, where part of the genes can determine the sample set and vice versa. Then, the blocks are clustered by some pre-specified search methods such that the mean squared residue or the corresponding p-value is minimized.

Bicluster. In biclustering, we call each cluster with the same features as a bicluster. According to the features of the biclusters, we can divide the biclusters into the following four classes (Figure 4.14.2): (1) Constant values, as seen in (*a*); (2) Constant values on rows or columns, as seen in (*b*) or (*c*); (3) Coherent values on both rows and columns either in an additive (*d*) or multiplicative (*e*) way; (4) Coherent evolutions, that is, subset of columns (e.g. genes) is increased (up-regulated) or decreased (down-regulated) across a subset of rows (sample) without taking into account their actual values,

0.2	0.2	0.2	0.2
0.2	0.2	0.2	0.2
0.2	0.2	0.2	0.2
0.2	0.2	0.2	0.2

(a)

0.2	0.2	0.2	0.2
0.4	0.4	0.4	0.4
0.6	0.6	0.6	0.6
0.8	0.8	0.8	0.8

(b)

0.2	0.4	0.6	0.8
0.2	0.4	0.6	0.8
0.2	0.4	0.6	0.8
0.2	0.4	0.6	0.8

(c)

0.1	0.2	0.5	0.6
0.2	0.3	0.6	0.7
0.4	0.5	0.8	0.9
0.5	0.6	0.9	1.0

(d)

0.1	0.2	0.1	0.3
0.2	0.4	0.2	0.6
0.4	0.8	0.4	1.2
0.5	1.0	0.5	1.5

(e)

↗	↗	↘	↗
↘	↘	↗	↘
↗	↗	↘	↗
↘	↘	↗	↘

(f)

Fig. 4.14.2. Different types of biclusters.

as seen in (f). In this situation, data in the bicluster does not follow any mathematical model.

The basic structures of biclusters include the following: single biclusters, exclusive row and column biclusters, rows exclusive biclusters, column exclusive biclusters, non-overlapping checkerboard biclusters, non-overlapping and non-exclusive biclusters, non-overlapping biclusters with tree structure, no-overlapping biclusters with hierarchical structure, and randomly overlapping biclusters, among others.

The main algorithms of biclustering include δ-Biclustering proposed by Cheng and Church, the coupled two-way clustering (CTWC), the spectral biclustering, ProBiclustering, etc.

The advantage of biclustering is that it can solve many problems that cannot be solved by the one-way clustering. For example, the related genes may have similar expressions only in part of the samples; one gene may have a variety of biological functions and may appear in multiple functional clusters.

4.15. Discriminant Analysis[1,41,42]

Discriminant analysis, also called supervised classification or class prediction, is a statistical method to build a discriminant criterion by the training samples and predict the categories of the new samples. In cluster analysis, however, there is no prior information about the number of clusters or cluster membership of each sample. Although discriminant analysis and cluster analysis have different goals, the two procedures have complementary

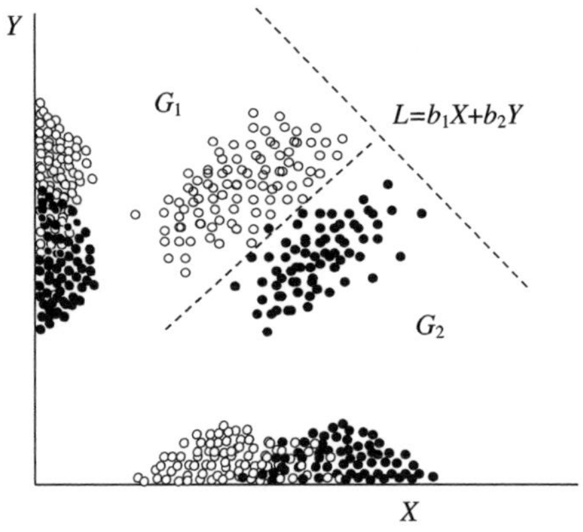

Fig. 4.15.1. The Fisher discriminant analysis for two categories

functionalities, and thus they are frequently used together: obtain cluster membership in cluster analysis first, and then run discriminant analysis.

There are many methods in the discriminant analysis, such as the distance discriminant analysis, Fisher discriminant analysis, and Bayes discriminant analysis.

(a) Distance discriminant analysis: The basic idea is to find the center for each category based on the training data, and then calculate the distance of a new sample with all centers; then the sample is classified to the for which the distance is shortest. Hence, the distance discriminant analysis is also known as the nearest neighbor method.
(b) Fisher discriminant analysis: The basic idea is to project the m-dimensional data with K categories into some direction(s) such that after the projection, the data in the same category are grouped together and the data in the different categories are separated as much as possible.

Figure 4.15.1 demonstrates a supervised classification problem for two categories. Category G_1 and G_2 are hard to discriminate when the data points are projected to the original X and Y axes; however, they can be well distinguished when data are projected to the direction L. The goal of Fisher discriminant is to find such a direction (linear combination of original variables), and establish a linear discriminant function to classify the new samples.

(c) Bayes discriminant analysis: The basic idea is to consider the prior probabilities in the discriminant analysis and derive the posterior probabilities using the Bayes' rule. That is, we can obtain the probabilities that the samples belong to each category and then these samples are classified to the category with the largest probability.

The distance discriminant analysis and Fisher discriminant analysis do not require any conditions on the distribution of the population, while Bayes discriminant analysis requires the population distribution to be known. However, the distance discriminant and Fisher discriminant do not consider the prior information in the model, and thus cannot provide the posterior probabilities, the estimate of the mis-classification rate, or the loss of the misclassification.

There are many other methods for discriminant analysis, including logistic discriminant analysis, probabilistic model-based methods (such as Gaussian mixed-effects model), tree-based methods (e.g., the classification tree, multivariate adaptive regression splines), machine learning methods (e.g., Bagging, Boosting, support vector machines, artificial neural network) and so on.

To evaluate the performance of discriminant analysis, we mainly consider two aspects: the discriminability of the new samples and the reliability of the classification rule. The former is usually measured by the misclassification rate (or prediction rate), which can be estimated using internal (or external) validation method. When there are no independent testing samples, we can apply the k-fold cross-validation or some resampling-based methods such as Bootstrap to estimate the rate. The latter usually refers to the accuracy of assigning the samples to the category with the largest posterior probability according to Bayes' rule. Note that the true posterior probabilities are usually unknown and some discriminant analysis methods do not calculate the posterior probabilities, thus the receiver operating characteristic curve (ROC) is also commonly used for the evaluation of the discriminant analysis.

4.16. Multidimensional Scaling (MDS)[43–45]

MDS, also called multidimensional similarity structure analysis, is a dimension reduction and data visualization technique for displaying the structure of multivariate data. It has seen wide application in behavior science and has led to a better understanding of complex psychological phenomena and marketing behaviors.

4.16.1. *Basic idea*

When the dissimilarity matrix of n objects in a high-dimensional space is given, we can seek the mapping of these objects in a low-dimensional space such that the dissimilarity matrix of the objects in the low-dimensional space is similar to or has the minimal difference with that in the original high-dimensional space.

The dissimilarity can be defined either by distance (like Euclidean distance, the weighted Euclidean distance), or by similarity coefficient using the formula:

$$d_{ij} = \sqrt{c_{ii} - 2c_{ij} + c_{jj}}, \tag{4.16.1}$$

where d_{ij} is a dissimilarity, and c_{ij} is a similarity between object i and object j.

Suppose that there are n samples in a p-dimensional space, and that the dissimilarity between the ith point and the j-th point is δ_{ij}, then the MDS model can be expressed as

$$\tau(\delta_{ij}) = d_{ij} + e_{ij}, \tag{4.16.2}$$

where τ is a monotone linear function of δ_{ij}, and d_{ij} is the dissimilarity between object i and j in the space defined by the t dimensions ($t < p$). We want to find a function τ such that $\tau(\delta_{ij}) \approx d_{ij}$, so that (x_{ik}, x_{jk}) can be displayed in a low-dimensional space. The general approach for solving the function τ is to minimize the stress function

$$\sum_{(i,j)} e_{ij} = \sum [\tau(\delta_{ij}) - d_{ij}]^2, \tag{4.16.3}$$

and we call this method LS scaling.

When d_{ij} are measurable values (such as physical distances), we call the method metric scaling analysis; when d_{ij} only keeps the order information which are not measurable, we call the method non-metric scaling analysis, or ordinal scaling analysis. Note that non-metric scaling can be solved by the isotonic regression.

Sometimes, for the same sample, we may have several dissimilarity matrices, i.e. these matrices are measured repeatedly. Then, we need to consider how to pool these matrices. Depending on the number of the matrices and how the matrices were pooled, we can classify the MDS analysis into classical MDS analysis (single matrix, unweighted model), repeated MDS analysis (multiple matrices, unweighted model) and weighted MDS analysis (multiple matrices, weighed model).

The classical MDS, is a special case of the LS MDS by using the Euclidean distance to measure the dissimilarity and setting the function τ to be an identity function. The basic idea is to find the eigenvectors of the matrices, thereby obtaining a set of coordinate axes, which is equivalent to the PCA.

The WLS MDS analysis is actually the combination of the weighted model and the LS approach, such as the Sammon mapping,[37] which assigns more weights to smaller distances.

4.16.2. *Evaluation*

The evaluation of the MDS analysis mainly considers three aspects of the model: the goodness-of-fit, the interpretability of the configuration, and the validation.

4.16.3. *Application*

(1) Use distances to measure the similarities or the dissimilarities in a low-dimensional space to visualize the high-dimensional data (see Sec. 4.20); (2) Test the structures of the high-dimensional data; (3) Identify the dimensions that can help explain the similarity (dissimilarity); (4) Explore the psychology structure in the psychological research.

It is worth mentioning that the MDS analysis is connected with PCA, EFA, canonical Correction analysis and the CA, but they have different focuses.

4.17. Generalized Estimating Equation (GEE)[46–52]

Developed by Liang and Zeger,[47] GEE is an extension of GLM to the analysis of longitudinal data using quasi-likelihood methods. Qusi-likelihood methods were introduced by Nelder and Wedderburn (1972),[49] and Wedderburn (1974),[50] and later developed and extended by McCullagh (1983),[48] and McCullagh and Nelder (1986)[16] among others. GEE is a general statistical approach to fit a marginal (or population-averaged) model for repeated measurement data in longitudinal studies.

4.17.1. *Key components*

Three key components in the GEE model are:

(1) Generalized linear structure (see Sec. 3.2). Suppose that Y_{ij} is the j-th ($j = 1, \ldots, t$) response of subject i at time j ($i = 1, \ldots, k$), $\boldsymbol{X}$ is a $p \times 1$ vector of covariates, and the marginal expectation of Y_{ij} is $\mu_{ij}[E(Y_{ij}) = \mu_{ij}]$. The marginal model that relates μ_{ij} to a linear combination of the covariates can be written as:

$$g(\mu_{ij}) = \boldsymbol{X}'\boldsymbol{\beta}, \tag{4.17.1}$$

where $\boldsymbol{\beta}$ is unknown $p \times 1$ vector of regression coefficients and g(.) is known linkage function, which could be identity linkage, logit linkage, log linkage, etc.

(2) Marginal variance. According to the theory of GLM, if the marginal distribution of Y_{ij} belongs to the exponential distribution family, then the variance of Y_{ij} can be expressed by the function of its marginal expectation

$$\mathrm{Var}(Y_{ij}) = V(\mu_{ij}) \cdot \varphi, \tag{4.17.2}$$

where $V(\cdot)$ is known variance function, and φ is a scale parameter denoting the deviation of $\mathrm{Var}(Y_{ij})$ from $V(\mu_{ij})$, which equals 1 when Y_{ij} has a binomial or Poisson distribution.

(3) Working correlation matrix. Denoted as $\boldsymbol{R}_i(\alpha)$, it is a $t \times t$ correlation matrix of the outcome measured at different occasions, which describes the pattern of measurements within subject. It depends on a vector of parameters denoted by α. Since different subjects may have different occasions of measurement and different within-subject correlations, $\boldsymbol{R}_i(\alpha)$ approximately characterizes the average correlation structure of the outcome across different measurement occasions.

4.17.2. *GEE modeling*

GEE yields asymptotically consistent estimates of regression coefficients even when the "working" correlation matrix $\boldsymbol{R}_i(\alpha)$ is misspecified, and the *quasi*-likelihood estimate of $\boldsymbol{\beta}$ is obtained by solving a set of p "quasi-score" differential equations:

$$U_p(\beta) = \sum_{i=1}^{k} \frac{\partial \mu_i}{\partial \beta} V_i^{-1}(Y_i - \mu_i) = 0, \tag{4.17.3}$$

where $\boldsymbol{V}_i$ is the "working" covariance matrix, and

$$V_i = \phi \boldsymbol{A}_i^{1/2} \boldsymbol{R}_i(\alpha) \boldsymbol{A}_i^{1/2}. \tag{4.17.4}$$

$\boldsymbol{R}_i(\alpha)$ is the "working" correlation matrix, and A_i is $t \times t$ diagonal matrix with $V(\mu_{it})$ as its t-th diagonal element.

4.17.3. *GEE solution*

There are three types of parameters that need to be estimated in the GEE model, i.e. regression coefficient vector $\boldsymbol{\beta}$, scale parameter φ and association parameter α. Since φ and α are both functions of $\boldsymbol{\beta}$, estimation is typically accomplished by using *quasi*-likelihood method, an interative procedure: (1) Given the estimates of φ and α from Pearson residuals, calculate $\boldsymbol{V}_i$ and an updated estimate of $\boldsymbol{\beta}$ as an solution of GEEs given by (4.17.3), using iteratively re-weighted LS method; (2) Given the estimate of $\boldsymbol{\beta}$, calculate Pearson (or standardized) residuals; (3) Obtain the consistent estimates of φ and α from Pearson residuals; (4) Repeat step (1)–(3) till the estimates are converged.

4.17.4. *Advantages and disadvantages*

The GEE model has a number of appealing properties for applied researchers: (1) Similar to GLM, GEE is applicable to a wide range of outcome-variables such as continuous, binary, ordered and unordered polychotomous, and an event count that is because GEE can flexibly specify various link functions; (2) It takes the correlation across different measurements into account; (3) It behaves robustly against misspecification of the working correlation structure, especially under large sample size; (4) It yields robust estimates even when the data is imbalanced due to missing values.

GEE does have limitations. First, GEE can handle hierarchical data with no more than two levels; Second, traditional GEE assumes missing data to be missing completely at random (MCAR), which is more stringent than missing at random (MAR) required by mixed-effects regression model.

4.18. Multilevel Model (MLM)[53–55]

Multilevel model, also known as hierarchical linear model (HLM) or random coefficient model, is a specific multivariate technique for modeling data with hierarchical, nested or clustered structures. It was first proposed by Goldstein H. (1986),[53] a British statistician in education research. Its basic idea lies in partitioning variances at different levels while considering the influence of independent variables on variance simultaneously; it makes full use of the interclass correlation at difference levels, and thus get reliable estimations of regression coefficients and theirs standard errors, which leads to more reliable statistical inferences.

4.18.1. *Multilevel linear model (MLLM)*

For simplicity, we use a 2-level model as an example

$$y_{ij} = \beta_{0j} + \beta_{1j}x_{1ij} + \cdots + e_{ij}, \tag{4.18.1}$$

where $i(i = 1, \ldots, n_j)$ and $j(j = 1, \ldots, m)$ refer to level-1 unit (e.g. student) and level-2 unit (e.g. class), respectively.

Here, β_{0j} and β_{1j} are random variables, which can be re-written as

$$\beta_{0j} = \beta_0 + u_{0j}, \quad \beta_{1j} = \beta_1 + u_{1j}, \tag{4.18.2}$$

where β_0 and β_1 are the fixed effects for the intercept and slopes, and u_{0j}, u_{1j} represent random individual variation around the population intercept and slope, respectively. More precisely,

$$\begin{aligned} E(u_{0j}) &= E(u_{1j}) = 0, \\ \text{var}(u_{0j}) &= \sigma_{u0}^2, \text{var}(u_{1j}) = \sigma_{u1}^2, \\ \text{cov}(u_{0j}, u_{1j}) &= \sigma_{u01}. \end{aligned}$$

Then, we can re-write the model (4.18.1) as the combined model

$$y_{ij} = \beta_0 + \beta_1 x_{1ij} + (u_{0j} + u_{1j} x_{1ij} + e_{ij}), \tag{4.18.3}$$

where e_{ij} is the residual at level 1 with parameter

$$E(e_{ij}) = 0, \ \text{var}(e_{ij}) = \sigma_0^2.$$

We also assume $\text{cov}(e_{ij}, u_{0j}) = \text{cov}(e_{ij}, u_{1j}) = 0$.

Obviously, model (4.18.3) has two parts, i.e. the fixed effect part and the random effect part. We can also consider adjusting covariates in the random part. The coefficient u_{1j} is called random coefficient, which is why MLM is also known as random coefficient model.

4.18.2. *Multilevel generalized linear model (ML-GLM)*

ML-LM can be easily extended to ML-GLM when the dependent variable is not normally distributed. ML-GLM includes a wide class of regression models such as multilevel logistic regression, multilevel probit regression, multilevel Poisson regression and multilevel negative binomial regression.

MLM can also be extended to other models in special situations: (1) Multilevel survival analysis model, which can be used to treat event history or survival data; (2) Multivariate MLM, which allows multiple dependent variables being simultaneously analyzed in the same model. The multiple dependent variables can either share the same distribution (e.g. multivariate normal distribution) or have different distributions. For example, some variables may be normally distributed, while others may have binomial distributions; as another example, or one variable may have binomial distribution and the other variable has a Poisson distribution.

Parameter estimation methods in MLM include iterative generalized least squares (IGLS), restricted iterative generalized least squares (RIGLS), restricted maximum likelihood (REML) and quasi-likelihood, etc.

The main attractive features of MLM are: (1) It can make use of all available information in the data for parameter estimation, and can get robust estimation even when missing values exist. (2) It can treat data with any levels, and fully consider errors as well as covariates at different levels.

4.19. High-Dimensional Data (HDD)[56–59]

HDD in general refers to data that have much larger dimensions p than the sample size $n(p \gg n)$. Such data are commonly seen in biomedical sciences, including microarray gene expression data, genome-wide association study (GWAS) data, next-generation high-throughput RNA sequencing data and CHIP sequencing data, among others.

The main features of HD are high dimensionality and small sample size, i.e. large p and small n. Small sample size results in stochastic uncertainty when making statistical inference about the population distribution; high dimension leads to increased computational complexity, data sparsity and empty space phenomenon, which incurs a series of issues in data analysis.

Curse of dimensionality, also called dimensionality problem, was proposed by R. Bellman in 1957 when he was considering problems in dynamic optimization.[56] He noticed that the complexity of optimizing a multivariate function increases exponentially as dimension grows. Later on, the curse of dimensionality was generalized to refer to virtually all the problems caused by high dimensions.

High dimensionality brings a number of challenges to traditional statistical analysis: (1) Stochastic uncertainty is increased due to "accumulated errors"; (2) "False correlation" leads to false discovery in feature screening, higher false positive rate in differential expression analysis, as well as other errors in statistical inference; (3) Incidental endogeneity causes inconsistency in model selection; (4) Due to data sparsity induced by high-dimensions, traditional L_k-norm is no longer applicable in high-dimensional space, which leads to the failure of traditional cluster analysis and classification analysis. To overcome these challenges, new strategies have been proposed, such as dimension reduction, reconstruction of the distance or similarity functions in high-dimensional space, and penalized *quasi*-likelihood approaches.

Dimension reduction. The main idea of dimension reduction is to project data points from a high-dimensional space into a low-dimensional space, and then use the low-dimensional vectors to conduct classification or other analysis. Depending on whether the original dimensions are transformed or not, the strategy of dimension reduction can be largely divided into two categories: (1) Variable selection, i.e. directly select the important variables; (2) Dimension reduction, i.e. reducing the dimension of the data space by projection, transformation, etc. There are many dimension reduction approaches, such as the traditional PCA (see Sec. 4.9) and multidimensional scaling analysis (MDS) (see Sec. 4.16). Modern dimension reduction approaches have also been developed, such as the LASSO regression (see Sec. 3.17), sliced inverse regression (SIR), projection pursuit (PP), and iterative sure independence screening (ISIS).

In practice, both variable selection and dimension reduction should be considered. The overall goal is to maximize the use of data and to benefit the subsequent data analysis, i.e. "Target-driven dimension reduction".

Sufficient dimension reduction refers to a class of approaches and concepts for dimension reduction. It shares similar spirit with Fisher's sufficient statistics (1922),[59] which aims to condense data without losing important information. The corresponding subspace's dimension is called the "intrinsic dimension". For example, in regression analysis, one often conducts the projection of a p-dimensional vector $\boldsymbol{X}$ into lower dimensional vector $\boldsymbol{R}(\boldsymbol{X})$; as long as the conditional distribution of $\boldsymbol{Y}$ given $\boldsymbol{R}(\boldsymbol{X})$ is the same as the conditional distribution of $\boldsymbol{Y}$ given $\boldsymbol{X}$, the dimension reduction from $\boldsymbol{X}$ to $\boldsymbol{R}(\mathrm{X})$ is considered to be sufficient.

To overcome the distance (similarity) problem in high-dimensional analysis such as clustering and classification, reconstruction of distance (similarity) function has become an urgent need. Of note, when reconstructing distance (dissimilarity) function in high-dimensional space, the following are suggested: (1) Using "relative" distance (e.g. statistical distance) instead of "absolute" distance (e.g. Minkowski distance) to avoid the influence of measure units or scales of the variables; (2) Giving more weights to the data points closer to the "center" of the data, and thus to efficiently avoid the influence of noisy data far away from the "center".

Typical statistical analysis under high dimensions includes differential expression analysis, cluster analysis (see Sec. 4.13), discriminant analysis (see Sec. 4.15), risk prediction, association analysis, etc.

4.20. High-Dimensional Data Visualization (HDDV)[60–63]

HDDV is to transform high-dimensional data into low-dimensional graphic representations that human can view and understand easily. The transformation should be as faithful as possible in preserving the original data's characteristics, such as clusters, distance, outliers, etc. Typical transformation includes direct graphic representation (such as scatter plot, constellation diagram, radar plot, parallel coordinate representation, and Chernoff face), statistical dimension reduction, etc.

Scatter plot is probably the most popular approach for projecting high-dimensional data into two-dimensional or three-dimensional space. Scatter plot shows the trend in the data and correlation between variables. By analyzing scatter plot or scatter plot matrix, one may find the subset of dimensions to well separate the data points, and find outliers in the data. The disadvantage of scatter plot is that it can easily cause dimension explosion. To improve scatter plot for high-dimensional data, one can seek to simplify its presentation by focusing on the most important aspects of the data structure.

Constellation diagram was proposed by Wakimoto K. and Taguri M. in 1978,[63] and was named so due to its similarity to the constellation graph in astronomy. The principle of this approach is to transform high-dimensional data into angle data, add weights to data points, and plot each data point by a dot in a half circle. Points that are in proximity are classified as a cluster. The purpose is to make it easy to recognize different clusters of data points. How to set the weights for data points can be critical for constellation plot.

Radar plot is also called spider plot. The main idea is to project the multiple characteristics of a data point into a two-dimensional space, and then connect those projections into a closed polygon. The advantage of radar plot is to reflect the trend of change for variables, so that one can make classification on the data. The typical approach for optimization of radar plot is based on the convex hull algorithm.

Parallel coordinate is a coordinate technique to represent high-dimensional data in a visualizable plane. The fundamental idea is to use a series of continuous line charts to project high-dimensional data into parallel coordinates. The merits of parallel coordinate lie in three aspects: they are easy to plot, simple to understand, and mathematically sound. The disadvantage is that when sample size is large, data visualization may become difficult due to overlapping of line charts. Furthermore, because the width of the parallel coordinate is determined by the screen, graphic presentation can become challenging when dimension is very high. The convex hull algorithm can also be used for its optimization.

Chernoff face was first proposed by statistician Chernoff H. in 1970s,[61] and is an icon-based technique. It represents the p variables by the shape and size of different elements of a human face (e.g. the angle of eyes, the width of the nose, etc.), and each data point is shown as a human face. Similar data points will be similar in their face representations, thus the Chernoff face was initially used for cluster analysis. Because different analysts may choose different elements to represent the same variable, it follows that one data may have many different presentations. The naïve presentation of Chernoff faces allows the researchers to visualize data with at most 18 variables. And an improved Chernoff faces, which is often plotted based on principle components, can overcome this limitation.

Commonly used statistical dimension reduction techniques include PCA (see Sec. 4.9), cluster analysis (see Sec. 4.13), partial least square (PLS), self-organizing maps (SOM), PP, LASSO regression (see Sec. 3.17), MDS analysis (see Sec. 4.16), etc.

HDDV research also utilizes color, brightness, and other auxiliary techniques to capture information. Popular approaches include heat map, height map, fluorescent map, etc.

By representing high-dimensional data in low dimensional space, HDDV assists researchers to gain insight of the data, and provides guidelines for the subsequent data analysis and policymaking.

References

1. Chen, F. *Multivariate Statistical Analysis for Medical Research.* (2nd edn). Beijing: China Statistics Press, 2007.
2. Liu, RY, Serfling, R, Souvaine, DL. *Data Depth: Robust Multivariate Analysis, Computational Geometry and Applications.* Providence: American Math Society, 2006.
3. Anderson, TW. *An Introduction to Multivariate Statistical Analysis.* (3rd edn). New York: John Wiley & Sons, 2003.
4. Hotelling, H. The generalization of student's ratio. *Ann. Math. Stat.*, 1931, 2: 360–378.
5. James, GS. Tests of linear hypotheses in univariate and multivariate analysis when the ratios of the population variances are unknown. *Biometrika*, 1954, 41: 19–43.
6. Warne, RT. A primer on multivariate analysis of variance (MANOVA) for behavioral scientists. *Prac. Assess. Res. Eval.*, 2014, 19(17):1–10.
7. Wilks, SS. Certain generalizations in the analysis of variance. *Biometrika*, 1932, 24(3): 471–494.
8. Akaike, H. Information theory and an extension of the maximum likelihood principle, in Petrov, B.N.; & Csáki, F., *2nd International Symposium on Information Theory*, Budapest: Akadémiai Kiadó, 1973: 267–281.
9. Breusch, TS, Pagan, AR. The Lagrange multiplier test and its applications to model specification in econometrics. *Rev. Econo. Stud.*, 1980, 47: 239–253.
10. Zhang, YT, Fang, KT. *Introduction to Multivariate Statistical Analysis.* Beijing: Science Press, 1982.
11. Acock, AC. *Discovering Structural Equation Modeling Using Stata.* (Rev. edn). College Station: Stata Press, 2013.

12. Bollen, KA. *Structural Equations with Latent Variables.* New York: Wiley, 1989.
13. Hao, YT, Fang JQ. The structural equation modelling and its application in medical researches. *Chinese J. Hosp. Stat.*, 2003, 20(4): 240–244.
14. Berkson, J. Application of the logistic function to bio-assay. *J. Amer. Statist. Assoc.*, 1944, 39(227): 357–365.
15. Hosmer, DW, Lemeshow, S, Sturdivant, RX. *Applied Logistic Regression.* (3rd edn). New York: John Wiley & Sons, 2013.
16. McCullagh P, Nelder JA. *Generalized Linear Models.* (2nd edn). London: Chapman & Hall, 1989.
17. Chen, F., Yangk, SQ. On negative binomial distribution and its applicable assumptions. *Chinese J. Health Stat.*, 1995, 12(4): 21–22.
18. Hardin, JW, Hilbe, JM. *Generalized Linear Models and Extensions.* (3rd edn). College Station: Stata Press, 2012.
19. Hilbe, JM. *Negative Binomial Regression.* (2nd edn). New York: Cambridge University Press, 2013.
20. Hastie, T. *Principal Curves and Surfaces.* Stanford: Stanford University, 1984.
21. Hotelling, H. Analysis of a complex of statistical variables into principal components. *J. Edu. Psychol.*, 1933, 24(6): 417–441.
22. Jolliffe, IT. *Principal Component Analysis.* (2nd edn). New York: Springer-Verlag, 2002.
23. Pearson, K. On lines and planes of closest fit to systems of points is space. *Philoso. Mag.*, 1901, 2: 559–572.
24. Bartlett, MS. The statistical conception of mental factors. *British J. Psychol.*, 1937, 28: 97–10.
25. Bruce, T. *Exploratory and Confirmatory Factor Analysis: Understanding Concepts and Applications.* Washington, DC: American Psychological Association, 2004.
26. Spearman, C. "General intelligence," objectively determined and measured. *Am. J. Psychol.*, 1904, 15 (2): 201–292.
27. Thomson, GH. *The Factorial Analysis of Human Ability.* London: London University Press, 1951.
28. Hotelling, H. The most predictable criterion. *J. Edu. Psychol.*, 1935, 26(2): 139–142.
29. Hotelling, H. Relations between two sets of variates. *Biometrika*, 1936, 28: 321–377.
30. Rencher, AC, Christensen, WF. *Methods of Multivariate Analysis.* (3rd edn). Hoboken: John Wiley & Sons, 2012.
31. Benzécri, JP. *The Data Analysis.* (Vol II). *The Correspondence Analysis.* Paris: Dunod, 1973.
32. Greenacre, MJ. *Correspondence Analysis in Practice.* (2nd edn). Boca Raton: Chapman & Hall/CRC, 2007.
33. Hirschfeld, HO. A connection between correlation and contingency. *Math. Proc. Cambridge*, 1935, 31(4): 520–524.
34. Blashfield, RK, Aldenderfer, MS. The literature on cluster analysis. *Multivar. Behavi. Res.*, 1978, 13: 271–295.
35. Everitt, BS, Landau, S, Leese, M, Stahl, D. *Cluster Analysis.* (5th edn). Chichester: John Wiley & Sons, 2011.
36. Kaufman, L, Rousseeuw, PJ. *Finding Groups in Data: An Introduction to Cluster Analysis.* New York: Wiley, 1990.
37. Cheng, YZ, Church, GM. Biclustering of expression data. *Proc. Int. Conf. Intell. Syst. Mol. Biol.*, 2000, 8: 93–103.
38. Hartigan, JA. Direct clustering of a data matrix. *J. Am. Stat. Assoc.*, 1972, 67 (337): 123–129.

39. Liu, PQ. *Study on the Clustering Algorithms of Bivariate Matrix.* Yantai: Shandong University, 2013.
40. Mirkin, B. *Mathematical Classification and Clustering.* Dorderecht: Kluwer Academic Press, 1996.
41. Andrew, RW, Keith, DC. *Statistical Pattern Recognition.* (3rd edn). New York: John Wiley & Sons, 2011.
42. Hastie, T., Tibshirani, R., Friedman, J. *The Elements of Statistical Learning: Data Mining, Inference, and Prediction.* (2nd edn). Berlin: Springer Verkag, 2009.
43. Borg, I., Groenen, PJF. *Modern Multidimensional Scaling: Theory and Applications.* (2nd edn). New York: Springer Verlag, 2005.
44. Sammon, JW Jr. A nonlinear mapping for data structure analysis. *IEEE Trans. Comput.*, 1969, 18: 401–409.
45. Torgerson, WS. Multidimensional scaling: I. Theory and method. *Psychometrika,* 1952, 17: 401–419.
46. Chen, QG. Generalized estimating equations for repeated measurement data in longitudinal studies. *Chinese J. Health Stat.*, 1995, 12(1): 22–25, 51.
47. Liang, KY, Zeger, SL. Longitudinal data analysis using generalized linear models. *Biometrics*, 1986, 73(1): 13–22.
48. McCullagh, P. Quasi-likelihood functions. *Ann. Stat.*, 1983, 11: 59–67.
49. Nelder, JA, Wedderburn, RWM. Generalized linear models. *J. R. Statist. Soc. A*, 1972, 135: 370–384.
50. Wedderburn, RWM. Quasi-likelihood functions, generalized linear model, and the gauss-newton method. *Biometrika,* 1974, 61: 439–447.
51. Zeger, SL, Liang, KY, Albert, PS. Models for longitudinal data: a generalized estimating equation approach. *Biometrics*, 1988, 44: 1049–1060.
52. Zeger, SL, Liang, KY, An overview of methods for the analysis of longitudinal data. *Stat. Med.*, 1992, 11: 1825–1839.
53. Goldstein, H. Multilevel mixed linear model analysis using iterative generalized least squares. *Biometrika*, 1986; 73: 43–56.
54. Goldstein, H, Browne, W, Rasbash, J. Multilevel modelling of medical data. *Stat. Med.*, 2002, 21: 3291–3315.
55. Little, TD, Schnabel, KU, *Baumert, J. Modeling Longitudinal and Multilevel Data: Practical Issues, Applied Approaches, and Specific Examples.* London: Erlbaum, 2000.
56. Bellman, RE. *Dynamic programming.* New Jersey: Princeton University Press, 1957.
57. Bühlmann, P, van de Geer, S. *Statistics for High-Dimensional Data: Methods, Theory and Applications.* Berlin, New York, and London: Springer Verlag, 2011.
58. Fan, J, Han, F, Liu, H. Challenges of big data analysis. *Natl. Sci. Rev.*, 2014, 1: 293–314.
59. Fisher, RA. On the mathematical foundation of theoretical statistics. *Philos. Trans. Roy. Soc. serie A.*, 1922, 222: 309–368.
60. Andrews, DF. Plots of high-dimensional data. *Biometrics*, 1972, 28(1): 125–136.
61. Chernoff, H. The use of faces to represent points in k-dimensional space graphically. *J. Am. Stat. Assoc.*, 1973, 68(342): 361–368.
62. Dzemyda, G., Kurasova, O., Žilinskas, J. *Multidimensional Data Visualization: Methods and Applications.* New York, Heidelberg, Dordrecht, London: Springer, 2013.
63. Wakimoto, K., Taguri, M. Constellation graphical method for representing multidimensional data. *Ann. Statist. Math.*, 1978; 30(Part A): 77–84.

About the Author

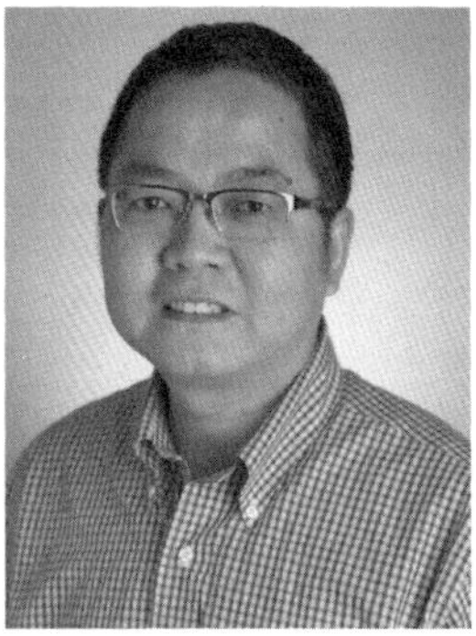

Pengcheng Xun obtained his PhD degree in Biostatistics from the School of Public Health, Nanjing Medical University, Jiangsu, China (2007), and his PhD dissertation mainly studied Target-driven Dimension Reduction of High-dimensional Data under the guidance of Professor Feng Chen. He got his postdoctoral research training in Nutrition Epidemiology (mentor: Professor Ka He) from the School of Public Health, University of North Carolina (UNC) at Chapel Hill, NC, the USA (2008–2012). He is currently Assistant Scientist at Department of Epidemiology & Biostatistics, School of Public Health, Indiana University at Bloomington, IN, the USA. He has rich experience in experimental design and statistical analysis, and has been involved in more than 20 research grants from funding agencies in both America (such as "National Institute of Health [NIH]", "America Cancer Association", and "Robert Wood Johnson Foundation") and China (such as "National Natural Science Foundation" and "Ministry of Science and Technology") as Biostatistician, sub-contract PI, or PI. He has published 10 books and ~120 peer-reviewed articles, in which ~70 articles were in prestigious English journals (e.g. *Journal of Allergy and Clinical Immunology, Diabetes Care, American Journal of Epidemiology, American Journal of Clinical Nutrition*, etc.). He obtained the Second Prize of "Excellent Teaching Achievement Award of Jiangsu Province" in 2005, and the "Postdoctoral Award for Research Excellence" from UNC in 2011. He is now an invited peer reviewer from many prestigious journals (e.g. *British Medical Journal, Annals of Internal Medicine, American Journal of Epidemiology, Statistics in Medicine*, etc.) and a reviewer of NIH Early Career Reviewer (ECR) program. His current research interest predominantly lies in applying modern statistical methods into the fields of public health, medicine, and biology.

CHAPTER 5

NON-PARAMETRIC STATISTICS

Xizhi Wu*, Zhi Geng and Qiang Zhao

5.1. Non-parametric Statistics[1,2]

Normally, traditional statistics makes different assumptions on probable distributions, which may contain various parameters, such as the mean, the variance and the degrees of freedom, etc. And that is the reason why the traditional statistics is called parametric statistics. In fact, it is inappropriate or even absurd to draw any conclusions by these inaccurate mathematical models, because the existence of world does not rely on the math formulas. Unlike parametric statistics, which makes so accurate mathematical model with assumptions on the type and number of parameters, non-parametric statistics at most make assumptions on the shape of distributions. Thus, non-parametric statistics is more robust. In other words, when nothing is known concerning about the distribution, non-parametric statistics may come to the reasonable conclusion, while traditional statistics would not work completely.

According to its definition, non-parametric statistics cover a large part of statistics, such as machine learning, non-parametric regression and density estimation. However, machine learning, covering a wide range of subjects, exists completely independent, and does not belong to the field of non-parametric statistics. Although the new emerging non-parametric regression and density estimation are supposed to be involved in non-parametric statistics, they are different from the traditional non-parametric statistics in method, training and practical application, and therefore, they have been listed into the field of single subject. An important characteristic of non-parametric statistics, which is not to rely on assumptions of accurate

*Corresponding author: xizhi_wu@163.com

population distribution, is that statistical inference is concluded by the character of the order statistics of observations.

How to make use of the information involved in the data when we do not know the population distribution of the variables? The most fundamental information of data is their orders. If we can order the data point from the small one to the large one, each specific data point has its own position or order (generally sorted from the smallest or by ascending order) in the entire data, which is called the rank of each data point in the entire data. The number of ranks about the data is as same as the number of the observed values. We can carry out the rank and the distribution of the related statistics under certain assumptions, and in this way, we can make statistical inference that we need.

Here is the definition of rank, which is a fundamental notion in parametric statistics. For a sample, $X_1, \ldots, X_n, X_{(1)} \leq X_{(2)} \leq \cdots \leq X_{(n)}$, which is numbered in increasing order and remarked again, is the ordered statistics, and $X_{(i)}$ is the ith ordered statistic. The study of the properties of the ordered statistics is one of the basic theories of non-parametric statistics. Although, non-parametric statistics do not rely on the population distribution of the variables, it makes large use of the distribution of the ordered statistics. The following are some examples.

There are many elementary statistical definitions based on the ordered statistics, such as the definition of the range and the quantile like the median. We can work out the distribution function of the ordered statistics in the case of knowing the population distribution. And if the population density exists, we can deduce the density functions of the ordered statistics, all kinds of joint density functions, and distributions of many frequently-used functions of the ordered statistics. As for the independent identically distributed samples, the rank's distribution has nothing to do with the population distribution. In addition, a very important non-parametric statistic is U-statistic proposed by Hoeffding. U-statistic is a symmetric function, which can deduce many useful statistics, and lots of key statistics are its special cases. U-statistic has very important theoretical significance to both non-parametric statistics and parametric statistics.

Textbooks in traditional statistics have contacted with many contents of non-parametric statistics, such as the histogram in descriptive statistics. Various analyses of contingency tables, such as the Pearson χ^2 testing, the log-linear models, the independence test for the high-dimensional contingency tables, and so on, all belong to non-parametric statistics.

The methods based on ranks are mainly used in various non-parametric tests. For single-sample data, there are various tests (and estimations), such as the sign test, the Wilcoxon signed rank test and the runs test for randomness. The typical tests for two-sample data are the Brown–Mood median test and the Wilcoxon rank sum test. And tests for multi-sample data cover the Kruskal–Wallis rank sum test, the Jonckheere–Terpstra test, various tests in block design and the Kendall's coefficient of concordance test. There are five specialized tests about scaling test: the Siegel–Tukey variance test, the Mood test, the square rank test, the Ansari–Bradley test, and the Fligner–Killeen test. In addition, there are normal score tests for a variety of samples, the Pearson χ^2 test and the Kolmogorov–Smirnov test about the distributions and so on.

5.2. Asymptotic Relative Efficiency (ARE)[2–4]

In which way are non-parametric tests superior to traditional parametric statistical tests? This requires criterion to compare differences with qualities of different tests.

The ARE, also called the Pitman efficiency, was proposed in 1948 by Pitman.

For any test T, assume that α represents the probability of committing a type I error, while β represents the probability of committing a type II error (the power is $1-\beta$). In theory, you can always find a sample size n to make the test meet fixed α and β. Obviously, in order to meet that condition, the test requiring large sample size is not as efficient as that requiring small sample size. To get the same α and β, if n_1 observations are needed in T_1, while n_2 observations are needed $T_2, n_1/n_2$ can be defined as the relative efficiency of T_2 to T_1. And the test with high relative efficiency is what we want. If we let α fix and $n_1 \to \infty$ (the power $1-\beta$ keeps getting larger), then the sample size n_2 also should increase (to ∞) in order to keep the same efficiency of the two tests. Under certain conditions, there is a limit for relative efficiency n_1/n_2. This limit is called the ARE of T_2 to T_1.

In practice, when the small sample size takes a large proportion, people would question whether the ARE is suitable or not. In fact, the ARE is deduced in large samples, but when comparing different tests, the relative efficiency with small sample size is usually close to the ARE. When comparing the results of non-parametric methods with traditional methods, the relative efficiency of small sample size tends to be higher than the ARE. As a result, a higher ARE of non-parametric test should not be overlooked.

The following table lists four different population distributions with the related non-parametric tests, such as the sign test (denoted by S) and the Wilcoxon signed rank test (denoted by W^+). Related to the t-test (denoted by t), which is a traditional test based on the assumption of normal population, we use ARE(S,t) and ARE(W^+,t) to denote the two AREs, from the fact that ARE(S,W^+) of the Wilcoxon signed rank test to the sign test can be calculated easily.

Distribution and density function	$U(-1,1)$ $\frac{1}{2}I(-1,1)$	$N(0,1)$ $\frac{1}{\sqrt{2\pi}}e^{-x^2/2}$	log *istic* $e^{-x}(1+e^{-x})^{-2}$	Double exponential $\frac{1}{2}e^{-\lvert x\rvert}$
ARE(W^+,t)	1	$3/\pi$ (≈ 0.0955)	$\pi^2/9$ (≈ 1.097)	$3/2$
ARE(S,t)	1/3	$2/\pi$ (≈ 0.637)	$\pi^2/12$ (≈ 0.822)	2
ARE(W^+,S)	3	3/2	4/3	3/4

Obviously, when the population is normal distribution, t-test is the best choice. But the advantage to the Wilcoxon test is not large ($\pi/3 \approx 1.047$). However, when the population is not normal, the Wilcoxon test is equal to or better than t-test. For double exponential distribution, the sign test is better than t-test. Now move to the standard normal population $\Phi(x)$, which is partially polluted (the ratio is ε) by normal distribution $\Phi(x/3)$. The population distribution function after being polluted is $F_\varepsilon(x) = (1-\varepsilon)\Phi(x) + \varepsilon\Phi(x/3)$. With this condition, for different ε, the AREs of the Wilcoxon test to t-test are

ε	0	0.01	0.03	0.05	0.08	0.10	0.15
ARE(W^+,t)	0.955	1.009	1.108	1.196	1.301	1.373	1.497

that is, the AREs under special conditions. Under common conditions, is there a range for the AREs? The following table lists the range of the AREs among the Wilcoxon test, the sign test and t-test.

ARE(W^+,t)	ARE(S,t)	ARE(W^+,S)
$\left(\frac{108}{125},\infty\right)$ $\approx (0.864,\infty)$	$\left[\frac{1}{3},\infty\right)$ non-single peak : $(0,\infty)$	$(0,3]$ non-single peak : $(0,\infty)$

From the former discussion of the ARE, we can see that non-parametric statistical tests have large advantages when not knowing the population distributions. Pitman efficiency can be applied not only to hypothesis testing, but also to parameter estimation.

When comparing efficiency, it is sometimes compared with the uniformly most powerful test (UMP test) instead of the test based on normal theory. Certainly, for normal population, many tests based on normal theory are UMP tests. But in general, the UMP test does not necessarily exist, thus we get the concept of the locally most powerful test (LMP test) ([3]), which is defined as: to testing $H_0\colon \Delta = 0 \Leftrightarrow H_1 : \Delta > 0$, if there is $\varepsilon > 0$, such that a test is the UMP test to $0 < \Delta < \varepsilon$, then the test is a LMP test. Compared with the UMP test, the condition where the LMP test exists is weaker.

5.3. Order Statistics[2,5]

Given the sample $X_1, \ldots, X_n$, is the ordered statistics that are $X_{(1)} \leq X_{(2)} \leq \cdots \leq X_{(n)}$. If the population distribution function is $F(x)$, then

$$F_r = P(X_{(r)} \leq x) = P(\#(X_i \leq x) \geq r) = \sum_{i=r}^{n} \binom{n}{i} F^i(x)[1 - F(x)]^{n-i}.$$

If the density function of a population exists, the density function of the rth ordered statistic $X_{(\tau)}$ is

$$f_r(x) = \frac{n!}{(r-1)(n-r)} F^{r-1}(x) f(x)[1 - F(x)]^{n-r}.$$

The joint density function of the order statistics $X_{(r)}$ and $X_{(s)}$ is

$$f_{r,s}(x, y) = C(n, r, s) F^{r-1}(x) f(x)[F(y) - F(x)]^{s-r-1} f(y)[1 - F(y)]^{n-s},$$

where

$$C(n, r, s) = \frac{n!}{(r-1)!(s-r-1)!(n-s)!}.$$

From the above joint density function, we can get the distributions of many frequently-used functions of the ordered statistics. For example, the distribution function of the range $W = X_{(n)} - X_{(1)}$ is

$$F_W(\omega) = n \int_{-\infty}^{\infty} f(x)[F(x + \omega) - F(x)]^{n-1} dx.$$

Because the main methods of the book are based on ranks, it is natural to introduce the distribution of ranks.

For an independent identically distributed sample $X_1, \ldots, X_n$, the rank of X_i is denoted by R_i, which is the number of sample points who are less than or equal to X_i, that is $R_i = \sum_{j=1}^{n} I(X_j \le X_i)$. Denote $R = (R_1, \ldots, R_n)$. It has been proved that for any permutation of $(1, \ldots, n)$, the joint distribution of $R_1, \ldots, R_n$ is

$$P(R = (i_1, \ldots, i_n)) = \frac{1}{n!}.$$

From which we can get

$$P(R_i = r) = \frac{1}{n}; \quad P(R_i = r, R_j = s) = \frac{1}{n(n-1)},$$

$$E(R_i) = \frac{n+1}{2}, \quad \mathrm{Var}(R_i) = \frac{(n+1)(n-1)}{12},$$

$$\mathrm{Cov}(R_i, R_j) = -\frac{n+1}{12}.$$

Similarly, we can get a variety of possible joint distributions and moments of $R_1, \ldots, R_n$. As for the independent identically distributed samples, the distribution of ranks has nothing to do with the population distribution.

We introduce the linear rank statistics below. First of all, we assume that R_i^+ is the rank of $|X_i|$ in $|X_1|, \ldots, |X_n|$. If $a_n^+(\cdot)$ is a non-decreasing function with domain $1, \ldots, n$, and satisfies

$$0 \le a_n^+(1) \le \cdots \le a_n^+(n), a_n^+(n) > 0,$$

the linear rank statistic is defined as

$$S_n^+ = \sum_{i=1}^{n} a_n^+(R_i^+) I(X_i > 0).$$

If $X_1, \ldots, X_n$ are independent identically distributed random variables with the distribution symmetrical about 0, then

$$E(S_n^+) = \frac{1}{2} \sum_{i=1}^{n} a_n^+(i); \quad \mathrm{Var}(S_n^+) = \frac{1}{4} \sum_{i=1}^{n} \{a_n^+(i)\}^2.$$

The famous Wilcoxon signed rank statistics W^+ and the sign statistics S^+ are special cases of linear rank statistics. For example, S_n^+ is equal to the Wilcoxon signed rank statistic W^+ when $a_n^+(i) = i$, and S_n^+ is equal to the sign statistics S^+ when $a_n^+(i) \equiv 1$.

Compared with the above statistics, $S_n = \sum_{i=1}^{n} c_n(i) a_n(R_i)$, is more common, where R_i is the rank of $X_i (i = 1, \ldots, n), a_n(\cdot)$ is a function of one variable and does not have to be non-negative. Both $a_n(\cdot)$ and $a_n^+(\cdot)$ are called score functions while $c_n(\cdot)$ is called regression constant. If $X_1, \ldots, X_n$ are independent identically distributed continuous random variables, in other words, $R_1, \ldots, R_n$ is uniformly distributed over $1, \ldots, n$, then

$$E(S_n) = n\bar{c}\bar{a}; \quad Var(S_n) = \frac{1}{n-1}\sum_{i=1}^{n}(c_n(i) - \bar{c})^2(a_n(i) - \bar{a})^2,$$

where $\bar{a} = \frac{1}{n}\sum_{i=1}^{n} a_n(i), \bar{c} = \frac{1}{n}\sum_{i=1}^{n} c_n(i)$.

When $N = m+n, a_N(i) = i, c_N(i) = I(i > m), S_n$ is the Wilcoxon signed rank statistic for two-sample data. In addition, if we let the normal quantile $\Phi^{-1}(i/(n+1))$, take the place of the score $a_n(i)$, the linear rank statistic is called the normal score.

5.4. U-statistics[6,7]

U-statistics plays an important role in estimation, and the U means unbiased.

Let P be a probability distribution family in any metric space. The family meets simple limitation conditions such as existence or continuity of moments. Assume that the population $P \in$ P, and $\theta(P)$ is a real-valued function. If there is a positive integer m and a real-valued measurable function $h(x_1, \ldots, x_m)$, such that

$$E_P(h(X_1, \ldots, X_m)) = \theta(P)$$

for all samples $X_1, \ldots, X_m$ from $P \in$ P, we call $\theta(P)$ an estimable parameter or rule parameter. The least positive integer m which meets the property above is called the order of $\theta(P)$. If f is an unbiased estimator for $\theta(P)$, the average of f about all the permutations of the variables is also unbiased. Thus, the function h should be assumed to be symmetric, that is

$$h(x_1, \ldots, x_m) = \frac{1}{m!}\sum_{P_m} f(x_{i1}, \ldots, x_{im}),$$

where the summation is concerning all the permutations of the m-dimensional vector, such that h is symmetric. For samples $X_1, \ldots, X_n$, (coming from P) and an essence measurable function $h(x_1, \ldots, x_n)$, the U-statistic is defined as

$$U_n = U_n(h) = \frac{(n-m)!}{n!}\sum_{P_{n,m}} h(X_{i1}, \ldots, X_{im}),$$

where $P_{n,m}$ is any possible permutation $(i_1, \ldots, i_m)$ from $(1, \ldots, n)$ such that the summation contains $n!/(n-m)!$ items. And the function h is called the m-order kernel of the U-statistic. If kernel h is symmetric with its all arguments, the equivalent form of the U-statistic is

$$U_n = U_n(h) = \binom{n}{m}^{-1} \sum_{C_{m,n}} h(X_{i1}, \ldots, X_{im}),$$

where this summation gets all possible $\binom{n}{m}$ kinds of combination $C_{n,m}$ of $(i_1, \ldots, i_m)$ from $(1, \ldots, n)$.

Using U-statistics, the unbiased statistics can be exported effectively. A U-statistics is the usual UMVUE in the non-parametric problems. In addition, we can make the advantage of U-statistics to export more effective estimations in the parametric problems. For example, U_n is the mean value when $m = 1$. Considering the estimation of $\theta = \mu^m$, where $\mu = E(X_1)$ is the mean, and m is a positive integer, the U-statistic

$$U_n = \binom{n}{m}^{-1} \sum_{C_{m,n}} X_{i1} \cdots X_{im}$$

is the unbiased estimation of $\theta = \mu^m$ when using

$$h(x_1, \ldots, x_m) = x_1 \cdots x_m.$$

Considering the estimation of $\theta = \sigma^2 = \text{Var}(X_1)$, the U-statistic is

$$U_n = \frac{2}{n(n-1)} \sum_{1 \le i < j \le n} \frac{(X_i - X_j)^2}{2} = \frac{1}{n-1} \left(\sum_{i=1}^{n} X_i^2 - n\bar{X}^2 \right) = S^2,$$

with the kernel function $h(x_1, x_2) = (x_1 - x_2)^2/2$, and it is just the sample variance.

Considering $\theta = P(X_1 + X_2 \le 0)$, we get the unbiased U-statistic

$$U_n = \frac{2}{n(n-1)} \sum_{1 \le i < j \le n} I_{(-\infty,0]}(X_i + X_j),$$

based on the kernel function $h(x_1, x_2) = I_{(-\infty,0]}(x_1 + x_2)$, which is just the Wilcoxon statistic for single-sample.

Here, Hoeffding Theorem is given. For a U-statistic, if $E[h(X_1, \ldots, X_m)]^2 < \infty$, then

$$\text{Var}(U_n) = \binom{n}{m}^{-1} \sum_{k=1}^{m} \binom{m}{k} \binom{nCm}{mCk} \zeta_k,$$

where $\zeta_k = \text{Var}(h_k(X_1, \ldots, X_k))$. Under the same condition, we can get the following three corollaries:

1. $\frac{m^2}{n}\zeta_1 \leq \text{Var}(U_n) \leq \frac{m}{n}\zeta_m$.
2. $(n+1)\text{Var}(U_n) \leq n\text{Var}(U_n)$ for any $n > m$.
3. For any m and $k = 1, \ldots, m$, if $j < k, \zeta_j = 0$, and $\zeta_k > 0$, then $\text{Var}(U_n)$
$$= \frac{k!\binom{m}{k}^2 \zeta_k}{n^k} + O\left(\frac{1}{n^{k+1}}\right).$$

5.5. The Sign Test[2,8]

There are many kinds of non-parametric tests for a single sample, and here are two representative tests: the sign test and the Wilcoxon sign rank test.

The thought of the sign test is very simple. The most common sign test is the test to the median. The test to the quantiles is rather too generalized. Considering the test to π-quantile Q_π of a continuous variable, the null hypothesis is $H_0\colon Q_\pi = q_0$, and the alternative hypothesis may be $H_1\colon Q_\pi > q_0, H_1\colon Q_\pi < q_0$, or $H_1\colon Q_\pi \neq q_0$. The test to the median is only a special example of $\pi = 0.5$. Let S^- denote the number of individuals which is less than q_0 in the sample, S^+ denotes the number of individuals which is greater than q_0 in the sample, and small letter s^- and s^+ represents the realization of S^- and S^+, respectively. Note that $n = s^+ + s^-$. According to the null hypothesis, the ratio of s^- to n is approximately equal to π, i.e. s^- is approximately equal to $n\pi$. While the ration of s^+ to n may be equal to about $1 - \pi$, in other words, s^+ is approximately equal to $n(1-\pi)$. If the values of s^- or s^+ is quite far away from the values above, the null hypothesis may be wrong. Under the null hypothesis $H_0\colon Q_\pi = q_0, S^-$ should comply with the binomial distribution $\text{Bin}(n, \pi)$. Because of $n = s^+ + s^-$, n is equal to the sample size when none of the sample point is equal to q_0. But when some sample points are equal to q_0, the sample points should not be used in the inference (because they can not work when judge the position of quantile). We should remove them from the sample, and n is less than the sample size. However, as for continuous variables, there is less possible that some sample points are equal to q_0 (note that, because of rounding, the sample of continuous variables is also be discretized in fact). We can get the p-value and make certain conclusions easily once we get the distribution of S^-.

Now we introduce the Wilcoxon sign rank test for a single sample. As for single-sample situation, the sign test only uses the side of the median or the quantile the data lies in, but does not use the distance of the data from the median or the quantile. If we use these information, the test may be more effective. That is the purpose of Wilcoxon sign rank test. This test needs a condition for population distribution, which is the assumption that the population distribution is symmetric. Then the median is equal to the mean, so the test for the median is equal to the test for the mean. We can use $X_1, \ldots, X_n$ to represent the observed values. If people doubt that the median M is less than M_0, then the test is made.

$$H_0\colon M = M_0 \Leftrightarrow H_1\colon M < M_0,$$

In the sign test, we only need to calculate how many plus or minus signs in $X_i - M_0 (i = 1, \ldots, n)$, and then use the binomial distribution to solve it. In the Wilcoxon sign rank test, we order $|X_i - M_0|$ to get the rank of $|X_i - M_0| (i = 1, \ldots, n)$, then add every sign of $X_i - M_0$ to the rank of $|X_i - M_0|$, and finally get many ranks with signs. Let W^- represent the sum of ranks with minus and W^+ represent the sum of ranks with plus. If M_0, is truly the median of the population, then W^- is approximately equal to W^+. If one of the W^- and W^+ is too big or too small, then we should doubt the null hypothesis $M = M_0$. Let $W = \min(W^-, W^+)$, and we should reject the null hypothesis when W is too small (this is suitable for both the left-tailed test and the right-tailed). This W is Wilcoxon sign rank statistic, and we can calculate its distribution easily in R or other kinds of software, which also exists in some books. In fact, because the generating function of W^+ has the form $M(t) = \frac{1}{2^n} \prod_{j=1}^{n} (1 + e^{tj})$. we can expand it to get $M(t) = a_0 + a_1 e^t + a_2 e^{2t} + \cdots$, and get $P_{H_0}(W^+ = j) = a_j$. according to the property of generating functions. By using the properties of exponential multiplications, we can write a small program to calculate the distribution table of W^+. We should pay attention to the relationship of the Wilcoxon distribution of W^+ and W^-

$$P(W^+ \le k - 1) + P\left(W^- \le \frac{n(n+1)}{2} - k\right) = 1,$$

$$P(W^+ \le k) + P\left(W^- \le \frac{n(n+1)}{2} - k - 1\right) = 1.$$

In fact, these calculations need just a simple command in computer software (such as R).

In addition to using software, people used to get the p-value by distribution tables. In the case of large sample, when n is too big to calculate or beyond distribution tables, we can use normal approximation. The Wilcoxon sign rank test is a special case of linear sign rank statistics, about which we can use the formulas to get the mean and variance of the Wilcoxon sign rank test:

$$E(W) = \frac{n(n+1)}{4};$$

$$\text{Var}(W) = \frac{n(n+1)(2n+1)}{24}.$$

Thus, we can get the asymptotically normal statistic constructing large sample, and the formula is (under the null hypothesis):

$$Z = \frac{W - n(n+1)/4}{\sqrt{n(n+1)(2n+1)/24}} \to N(0,1).$$

After calculating the value of Z, we can calculate the p-value from the normal distribution, or look it up from the table of normal distribution.

5.6. The Wilcoxon Rank Sum Test[2,8,9]

We'd like to introduce the Wilcoxon rank sum test for two samples.

For two independent populations, we need to assume that they have the similar shapes. Suppose that M_1 and M_2 are medians of the two populations, respectively, the Wilcoxon rank sum test is the non-parametric test that is to compare the values of M_1 with M_2. The null hypothesis is H_0: $M_1 = M_2$, and without loss of generality, it assumes that the alternative hypothesis is H_1: $M_X > M_Y$. The sample coming from the first population contains observations $X_1, X_2, \ldots, X_m$, and the sample coming from the second population contains observations $Y_1, Y_2, \ldots, Y_m$. Mixing the two samples and sorting the $N(= m + n)$ observations in the ascending order, every observation Y has a rank in the mixed observations. Denote R_i as the rank of Y_i in the N numbers (Y_i is the R_ith smallest). Obviously, if the sum of the rank of Y_i in these numbers $W_Y = \sum_{i=1}^{n} R_i$ is small, the sample values of Y will be small, and we will suspect the null hypothesis. Similarly, we can get the sum of the ranks of X's sample W_X, in the mixed samples. We call W_Y and W_X the Wilcoxon rank sum statistics.

Therefore, we can make test once we have discovered the distribution of the statistics. In fact, there are some other properties. Let W_{XY} be the number that observations of Y are greater than observations of X, that W_{XY} is the number of the pairs satisfying the following inequality $X_i < Y_j$ in the all possible pairs (X_i, Y_j). Then W_{XY} is called the Mann–Whitney statistic and satisfies the following relationship with W_Y,

$$W_Y = W_{XY} + \frac{1}{2}n(n+1).$$

Similarly, we can define W_X and W_{YX}, and we get

$$W_X = W_{YX} + \frac{1}{2}m(m+1).$$

Thus, the following equality is established.

$$W_{XY} + W_{YX} = nm.$$

The statistic W_Y was proposed by Wilcoxon,[8] while W_{XY} was proposed by Mann and Whitney.[9] Because these statistics are equivalent in tests, we call them Mann–Whitney–Wilcoxon statistics. For the null hypothesis and the alternative hypothesis above

$$H_0\colon M_X = M_Y \Leftrightarrow H_1\colon M_X > M_Y,$$

we can suspect the null hypothesis if W_{XY} is small (i.e. W_Y is small). Similarly, for hypotheses

$$H_0\colon M_X = M_Y \Leftrightarrow H_1\colon M_X > M_Y,$$

we can suspect the null hypothesis when W_{XY} is great (i.e. W_Y is great).

Here are some properties of the statistic R_i, and their proofs are simple. We'd like to leave them to the readers who are interested. Under the null hypothesis, we have

$$P(R_i = k) = \frac{1}{N}, \quad k = 1, \ldots, N; \quad P(R_i = k, R_j = l) = \begin{cases} \frac{1}{N(N-1)}, & k \neq l, \\ 0, & k = l. \end{cases}$$

Thus, the following formulas are available.

$$E(R_i) = \frac{N+1}{2}, \quad \mathrm{Var}(R_i) = \frac{N^2-1}{12}, \quad \mathrm{Cov}(R_i, R_j) = -\frac{N+1}{12}, \quad (i \neq j),$$

Because $W_Y = \sum_{i=1}^{n} R_i$; $W_Y = W_{XY} + n(n+1)/2$,
we can get

$$E(W_Y) = \frac{n(N+1)}{2}, \quad \mathrm{Var}(W_Y) = \frac{mn(N+1)}{12},$$

and

$$E(W_{XY}) = \frac{mn}{2}, \quad \mathrm{Var}(W_{XY}) = \frac{mn(N+1)}{12}.$$

These formulas are the foundations for calculating the probabilities of the Mann–Whitney–Wilcoxon statistics.

When the sample size is large, we can use the normal approximation. Under the null hypothesis, W_{XY} satisfies the following formula,

$$Z = \frac{W_{XY} - mn/2}{\sqrt{mn(N+1)/12}} \to N(0,1).$$

Because there is only one constant between W_{XY} and W_Y, we can use normal approximation for W_Y, i.e.

$$Z = \frac{W_Y - n(N+1)/2}{\sqrt{mn(N+1)/12}} \to N(0,1).$$

Just like the Wilcoxon sign rank test, the large sample approximate formula should be corrected if some ties happened.

The Kruskal–Wallis rank sum test for multiple samples is the generation of the Wilcoxon rank sum test for two samples.

5.7. The Kruskal–Wallis Rank Sum Test[2,10,11]

In the general case of multiple samples, the data has the form below,

1	2	$\cdots$	k
x_{11}	x_{21}	$\cdots$	x_{k1}
x_{12}	x_{22}	$\cdots$	x_{k2}
$\vdots$	$\vdots$	$\vdots$	$\vdots$
x_{1n_1}	x_{2n_1}	$\cdots$	x_{kn_1}

The sizes of the samples are not necessarily same, and the number of the total observations is $N = \sum_{i=1}^{k} n_i$.

The non-parametric statistical method mentioned here just assumes that k samples have the same continuous distribution (except that the positions may be different), and all the observations are independent not only within the samples but also between the samples. Formally, we assume that the k independent samples have continuous distribution functions $F_1, \ldots, F_k$, and the null hypothesis and the alternative hypothesis are as follows,

$$H_0\colon F_1(x) = \cdots = F_k(x) = F(x),$$

$$H_1\colon F_i(x) = F(x - \theta_i) i = 1, \ldots, k,$$

where F is some continuous distribution function, and the location parameters θ_i are not same. This problem can also be written in the form of a linear model. Assume that there are k samples and the size of each sample is $n_i, i = 1, \ldots, k$. The observation can be expressed as the following linear model,

$$x_{ij} = \mu + \theta_i + \varepsilon_{ij}, \quad j = 1, \ldots, n_i, \quad i = 1, \ldots, k,$$

where the errors are independent and identically distributed. What we need to test is the null hypothesis $H_0: \theta_1 = \theta_2 = \cdots = \theta_k$ versus the alternative hypothesis H_1: There is at least an inequality in H_0.

We need to build a test statistic which is similar to the previous two -sample Wilcoxon rank sum tests, where we first mix the two samples, and then find each observations' rank in the mixed samples and sum the ranks according to each sample. The solution for multiple samples is as same as that for two samples. We mix all the samples and get the rank of each observation, and get the sum of order for each sample. When calculate the rank of each observation in the mixed sample, we can average the rank of observations with the same value. Denote R_{ij} as the rank of jth observation x_{ij} of the ith sample. Summing up the observations' rank for each sample, we get $R_i = \sum_{j=1}^{n_i} R_{ij}, i = 1, \ldots, k$, and the average $\bar{R}_i = R_i/n_i$ of each sample. If these $\bar{R}_i$ are very different from each other, we can suspect the null hypothesis. Certainly, we need to build statistics, which reflects the difference among the position parameters of each samples and have precise distributions or approximate distributions.

Kruskal–Wallis[11] generalized the two-sample Mann–Wilcoxon statistic to the following multi-sample statistic (Kruskal-Wallis statistic)

$$H = \frac{12}{N(N+1)} \sum_{i=1}^{k} n_i(\bar{R}_i - \bar{R})^2 = \frac{12}{N(N+1)} \sum_{i=1}^{k} \frac{R_i^2}{n_i} - 3(N+1),$$

where $\bar{R}$ is the average rank of all observations,

$$\bar{R} = \sum_{i=1}^{k} R_i/N = (N+1)/2.$$

The second formula of H is not as intuitive as the first one, but it is more convenient for calculation. For the fixed sample sizes $n_1, \ldots, n_k$, there are $M = N!/\prod_{i=1}^{k} n_i!$ ways to assign N ranks to these samples. Under the null hypothesis, all the assignments have the same probability $1/M$. The Kruskal–Wallis test at the α level is defined as below: if the allocated number which makes the value of H greater than its realization is less than $m (m/M = \alpha)$, the null hypothesis will be rejected. When $k = 3, n_i \leq 5$ is satisfied, its distribution under the null hypothesis can be referred to the distribution tables (certainly, it is more convenient and accurate to use the statistical software), where the critical value α can be found by (n_1, n_2, n_3) (the order are unconcerned) and level α such that $P(H \geq c) = \alpha$.

If N is large, and n_i/N tends to a nonzero number $\lambda_i \neq 0$ for each i, H approximately complies with the $\chi^2_{(k-1)}$ distribution with $(k-1)$ degrees of freedom under the null hypothesis. In addition, when the sample is large, there is a statistic,

$$F^* = \frac{(N-k)H}{(k-1)(N-1-H)},$$

which approximately complies with the $F(k-1, N-k)$ distribution under the null hypothesis.

5.8. The Jonckheere–Terpstra Trend Test[2,10,12,13]

Similar with the Kruskal–Wallis rank sum, we assume there are k independent samples that have continuous distribution functions with the same shape and the location parameters (e.g. the medians) $\theta_1, \ldots, \theta_k$. Let x_{ij} denote the jth independent observation of the ith sample $(i = 1, \ldots, k, j = 1, \ldots, n_i)$. We assume that the k sample sizes are $n_i, i = 1, \ldots, k$, respectively, and the observations can be described with the following linear model,

$$\mathrm{x}_{ij} = \mathrm{u} + \theta_{ij} + \varepsilon_{ij}, \quad j = 1, \ldots, n_i, \quad i = 1, \ldots, k,$$

where the errors are independent identically distributed.

The Kruskal–Wallis test is to test whether the positions are the same or not. If the positions of samples show a rising tendency, the null hypothesis is

$$H_0: \theta_1 = \cdots = \theta_k,$$

and the alternative hypothesis is

$H_1: \theta_1 \leq \cdots \leq \theta_k$, and there is at least one strict inequality. Similarly, if the positions of samples show a descending tendency, the null hypothesis stays the same, while the alternative hypothesis is

$H_1: \theta_1 \geq \cdots \geq \theta_k$, and there is at least one strict inequality.

In the Mann–Whitney statistic, we have calculated the number whose observations of one sample are less than the observations of the other sample. With the similar thinking, we need to test every pair of samples (to make one-side test), and have to make

$$\binom{k}{2} = \frac{k(k-1)}{2}$$

tests. The sum of $k(k-2)/2$ statistics is supposed to be excellent if every statistic of the paired test is great. This is the motivation of the Jonckheere–Terpstra statistic. Making Mann–Whitney statistic for every pair of parameters, the Jonckheere–Terpstra statistic is the sum of the paired Mann–Whitney statistics concerning one-side tests. Specifically, first of all, calculate

$$U_{ij} = \#(X_{ik} < X_{jl}, k = 1, \ldots, n_i, l = 1, \ldots, n_j),$$

where #() resembles the number of the expressions meeting the conditions in the bracket. And the Jonckheere–Terpstra statistic is available by summing up all U_{ij} for $i < j$, i.e.

$$J = \sum_{i<j} U_{ij},$$

which ranges from 0 to $\sum_{i<j} n_i n_j$. When some ties happen, U_{ij} can be revised as

$$U_{ij}^* = \#(X_{ik} < X_{jl} k \in K, l \in L) + \frac{1}{2}\#(X_{ik} = X_{jl} k \in K, l \in L),$$

where $K = 1, \ldots, n_i, L = 1, \ldots, n_j$. And J can be revised as $J^* = \sum_{i<j} U_{ij}^*$ correspondingly. Similar with the Wilcoxon–Mann–Whitney statistic for two samples, when J or J^* is great, the null hypothesis should be rejected. Except using software, we can get the critical value c under the null hypothesis by searching the distribution table according to (n_1, n_2, n_3) and the test level α, which meets $P(J \geq c) = \sigma$.

But the table is inaccurate when ties exist (it works well when the sample size is large). While the sample size is beyond the table's limitation and there is no tie, normal approximation can be used, i.e. when $\min_i\{n_i\} \to \infty$,

$$Z = \frac{J - (N^2 - \sum_{i=1}^k n_i^2)/4}{\sqrt{[N^2(2N+3) - \sum_{i=1}^k n_i^2(2n_i+3)]/72}}$$

tends to be standard normal distribution.

When ties exist, the formula is more complex if the sample size is large. So we do not talk it over here. In fact, many software and programs can finish the Joncheere–Terpstra test, instead of manual calculation. The reason why we introduce the formula here is to learn its mathematical thought and background.

The Jonckheere–Terpstra test was proposed independently by Terpstra[13] and Jonckheere,[12] and Daniel[10] explained it carefully. It is more powerful than the Kruskal–Wallis test.

5.9. The Friedman Rank Sum Test[2,14–17]

At first, the complete block design is considered. There is exactly one observation in each block for each treatment. The null hypothesis of location parameters is

$$H_0\colon \theta_1 = \cdots = \theta_k$$

and the alternative hypothesis is

$$H_1\colon \text{not all of the location parameters are equal,}$$

which is as same as the Kruskal–Wllis test.

Due to the effects of blocks, we have to work out the ranks of every treatment in each block, and then sum them up for each treatment. If we denote R_{ij} as the rank of the ith treatment in the jth block, the sum of ranks according to treatment is

$$R_i = \sum_{i=1}^{b} R_{ij}, \quad i = 1, \ldots, k.$$

The aim is to compare the treatments in each block. For example, comparing the efficacy of medicines in the same age group is more reasonable than comparing them regardless of age, and comparing different materials in the same part is more reasonable than comparing them in the mixture. Here is the definition of the Friedman statistic, i.e.

$$Q = \frac{12}{bk(k+1)} \sum_{i=1}^{k} \left(R_i - \frac{b(k+1)}{2} \right)^2 = \frac{12}{bk(k+1)} \sum_{i=1}^{k} R_i^2 - 3b(k+1).$$

The second formula is not as intuitive as the first one, but it is more convenient for manual calculation. This statistic was proposed by Friedman,[14] and had been developed by Kendall[15,16] and Kendall and Smith[17] to the coefficient of concordance for multiple variables. When k and b are finite, the distribution table is available under the null hypothesis. And when looked up in the table, Q should be turned into $W = \frac{Q}{b(k-1)}$. If it is difficult to look Q up, the χ^2 distribution with $(k-1)$ degrees of freedom can be used approximately. Under the null hypothesis,

$$Q \to \chi^2_{k-1}$$

for fixed k and $b \to \infty$.

When some ties exist in the block, Q is corrected to be

$$Q_c = \frac{C}{1-Q}, \quad C = \frac{\sum_{i,j} t_{ij}^3 - t_{ij}}{bk(k^2-1)},$$

where τ_{ij} is ith tie statistic in the jth block. Under the null hypothesis, there is no distribution table for Q_c when the sample size is small, but the limiting distribution of Q_c is the same as Q.

Now let us discuss the approximate relative efficiency (ARE) of the Friedman test versus the analysis of variance under the normal assumption.

Denote the distribution of x_{ij} as $F((x-\theta_i)/\sigma_j)$. If the scale parameter σ_j is different because of the block effect, the ARE of the Friedman test versus the analysis of variance can be greater than 1 for normal distributions. If both the scale parameters and the location parameters are different because of the block effect, the ARE has the lower boundary $0.864k/(k+1)$. If the normal assumption is valid and the variances are equal, the ARE can reach $0.955k/(k+1)$. Thus, even if the normal assumption is valid, the Friedman test can be used to antagonize the heteroscedasticity in the analysis of variance, which is safe and has reasonable efficiency.

Now we compare each pair of treatment. The null hypothesis and the alternative hypothesis above are suitable to all treatments, but sometimes we want to compare two treatments. Below we introduce the method based on the Friedman rank sum test for large samples. If the null hypothesis is that there is no difference between the ith treatment and the jth treatment, the statistic of the two-sided test is $|R_j - R_i|$. If

$$|R_j - R_i| > Z_{\frac{*2}{2}} \sqrt{b(k+1)k/6},$$

the null hypothesis should be rejected with confidence level α, where

$$\alpha^* = \frac{\alpha}{k(k-1)/2} = \frac{2\alpha}{k(k-1)}.$$

The denominator here is the total number of the pairs of treatment to be compared. Obviously, the test is conservative, that is, it is difficult to reject the null hypothesis.

5.10. The Kendall Test of Coefficient of Concordance[2,14–17]

In practice, we often need to evaluate or order n individuals for many times (m times) according to some special character, e.g. m judges sorting n brand of wines, m voters evaluating n candidates, m consultancies estimating n enterprises, and gymnastics referees giving scores to the players and so on.

What we want to know is whether the m results are more or less concordant with each other. If it is very discordant, the evaluation is more or less random such that it is meaningless. We show how to judge by the following examples.

Here are 10 city ranks of air quality levels from four independent environmental research institutes.

Institute	Ranking of 10 cities(A–J) ($n = 10$)									
($m = 4$)	A	B	C	D	E	F	G	H	I	J
A	9	2	4	10	7	6	8	5	3	1
B	10	1	3	8	7	5	9	6	4	2
C	8	4	2	10	9	7	5	6	3	1
D	9	1	2	10	6	7	4	8	5	3
	36	8	11	38	29	25	26	25	15	7

There are $m = 4$ assessment agencies, which are marked with A,B,C, and D, and there are $n = 10$ cities to be assessed, which are marked from A to J. The corresponding scores are expressed in the table, and the last line is the sum of the scores (ranks) from every agency. The null hypothesis is

H_0: these assessments towards different individuals are uncorrelated or random,

and the alternative hypothesis is

H_1: these assessments towards different individuals are positively correlated or somewhat consistent.

It is reasonable to use the Friedman method[14] to test the hypothesis, and Kendall also did like that at first. Then Kendall and Smith[17] proposed the coefficient of concordance to measure the association of two variables. The coefficient of concordance can be seen as the generalization of Kendall's τ for binary variables in the multivariate case. The Kendall coefficient of concordance, which is also known as the Kendall's W, is defined as

$$W = \frac{12S}{m^2(n^3 - n)},$$

where S is the sum of squared deviations of the individual rank and the average rank. For all participating individuals (m), each assessor has an order (rank) from 1 to n, while each individual has m scores (ranks). Let R_i

be the sum of ranks of the i-th individual ($i = 1, \ldots, n$) we can get that

$$S = \sum_{i=1}^{n} \left(R_i - \frac{m(n+1)}{2} \right)^2,$$

because the sum of the ranks is $m(1 + \cdots + n) = mn(n+1)/2$, and the average rank is $m(n+1)/2$.

The Kendall coefficient of concordance can be expressed as the following form

$$W = \sum_{i=1}^{n} \frac{(R_i - m(n+1)/2)^2}{[m^2 n(n^2 - 1)]/12} = \frac{12 \sum_{i=1}^{n} R_i^2 - 3m^2 n(n+1)^2}{m^2 n(n^2 - 1)}.$$

The second expression is very convenient to calculate. The range of W is from 0 to 1 ($0 \leq W \leq 1$), and there are tables available for W and S. When n is great, we can use the large sample properties. Under the null hypothesis, m is fixed, and n tends to infinity, we have

$$m(n-1)W = \frac{12S}{mn(n+1)} \to \chi^2_{(n-1)}.$$

It means that every individual is significantly different from each other in the assessment if W is great, and the result of the assessment is reasonable. Otherwise, it means there are big differences among assessors' opinions towards all individuals, and there is no reason to reach a common assessment result.

Here is the result of the former example.

$$W = 0.8530, \quad m(n-1)W = 30.70909.$$

Under the null hypothesis, the p-value is 0.000332 by using $\chi^2(9)$ approximately. And as a result, the null hypothesis should be rejected when the value is greater than or equal to that of p, that is, the assessment is not random.

5.11. The Cochran Test[2,18,19]

Sometimes, the observations are expressed in binary response data such as "yes" or "no", "be for" or "be against", and "+" or "−". There is an investigation about villagers' opinions towards the four candidates (A, B, C, D), and 1 represents consent while 0 represents dissent. We can obtain a 4×20 matrix which only contains 0 and 1 (not shown here). If we add a column (composed of R_i) to be the sum of each row, and add a row (composed of L_j) to be the sum of each column($k = 4, b = 20$), the sum of consent "1" is $N = \sum_i N_i = \sum_j L_j = 42$.

What we concern about is to see if there are differences among the four candidates in the villagers' opinions. That is to test $H_0: \theta_1 = \cdots = \theta_k (k = 4)$, and the alternative hypothesis is H_1: all of the location parameters are not equal. If we use the Friedman test, there will be a lot of ties, and there will be many ranks which are the same. The Cochran test can solve this problem. Cochran[18] regarded L_j to be fixed, and he proposed that under the null hypothesis, L_j "1"s are equivalent in probability for each treatment j. It means that every treatment shares the same probability to get "1", and the probability relies on the fixed L_j. The value of L_j varies with the different observation j. The Cochran test statistic is defined as

$$Q = \frac{k(k-1)\sum_{i=1}^{k}(N_i - \bar{N})^2}{kN - \sum_{j=1}^{b} L_j^2} = \frac{k(k-1)\sum_{i=1}^{k} N_i^2 - (k-1)N^2}{kN - \sum_{j=1}^{b} L_j^2},$$

where $\bar{N} = \frac{1}{k}\sum_{i=1}^{k} N_i$. It is obvious that the value of Q keeps invariant no matter what we add or delete in the situation $L_j = 0$ or $L_j = k$. That is to say, the observations can be canceled when L_j is equal to 0 or k in the Cochran test. In this example, if some villagers' evaluations towards the four candidates are all 0 or all 1, these assessments will be canceled in the Cochran test.

Under the null hypothesis,

$$Q \to \chi^2_{(k-1)}$$

for the fixed k and when $b \to \infty$. Thus, we can obtain the p value by χ^2 tables when there are many blocks.

Take the incomplete block designs BIBD(k, b, r, t, λ) into consideration. We assume that the population distribution is continuous, so there is no tie. Furthermore, we assume that the blocks are independent of each other. Consider the test

$$H_0: q_1 = \cdots = q_k$$

versus

H_1: not all of the location parameters are the same.

Like the Friedman test above, order the treatments in every block, and sum up the ranks of the observations in each block for every treatment. Denote R_{ij} as the rank of the ith treatment in the jth block, sum them up according to each treatment, and we get $R_i = \sum_j R_{ij}, i = 1, \ldots, k$. The

Durbin[19] test statistic is

$$D = \frac{12(k-1)}{rk(t^2-1)} \sum_{i=1}^{k} \left\{ R_i - \frac{r(t+1)}{2} \right\}^2$$

$$= \frac{12(k-1)}{rk(t^2-1)} \sum_{i=1}^{k} R_i^2 - \frac{3r(k-1)(t+1)}{t-1}.$$

The second expression is very convenient to calculate. Obviously, the above statistic is the same as the Friedman statistic with complete block designs ($t = k, r = b$). For the test level α, if D is very large such that it is larger than or equal to $D_{1-\alpha}$, which is the minimal value satisfying $P_{H_0}(D \geq D_{1-\alpha}) = \alpha$, the null hypothesis will be rejected based on level α. The accurate distribution under the null hypothesis can only be calculated for several groups with limited k and b. The large sample approximation is often used in practice. Under the null hypothesis, for the fixed k and t, when $r \to \infty, D \to \chi^2_{(k-1)}$. The related formula when ties exist is

$$D = \frac{(k-1)\sum_{i=1}^{k} \{R_i - \frac{r(t+1)}{2}\}^2}{A - C},$$

where

$$A = \sum_{i=1}^{k} \sum_{j=1}^{b} R_{ij}^2; \quad C = \frac{bt(t+1)^2}{4}.$$

According to this formula, D is the same as the above one when no tie exists.

5.12. The Log-linear Model for Contingency Tables[2,21,22]

Suppose that the three variables in the contingency table are X_1, X_2, and X_3, which have I, J, K levels, respectively, and the frequency of the (i, j, k) lattice in the contingency table is n_{ijk}, where $i = 1, \ldots, I, j = 1, \ldots, J, k = 1, \ldots, K$ (they have the same range, when i, j, k appear in the rest of this section). Let $n_{.jk} = \sum_{i=1}^{I} n_{ijk}, n_{..k} = \sum_{j=1}^{J} n_{.jk}$ and so on.

The expected frequency is defined as $m_{ijk} = E(n_{ijk})$, then $p_{ijk} = m_{ijk} / n_{...}$. Applying the similar marks, we get $m_{.jk} = \sum_{i=1}^{I} m_{ijk}$, $m_{..k} = \sum_{j=1}^{J} m_{.jk}$, $p_{.jk} = \sum_{i=1}^{I} p_{ijk}$, $p_{..k} = \sum_{j=1}^{J} p_{.jk}$ and so on.

Let $\boldsymbol{n}$ be a vector with length IJK, whose $(i \times I + j \times J + k)$th element is n_{ijk}. Similarly, $\boldsymbol{m}$ and $\boldsymbol{p}$ are two vectors, whose $(i \times I + j \times J + k)$th elements are m_{ijk} and p_{ijk}, respectively.

Considering the complete random sampling for the fixed sample size $n_{...}$, if the population is great, the probability of one of the $n_{...}$ observations falling into the (i, j, k)th lattice is equal to p_{ijk}. Thus $\mathbf{n} \sim M(n_{...}, \mathbf{m}/n_{...})$ ($M(N, \pi)$ is the multinomial distribution with parameters N and π, N is the sample size and the sum of the elements of π is 1). The parameter space Q of parameter $\boldsymbol{m}$ is

$$\{\boldsymbol{m}|1\boldsymbol{m} = n_{...}, \boldsymbol{m} \in (\mathbb{R}^+)^{JIK}\}, \tag{5.12.1}$$

We can infer the parameter m_{ijk} based on data.

Let us think about the hypothesis testing problem. Suppose the null hypothesis H_0 is $m_{ijk}m_{...} = m_{i.k}m_{.j.}$, which is equivalent to $p_{ijk} = p_{i.k}p_{.j.}$, i.e. X_2 and (X_1, X_3) are independent. Under the null hypothesis, the parameter space of $\boldsymbol{m}$ is

$$\boldsymbol{Q}_0 = \{\boldsymbol{m}|1\boldsymbol{m} = n_{...}, \boldsymbol{m} \in (\mathbb{R}^+)^{JIK}, m_{ijk}m_{...} = m_{i.k}m_{.j.}\}.$$

The alternative hypothesis H_1 is $\boldsymbol{m} \in Q - Q_0$. Defining $\mu = \log \boldsymbol{m}$, when $\boldsymbol{m} \in Q$, we have

$$\mu_{ijk} = l + l_i^{(1)} + l_j^{(2)} + l_k^{(3)} + l_{ij}^{(12)} + l_{jk}^{(23)} + l_{ik}^{(13)} + l_{ijk}^{(123)}. \tag{5.12.2}$$

Obviously, the coefficients of formula (5.12.2) cannot be uniquely determined, that is to say, these coefficients are not estimable. In order to obtain specific numerical results, we must make some kind of constrain towards β, and there are many constraint methods (they are a variety of options in software). For example, the following constraint is selected

$$\begin{cases} \sum_{i=1}^{I} \lambda_i^{(1)} = \sum_{i=1}^{I} \lambda_{ij}^{(12)} = \sum_{i=1}^{I} \lambda_{ik}^{(13)} = \sum_{i=1}^{I} \lambda_{ijk}^{(123)} \\ \sum_{j=1}^{J} \lambda_j^{(2)} = \sum_{j=1}^{J} \lambda_{ij}^{(12)} = \sum_{j=1}^{J} \lambda_{jk}^{(23)} = \sum_{j=1}^{J} \lambda_{ijk}^{(123)} \\ \sum_{k=1}^{K} \lambda_k^{(3)} = \sum_{k=1}^{K} \lambda_{ik}^{(13)} = \sum_{k=1}^{K} \lambda_{jk}^{(23)} = \sum_{k=1}^{K} \lambda_{ijk}^{(123)} \end{cases}. \tag{5.12.3}$$

Then we can calculate these coefficient (in other words, under the condition (3), the definition from (5.12.2) definite a 1-1 mapping). If the null hypothesis is true, formula (2) will degenerate to

$$\mu_{ijk} = \lambda + \lambda_i^{(1)} + \lambda_j^{(2)} + \lambda_k^{(3)} + \lambda_{ik}^{(13)}. \tag{5.12.4}$$

We can also calculate these coefficients (output of computer software) by making appropriate constraints. For different constraints, the calculated values of the coefficients are different. That is why they are inestimable. However, under different constraints (also statistical software options), the variables' linear combinations are unchanged, so they can be said estimable.

The following table shows the corresponding log-linear models for different tests of hypothesis.

Type	Number	Sign	Model	Statistical meaning
1	(8)	(X_1, X_2, X_3)	$\mu_{ijk} = \lambda + l_i^{(1)} + \lambda_j^{(2)} + \lambda_k^{(3)} + \lambda_{ik}^{(13)}$	X_1, X_2, X_3 are independent
2	(7)	(X_3, X_1X_2)	$m_{ijk} = \lambda + l_i^{(1)} + \lambda_j^{(2)} + \lambda_k^{(3)} + \lambda_{ij}^{(12)}$	(X_1, X_2) and X_3 are independent
	(6)	(X_2, X_1X_3)	$m_{ijk} = \lambda + l_i^{(1)} + \lambda_j^{(2)} + \lambda_k^{(3)} + \lambda_{ik}^{(13)}$	(X_1, X_3) and X_2 are independent
	(5)	(X_1, X_2X_3)	$m_{ijk} = \lambda + \lambda_i^{(1)} + \lambda_j^{(2)} + \lambda_k^{(3)} + \lambda_{jk}^{(23)}$	(X_2, X_3) and X_1 are independent
3	(4)	(X_1X_3, X_2X_3)	$\lambda_{ij}^{(12)} = 0, \lambda_{ijk}^{(123)} = 0$	X_1, X_2 are independent given X_3
	(3)	(X_1X_2, X_2X_3)	$\lambda_{ik}^{(13)} = 0, \lambda_{ijk}^{(123)} = 0$	X_1, X_3 are independent given X_2
	(2)	(X_1X_2, X_1X_3)	$\lambda_{jk}^{(23)} = 0, \lambda_{ijk}^{(123)} = 0$	X_2, X_3 are independent given X_1
4	(1)	(X_1X_2, X_2X_3, X_1X_3)	$\lambda_{ijk}^{(123)} = 0$	All odd ratios are the same

The statistical meaning in the table is based on the tests which correspond to the previous models.

Because there is an interaction term, the model above is called as a hierarchical log-linear model. For example, if the interaction term $\lambda_{jk}^{(23)}$ exists,

$l_j^{(2)}, l_k^{(3)}$ must be contained in the model. The model defined by formula (3) is called a saturate model, whose number of free parameters is equal to the number of lattices in the contingency table, and the number cannot be increased.

The log-linear model for multinomial distribution associates the contingency tables with the linear models, so it is convenient for us to use a lot of linear model theories and methods we have learned. The contents of the contingency tables or the log-linear models are very rich.

5.13. Non-parametric Density Estimation[21,23,25]

The simplest estimation method of cumulative distribution function (CDF) is the empirical distribution. Let $X_1, \ldots, X_n \sim F$, where $F(x) = P(X \leq x)$ is a distribution function in the real number field. We use the empirical distribution function to estimate F. The empirical distribution function $\hat{F}_n$ is the CDF which has probability $1/n$ at each data point X_i. Formally,

$$\hat{F}_n(x) = \frac{1}{n}\sum_{i=1}^{n} I(X_i \leq x),$$

where

$$I(X_i \leq x) = \begin{cases} 1 & X_i \leq x, \\ 0 & X_i > x. \end{cases}$$

Here are some properties of the empirical distributions. For each fixed value of x, we have

$$\mathrm{E}(\hat{F}_n(x)) = F(x), \mathrm{V}(\hat{F}_n(x)) = \frac{F(x)(1 - F(x))}{n}.$$

The Glivenko–Cantelli theory shows that

$$\sup_x |\hat{F}_n(x) - F(x)| \overset{a.s.}{\to} 0.$$

And the Dvoretzky–Kiefer–Wolfowitz (DKW) inequality shows that for any $\varepsilon > 0$,

$$P(\sup_x |F(x) - \hat{F}_n(x)| > \varepsilon) \leq 2e^{-2n\varepsilon^2}.$$

(1) The principle of the kernel estimation is somewhat similar to the histogram's. The kernel estimation also calculates the number of points around a certain point, but the near points get more consideration while

the far points get less consideration (or even no consideration). Specifically, if the data are x_1, L, x_n, the kernel density estimation at any point x is

$$f(x) = \frac{1}{nh} \sum_{i=1}^{n} K\left(\frac{x - x_i}{h}\right),$$

where $K(\cdot)$ is the kernel function, which is usually symmetric and satisfies $\int K(x)dx = 1$. From that, we can find that the kernel function is one of weighted functions. The estimation uses the distance $(x - x_i)$ from point x_i to point x to determine the role of x_i when the density at the point x is estimated. If we take the standard normal density function $f(\cdot)$ as the kernel function, the closer the sample point is to x, the greater weight the sample point has. The condition that the above integral equals 1 is to make $f(\cdot)$ be a density whose integral is 1 in the expression, h in the formula is called bandwidth. In general, the larger the bandwidth, the smoother the estimated density function, but the deviations may be larger. If h is too small, the curve of the estimated density will fit the sample well, but it will not be smooth enough. In general, we choose h such that it could minimize the mean square error. There are many methods to choose h, such as the cross-validation method, the direct plug-in method, choosing different bandwidths in each part or estimating a smooth bandwidth function $\hat{h}(x)$ and so on.

(2) The local polynomial estimation is a popular and effective method to estimate the density, which estimates the density at each point x by fitting a local polynomial.

(3) The k-nearest neighbor estimation is a method which uses the k nearest points no matter how far the Euclidean distances are. Below is a specific k-nearest neighbor estimation,

$$f(x) = \frac{k - 1}{2nd_k(x)}.$$

Let $d_1(x) \leq d_2(x) \leq \cdots \leq d_n(x)$ be the Euclidean distances from x to n sample points in the ascending order. Obviously, the value of k determines the smoothness of the estimated density curve. The larger the K, the smoother the curve. Combining with the kernel estimation, we can define the generalized k-nearest neighbor estimation, i.e.

$$f(x) = \frac{1}{nd_k(X)} \sum_{i=1}^{n} K\left(\frac{x - x_i}{d_k(X)}\right).$$

The multivariate density estimation is a generalization of the unary density estimation. For the binary data, we can use the two-dimension histogram and the multivariate kernel estimation. Supposing that x is a d-dimensional vector, the multivariate density estimation is

$$f(\mathbf{x}) = \frac{1}{nh^d}\sum_{i=1}^{n} K\left(\frac{x - x_i}{h}\right),$$

where h does not have to be the same for each variable, and each variable often chooses a proper h for itself. The kernel function should meet

$$\int_{R^d} K(\mathbf{x})d\mathbf{x} = 1.$$

Similar to the unary case, we can choose the multivariate normal distribution function or other multivariate distribution density functions as the kernel function.

5.14. Non-parametric Regression[2,24]

There are several non-parametric regressions.

(1) The basic idea of Kernel regression smoothing is similar to descriptive three-point (or five-point) average, and the only difference is that we get the weighted average according to the kernel function. The estimation formula is similar to the density estimation. Here is a so-called Nadaraya–Watson form of the kernel estimation

$$\hat{m}(x) = \frac{\frac{1}{nh}\sum_{i=1}^{n} K(\frac{x-x_i}{h})y_i}{\frac{1}{nh}\sum_{i=1}^{n} K(\frac{x-x_i}{h})}.$$

Like the density estimation, the kernel function $K(\cdot)$ is a function whose integral is 1. The positive number $h > 0$ is called a bandwidth, which plays a very important role in the estimation. When the bandwidth is large, the regression curve is smooth, and when the bandwidth is relatively small, it is not so smooth. The role of bandwidths to the regression result is often more important than the choice of the kernel functions.

In the above formula, the denominator is a kernel estimation of the density function $f(x)$, and the numerator is an estimation of $\int yf(x)dx$. Just like the kernel density estimation, the choice of the bandwidth h is very important. Usually, we apply cross-validation method. Besides the Nadaraya–Watson kernel, there are other forms of kernels which have their own advantages.

(2) The k-nearest smoothing

Let J_x be the set of the k points that are nearest to x. Then we can get

$$\hat{m}_k(x) = \frac{1}{n}\sum_{i=1}^{n} W_k(x)y_i,$$

where the weight $W_k(x)$ is defined as

$$W_k(x) = \begin{cases} \frac{n}{k} & i \in J_x, \\ 0 & i \notin J_x. \end{cases}$$

(3) The local polynomial regression

In the local neighborhood of x, suppose that the regression function $m(g)$, at z, could be expanded by Taylor series as

$$m(z) \approx \sum_{j=0}^{p} \frac{m^{(j)}(x)}{j!}(z-x)^j \equiv \sum_{j=0}^{p} \beta_j (z-x)^j.$$

Thus, we need to estimate $m^{(j)}, j = 0, \ldots, p$. and then get the weighted sum. It comes to the local weighted polynomial regression, which needs to choose $\beta_j, j = 0, \mathrm{L}, p$ to minimize the following formula,

$$\sum_{i=1}^{n} \left\{ y_i - \sum_{j=0}^{p} \beta_j (x_i - x)^j \right\}^2 K\left(\frac{x_i - x}{h}\right).$$

Denote this estimation of β_j as $\hat{\beta}_j$, and we get the estimation of $m^{(v)}$, i.e. $\hat{m}_v(x) = v!\hat{\beta}_v$. That is to say, in the neighborhood of each point x, we can use the following estimation

$$\hat{m}(z) = \sum_{j=0}^{p} \frac{\hat{m}_j(x)}{j!}(z-x)^j.$$

When $p = 1$, the estimation is called a local linear estimation. The local polynomial regression estimation has many advantages, and the related methods have many different forms and improvements. There are also many choices for bandwidths, including the local bandwidths and the smooth bandwidth functions.

(4) The local weighted polynomial regression is similar to the LOWESS method. The main idea is that at each data point, it uses a low-dimensional polynomial to fit a subset of data, and to estimate the dependent variables corresponding to the independent variables near this point. This polynomial regression is fitted by the weighted least square method, and the further the point, the lighter the weight. The regression function value is got by this local

polynomial regression. And the data subset which is used in the weighted least square method is determined by the nearest neighbor method. The best advantage is that it does not need to set a function to fit a model for all data. In addition, LOESS is very flexible and applicable to very complex situation where there is no theoretical model. And its simple idea makes it more attractive. The denser the data, the better the results of LOESS. There are also many improved methods of LOESS to make the results better or more robust.

(5) The principle of the smoothing spline is to reconcile the degree of fitness and smoothness. The selected approximate function $f(\cdot)$ tries to make the following formula, as small as possible,

$$\sum_{i=1}^{n} [y_i - f(x_i)]^2 + \lambda \inf(f''(x))^2 dx.$$

Obviously, when $\lambda(> 0)$ is great, the second-order derivative should be very small, which makes the fitting very smooth, but the deviation of the first item may be great. If l is small, the effect is opposite, that is, the fitting is very good but the smoothness is not good. This also requires the cross-validation method to determine the appropriate value of l.

(6) The Friedman super smoothing will make the bandwidth change with x. For each point, there are three bandwidths to be automatically selected, which depend on the number of points (determined by cross validation) in the neighborhood of the point. And it needs not iterations.

5.15. The Smoothing Parameters[24,25]

The positive bandwidth ($h > 0$) of the non-parametric density estimation and the non-parametric regression is a smoothing parameter, which needs a method to select h. Consider the general linear regression (also known as linear smoothing)

$$\hat{m}_n(x) = \frac{1}{n} \sum_{i=1}^{n} W_n(x) y_i.$$

If the fitted value vector is denoted as

$$\hat{\mathbf{m}} = (\hat{m}_n(x_1), \ldots, \hat{m}_n(x_n))^{\mathrm{T}},$$

and $\mathbf{y} = (y_1, \ldots, y_n)^{\mathrm{T}}$, we get

$$\boldsymbol{m} = \boldsymbol{W}\boldsymbol{y},$$

where $\boldsymbol{W}$ is a $n \times n$ matrix, whose ith row is $W(x_i)^{\mathrm{T}}$. Thus, $W_{ij} = W_j(x_i)$, Then elements of the ith row show the weights of each y_i when forming the estimation $\hat{m}_n(x_i)$.

The risk (the mean square error) is defined as

$$R(h) = \mathbf{E}\left(\frac{1}{n}\sum_{i=1}^{n}(\hat{m}_n(x_i) - m(x_i))^2\right).$$

The ideal situation is that we would like to choose h to minimize $R(h)$, but $R(h)$ depends on the unknown function $m(x)$. People might think up to make the estimation $\hat{R}(h)$ of $R(h)$ be the smallest, and use the mean residual sum of squares (the training error),

$$\frac{1}{n}\sum_{i=1}^{n}(y_i - \hat{m}_n(x_i))^2$$

to estimate $R(h)$. It is not a good estimation for $R(h)$, because the data is used twice (the first time is to estimate the function, and the second time is to estimate the risk). Using the cross-validation score to estimate the risk is more objective.

The Leave-one cross-validation, is a cross-validation, whose testing set only has one observation, and the score is defined as

$$\mathrm{CV} = \hat{R}(h) = \frac{1}{n}\sum_{i=1}^{n}(y_i - \hat{m}_{(-i)}(x_i))^2,$$

where $\hat{m}_{(-i)}$ is the estimation when the ith data point (x_i, y_i) is not used. That is,

$$\hat{m}_{(-i)}(x) = \sum_{j=1}^{n} y_j W_{j,(-i)}(x),$$

where

$$W_{j,(-i)}(x) = \begin{cases} 0, & j = i \\ \frac{W_j(x)}{\sum_{k\neq i} W_k(x)}, & j \neq i \end{cases}.$$

In other words, the weight on the point x_i is 0, and the other weights are re-regularized such that the sum of them is 1.

Because

$$\begin{aligned} E(y_i - \hat{m}_{(-i)}(x_i))^2 &= E(y_i - m(x_i) + m(x_i) - \hat{m}_{(-i)}(x_i))^2 \\ &= \sigma^2 + E(m(x_i) - \hat{m}_{(-i)}(x_i))^2 \approx \sigma^2 \\ &\quad + E(m(x_i) - \hat{m}_n(x_i))^2, \end{aligned}$$

we have $E(\hat{R}) \approx R + \sigma^2$, which is the predictive risk. So the cross-validation score is the almost unbiased estimation of the risk.

In the generalized cross-validation (GCV), it is needed to minimize the following formula

$$\mathrm{GCV}(h) = \frac{1}{n}\sum_{i=1}^{n}\left(\frac{m_i - \hat{m}_n(x_i)}{1 - v/n}\right)^2,$$

where $n^{-1}\sum_{i=1}^{n} W_{ii} = v/n$, and $v = tr(W)$ is the effective degree of freedom. Usually, the bandwidth which minimizes the generalized cross-validation score is close to the bandwidth which minimizes the cross-validation score.

Using approximation $(1-x)^{-1} \approx 1 + 2x$, we can get

$$\mathrm{GCV}(h) \approx \frac{1}{n}\sum_{i=1}^{n}(y_i - \hat{m}_n(x_i))^2 + \frac{2v\hat{s}^2}{n},$$

where $\hat{s}^2 = n^{-1}\sum_{i=1}^{n}(y_i - \hat{m}_n(x_i))^2$. Sometimes, $\mathrm{GCV}(h)$ is called the C_p statistic, which was originally proposed by Colin Mallows as a criterion for variable selection of the linear regression. More generally, for some selected functions $\mathrm{E}(n, h)$, many criteria for bandwidth selection can be written as

$$B(h) = \mathrm{E}(n, h) \times \frac{1}{n}\sum_{i=1}^{n}(y_i - \hat{m}_n(x_i))^2.$$

Under appropriate conditions, Hardle *et al.* (1988) proved some results about $\hat{h}$ minimizing $B(h)$. Let $\hat{h}_0$ make the loss $L(\hat{h}) = n^{-1}\sum_{i=1}^{n}(\hat{m}_n(x_i) - m(x_i))^2$ and the risk minimal, then all of the $\hat{h}, \hat{h}_0$ and h_0 tend to be 0 at a rate of $n^{-1/5}$.

5.16. Spline Regression[26,27]

Spline is a piece wise polynomial function and has a very simple form in local neighborhood. It is very flexible and smooth in general, and especially sufficiently smooth at knots where two polynomials are pieced together. On issues of interpolation, a typically used spline interpolation is the polynomial interpolation, because it can produce similar results that occur when using polynomial interpolation with polynomials of high degree and avoid oscillation at the edges of an interval due to the emergence of Runge phenomenon. In computer drawing, it commonly uses spline coordination to draw the parameters curve, because it is simple, easy to evaluate and accurate, as well as it can approximate complex graphics.

The most commonly used spline is the cubic spline, especially the cubic B-spline, which is equivalent to a C2_ continuous composite Bézier curve. A quadratic Bézier curve is the track of a function $B(x)$ that is based on the given $\beta_0, \beta_1, \beta_2$.

$$B(x) = \beta_0(1-x)^2 + 2\beta_1(1-x)x + \beta_2 x^2 = \sum_{i=0}^{2} \beta_i B_i(x), \quad x \in [0,1],$$

where $B_0(x) = (1-x)^2, B_1(x) = 2(1-x)x, B_2(x) = x^2$ are basis. The more general Bézier curve with degree n (order m) is composed by $m = n+1$ components:

$$B(x) = \textstyle\sum_{i=0}^{n} \beta_i \binom{n}{i} (1-x)^{n-i} x^i = \sum_{i=0}^{n} \beta_i B_{i,n}(x).$$

It can be expressed as a recursive form:

$$B(x) = (1-x)\left(\sum_{i=0}^{n} \beta_i B_{i,n-1}(x)\right) + x\left(\sum_{i=1}^{n} \beta_i B_{i,n-1}(x)\right).$$

A Bézier curve with degree n is the interpolation of two Bézier curves with degree $n-1$. Notice that $B_{i,n}(x) = \binom{n}{i}(1-x)^{n-i}x^i$ and $\sum_{i=0}^{n} B_{i,n}(x) = 1$, it is called the Bernstein polynomial with degree n.

Let $t = \{t_i | i \in Z\}$ be a non-decreasing real numbers sequence of knots:

$$t_0 \le t_1 \le \cdots \le t_{N+1}.$$

The collection of augmented knots for the need of recursion is:

$$t_{-(m-1)} = \cdots = t_0 \le \cdots \le t_{N+1} = \cdots = t_{N+m}.$$

These knots are relabeled as $i = 0, \ldots, N+2m-1$, and they recursively define the essence functions $B_{i,j}$ for the ith B-spline base function of degree $j, j = 1, \ldots, n$, (n is the degree of the B-spline)

$$B_{i,0} = \begin{cases} 1, & x \in [t_i, t_{i+1}] \\ 0, & x \notin [t_i, t_{i+1}] \end{cases}$$

$$B_{i,j+1}(x) = \alpha_{i,j+1}(x) B_{i,j}(x) + [1 - \alpha_{i+1,j+1}(x)] B_{i+1,j}(x),$$

(define 0/0 as 0).

$$\alpha_{i,j}(x) = \begin{cases} \frac{x - t_i}{t_{i+j} - t_i}, & t_{i+j} \ne t_i, \\ 0, & t_{i+j} = t_i. \end{cases}$$

For any given non-negative integer j, the vector $V_j(t)$ defined on $\mathbb{R}$, which is produced by the set of all the B-spline basis functions with degree j, and is called B-spline of orders j, or in other words, the definition of B-spline based on $\mathbb{R}$ is defined by

$$V_j(t) = \text{span}\{B_{i,j}(x)|i = 0, 1, \ldots\}.$$

Any elements of $V_j(t)$ are the B-spline function of order j.

A B-spline of degree n (of order $m = n+1$) is the parameter curve which is a linear combination of B-spline basis $B_{i,n}(x)$ of degree n, that is:

$$B(\mathbf{x}) = \sum_{i=0}^{N+n} \beta_i B_{i,n}(x), \quad x \in [t_0, t_{N+1}],$$

β_i is called de Boor point or control point. For a B-spline of order m with N interior knots, there are $K = N + m = N + n + 1$ control points. When $j = 0$, there is only one control point. The number of order m for the B-spline should be 2 at least, that is to say, the degree has to be 1 at least, where linear and interior knots are non-negative, meaning $N \geq 0$.

The above figure shows B-spline basis, and the below one shows the fits by using the above spline basis to a group of simulated points.

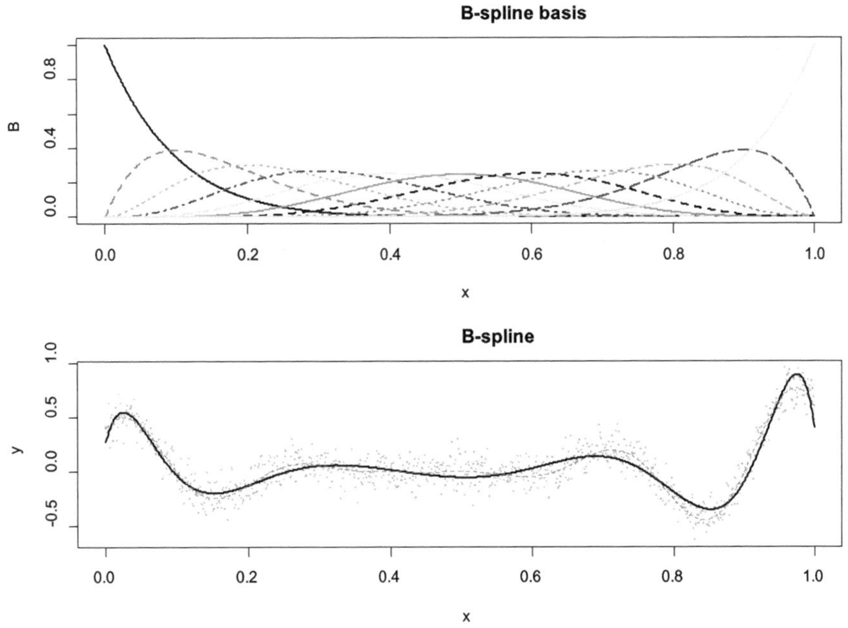

5.17. Measure of Association[13,14]

Association is used to measure the relationship between variables. The Pearson correlation coefficient is the commonest measure of association, which describes the linear relationship between two variables. But when there is strong interdependence rather than linear relationship between variables, the Pearson correlation coefficient can't work well. In this situation, the non-parametric measure is considered, in which the Spearman rank correlation coefficient and the Kendall rank correlation coefficient are commonly used. These coefficients measure the tendency of change of one variable with the change of the other variable.

The Spearman rank correlation coefficient. Suppose there are n observations, which is denoted as $(X_1, Y_1), (X_2, Y_2), \ldots, (X_n, Y_n)$, of two variables (X, Y). Sorting $(X_1, X_2, \ldots, X_n)$ according to the ascending order, the order number of X_i is called the rank of X_i, which is denoted as U_i. The rank of vector $(X_1, X_2, \ldots, X_n)$ is $U = (U_1, U_2, \ldots, U)$, and similarly, the rank of vector $(Y_1, Y_2, \ldots, Y_n)$ is $V = (V_1, V_2, \ldots, V)$. If $(U_i = V_i)$ for $i = 1, 2, \ldots, n$, it shows that Y becomes larger (smaller) as X gets larger (smaller), such that X and Y have strong association. Let $D_i = U_i - V_i$, the Spearman rank correlation coefficient can be defined as

$$R = 1 - \frac{6\sum_{i=1}^{n} D_i^2}{n(n^2 - 1)}.$$

When $U = V$, $R = 1$, and we say that there are completely positive correlation between these two groups of data. When the orders of U and V are completely inconsistent, such as when $U = (1, 2, \ldots, n)$ and $V = (n, n-1, \ldots, 1)$, $R = -1$, and we say that there are completely negative correlation between these two groups of data. In general, $-1 \leq R \leq 1$, and when $R = 0$, we say that these two groups of data are uncorrelated. When there are ties in data, i.e. some values of X or Y are equal, some correlations should be made when calculating R.

The Kendall rank correlation coefficient. Consider n observations of two variables (X, Y) again. Suppose that $X_i \neq X_j$ and $Y_i \neq Y_j$. A pair of observations (X_i, Y_i) and (X_j, Y_j), where $i \neq j$, are said to be concordant if both $X_i > X_j$ and $Y_i > Y_j$, or if both $X_i < X_j$ and $Y_i < Y_j$. In other words, if a pair of observations (X_i, Y_i) and (X_j, Y_j) are concordant, $(X_i - X_j)(Y_i - Y_j) > 0$. Otherwise, this pair of observations are said to be discordant if $(X_i - X_j)(Y_i - Y_j) < 0$. The Kendall rank correlation coefficient is defined as:

$$\tau = \frac{(number\ of\ concordant\ pairs) - (number\ of\ discordant\ pairs)}{0.5n(n-1)}.$$

Obviously, $-1 \leq \tau \leq 1$.

To judge whether two variables are correlated, we can test whether the Spearman rank correlation coefficient or the Kendall rank correlation coefficient equals to 0.

Reshef *et al.* (2011) defined a new measure of association, which is called the maximal information coefficient (MIC). The maximal information coefficient can even measure the association between two curves. The basic idea of the maximal information coefficient is that if there is some association between two variables, we can divide the two-dimensional plane such that the data are very concentrate on a small region. Based on this idea, the maximal information coefficient can be calculated by the following steps:

(1) Give a resolution, and consider all the two-dimensional grids within this resolution.
(2) For any pair of positive integers (x, y), calculate the mutual information of data which fall into the grid whose resolution is $x \times y$, and get the maximal mutual information of the $x \times y$ grid.
(3) Normalize the maximal mutual information.
(4) Get the matrix $M = (M_{x,y})$, where $M_{x,y}$ denotes the normalized maximal mutual information for the grid whose resolution is $x \times y$, and $-1 \leq M_{x,y} \leq 1$.
(5) The maximal element of matrix M is called the maximal information coefficient.

References

1. Lehmann, EL. *Nonparametrics: Statistical Methods Based on Ranks.* San Francisco: Holden-Day, 1975.
2. Wu, XZ, Zhao, BJ. *Nonparametric Statistics* (4th edn.), Beijing: China Statistics Press, 2013.
3. Hoeffding, W. Optimum nonparametric tests. *Proceedings of the Second Berkeley Symposium on Mathematical Statistics and Probability.* pp. 83–92, University of California Press, Berkeley, 1951.
4. Pitman, EJG. Mimeographed Lecture notes on nonparametric statistics, Columbia University, 1948.
5. Hajek, J, Zbynek, S. *Theory of Rank Tests.* New York: Academic Press, 1967.

6. Hoeffding, W. A class of statistics with asymptotically normal distribution. *Ann. Math. Statist.*, 1948a, 19: 293–325.
7. Hoeffding, W. A non-parametric test for independence. *Ann. Math. Statist.*, 1948b, 19: 546–557.
8. Wilcoxon, F. Individual comparisons by ranking methods. *Biometrics*, 1945, 1: 80–83.
9. Mann, HB. Whitney, DR. On a test of whether one of two random variables is stochastically larger than the other. *Ann. Math. Statist.*, 1947, 18: 50–60.
10. Daniel, WW. *Applied Nonparametric Statistics.* Boston: Houghton Mifflin Company, 1978.
11. Kruskal, WH, Wallis, WA. Use of ranks in one-criterion variance analysis. *J. Amer. Statist. Assoc.*, 1952, 47(260): 583–621.
12. Jonckheere, AR. A distribution free k-sample test against ordered alternatives. *Biometrika*, 1954, 41: 133–145.
13. Terpstra, TJ. The asymptotic normality and consistency of Kendall's test against trend, when ties are present in one ranking. *Indag. Math.*, 1952, 14: 327–333.
14. Friedman, MA. The use of ranks to avoid the assumptions of normality implicit in the analysis of variance. *J. Amer.Statist. Assoc.* 1937, 32: 675–701.
15. Kendall, MG. A new measure of rank correlation. *Biometrika*, 1938, 30: 81–93.
16. Kendall, MG. *Rank Correlation Methods* (3rd edn.), London: Griffin, 1962.
17. Kendall, MG, Smith, BB. The problem of m rankings. *Ann. Math. Statist.* 1939, 23: 525–540.
18. Cochran, WG. The comparison of percentages in matched samples. *Biometrika*, 1950, 37: 256–266.
19. Durbin, J. Incomplete blocks in ranking experiments. *Brit. J. Psychol.* (Statistical Section), 1951, 4: 85–90.
20. Yates, F. Contingency tables involving small numbers and the χ^2 test. *J. R. Statist. Soc. Suppl.*, 1934, 1: 217–235.
21. Bishop, YMM, Fienberg, SE, Holland, PW. *Discrete Multivariate Analysis Theory and Practice.* Cambridge, MA: MIT Press, 1975.
22. Zhang, RT. *Statistical Analysis of Qualitative Data.* Guilin: Guangxi Normal University Press, 1991.
23. Silverman, BW. *Density Estimation for Statistics and Data Analysis.* London: Chapman & Hall/CRC, 1998.
24. Wasserman, L. *All of Nonparametric Statistics*, Berlin: Springer, 2006.
25. Hardle, W. *Applied Nonparametric Regression.* Cambridge: Cambridge University Press, 1990.
26. Judd, Kenneth L. *Numerical Methods in Economics.* Cambridge, MA: MIT Press, 1998.
27. Ma, S, Racine, JS. Additive regression splines with irrelevant categorical and continuous regressors. *Stat. Sinica.*, 2013, 23: 515–541.

About the Author

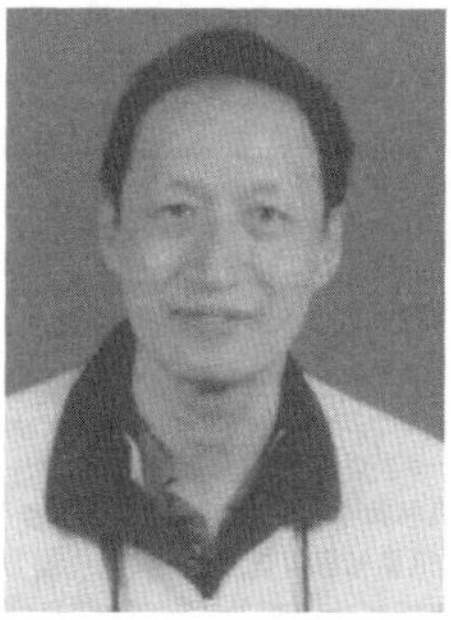

Xizhi Wu is a Professor at Renmin University of China and Nankai University. He taught at Nankai University, University of California and University of North Carolina at Chapel Hill. He graduated from Peking University in 1969 and got his Ph.D. from the University of North Carolina at Chapel Hill in 1987. He has published 10 papers and more than 20 books so far. His research interests are statistical diagnosis, model selection, categorical data analysis, longitudinal data analysis, component data analysis, robust statistics, partial least square regression, path analysis, Bayesian statistics, data mining, and machine learning.

CHAPTER 6

SURVIVAL ANALYSIS

Jingmei Jiang*, Wei Han and Yuyan Wang

6.1. Survival Analysis[1]

Survival analysis, which has rapidly developed and flourished over the past 30 years, is a set of methods for analyzing survival time. Survival time, also known as failure time, is defined as the time interval between the strictly defined and related initial observation and endpoint event. It has two important characteristics: (1) Survival time is non-negative and generally positively skewed; and (2) Individuals often have censored survival times. These features have impeded the application of traditional statistical methods when analyzing survival data. Nowadays, survival analysis has become an independent branch of statistics and plays a decisive role in analyzing follow-up data generated during studies on human life that track for chronic diseases.

Censoring is a key analytical problem that most survival analysts must take into consideration. It occurs when the endpoint of interest has not been observed during the follow-up period and therefore the exact survival time cannot be obtained. There are generally three reasons why censoring may occur: (1) An individual does not experience the endpoint event before the study ends; (2) An individual is lost to follow-up during the study period; and (3) An individual withdraws from the study because of some other reason (e.g. adverse drug reaction or other competing risk). Censored data can be classified into right-censored, left-censored, and interval-censored. The focus of this section is on right-censored data because it occurs most frequently in the field of medical research. Let survival time $T_1, T_2, \dots, T_n$ be random variables, which are non-negative, independent, and identically distributed with

*Corresponding author: jingmeijiang@ibms.pumc.edu.cn

distribution function F, and $G_1, G_2, \ldots, G_n$ be random censoring variables, which are non-negative, independent, and identically distributed with distribution function G. In the random right-censored model, we cannot observe actual survival time T_i, but only the following descriptions

$$X_i = \min(T_i, G_i), \quad \delta_i = I[T_i \leq G_i], \quad i = 1, 2, \ldots, n,$$

where $I[.]$ denotes the indicative function that indicates whether the event has occurred. Clearly, δ contains censored information. In the case of right-censored data, the actual survival time for study object is longer than the observed time.

Survival analysis is a collection of statistical procedures that mainly include describing the survival process, comparing different survival processes, and identifying the risk and/or prognostic factors related to the endpoint of interest. Corresponding analysis methods can be divided into three categories as follows:

(1) Non-parametric methods: They are also called distribution-free because no specific assumption of distribution is required. The product-limit method and life-table method are the popular non-parametric methods in survival analysis.
(2) Parametric methods: It is assumed that the survival time follows a specific distribution, such as the exponential distribution or Weibull distribution. They explore the risk and/or prognostic factors related to survival time according to the characteristics of a certain distribution. The corresponding popular parametric models include exponential regression, Weibull regression, log-normal regression, and log-logistic regression.
(3) Semi-parametric methods: They generally combine the features of both the parametric and non-parametric methods, and mainly used to identify the risk and/or prognostic factors that might relate to survival time and survival rate. The corresponding typical semi-parametric model is the Cox proportional hazards model.

6.2. Interval-Censoring[2]

Interval-censoring refers to the situation where we only know the individuals have experienced the endpoint event within a time interval, say time $(L, R]$, but the actual survival time T is unknown. For example, an individual had two times of hypertension examinations, where he/she had a normal blood pressure in the first examination (say, time L), and was found to be hypertensive in the second time (time R). That is, the individual developed hypertension between time L and R. One basic and important assumption is that the censoring mechanism is independent of or non-informative about the failure time of interest, which can be expressed as

$$P(T \leq t|L = l, R = r, L < T \leq R) = P(T \leq t|l < T \leq r).$$

That means, a single L or R is independent of the survival time T.

Interval-censored data actually incorporate both right-censored and left-censored data. Based on the above definition, $L = 0$ implies left-censored, which means that the actual survival time is less than or equal to the observed time. For example, individuals who had been diagnosed with hypertension in the first examination had the occurring time $t \in (0, R]$, with R representing the first examination time; $L \neq 0$ but $R = \infty$ represents right-censored, which means the endpoint event occurred after a certain moment. For example, individuals who had not been diagnosed as hypertension until the end of the study had occurring time $t \in (L, \infty]$, with L representing the last examination time.

Survival function can be estimated based on interval-censored data. Suppose there are n independent individuals, the interval-censored data can be expressed as $\{I_i\}_{i=1}^n$, in which $I_i = (L_i, R_i]$ denotes the interval including survival time T_i for individual i, and the corresponding partial likelihood function can be written as

$$L = \prod_{i=1}^{n} [S(L_i) - S(R_i)].$$

The maximum likelihood (ML) estimate of the survival function is only determined by the observed interval $(t_{j-1}, t_j]$, defined as a right-continuous piecewise function with its estimate denoted as $\hat{S}(\cdot)$. When $t_{i-1} \leq t < t_i$, we have $\hat{S}(t) = \hat{S}(t_{i-1})$. Several methods can be employed to realize the maximization process, such as the consistency algorithm, iterative convex minorant (ICM) algorithm, and expectation maximization-ICM algorithm.

To compare survival functions among different groups with interval-censored data, a class of methods is available based on an extension of those for right-censored data, such as weighted log-rank test, weighted Kolmogorov test, and weighted Kaplan–Meier method. An alternative class of methods is the weighted imputation methods, which can be applied for interval-censored data by imputing the observed interval in the form of right-censored data.

Most models suitable for right-censored data can also be used to analyze interval-censored data after being generalized in model fittings, such as the proprotional hazards (PH) model and accelerated failure time (AFT) model. However, it is not the case for all the models. For instance, the counting process method is only suitable for right-censored data.

6.3. Functions of Survival Time[3]

In survival analysis, the distribution of survival time can be summarized by functions of survival time, which also plays an important role in inferring the overall survival model.

Let T be a non-negative continuous random variable with its distribution completely determined by the probability density function $f(t)$, which can be expressed as

$$f(t) = \lim_{\Delta t \to 0} \frac{P\left\{\begin{matrix}\text{endpoint event occurs for individuals} \\ \text{in the interval } (t, t+\Delta t)\end{matrix}\right\}}{\Delta t}.$$

The cumulative form of $f(t)$ is known as the distribution function or cumulative probability function and denoted as $F(t) = \int_0^t f(x)dx$. Then, $1 - F(t)$ is called the survival function and denoted as $S(t)$, which is also known as the cumulative survival probability. As the most instinctive description of the survival state, $S(t)$ describes the probability that survival is greater than or equal to time t. It can be expressed as

$$S(t) = P(T \geq t) = \int_t^{\infty} f(x)dx.$$

In practice, if there are no censored observations, $S(t)$ is estimated by the following formula

$$\hat{S}(t) = \frac{\text{Number of individuals with survival time} \geq t}{\text{Total number of follow-up individuals}}.$$

The graph of $S(t)$ is called survival curve, which can be used to compare survival distributions of two or more groups intuitively, and its median survival time can be easily determined, as shown in Figure 6.3.1.

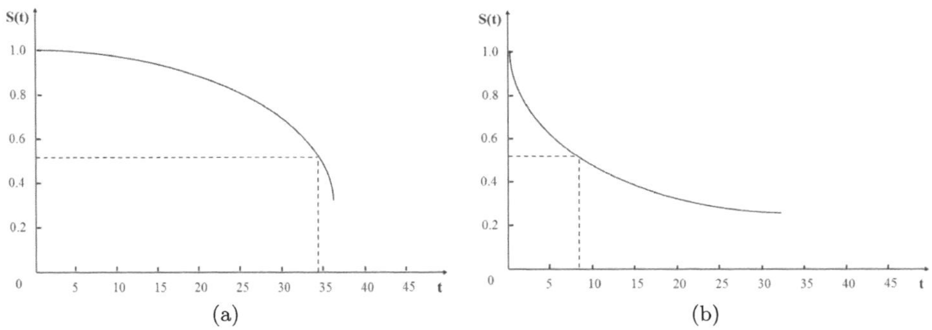

Fig. 6.3.1. Two examples of survival curve

The $S(t)$ has two important properties: (1) monotone non-increasing; and (2) $S(0) = 1$, and $S(\infty) = 0$, in theory.

The hazard function of survival time T, usually denoted as $h(t)$, gives an instantaneous failure rate, and can be expressed as

$$h(t) = \lim_{\Delta t \to 0} \frac{P(t \leq T < t + \Delta t | T \geq t)}{\Delta t},$$

where Δt denotes a small time interval. The numerator of the formula is the conditional probability that an individual fails in the interval $(t, t+\Delta t)$, given that the individual has survived up to time t. Unlike $S(t)$, which concerns the process of "surviving", $h(t)$ is more concerned about "failing" in survival process.

In practice, when there are no censored observations, $h(t)$ can be estimated by the following formula

$$\hat{h}(t) = \frac{\begin{array}{c}\text{Number of the individuals who had}\\ \text{endpoint event within } (t, t + \Delta t)\end{array}}{\text{Number of alive individuals at } t \times \Delta t}.$$

The relationship between these functions introduced above can be clearly defined; that is, if one of the above three functions is known, the expressions of the remaining two can be derived. For example, it is easy to obtain $f(t) = -S'(t)$ by definition, and then the associated expression for $S(t)$ and $h(t)$ can be derived as

$$h(t) = -\frac{d}{dt} \ln S(t) \Leftrightarrow S(t) = \exp\left(-\int_0^t h(x)dx\right).$$

When survival time T is a discrete random variable, the above functions can be defined in a similar manner by transforming the integral into the sum of the approximate probabilities.

6.4. Product-Limit Method[4, 22]

In survival analysis, the survival function is usually estimated using "product-limit" method, which was proposed by Kaplan and Meier (KM) (1958), and also known as KM method. As a non-parametric method, it calculates product of a series of conditional survival probabilities up to a specified time, and the general formula is

$$\hat{S}_{\text{KM}}(t) = \prod_{t_i \leq t} \left(1 - \frac{1}{n_i}\right)^{\delta_i} = \prod_{t_i \leq t} \left(1 - \frac{1}{n - i + 1}\right)^{\delta_i},$$

where n_i denotes the number of survival individuals with observed survival time arranged in ascending order $t_1 \leq t_2 \leq \cdots \leq t_n$, i is any positive integer that satisfies the non-censored observation $t_i \leq t$, and δ_i is the indicative function that represents whether censoring happened. In above formula, the estimate at any time point is obtained by multiplying a sequence of conditional probability estimates.

Example 6.4.1. Take regular follow-up tracks for five patients suffering from esophageal cancer after resection, and their survival times (months) are shown as follows

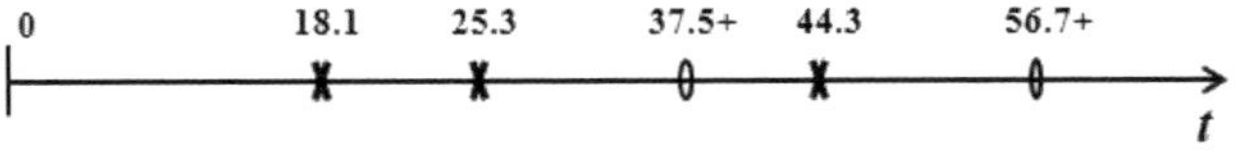

where "×" represents non-censored and "o" represents censored. The survival function value for every fixed time can be obtained as

$$\begin{aligned}\hat{S}(0) &= 1,\\ \hat{S}(18.1) &= \hat{S}(0) \times \frac{4}{5} = 0.8,\\ \hat{S}(25.3) &= \hat{S}(18.1) \times \frac{3}{4} = 0.6,\\ \hat{S}(44.3) &= \hat{S}(25.3) \times \frac{1}{2} = 0.3.\end{aligned}$$

For example, $\hat{S}(18.1)$ denotes the probability that all follow-up individuals survive to the moment $t = 18.1$. Graph method is an effective way to display the estimate of the survival function. Let t be the horizontal axis and $S(t)$ the vertical axis, an empirical survival curve is shown in Figure 6.4.1.

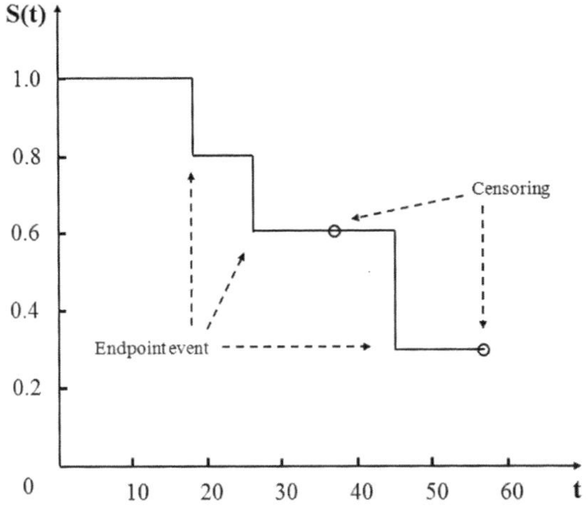

Fig. 6.4.1. Survival curve for Example 6.4.1

In practice, $\hat{S}(t)$ can be plotted as a step function since it remains constant between two observed exact survival times. For instance, the above KM survival curve for five individuals starts at time 0 with a value of 1 (or 100% survival), continues horizontally until the time death occurs, and then drops by 1/5 at $t = 18.1$. The three steps in the figure show the death event of three individuals. There is no step for censoring, such as $t = 37.5$, and "o" represents the censoring of two patients in order.

When calculating confidence intervals (CIs), it is convenient to assume $\hat{S}(t)$ approximately follows a normal distribution, and then the 95% CI of the KM curve can be expressed as

$$\hat{S}_{\text{KM}}(t) \pm 1.96\sqrt{\text{Var}[\hat{S}_{\text{KM}}(t)]}.$$

The most common approach to calculate the variance of $\hat{S}_{\text{KM}}(t)$ is employing Greenwood's formula, which is

$$\text{Var}[\hat{S}_{\text{KM}}(t)] = [\hat{S}_{\text{KM}}(t)]^2 \sum_{t_i \le t} \left[\frac{m_i}{n_i(n_i - m_i)}\right]$$

where n_i denotes the number of individuals who are still in the risk set before t, and m_i denotes the number of individuals who experienced the endpoint event before t. Moreover, the interval estimate for the median survival time can be obtained by solving the following equations

$$\hat{S}_{\text{KM}}(t) \pm 1.96\sqrt{\text{Var}[\hat{S}_{\text{KM}}(t)]} = 0.5.$$

That is, the upper limit and lower limit of the 95% CI are set to be 0.5, respectively. When the sample size is large enough, a series of sub-intervals can be constructed covering all the observed failure times, then, the life-table method can be used to calculate the survival function.

The survival functions estimated by product-limit method can also be accomplished by life-table method. The difference is that the conditional probabilities are estimated on the sub-intervals by the life-table method, whereas the conditional probabilities are estimated at each observed time point by the KM method, and the observed time point can be regarded as the limits of the sub-intervals indeed. Thus, the KM method is an extension of the life-table method in terms of two aspects: product of the conditional probabilities, and limit of the sub-interval.

6.5. Log-Rank Test[5, 23]

Since any survival function corresponding to the survival process can be expressed by a monotonic decreasing survival curve, a comparison between two or more survival processes can be accomplished by evaluating whether they are "statistically equivalent". The log-rank test, which was proposed by Mantel *et al.* in 1966, is the most popular method to compare two KM survival curves.

The null hypothesis for two-sample log-rank test is $H_0: S_1(t) = S_2(t)$. The test statistic can be computed using the following steps.

Step 1: Calculate the expected number of events for each survival curve at each ordered failure time, which can be expressed as

$$e_{1j} = \left(\frac{n_{1j}}{n_{1j} + n_{2j}}\right) \times (m_{1j} + m_{2j})$$

$$e_{2j} = \left(\frac{n_{2j}}{n_{1j} + n_{2j}}\right) \times (m_{1j} + m_{2j}),$$

where n_{kj} denotes the number of individuals in the corresponding risk set at that time in group $k (k = 1, 2)$, and m_{kj} denotes the number of individuals that failed at time j in group k.

Step 2: Sum up the differences between the expected number and observed number of individuals that fail at each time point, which is

$$O_k - E_k = \sum (m_{kj} - e_{kj}), \quad k = 1, 2$$

and its variance can be estimated by

$$\mathrm{Var}(O_k - E_k) = \sum_j \frac{n_{1j} n_{2j} (m_{1j} + m_{2j})(n_{1j} + n_{2j} - m_{1j} - m_{2j})}{(n_{1j} + n_{2j})^2 (n_{1j} + n_{2j} - 1)}.$$

For group two, the log-rank test statistic can be formed as follows

$$\text{Test Statistics} = \frac{(O_2 - E_2)^2}{\mathrm{Var}(O_2 - E_2)}.$$

In the condition of large sample size, the log-rank statistic approximately equals to the following expression

$$\chi^2 = \sum \frac{(O_k - E_k)^2}{E_k}$$

and follows χ^2 distribution with one degree of freedom when H_0 holds.

The log-rank test can also be used to test the difference in survival curves among three or more groups. The null hypothesis is that all the survival curves among k groups $(k \geq 3)$ are the same. The rationale for computing the test statistic is similar in essence, with test statistic following $\chi^2(k-1)$ distribution.

Moreover, different weights at failure time can be applied in order to fit survival data with different characteristics, such as the Wilcoxon test, Peto test, and Tarone–Ware test. Details of test statistics and methods are as follows

$$\frac{(\sum w(t_j)(m_{ij} - e_{ij}))^2}{\text{Var}(\sum w(t_j)(m_{ij} - e_{ij}))}.$$

Test Statistics	Weight $w(t_j)$
Log-rank Test	1
Wilcoxon Test	n_j
Tarone–Ware Test	$\sqrt{n_j}$
Peto Test	$\hat{S}(t_j)$
Flemington–Harrington Test	$\hat{S}(t_{j-1})^p[1 - \hat{S}(t_{j-1})]^q$

6.6. Trend Test for Survival Data[6, 24]

Sometimes natural order among groups might exist for survival data, for example, the groups may correspond to increasing doses of a treatment or the stages of a disease. In comparing these groups, insignificant difference might be obtained using the log-rank test mentioned previously, even though an increase or decrease hazard of the endpoint event exist across the groups. In such condition, it is necessary to undergo trend test, which takes the ordering information of groups into consideration and is more likely to lead to a trend identified as significant.

Example 6.6.1. In a follow-up study of larynx cancer, the patients who received treatment for the first time were classified into four groups by the stage of the disease to test whether a higher stage accelerated the death rate. (Data are sourced from the reference by Kardaun in 1983.)

Assume there are g ordered groups, the trend test can be carried out by the following steps. First, the statistic U_T can be calculated as

$$U_T = \sum_{k=1}^{g} w_k(o_k - e_k), \quad o_k = \sum_{j=1}^{r_k} o_{kj} \quad e_k = \sum_{j=1}^{r_k} e_{kj}, \quad k = 1, 2, \ldots, g,$$

where o_k and e_k denote the observed and expected number of events that occurred over time r_k in kth group, and w_k denotes the weight for kth group, which is often taken an equally spaced to reflect a linear trend across the groups. For example, codes might be taken as (1, 2, 3) or $(-1, 0, 1)$ for

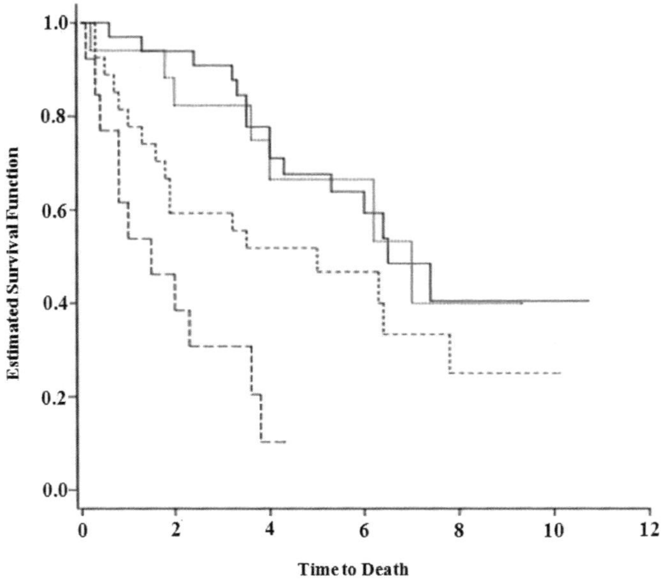

Fig. 6.6.1. Survival curves in Example 6.6.1

three groups to simplify the calculation. The variance of statistic U_T can be defined as

$$V_T = \sum_{k=1}^{g} (w_k - \bar{w})^2 e_k, \quad \bar{w} = \sum_{k=1}^{g} w_k e_k \bigg/ \sum_{k=1}^{g} e_k.$$

The test statistic W_T approximately follows a χ^2 distribution with one degree of freedom under H_0 as

$$W_T = \frac{U_T^2}{V_T}.$$

The trend test can also be done by other alternative methods. For example, when modeling survival data based on a PH regression model, the significance of the regression coefficient can be used to test whether a trend exist across the ordered groups. Then, a significant linear trend can be verified if the null hypothesis (H_0: $\beta = 0$) is rejected, with the size and direction of the trend determined by the absolute value and symbol of the coefficient.

6.7. Exponential Regression[7]

In modeling survival data, some important theoretical distribution are widely used to describe survival time. The exponential distribution is one of the basic distributions in survival analysis. Let T denote the survival time with the probability density function defined as

$$f(t) = \begin{cases} \lambda e^{-\lambda t} & t \geq 0, \quad \lambda > 0 \\ 0 & t < 0 \end{cases}.$$

Then T follows the exponential distribution with scale parameter λ. The corresponding survival function $S(t)$ and hazard function $h(t)$ can be specified respectively by

$$S(t) = \int_t^{\infty} f(x)dx = e^{-\lambda t}, \quad t \geq 0$$

$$h(t) = f(t)/S(t) = \lambda, \quad t \geq 0.$$

The above formulas indicate that the parameter λ is related to the value of $S(t)$, with a larger λ means a shorter average survival time. Moreover, $h(t)$ is a constant λ, which means that the hazard is irrelevant to the survival time.

Let T follow the exponential distribution, $X_1, X_2, \ldots, X_p$ be covariates, and the log-survival time regression model can be expressed as

$$\log T_i = \alpha_0 + \alpha_1 X_{1i} + \cdots + \alpha_p X_{pi} + \sigma\varepsilon_i,$$

where $\sigma = 1$, and ε_i denotes the random error term, $i = 1, 2, \ldots, n$ which follows the double exponential distribution with probability density function $f(\varepsilon) = \exp\{\varepsilon - \exp(\varepsilon)\}$. It is worth noting that an exponential distribution for T corresponds to a constant hazard function, which is the most striking feature of this model. Therefore, we have

$$h(t, \lambda_i) = \lambda_i = \exp\left\{\beta_0 + \sum_{j=1}^{p} \beta_j X_{ji}\right\}.$$

In essence, the above two models are completely equivalent.

Let $h_i(t, \lambda_i)$ and $h_l(t, \lambda_l)$ be the risk for observed individuals i and l, respectively, then the hazard ratio (HR) can be expressed as

$$\text{HR} = \frac{h_i(t, \lambda_i)}{h_l(t, \lambda_l)} = \frac{\lambda_i}{\lambda_l} = \exp\left\{-\sum_{j=1}^{p} \beta_j (X_{ji} - X_{jl})\right\}.$$

Since HR is irrelevant to survival time, which means that the exponential regression model is a PH model.

Methods to test the hypotheses for models and parameters include the likelihood ratio (LR) test, Wald test, and score test, of which the LR test is the most common used. For large sample, all of the three test statistics approximately follow a χ^2 distribution under H_0 as

$$X^2 \sim \chi^2(p-1).$$

To assess whether T follows the exponential distribution, an applicable and simple method is graphing, that is, by log-transforming the survival function under the exponential distribution $\ln S(t,\lambda) = -\lambda t$, a unary linear regression equation can be fitted with $-\lambda$ as slope. In practice, $S(t)$ is usually estimated by KM method. If the scatter spots present an approximate straight line, we can initially conclude that the T approximately follows an exponential distribution.

6.8. Weibull Regression[8]

The Weibull distribution is also one of the basic distributions in survival analysis, which was firstly proposed by Weibull in 1939 and can be considered as a generalization of the exponential distribution. Suppose T has the probability density function

$$f(t) = \lambda\gamma t^{\gamma-1}\exp\{-\lambda t^{\gamma}\}, \quad t \geq 0, \lambda > 0, \gamma > 0.$$

Then, survival time T follows the Weibull distribution with scale parameter λ and shape parameter γ. The involving of γ makes the Weibull regression more flexible and applicable to various failure situations comparing with exponential regression.

The corresponding survival function $S(t)$ and hazard function $h(t)$ can be specified by

$$S(t) = \exp\{-\lambda t^{\gamma}\}, \quad t \geq 0$$
$$h(t) = f(t)/S(t) = \lambda\gamma t^{\gamma-1}, \quad t \geq 0,$$

where λ denotes the average hazard and γ denotes the change of hazard over time. The hazard rate increases when $\gamma > 1$ and decreases when $\gamma < 1$ as time increases. When $\gamma = 1$, the hazard rate remains constant, which is the exponential case.

Let T follow the Weibull distribution, $X_1, X_2, \ldots, X_p$ be covariates, and the log-survival time regression model can be expressed as

$$\log T_i = \alpha_0 + \alpha_1 X_{1i} + \cdots + \alpha_p X_{pi} + \sigma\varepsilon_i.$$

The random error term ε_i also follows the double exponential distribution. Here, we relax the assumption of $\sigma = 1$, with $\sigma > 1$ indicating decreasing hazard, while $\sigma < 1$ increasing hazard with time.

Moreover, the hazard form, which is equivalent to the log-survival time form, can be defined as

$$h(t, \lambda_i, \gamma) = \lambda_i \gamma t^{\gamma-1} = \exp\left\{\beta_0 + \sum_{j=1}^{p} \beta_j X_{ji}\right\}.$$

Let $h_i(t, \lambda_i, \gamma)$ and $h_l(t, \lambda_l, \gamma)$ be the hazard functions for observed individuals i and l, respectively, then the HR can be expressed as

$$\text{HR} = \frac{h_i(t, \lambda_i, \gamma)}{h_l(t, \lambda_l, \gamma)} = \exp\left\{-\sum_{j=1}^{p} \beta_j (X_{ji} - X_{jl})\right\}.$$

Because HR is irrelevant to survival time, we can say that the Weibull regression model is also a PH model.

Parameters λ and γ are often estimated using ML method and Newton–Raphson iterative method. Moreover, approximate estimate can also be conveniently obtained by transforming the formula $S(t) = \exp\{-\lambda t^{\gamma}\}$ into

$$\ln[-\ln S(t)] = \ln \lambda + \gamma \ln t.$$

The intercept $\ln \lambda$ and slope γ can be estimated by least square method. Similar with exponential regression, the LR test, Wald test, or score test can be adopted to test the hypotheses of the parameters and models.

According to the above formula, we can assess whether T follows the Weibull distribution. If the plot presents an approximate straight line indicating T approximately follows the Weibull distribution.

6.9. Cox PH Model[9, 25]

The parametric models introduced previously assume survival time T follows a specific distribution. In practice, we may not be able to find an appropriate distribution, which impedes the application of the parameter model. Cox (1972) proposed the semiparametric PH model with no specific requirements for the underlying distribution of the survival time when identifying the prognostic factors related to survival time. In view of this, the Cox PH model is widely employed in survival analysis and can be defined as

$$h(t|X) = h_0(t)g(X), \quad g(X) = \exp\left(\sum_{j=1}^{p} \beta_j X_j\right).$$

Obviously, $h(t|X)$ is the product of two functions, where $h_0(t)$ is a baseline hazard function that can be interpreted as the hazard change with time when all covariates are ignored or equal to $0, g(X)$ is a linear function of a set of p fixed covariates, and $\beta = (\beta_1, \ldots, \beta_p)^T$ is the vector of regression coefficients.

The key assumption for Cox regression is the PH.

Suppose there are two individuals with covariates of X_1 and X_2, respectively, and no interaction effect exist between them, the ratio between the hazard functions of the two individuals is known as the HR, which can be expressed as,

$$\frac{h(t|X_1)}{h(t|X_2)} = \frac{h_0(t)g(X_1)}{h_0(t)g(X_2)} = \exp\{\beta^T(X_1 - X_2)\}.$$

Clearly, irrespective of how $h_0(t)$ varies over time, the ratio of one hazard to the other is $\exp\{\beta^T(X_1 - X_2)\}$, that is, the hazards of the two individuals remain proportional to each other.

Because of the existence of censoring, the regression coefficients of the Cox model should be estimated by constructing partial likelihood function. Additionally, the LR test, Wald test, and score test are often used to test the goodness-of-fit of the regression model, and for large-sample all these test statistics approximately follow a χ^2 distribution, with the degrees of freedom related to the number of covariates involved in the model. For covariates selection in the model fitting process, the Wald test is often used to remove the covariates already in the model, the score test is often used to select new covariates that are not included in the model, and the LR test can be used in both of the conditions mentioned above, which makes it the most commonly used in variable selection and model fitting.

There are two common methods to assess the PH assumption: (1) Graphing method: the KM survival curve can be drawn, and parallel survival curves indicate that PH assumption is satisfied initially. Moreover, the Schoenfeld residuals plot and martingale residuals plot can also be used, and PH assumption holds with residual irrelevant to time t; (2) Analytical method: the PH assumption is violated if any of the covariates varies with time. Thus, the PH assumption can be tested by involving a time-covariate interaction term in the model, with a significant coefficient indicating a violation of PH assumption.

6.10. Partial Likelihood Estimate[10,11,26,27]

In the Cox PH model, regression coefficients are estimated by partial likelihood function. The term "partial" likelihood is used because likelihood formula does not explicitly include the probabilities for those individuals that are censored.

The partial likelihood function can be constructed by the following steps. First, let $t_1 \le \cdots \le t_i \le \cdots \le t_n$ be the ordered survival time of n independent individuals. Let R_i be the risk set at time t_i and it consists of those individuals whose $T \ge t_i$, and individuals in set R_i are numbered $i, i+1, i+2, \ldots, n$. Thus, the conditional probability of endpoint event for individual i is defined as

$$L_i = \frac{h_0(t_i)\exp\{\beta_1 X_{i1} + \cdots + \beta_p X_{ip}\}}{\sum_{m=i}^{n} h_0(t_i)\exp\{\beta_1 X_{m1} + \cdots + \beta_p X_{mp}\}} = \frac{\exp\{\beta^T X_i\}}{\sum_{m \in R_i} \exp\{\beta^T X_m\}},$$

where $X_{i1}, X_{i2}, \ldots, X_{ip}$ denote the covariates. According to the probability multiplication principle, the probability of the endpoint event for all individuals is the continuous product of the conditional probabilities over the survival process. Therefore, the partial likelihood function can be expressed as

$$L(\beta) = \prod_{i=1}^{n} L_i = \prod_{i=1}^{n} \left[\frac{\exp\{\beta^T X_i\}}{\sum_{m \in R_i} \exp\{\beta^T X_m\}} \right]^{\delta_i}$$

where δ_i is a function that indicates whether individual i has the endpoint event. Clearly, $L(\beta)$ only includes complete information of individuals experiencing endpoint event, and the survival information before censoring is still in L_i.

Once the partial likelihood function is constructed for a given model, the regression coefficients can be estimated by maximizing L, which is performed by taking partial derivatives with respect to each parameter in the model. The solution $\hat{\beta}_1, \hat{\beta}_2, \ldots, \hat{\beta}_p$ is usually obtained by the Newton–Raphson iterative method, which starts with an initial value for the solution and then successively modifies the value until a solution is finally obtained.

In survival analysis, if there are two or more endpoint events at a certain time t_i, then we say there is a tie at this moment. The above method assumes there are no tied values in the survival times; if ties do exist, the partial likelihood function needs to be adjusted to estimate the regression coefficients. There are usually three ways to make adjustment: First, make the partial likelihood function exact, which is fairly complicated; the remaining two are the approximate exact partial likelihood function methods proposed by Breslow (1974) and Efron (1977). Generally, the method proposed by Efron is more precise than Breslow's, but if there are few tie points, Breslow's method can also obtain satisfactory estimate.

6.11. Stratified Cox Model[12,28]

An important assumption for Cox PH model is that the ratio of the hazard functions between any two individuals is independent of time. This assumption may not always hold in practice. To accommodate the non-proportional situation, Kalbfeisch and Prentice (1980) proposed the stratified Cox (SC) model. Assuming k covariates $Z_1, \ldots, Z_k$ not satisfying the PH assumption and p covariates $X_1, \ldots, X_p$ satisfying the PH assumption, then the categories of each Z_i (interval variables should be categorized first) can be combined into a new variable Z^* with k^* categories. These categories are the stratum, and hazard function of each stratum in the SC model can be defined as

$$h_i(t|X) = h_{0i}(t) \exp\left\{\sum_{j=1}^{p} \beta_j X_j\right\},$$

where $i = 1, \ldots, k^*$ denotes the number of strata, $h_{0i}(t)$ denotes the baseline hazard function in stratum i, and $\beta_1, \ldots, \beta_p$ are the regression coefficients, which remain constant across different stratum.

The regression coefficients can be estimated by multiplying the partial likelihood function of each stratum and constructing the overall partial likelihood function, and then the Newton–Raphson iterative method can be employed for coefficient estimation. The overall likelihood function can be expressed as

$$L(\beta) = \prod_{i=1}^{k^*} L_i(\beta),$$

where $L_i(\beta)$ denotes the partial likelihood function of the ith stratum.

To assess whether coefficient of a certain covariate in X change with stratum, LR test can be done by

$$LR = -2 \ln L_R - (-2 \ln L_F),$$

where L_R denotes the likelihood function of the model that does not include interaction terms and L_F denotes the likelihood function of the model including the interaction term. For large-sample, the LR statistic approximately follows a χ^2 distribution, with the degrees of freedom equal to the number of interaction terms in the model.

Moreover, the no-interaction assumption can also be assessed by plotting curves of the double logarithmic survival function $\ln[-\ln S(t)] = \ln[-\ln S_0(t)] + \beta X$ and determining whether the curves are parallel between different strata.

Overall, the SC model is an extension of the Cox PH model, in which the variables not meeting the PH assumption are used for stratifying. However, because we cannot estimate the influence of stratified variables on the survival time under this condition, the application range of this model is restricted to stratified or multilevel data.

6.12. Extended Cox Model for Time-dependent Covariates[13]

In the Cox PH model, the HR for any two individuals is assumed to be independent of time, or the covariates are not time-dependent. However, in practice, the values of covariates for given individuals might vary with time, and the corresponding X are defined as time-dependent covariates. There are two kinds of time-dependent covariates: (1) Covariates that are observed repeatedly at different time points during the follow-up period; and (2) Covariates that change with time according to a certain mathematical function. By incorporating the time-dependent covariates, the corresponding hazard function is defined as

$$h(t, X) = h_0(t)\exp\left\{\sum_{k=1}^{p_1}\beta_k X_k + \sum_{j=1}^{p_2}\delta_j X_j(t)\right\}.$$

The above formula shows that the basic form of the Cox PH model remains unchanged. The covariates $X(t)$ can be classified into two parts: time-independent $X_k(k = 1, 2, \ldots, p_1)$ and time-dependent covariates $X_j(t)(j = 1, 2, \ldots, p_2)$. Although $X_j(t)$ might change over time, each $X_j(t)$ corresponds to the only regression coefficient δ_j, which remains constant and indicates the average effect of $X_j(t)$ on the hazard function in the model.

Suppose there are two sets of covariates $X^*(t)$ and $X(t)$, the estimate of the HR in the extended Cox model is defined as

$$\begin{aligned}\mathrm{HR}(t) &= \frac{\hat{h}(t, X^*(t))}{\hat{h}(t, X(t))},\\ &= \exp\left\{\sum_{k=1}^{p_1}\hat{\beta}_k[X_k^* - X_k] + \sum_{j=1}^{p_2}\hat{\delta}_j[X_j^*(t) - X_j(t)]\right\},\end{aligned}$$

where the HR changes over the survival time, that is, the model no longer satisfies the PH assumption.

Similar with Cox PH model, the estimates of the regression coefficients are obtained using the partial likelihood function, with the fixed covariates being changed into the function of survival time t. Therefore, the partial likelihood function can be expressed as

$$L(\beta) = \prod_{i=1}^{K} \frac{\exp\{\sum_{j=1}^{p} \beta_j X_{ji}(t_i)\}}{\sum_{l \in R(t_{(i)})} \exp\{\sum_{j=1}^{p} \beta_j X_{jl}(t_i)\}},$$

where K denotes the number of distinct failure times; $R(t_i)$ is the risk set at t_i; $X_{jl}(t_i)$ denotes the jth covariate of the lth individual at t_i; and β_j denotes the jth fixed coefficients. The hypothesis test of the extended Cox model is similar to that discussed in 6.10.

6.13. Counting Process[14]

In survival analysis, sometimes the survival data may involve recurrent events or events of different types. The counting process, which was introduced into survival analysis in the 1970s, is an effective method for complex stochastic process issues mentioned above by virtue of its flexibility in model fitting.

Suppose there are n individuals to follow up, and $\bar{T}_i$ denotes the follow-up time of individual i, which is either true survival time or the censoring time. Let $\delta_i = 1$, if $\bar{T}_i = T_i(T_i$ is the true survival time), and $\delta_i = 0$ otherwise, and the pairs (T_i, δ_i) are independent for individuals. Therefore, the counting process is defined as

$$N_i(t) = I(\bar{T}_i \leq t, \delta_i = 1),$$

where $N(t)$ represents the counting of the observed events up to time t, and $I(.)$ is the indicator function with its value equals 1 if the content in parentheses is true and 0 otherwise. Within a small interval approaching t, the conditional probability of observing $N_i(t)$ is approximate to 0 if the endpoint event or censor occurs, and the probability is near $h_i(t)dt$ if the individual is still in the risk set, where $h_i(t)$ is the hazard function for the ith individual at time t.

Whether the individual is still at risk before time t can be expressed as

$$Y_i(t) = I(\bar{T}_i \geq t)$$

and then the survival probability from the above definition can be specified as

$$P[\mathrm{d}N_i(t) = 1|\phi_{t-}] = h_i(t)Y_i(t)dt,$$

where $\mathrm{d}N_i(t)$ denotes the increment in a small interval near t, and ϕ_{t-} denotes that all the information on the course of the endpoint event up to time t is complete, which is called filtration.

In practice, the survival data can be expressed in the form of a counting process in which i denotes the individual, j denotes the number of recording data line for the ith subject, δ_{ij} indicates whether the censor occurs for the jth data line on the ith individual, t_{ij0} and t_{ij1} denote the start and end time for each data line, respectively, and X_{ijp} denotes the value for the pth covariate for the jth data line on the ith individual. The layout of the counting process can be expressed as

i	j	δ_{ij}	t_{ij0}	t_{ij1}	X_{ij1}	$\cdots$	X_{ijp}
1	1	δ_{11}	t_{110}	t_{111}	X_{111}	$\cdots$	X_{11p}
1	2	δ_{12}	t_{120}	t_{121}	X_{121}	$\cdots$	X_{12p}
$\vdots$	$\vdots$	$\vdots$	$\vdots$	$\vdots$	$\vdots$	$\vdots$	$\vdots$
n	r_n	δ_{nr_n}	t_{nr_n0}	t_{nr_n1}	X_{nr_n1}	$\cdots$	X_{nr_np}

From the above, we can determine that multiple data lines are allowed for the same individual in the counting process, with the follow-up process divided in more detail. Every data line is fixed by the start and end time, whereas the traditional form of recording includes the end time only.

The counting process has a widespread application, with different statistical models corresponding to different situations, such as the Cox PH model, multiplicative intensity model, Aalen's additive regression model, Markov process, and the special case of the competing risk and frailty model. The counting process can also be combined with martingale theory. The random process Y_i can be expressed as $\mathrm{d}M_i = \mathrm{d}N_i(t) - h_i(t)Y_i(t)\mathrm{d}t$ under this framework, with $\lambda_i(t) \equiv h_i(t)Y_i(t)$ denoting the intensity process for the counting process N_i.

6.14. Proportional Odds Model[15,29,30]

The proportional odds model, which is also known as the cumulative log-logistic model or the ordered logit model, was proposed by Pettitt and Bennett in 1983, and it is mainly used to model for the ordinal response variables.

The term "proportional odds" means that the survival odds ratio (SOR) remains constant over time, where survival odds are defined as the ratio of the probability that the endpoint event did not happen until t and the probability that the endpoint event happened before or at time t, which can be expressed as

$$\frac{S(t)}{1-S(t)} = \frac{P(T>t)}{P(T\leq t)}.$$

For two groups of individuals with survival function $S_1(t)$ and $S_2(t)$, respectively, the SOR is the ratio of survival odds in two groups, and can be written as

$$\text{SOR} = \frac{S_1(t)/(1-S_1(t))}{S_2(t)/(1-S_2(t))}.$$

Suppose Y denotes ordinal response with j categories ($j = 1,\ldots,k(k\geq 2)$), $\gamma_j = P(Y\leq j|X)$ represents the cumulative response probability conditional on X. The proportional odds model can be defined as

$$\text{logit}(\gamma_j) = \alpha_j - \beta^T X,$$

where the intercepts depend on j, with the slopes remaining the same for different j. The odds of the event $Y\leq j$ satisfies

$$\text{odds}(Y\leq j|X) = \exp(\alpha_j - \beta^T X).$$

Consequently, the ratio of the odds of the event $Y\leq j$ for X_1 and X_2 is

$$\frac{\text{odds}(Y\leq j|X_1)}{\text{odds}(Y\leq j|X_2)} = \exp(-\beta^T(X_1 - X_2)).$$

which is a constant independent of j and reflects the "proportional odds".

The most common proportional odds model is the log-logistic model, with its survival function expressed as

$$S(t) = \frac{1}{1+\lambda t^p},$$

where λ and p denote the scale parameter and shape parameter, respectively. The corresponding survival odds are written as

$$\frac{S(t)}{1-S(t)} = \frac{1/(1+\lambda t^p)}{(\lambda t^p)/(1+\lambda t^p)} = \frac{1}{\lambda t^p}.$$

The proportional odds form of the log-logistic regression model can be formulated by reparametrizing λ as

$$\lambda = \exp(\beta_0 + \beta^T X).$$

To assess whether the survival time follow log-logistic distribution, logarithmic transformation of survival odds can be used

$$\ln((\lambda t^p)^{-1}) = -\ln(\lambda) - p\ln(t).$$

Obviously, $\ln((\lambda t^p)^{-1})$ is a linear function of $\ln(t)$, where $-\ln(\lambda)$ is the intercept term and $-p$ is the slope. If the spots present a linear relationship approximately, we can conclude initially the data follow the log-logistic distribution. Additionally, if the curves from the two groups to be compared are parallel, the proportional odds assumption is satisfied.

Both the PH model and proportional odds model belong to the linear transformation model, which can be summarized as the linear relationship between an unknown function of the survival time and covariates X, and can be expressed as

$$H(T) = -\beta X + \varepsilon,$$

where $H(.)$ denotes the unknown monotone increasing function, β denotes the unknown regression coefficients, and ε denotes the random error term that follows the fixed parameter distribution. If ε follows the extreme value distribution, the model is the PH model; and if parameter ε follows the logistic distribution, the model is the proportional odds model.

6.15. Recurrent Events Models[16]

Thus far, we have introduced the analytical methods that allow endpoint event to occur only once, and the individuals are not involved in the risk set once the endpoint events of interest occur. However, in practice, the endpoint events can occur several times in the follow-up duration, such as the recurrence of a tumor after surgery or recurrence of myocardial infarction. In such conditions, a number of regression models are available, among which, Prentice, Williams, and Peterson (PWP), Anderson and Gill (AG), and Wei, Lin and Weissfeld (WLW) models are most common methods. All the three models are PH models, and the main difference lies in the definition of the risk set when constructing the partial likelihood function.

PWP proposed two extended models in 1981, in which the individuals are stratified by the number and time of the recurrent events. In the first PWP model, the follow-up time starts at the beginning of the study and the hazard function of the i-th individual can be defined as

$$h(t|\beta_s, X_i(t)) = h_{0s}(t)\exp\{\beta_s^T X_i(t)\},$$

where the subscript s denotes the stratum that the individual is at time t. The first stratum involves the individuals who are censored without recurrence or have experienced at least one recurrence of the endpoint events, and the second stratum involves individuals who have experienced at least two recurrences or are censored after experiencing the first recurrence. The subsequent strata can be defined similarly. The term $h_{0s}(t)$ denotes the baseline hazard function in stratum s. Obviously, the regression coefficient β_s is stratum-specific, and can be estimated by constructing the partial likelihood function and the ML method is applied in the estimation process. The partial likelihood function can be defined as

$$L(\beta) = \prod_{s\geq 1}\prod_{i=1}^{d_s} \frac{\exp\{\beta_s^T X_{si}(t_{si})\}}{\sum_{l\in R(t_{si},s)} \exp\{\beta_s^T X_{sl}(t_{si})\}},$$

where $t_{s1} < \cdots < t_{sd_s}$ represents the ordered failure times in stratum s; $X_{si}(t_{si})$ denotes the covariate vector of an individual in stratum s that fails at time t_{si}; $R(t,s)$ is the risk set for the s th stratum before time t; and all the follow-up individuals in $R(t,s)$ have experienced the first $s-1$ recurrent events.

The second model of PWP is different in the time point when defining the baseline hazard function, and it can be defined in terms of a hazard function as

$$h(t|\beta_s, X_i(t)) = h_{0s}(t - t_{s-1}) \exp\{\beta_s^T X_i(t)\},$$

where t_{s-1} denotes the time of occurrence of the previous event. This model is concerned more about the gap time, which is defined as the time period between two consecutive recurrent events or between the occurrence of the last recurrent event time and the end of the follow-up.

Anderson and Gill proposed the AG model in 1982, which assumes that all events are of the same type and are independent of each other. The risk set for the likelihood function construction contains all the individuals who are still being followed, regardless of how many events they have experienced before that time. The multiplicative hazard function for the ith individual can be expressed as

$$h(t, X_i) = Y_i(t) h_0(t) \exp\{\beta^T X_i(t)\},$$

where $Y_i(t)$ is the indicator function that indicates whether the ith individual is still at risk at time t. Wei, Lin, and Weissfeld proposed the WLW model in 1989, and applied the marginal partial likelihood to analyze recurrent events. It assumes that the failures may be recurrences of the same type of event or events of different natures, and each stratum in the model contains all the individuals in the study.

6.16. Competing Risks[17]

In survival analysis, there is usually a restriction that only one cause of an endpoint event exists for all follow-up individuals. However, in practice, the endpoint event for the individuals may have several causes. For example, patients who have received heart transplant surgery might die from heart failure, cancer, or other accidents with heart failure as the primary cause of interest. Therefore, causes other than heart failure are considered as competing risks. For survival data with competing risks, independent processes should be proposed to model the effect of covariates for the specific cause of failure.

Let T denote the survival time, X denote the covariates, and J denote competing risks. The hazard function of the jth cause of the endpoint event can be defined as

$$h_j(t, X) = \lim_{\Delta t \to 0} \frac{P(t \leq T < t + \Delta t, J = j | T \geq t, X)}{\Delta t},$$

where $h_j(t, x)(j = 1, \ldots, m)$ denotes the instantaneous failure rate at moment t for the jth cause. This definition of hazard function is similar to that in other survival models with only cause $J = j$. The overall hazard of the endpoint event is the sum of all the type-specific hazards, which can be expressed as

$$h(t, X) = \sum_j h_j(t, X).$$

The construction of above formula requires that the causes of endpoint event are independent of each other, and then the survival function for the jth competing risk can be defined as

$$S_j(t, X) = \exp\left\{ - \int_0^t h_j(u, X) du \right\}.$$

The corresponding hazard function in the PH assumption is defined as

$$h_j(t, X) = h_{0j}(t) \exp\{\beta_j^T X\}.$$

The expression can be further extended to time-dependent covariates by changing the fixed covariate X into the time-dependent $X(t)$. The partial likelihood function for the competing risks model can be defined as

$$L = \prod_{j=1}^{m} \prod_{i=1}^{k_j} \frac{\exp\{\beta_j^T X_{ji}(t_{ji})\}}{\sum_{l \in R(t_{ji})} \exp\{\beta_j^T X_l(t_{ji})\}},$$

where $R(t_{ij})$ denotes the risk set right before time t_{ij}. The coefficients estimation and significant test of covariates can be performed in the same way as described previously in 6.10, by treating failure times of types other than the jth cause as censored observations. The key assumption for a competing risks model is that the occurrence of one type of endpoint event removes the individual from the risk of all other types of endpoint events, and then the individual no longer contributes to the successive risk set. To summarize, different types of models can be fitted for different causes of endpoint event. For instance, we can build a PH model for cardiovascular disease and a parametric model for cancer at the same time in a mortality study.

The coefficient vector β_j in the model can only represent the effect of covariates for the endpoint event under the condition of the jth competing risk, with other covariates not related to the jth competing risk set to 0. If the coefficients β_j are equal for all competing risks, the competing risks model is degenerated as a PH model at this time.

6.17. AFT Models[18]

The AFT models are alternatives to the Cox PH model, and it assumes that the effect of the covariates is multiplicative (proportional) with respect to survival time.

Let T_0 represent the survival time under control condition, and T represent the survival time of exposure to a risk factor, which modifies the survival time T_0 to T for some fixed scaling parameter γ, and it can be expressed as

$$T = \gamma T_0,$$

where γ indicates the accelerated factor, through which the investigator can evaluate the effect of risk factor on the survival time. Moreover, the survival functions are related by

$$S(t) = S_0(\gamma t).$$

Obviously, the accelerated factor describes the "stretching" or "contraction" of survival functions when comparing one group to another.

AFT models can be generally defined in the form of

$$\log(T) = -\beta^T X + \varepsilon,$$

where ε denotes the random error term with un-specified distribution. Obviously, the logarithm of the survival time is linear to the covariates and applicable for comparison of survival times, and the parameter is easy to interpret because they directly refer to the level of $\log(T)$. However, the model is not quite as easy to fit as the regression model introduced previously (with censored observations), and the asymptotic properties of the estimate is also more difficult to obtain. Therefore, the specification can be presented using hazard function for T given X

$$h(t) = h_0(t\exp(\beta^T X))\exp(\beta^T X),$$

where $h_0(t)$ is the hazard associated with the un-specified error distribution $\exp(\varepsilon)$. Obviously, covariates or explanatory variables had been incorporated into γ, and $\exp\{\beta^T X\}$ is regarded as the accelerated factor, which acts multiplicatively on survival time so that the effect of covariates accelerates or decelerates time to failure relative to $h_0(t)$.

Due to the computational difficulties for $h_0(t)$, AFT models are mainly used based on parametric approaches with log-normal, gamma, and inverse Gaussian baseline hazards, and some of them can satisfy the AFT assumption and PH assumption simultaneously, such as the exponential model and Weibull model. Take the exponential regression as example, the hazard function and survival function in the PH model are $h(t) = \lambda = \exp\{\beta_0 + \beta^T X\}$ and $S(t) = \exp\{-\lambda t\}$, respectively, and the survival time is expressed as $t = [-\ln(S(t))] \times (1/\lambda)$. In the ART model, when we assume that $(1/\lambda) = \exp\{\alpha_0 + \alpha X\}$, the accelerated factor can be stated as

$$\gamma = \frac{[-\ln(S(t))]\exp\{\alpha_0 + \alpha\}}{[-\ln(S(t))]\exp\{\alpha_0\}} = \exp\{\alpha\}.$$

Based on the above expression, we can deduce that the HR and accelerated factor are the inverse of each other. For HR < 1, this factor is protective and beneficial for the extension of the survival time. Therefore, although differences in underlying assumptions exist between the PH model and AFT model, the expressions of the models are the same in nature in the framework of the exponential regression model.

6.18. Shared Frailty Model[19,31]

In survival analysis, covariates are not always measurable or predictable in all cases. The influence of these covariates is known as the hidden difference in the model, and Vaupel *et al.* (1979) defined it as the frailty of the sample individuals, which has the effect on the individual survival time in subgroups. When the frailty factor is considered in the survival model, the variance caused by a random effect should be reduced for the hidden differences to come out. Therefore, frailty models contain an extra component designed to account for individual-level differences in the hazard, and are widely used to describe the correlation of the survival time between different subgroup individuals.

Shared frailty model, as an important type of frailty model, is the extension of the PH model in the condition of the frailty, which assumes clusters of individuals share the same frailty. For example, individuals from the same family may share some unobserved genetic or environmental factors, and sharing the same frailty with family members accounts for such similarities.

In the shared frailty model, the hazard function of the ith individual in the jth subgroup is defined as

$$h_{ji}(t) = Z_j h_0(t) \exp\{\beta^T X_{ji}\},$$

where $h_0(t)$ denotes the baseline hazard function, which determines the property of the model (parametric or semi-parametric); X_{ji} denotes the main effects, β denotes the fixed coefficient; Z_j denotes the frailty value in the jth subgroup, and the individuals in the same subgroup share the same Z_j, so it is known as the shared frailty factor, which can reflect the effect of individual correlation in different subgroups. An important assumption here is that there is correlation of the survival time between different subgroups.

The survival function in the jth subgroup is defined as

$$\begin{aligned} S(t_{j1}, \ldots, t_{jn}|X_j, Z_j) &= S(t_{j1}|X_{j1}, Z_j) \cdots S(t_{jn}|X_{jn}, Z_j) \\ &= \exp\left\{-Z_j \sum_{i=1}^{n_i} M_0(t_{ji}) \exp\{\beta^T X_{ji}\}\right\}, \end{aligned}$$

where $M_0(t) = \int_0^t h_0(s)$ is the cumulated baseline hazard function.

The most common shared frailty model is the gamma model, in which the shared frailty factor Z_j follows an independent gamma distribution with parametric and non-parametric forms. The piecewise constant model is another type of shared frailty model, and there are two ways to divide the observed time: by setting the endpoint event as the lower of every interval or by making the observed interval independent of the observed time point. Moreover, shared frailty models include other forms, such as log-normal, positive stable, and compound Poisson model. The shared frailty model can also be used to analyze the recurrent event data with the frailty factor, and the shared frailty in the model represents the cluster of the observed individuals, which refers to the specific variance caused by an unobserved factor within the individual correlation.

6.19. Additive Hazard Models[20]

When fitting the Cox model in survival analysis, the underlying PH assumption might not always hold in practice. For instance, the treatment effect might deteriorate over time. In this situation, additive hazard model may provide a useful alternative to the Cox model by incorporating the time-varying covariate effect.

There are several forms for additive hazard model, among which Aalen's additive regression model (1980) is most commonly used. The hazard function for an individual at time t is defined as

$$h(t, X, \beta(t)) = \beta_0(t) + \beta_1(t)X_1 + \cdots + \beta_p(t)X_p,$$

where $\beta_j(t)(j = 0, 1, \ldots, p)$ is a vector of coefficients, can change over time and represent additive increase or decrease of HR from covariates that also can be time-dependent. The cumulated hazard function can be written as

$$\begin{aligned} H(t, X, B(t)) &= \int_0^t h(t, X, \beta(u))du, \\ &= \sum_{j=0}^{p} X_j \int_0^t \beta_j(u)du = \sum_{j=0}^{p} X_j B_j(t), \end{aligned}$$

where $B_j(t)$ denotes the cumulated coefficients up to time t for the jth covariate, which is easier to estimate compared with $\beta_j(t)$, and can be expressed as

$$\hat{B}(t) = \sum_{t_j \leq t} (X_j^T X_j)^{-1} X_j^T Y_j,$$

where X_j denotes the $n \times (p+1)$ dimension matrix, in which the ith line indicates whether the ith individual is at risk, which equals 1 if the individual is still at risk, and Y_j denotes the $1 \times n$ dimension vector that indicates whether the individual is censored. Obviously, the cumulated regression coefficients vary with time. The cumulated hazard function for ith individual up to time t can be estimated by

$$\hat{H}(t, X_i, \hat{B}(t)) = \sum_{j=0}^{p} X_{ij} \hat{B}_j(t).$$

Correspondingly, the survival function with covariates adjusted can be estimated

$$\hat{S}(t, X_i, \hat{B}(t)) = \exp\{\hat{H}(t, X_i, \hat{B}(t))\}.$$

The additive hazard regression model can be used to analyze recurrent events as well as the clustered survival data, in which the endpoint event is recorded for members of clusters. There are several extensions for Aalen's additive hazard regression model, such as extending $\beta_0(t)$ to be a non-negative function, or allowing the effect to be constant for one or several covariates in the model.

There are several advantages for additive hazard model over Cox PH model. First, the additive hazard model theoretically allows the effect of covariate change over time; second, the additive model can be adapted to the situation that uncertain covariates can be dropped from or added to the model, which is not allowed in Cox model. Moreover, the additive hazard model is more flexible and can be well combined with martingale theory, in which the accurate martingale value can be obtained during the process of estimating the parameter and residuals, and transforming the empirical matrix.

6.20. Marginal Model for Multivariate Survival[21]

Multivariate survival data arise in survival analysis when each individual may experience several events or artificial groups exist among individuals, thus dependence between failure times might be induced. For example, the same carcinogens influenced by many factors may result in different tumor manifestation times and stages, and the onset of diseases among family members. Obviously, in such cases, Cox PH model is no longer suitable, and a class of marginal models were therefore developed to process the multivariate survival data thus far, among which WLW is the most commonly used.

WLW model is a marginal model for multivariate survival data based on the Cox PH model. Assuming there are n individuals with K dimension survival time $T_{ki}(i = 1, \ldots, n; k = 1, \ldots, K)$, and let C_{ki} denote the random censoring variables corresponding to T_{ki}, then each record of multivariate survival data can be expressed as

$$(\tilde{T}_{ki}, \delta_{ki}, Z_{ki}\colon i = 1, \ldots, n;\ k = 1, \ldots, K),$$

where $\tilde{T}_{ki} = \min\{T_{ki}, C_{ki}\}$ denote the observed survival time, and $\delta_{ki} = I$ $(T_{ki} \leq C_{ki})$ represents non-censoring indicative variables, and vector $Z_{ki}(t)$ denotes p-dimensional covariates.

The marginal hazard function at T_{ki} for WLW regression model is defined as

$$h_{ki}(t|Z_{ki}) = h_{k0}(t)\exp\{\beta_k^T Z_{ki}(t)\}, \quad t \geq 0,$$

where $h_{k0}(t)$ denotes the baseline hazard function, and β_k denotes the regression coefficients of kth group, respectively.

The WLW model assumes that T_{ki} for n individuals satisfies PH assumption for each group. The covariance matrix of the regression coefficients represents the correlation between the survival data of K groups. Marginal partial likelihood function is used to estimate coefficients, which is expressed as

$$L_k(\beta_k) = \prod_{i=1}^{n} \left(\frac{\exp(\beta_k^T Z_{ki}(\tilde{T}_{ki}))}{\sum_{j \in R_k(\tilde{T}_{ki})} \exp(\beta_k^T Z_{ki}(\tilde{T}_{ki}))} \right)^{\delta_{ki}},$$

$$= \prod_{i=1}^{n} \left(\frac{\exp(\beta_k^T Z_{ki}(\tilde{T}_{ki}))}{\sum_{j=1}^{n} Y_{ki}(\tilde{T}_{ki}) \exp(\beta_k^T Z_{ki}(\tilde{T}_{ki}))} \right)^{\delta_{ki}}.$$

And then we take partial derivatives of the logarithm of L with respect to each parameter in the model to obtain

$$U_k(\beta_k) = \frac{\partial \log L_k(\beta_k)}{\partial \beta_k}.$$

The solutions of the above equations are denoted by $\hat{\beta}$.

Lee, Wei and Amato extended the WLW to LWA model by setting all K baseline hazard functions to the same value. Moreover, the mixed baseline hazard proportional hazard (MBH-PH) model is the marginal PH model based on a "mixed" baseline hazard function, which combines the WLW and LWA models regardless of whether the baseline hazard function is the same.

References

1. Wang, QH. *Statistical Analysis of Survival Data.* Beijing: Sciences Press, 2006.
2. Chen, DG, Sun, J, Peace, KE. *Interval-Censored Time-to-Event Data: Methods and Applications.* London: Chapman and Hall, CRC Press, 2012.
3. Kleinbaum, DG, Klein, M. *Survival Analysis: A Self-Learning Text.* New York: Spring Science+Business Media, 2011.
4. Lawless, JF. *Statistical Models and Methods for Lifetime Data.* John Wiley & Sons, 2011.
5. Bajorunaite, R, Klein, JP. Two sample tests of the equality of two cumulative incidence functions. *Comp. Stat. Data Anal.*, 2007, 51: 4209–4281.
6. Klein, JP, Moeschberger, ML. *Survival Analysis: Techniques for Censored and Truncated Data.* Berlin: Springer Science & Business Media, 2003.
7. Lee, ET, Wang, J. *Statistical Methods for Survival Data Analysis.* John Wiley & Sons, 2003.
8. Jiang, JM. *Applied Medical Multivariate Statistics.* Beijing: Science Press, 2014.
9. Chen, YQ, Hu, C, Wang, Y. Attributable risk function in the proportional hazards model for censored time-to-event. *Biostatistics*, 2006, 7(4): 515–529.
10. Bradburn, MJ, Clark, TG, Love, SB, *et al.* Survival analysis part II: Multivariate data analysis — An introduction to concepts and methods. *Bri. J. Cancer*, 2003, 89(3): 431–436.

11. Held, L, Sabanes, BD. *Applied Statistical Inference: Likelihood and Bayes.* Berlin: Springer, 2014.
12. Gorfine, M, Hsu, L, Prentice, RL. Nonparametric correction for covariate measurement error in a stratified Cox model. *Biostatistics*, 2004, 5(1): 75–87.
13. Fisher, LD, Lin, DY. Time-dependent covariates in the Cox proportional-hazards regression model. *Ann. Rev. Publ. Health.* 1999, 20: 145–157.
14. Fleming, TR, Harrington, DP. *Counting Processes & Survival Analysis, Applied Probability and Statistics.* New York: Wiley, 1991.
15. Sun, J, Sun, L, Zhu, C. Testing the proportional odds model for interval censored data. *Lifetime Data Anal.* 2007, 13: 37–50.
16. Prentice, RL, Williams, BJ, Peterson, AV. On the regression analysis of multivariate failure time data. Biometrika, 1981, 68: 373–379.
17. Beyersmann, J, Allignol, A, Schumacher, M. *Competing Risks and Multistate Models with R.* New York: Springer-Verlag 2012.
18. Bedrick, EJ, Exuzides, A, Johnaon, WO, *et al.* Predictive influence in the accelerated failure time model. *Biostatistics*, 2002, 3(3): 331–346.
19. Wienke A. *Frailty Models in Survival Analysis.* Chapman & Hall, Boca Raton, FL, 2010.
20. Kulich, M, Lin, D. Additive hazards regression for case-cohort studies. *Biometrika*, 2000, 87: 73–87.
21. Peng, Y, Taylor, JM, Yu, B. A marginal regression model for multivariate failure time data with a surviving fraction. *Lifetime Data Analysis*, 2007, 13(3): 351–369.
22. Kaplan EL, Meier P. Nonparametric estimation from incomplete observations. *Journal of the American Statistical Association*, 1958, 53(282): 457–481.
23. Mantel N, *et al.* Evaluation of survival data and two new rank-order statistics arising in its consideration. *Cancer Chemotherapy Reports*, 1966, 50, 163–170.
24. Kardaun O. Statistical analysis of male larynx cancer patients: A case study. *Statistical Nederlandica*, 1983, 37: 103–126.
25. Cox DR. Regression Models and Life Tables (with Discussion). Journal of the Royal Statistical Society, 1972, Series B, 34: 187–220.
26. Breslow NE, Crowley J. A large-sample study of the life table and product limit estimates under random censorship. *The Annals of Statistics*, 1974, 2, 437–454.
27. Efron B. The efficiency of Cox's likelihood function for censored data. *Journal of the Royal Statistical Society*, 1977, 72, 557–565.
28. Kalbfleisch JD, Prentice RL. *The Statistical Analysis of Failure Time Data.* New York: 1980.
29. Pettitt AN. Inference for the linear model using a likelihood based on ranks. *Journal of the Royal Statistical Society*, 1982, Series B, 44, 234–243.
30. Bennett S. Analysis of survival data by the proportional odds model. *Statistics in Medicine*, 1983, 2, 273–277.
31. Vaupel JW, Manton KG, Stallard E. The impact of heterogeneity in individual frailty on the dynamics of mortality. *Demography*, 1979, 16, 439–454.

About the Author

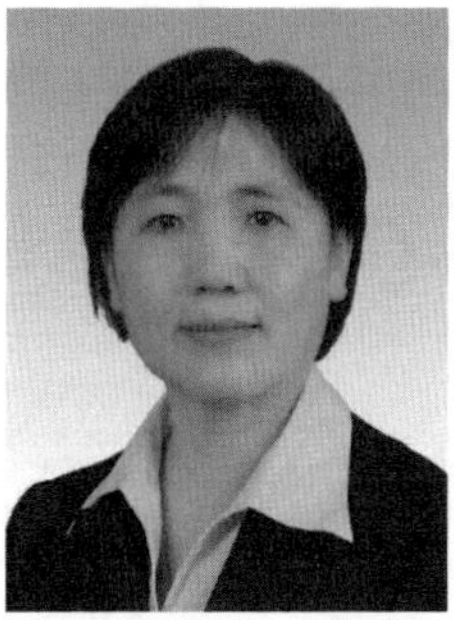

Jingmei Jiang, PhD, is Professor at the Department of Epidemiology and Biostatistics, Institute of Basic Medical Sciences Chinese Academy of Medical Sciences & School of Basic Medicine Peking Union Medical College. She is the current head of statistics courses and Principal Investigator of statistical research. She has been in charge of projects of the National Natural Science Foundation of China, the Special Program Foundation of Ministry of Health, and the Special Program Foundation for Basic Research of Ministry of Science and Technology of China. She has published one statistical textbook and more than 60 research articles since 2000.

CHAPTER 7

SPATIO-TEMPORAL DATA ANALYSIS

Hui Huang*

7.1. Spatio-Temporal Structure[1,2]

Data structure in real life can be very different from the independent and identically distributed (i.i.d.) assumption in conventional statistics. Observations are space- and/or time-dependent, and thus bear important spatial and/or temporal information. Ignoring such information in statistical analysis may lead to inaccurate or inefficient inferences. In recent years, with the fast development of Bio-medicine, Ecology, Environmental Science, and many other disciplines, there are growing needs to analyze data with complex spatio-temporal structures. New computational tools and statistical modeling techniques have been developed accordingly.

Suppose that an observation at spot (location) s and time point t belong to a random field, say $Z(s;t), s \in D \subset \mathbb{R}^d, t \in \mathcal{T}$. Here, $\mathbb{R}^d$ is a d-dimensional Euclidean space, usually, we use $d = 2$ to 3 indicate spaces; D is a subset of $\mathbb{R}^d$, and can be deterministic or random; $\mathcal{T}$ is usually used to denote a compact time interval. For any given s and t, $Z(s;t)$ is a random variable, either continuous or discrete. The randomness of $Z(s;t)$ characterizes uncertainties in real life or scientific problems.

If we ignore temporal variations, $Z(s;t)$ becomes $Z(s)$, a spatial process. Analysis and modeling methods of $Z(s)$ depend on the characteristics of D. In general, there are three categories of spatial analysis: geostatistics with continuous D, lattice data analysis with countable elements in D, and point pattern analysis where D is a spatial point process.

*Corresponding author: huanghui@math.pku.edu.cn

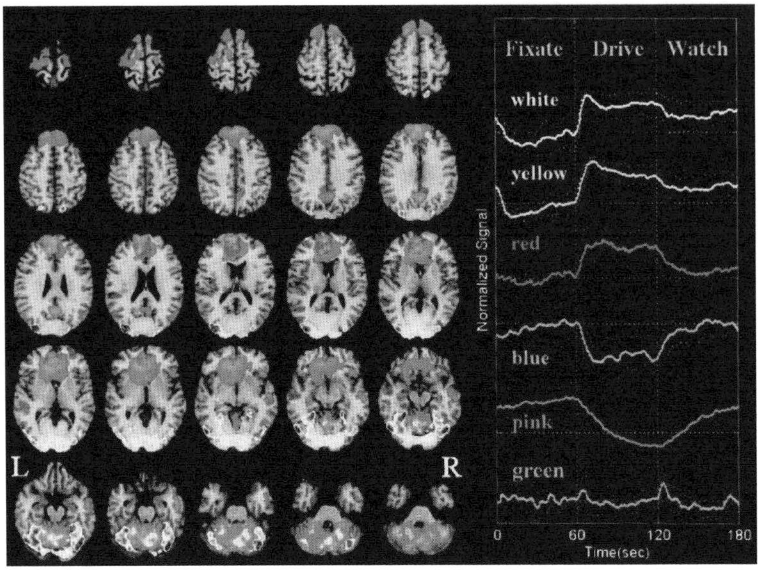

Fig. 7.2.1. fMRI signals of brain activities: *Source*: Ref. [1].

On the other hand, if we only consider temporal variations, $Z(s;t)$ reduces to a time-dependent process $Z(t)$. There are tons of literatures studying $Z(t)$. For example, if we treat $Z(t)$ as a time discrete process, tools of time series analysis or longitudinal data analysis can be used to investigate the dynamic natures or correlation patterns of $Z(t)$. If $Z(t)$ is more like a time-continuous process, methods in a recently booming area, functional data analysis (FDA), can be an option to analyze such data.

Datasets in the real world, however, are much more complicated. To make a comprehensive data analysis, one should take both spatial and temporal structures into consideration; otherwise, one may lose important information on the key features of data. Figure 7.2.1 is an illustration of functional magnetic resonance imaging (fMRI) data from a psychiatric study. One can see that various activation signals are observed from different brain regions, while the time courses of these signals also contain important features of brain activities. Therefore, a careful investigation on the interaction between spatial and temporal effects will enrich our knowledge of such dataset.

7.2. Geostatistics[3,4]

Geostatistics originally emerged from studies in geographical distribution of minerals, but now is widely used in atmospheric science, ecology and biomedical image analysis.

One basic assumption in geostatistics is the continuity of spatial index. That is, a random variable z is well defined on any point of D, the region of interest. Hence, the collection of all Z over D forms a spatial stochastic process, or random field:

$$\{Z(s), s \in D\}$$

Note that $D \subset \mathbb{R}^d$ is a fixed subset of the d-dimensional Euclidean space. The volume of D can be problem-specific. At any spatial point $s \in D, Z(s)$ can be a scalar or vector random variable. Denote the finite spatial sampling point as $\{s_1, \ldots, s_n\}$, the observations $\{Z(s_1), \ldots, Z(s_n)\}$ are called geostatistics data, or geo-information data. Different from conventional statistics, sample points $\{Z(s_1), \ldots, Z(s_n)\}$ are not independent, they have spatial correlations.

Studying an index-continuous random process based on its finite, dependent sample can be very hard. Therefore, before any statistical analysis, we need some reasonable assumptions about the data generation mechanism. Suppose that the first and second moments of $Z(s)$ exist, we consider a general model:

$$Z(s) = \mu(s) + \varepsilon(s),$$

where $\mu(s)$ is the mean surface, $\varepsilon(s)$ is a spatial oscillation bearing some spatial correlation structure. If we further assume that for all $s \in D, \mu(s) \equiv \mu, \mathrm{Var}[\varepsilon(s)] \equiv \sigma^2$, then we can use the finite sample to estimate parameters and make statistical inferences. For any two s points u, denote $C(s,u) := \mathrm{COV}(\varepsilon(s), \varepsilon(u))$ as the covariance function of spatial process $Z(s)$, features of $C(s,u)$ play an important role in statistical analysis.

A commonly used assumption on $C(s,u)$ in spatial analysis is the second-order stationarity or weak stationarity. Similar to the time series, any spatial process is second-order stationary if $\mu(s) \equiv \mu, \mathrm{Var}[\varepsilon(s)] \equiv \sigma^2$, and the covariance $C(s,u) = C(h)$ only depends on $h = \mathrm{s} - \mathrm{u}$. Another popular assumption is the Isotropy. For a second-order stationary process, if $C(h) = C(\|h\|)$, i.e. the covariance function only depends on the distance between two spatial points, then this process is isotropic. Accordingly, $C(\|h\|)$ is called an isotropic covariance. The isotropy assumption brings lots of convenience in modeling spatial data since it simplifies the correlation structure. In real life data analysis, however, this assumption may not hold, especially in problems of atmospheric or environmental sciences. There are growing research interests in anisotropic processes in recent years.

7.3. Variogram[3,5]

The most important feature in geostatistics data is the spatial correlation. Correlated data brings challenges in estimation and inference procedures, but is advantageous in prediction. Thus, it is essential to specify the correlation structure of the dataset. In spatial analysis, we usually use another terminology, variogram, rather than covariance functions or correlation coefficients, to describe the correlation between random variables from two different spatial points.

If we assume that for any two points s and u, we always have $E(Z(s) - Z(u)) = 0$, then a variogram is defined as

$$2\gamma(h) := \mathrm{Var}(Z(s) - Z(u)),$$

where $h = s - u$. One can see that a variogram is variance of the difference between two spatial random variables. To make this definition valid, we need to assume second-order stationarity of the process. In that case, we say the process has Intrinsic Stationarity.

To better understand the concept of the variogram, we briefly discuss its connection with the covariance function. By the definition, it is easy to show that $\gamma(h) = C(0) - C(h)$, where $C(h)$ is the covariance function which depends only on h. By this relationship, once the form of the covariance is determined, the variogram is determined, but not vice versa. Unless we assume $\lim_{\|h\|\to\infty} \gamma(h) = C(0)$, which means that the spatial correlation attenuates to zero as the distance $\|h\|$ gets large, otherwise $\gamma(h)$ cannot determine the form of $C(h)$. In fact, the assumption $\lim_{\|h\|\to\infty} \gamma(h) = C(0)$ is not always satisfied. If it is true, then the process $Z(s)$ must be second-order stationary. Thus, we have two conclusions:

Intrinsic stationarity contains second-order stationarity;

For a second-order stationary spatial process, the variogram and the covariance function equivalently reflect the correlation structure.

From the above discussions, we can see that the variogram is conceptually more general than the covariance. This is the reason why people use variograms more often in spatial statistics literatures. There are lots of important features about the variogram. The nugget effect could be the most famous one. The value of a variogram $2\gamma(h)$ may not be continuous at the initial point $h = 0$, i.e. $\lim_{\|h\|\to 0} 2\gamma(h) = c_0 > 0$, which means that the difference between two spatial random variables cannot be neglected, even when they are geographically very close. The limit c_0 is called a nugget effect. Main sources of the nugget effect include measurement error and microscale variation. In general, we assume that a nugget effect c_0 always exists, and it is an important parameter to be estimated.

By the definition of variogram, $2\gamma(h)$ is a non-decreasing function of $\|h\|$. But when $\|h\|$ is large enough, the variogram may reach an up limit. We call this limit the "sill", and the h of which $2\gamma(h)$ reaches the sill at the first time is called the "range".

7.4. Models of the Variogram[6,7]

The variogram is closely related to the covariance function. But the intuitions between these two terminologies are different. Generally speaking, a variogram describes the differences within a spatial process, while a covariance function illustrates the process's internal similarities. A valid covariance matrix must be symmetric and non-negative definite, that is, for any set of spatial points $\{s_1, \ldots, s_n\}$, we must have

$$\sum_{i=1}^{n}\sum_{j=1}^{n} a_i a_j C(s_i - s_j) \geq 0$$

for any real vectors $\{a_1, \ldots, a_n\}$. By considering the relationship between the variogram and the covariance function, a valid variogram must be conditionally negative definite, i.e.

$$\sum_{i=1}^{n}\sum_{j=1}^{n} a_i a_j \gamma(s_i - s_j) \leq 0,$$

subject to $\sum a_i = 0$.

In a one-dimensional analysis such as time series or longitudinal data analysis, we usually pre-specify a parametric correlation structure. Commonly used models for the covariance matrix include autoregressive model, exponential model, compound symmetry model, etc. Similarly, given validity, we can also specify some parametric models for the variogram.

Power Variogram: A variogram with the form

$$2\gamma(h) = c_0 + ah^{\alpha},$$

where c_0 is the nugget effect, $\alpha > 0$ is some constant to control the decay rate of the spatial correlation. A power variogram does not have a sill.

Spherical Variogram: We define

$$2\gamma(h) = \begin{cases} c_0 + c_s\{\frac{3}{2}(\frac{h}{a_s}) - \frac{1}{2}(\frac{h}{a_s})^3\}; & 0 < \|h\| \leq a_s \\ c_0 + c_s; & \|h\| \geq a_S, \end{cases}$$

where c_0 is the nugget effect, $c_0 + c_s$ is the sill, a_s is the range.

Matérn Class: Matérn class is probably the most popular variogram model in spatial statistics. It has a general form

$$2\gamma(h) = c_0 + c_1 \left\{ 1 - \frac{(\frac{h}{2\alpha})^v}{2\Gamma(v)} K_v(h/\alpha) \right\},$$

where c_0 is the nugget effect, $c_0 + c_1$ is the sill, v controls the smoothness of $Z(s)$, and K_v is a modified Bessel function of the second kind, Γ is the Gamma function. Many other models are special cases of the Matérn class. For example, when $v = 0.5$, it is an exponential variogram:

$$2\gamma(h) = c_0 + c_1\{1 - \text{Exp}(-\|h\|/\alpha)\}.$$

While when $v = \infty$, it becomes a Gaussian variogram:

$$2\gamma(h) = c_0 + c_1 \left\{ 1 - \text{Exp}\left(-\frac{\|h\|^2}{\alpha^2} \right) \right\}.$$

Anisotropic Variogram: When a variogram depends not only on the spatial lag $\|h\|$, but also on the direction, then it is an anisotropic variogram. In this case, the dynamic pattern of the spatial process varies for different directions. Specifically, if there exists an invertible matrix A such that

$$2\gamma(h) = 2\gamma_0(\|Ah\|)$$

for any $h \in \mathbb{R}^d$, then the variogram is said to be geometrically anisotropic.

Cross Variogram: For a k-variate spatial process $Z(s) = (Z_1(s), \ldots, Z_k(s))$, we can define a cross variogram to describe the spatial cross correlation. In particular, when $i = j$, we have

$$2\gamma_{ii}(h) = \text{Var}(\text{Z}_i(\text{s} + h) - \text{Z}_i(\text{s})).$$

When $i \neq j$, we can define

$$2\gamma_{ij}(h) = \text{Var}(\text{Z}_i(\text{s} + h) - \text{Z}_j(\text{s})).$$

This is a multivariate version of the regular variogram.

7.5. Estimation of the Variogram[4,6]

There are many methods to estimate the variogram. For convenience, we assume intrinsic stationarity of the spatial process $Z(s)$. Usually, the estimation starts with an empirical semi-variogram, which is an estimate by the method-of-moment. Then the plot of empirical semi-variogram is compared with several theoretical semi-variograms, the closest one is then picked as the parametric model for the variogram.

Specifically, given spatial data $\{Z(s_1), \ldots, Z(s_n)\}$, the empirical semi-variogram is

$$\hat{\gamma}(h) = \frac{1}{2N(h)} \sum_{s_i, s_j \in N(h)} [Z^2(s_i) - Z^2(s_j)],$$

where N(h) is the collection of all pairs satisfying $s_i - s_j = h$. In real data, for any fixed $h, N(h)$ can be very small in size, thus to increase sample sizes, an alternative way is to define $N(h)$ as the collection of all pairs satisfying $\mathrm{s}_i - \mathrm{s}_j \in h \pm \delta$, where δ is some pre-specified tolerance. In general, we can divide the real line by small regions $h \pm \delta$, and for each region, the estimates $\hat{\gamma}(h)$ are obtained. Theoretical works show that, by using this procedure, the estimated variogram has good asymptotic properties such as consistency and asymptotic normality. One issue to be emphasized is that there are two kinds of asymptotic theories in spatial statistics. If the region of interest D expands as the sample size $n \to \infty$, then we have increasing domain asymptotics; the consistency and asymptotic normality of the variogram belong to this class. If the region remains fixed, then we have infill asymptotics.

In real life data analysis, the sample size is always finite. The empirical variogram, though has some good asymptotic properties, is in fact a non-parametric estimator. Thus, we need a good parametric approximation to make things more convenient. Once the parametric form is determined, likelihood based methods or Bayesian methods can then be applied to estimate the parameters.

If we assume Gaussianity of the process $Z(s)$, given a parametric form of variogram, we can estimate parameters by maximizing the likelihood or restricted likelihood. Another way is using the least square method to minimize the square loss. In particular, select $\{h_1, \ldots, h_K\}$ as the interested distances and use them to divide the real line, we minimize

$$\sum_{j=1}^{K} \{\hat{\gamma}(h_j) - \gamma(h_j, \theta)\}^2$$

to estimate θ. If the variances of $\{\hat{\gamma}(h_j)\}$, $j = 1, \ldots, K$, are not equal, a weighted least square can be used.

7.6. Kriging I[8,9]

Kriging is a popular method for spatial interpolation. The name of Kriging came from D. G. Krige, a mining engineer in South Africa. The basic idea behind Kriging is to linearly predict the value of $Z(s_0)$ at an arbitrary spatial point s_0, based on a spatial sample $\{Z(s_1), \ldots, Z(s_n)\}$.

Suppose the spatial process $Z(s)$ has a model $Z(s) = \mu + \varepsilon(s)$, where μ is the common mean, $\varepsilon(s)$ is the random deviation at location s from the mean. The purpose of Kriging is to find coefficients $\lambda = \{\lambda_1, \dots, \lambda_n\}$ such that $\hat{Z}(s_0) = \sum \lambda_i Z(s_i)$ with two constraints: unbiasedness $E[\hat{Z}(s_0)] = Z(s_0)$ and the minimal mean squared error $\text{MSE}(\lambda) := E\{|\hat{Z}(s_0) - Z(s_0)|^2\}$. A constant mean leads to $\sum \lambda_i = 1$, and by simple steps, one can find that the mean square error is equivalent to

$$\text{MSE}(\lambda) = -\sum_{i=1}^{n}\sum_{j=1}^{n} \lambda_i \lambda_j \gamma(s_i - s_j) + 2\sum_{i=1}^{n} \lambda_i \gamma(s_i - s_0),$$

where $\gamma(\cdot)$ is the variogram. Hence, looking for λ becomes an optimization problem of the MSE subject to $\sum \lambda_i = 1$.

By using a Lagrange multiplier ρ, we can have $\tilde{\lambda} = \Gamma^{-1}\tilde{\gamma}$, where $\tilde{\lambda} = (\lambda_1, \dots, \lambda_n, \rho)'$,

$$\tilde{\gamma} = \begin{pmatrix} \gamma(s_1 - s_0) \\ \vdots \\ \gamma(s_n - s_0) \\ 1 \end{pmatrix},$$

$$\Gamma = \begin{cases} \gamma(s_i - s_j) & i = 1, \dots, n; \quad j = 1, \dots, n \\ 1 & i = n+1; \quad j = 1, \dots, n\,. \\ 0 & i = n+1; \quad j = n+1 \end{cases}$$

The coefficient λ is determined by the form of variogram γ, thus the correlation structure of $Z(s)$. In addition, we can also estimate the Kriging Variance:

$$\sigma_K^2(s_0) := \text{Var}(\hat{Z}(s_0)) = \rho + \sum_{i=1}^{n} \lambda_i \gamma(s_i - s_0).$$

The Kriging method above is called Ordinary Kriging. There are some important features about this interpolation technique:

(1) By definition, $\hat{Z}(s_0)$ is the best linear unbiased prediction (BLUP) of $Z(s_0)$.
(2) For any sample point $Z(s_i)$, the kriged value is the true value, i.e. $\hat{Z}(s_i) = Z(s_i)$.
(3) Except Gaussian variogram, Kriging is robust to the variogram model. In other words, even if the variogram model is misspecified, the kriged values will not be very different.
(4) The Kriging variance $\sigma_K^2(s_0)$, however, is sensitive to the underlying model of the variogram.

(5) Under Gaussianity assumption of $Z(s)$, the 95% confidence interval of $Z(s_0)$ is $\hat{Z}(s_0) \pm 1.96\sigma_K(s_0)$.

7.7. Kriging II[4,6]

The ordinary Kriging has many variations. Before we introduce other Kriging methods, one thing should be mentioned is that the Kriged value and Kriging variance can be represented by covariance functions. Specifically, if the mean surface $\mu(s)$ and the covariance function $C(s,u)$ are known, then we have

$$\hat{Z}(s_0) = \mu(s_0) + c' \sum^{-1} (Z - \mu),$$

where $c = (C(s_0, s_1), \ldots, C(s_0, s_n))'$, the sample covariance matrix $\Sigma = \{C(s_i, s_j)\}_{i,j=1,\ldots,n}$, $Z - \mu$ is the residual. A Kriging method based on known mean and covariance is called Simple Kriging.

The limitation of Simple Kriging or Ordinary Kriging is obvious, since in real data analysis, we rarely know the mean or the covariance structure. Now, we consider a more general model

$$Z(s) = \mu(s) + \varepsilon(s),$$

where $\mu(s)$ is an unknown surface. Moreover, $Z(s)$ can be affected by some covariates X, i.e.

$$\mu(s) = \beta_0 + X_1(s)\beta_1 + \cdots + X_p(s)\beta_p,$$

where $X_j(s)$, $j = 1, \ldots, p$ are observed processes for any arbitrary point s_0, β_js are regression coefficients. We still develop Kriging methods in the framework of BLUP. There are two constraints that must be fulfilled when optimizing the MSE(λ): $\sum \lambda_i = 1$ and $\sum_{i=1}^{n} \lambda_i \mathrm{X}_j(s_i) = X_j(s_0)$, $j = 1, \ldots, p$. Therefore, there are $p+1$ Lagrange multiplier in total. This method is called Universal Kriging, it can be seen as an extension of the linear regression since we need to fit a regression model of the mean surface. In particular, if the random error $\varepsilon(s)$ is a white noise process, then the Universal Kriging becomes a regular prediction procedure by a linear model.

Please note that the regression coefficients need to be estimated before prediction. By using conventional lease square method, the spatial structure of residual $\hat{\varepsilon}(s)$ may be very different from the true error $\varepsilon(s)$, which leads to serious bias in prediction. Iterative methods such as reweighted least square, general estimating equation (GEE), or profile likelihood can be used to improve the prediction bias, but the computation will be more intensive, especially when sample size n is large.

Other Kriging methods include:

Co-Kriging: If $Z(s)$ is a multivariate spatial process, the prediction of $\hat{Z}(s_0)$ not only depends on the spatial correlation, but also the cross-correlation among the random variables.

Trans-Gaussian Kriging: When $Z(s)$ is not Gaussian, it may be less efficient to predict $\hat{Z}(s_0)$ by regular Kriging methods. Transformation to Gaussian distribution can be a solution.

Indicator Kriging: A Kriging method for 0–1 discrete random field.

7.8. Bayesian Hierarchical Models (BHM)[5,10]

The complexity of spatial data comes from its correlation structure, and also from the data uncertainties (randomness). Therefore, the underlying model can be very complicated. With the fast development of other disciplines, there are more and more big and noisy spatial data coming up for analysis. To analyze spatial data, we need to quantify both its structure and uncertainties, which means to characterize the data generation mechanism.

BHM's have become popular in recent years, due to their ability to explain the uncertainties in all levels in a data generation procedure. Generally speaking, a BHM includes a data model, a (scientific) process model and a parameter model. Let Z denote the data, Y and θ, respectively be the underlying process and corresponding parameters, then the data model is $[Z|Y, \theta]$, the process model is $[Y|\theta]$ and the parameter model is $[\theta]$. Here, $[A|B, C]$ is the conditional distribution of random variable A given random variables B and C. In particular for a spatial process in Geostatistics, we usually represent the observed data as

$$Z(s) = Y(s) + \epsilon(s),$$

where $Y(s)$ is the true but unobserved process, $\epsilon(s)$ is a white noise causing the uncertainties in data. The process $Y(s)$ has its own model

$$Y(s) = \beta_0 + X_1(s)\beta_1 + \cdots + X_p(s)\beta_p + \delta$$

with Xs as covariates, βs as regression coefficients and δ the spatial random effect. The spatial correlation structure of Y inherits from the structure of δ. Please note that the relationship between Y and the covariates can also be nonlinear and non-parametric. If we further assume that all parameters in the data and process models are also random, then we have a probability model for the parameters at the bottom hierarchy. In this way, we quantify uncertainties of the data through parameters.

In the framework of BHM, we can still use Kriging methods to interpolate data. Specifically, if both the data $Z(s)$ and the process $Y(s)$ are Gaussian, then by the Bayesian formula, the posterior distribution of the Kriged value at point $s_0, Y(s_0)$, is also Gaussian. Under the square error loss, the prediction $\hat{Y}(s_0)$ is the posterior mean of $Y(s_0)$, and its variance can be written in an explicit form. If the data process is not Gasussian, especially when generalized linear models are used, then the posterior distribution of $Y(s_0)$ usually does not have a closed form. A Monte Carlo Markov Chain (MCMC) method, however, can be used to simulate the posterior distribution, which brings a lot more conveniences in computation than conventional Kriging methods. In fact, by using a BHM, the stationarity of the process $Y(s)$ is not required, since the model parameters are characterized by their prior distributions. There is no need to specify the correlation for any spatial lag h based on repeated measures.

In summary, the BHM is much more flexible and has wider applications, whereas Bayesian Kriging has many advantages in computing for non-Gaussian predictions.

7.9. Lattice Data[3,4]

Geostatistics data is defined on a fixed and space-continuous region D, then a geostatistical random field $Z(s)$ has definition on any arbitrary point $s \in D$. A lattice data, on the other hand, is defined on a discrete D, where $D = \{s_1, s_2, \ldots\}$ is finite or countably many. For example, if we are interested in the regional risk rate of some disease in Beijing, then central locations of all the 16 regions in Beijing are the entire D we consider. Usually, we use longitude and latitude to index these locations.

Before analyzing a lattice data, an important concept to be specified is how we define a "neighborhood". In mathematics, we can use a buffer circle with radius r. Then the neighbors of any lattice s are all the lattices within the buffer of s. In real data analysis, neighbors may also be defined as actual regions, such as administrative or census divisions that have common borders.

We usually have lattice data in remote sensing or image analysis problems. They can be regular, such as pixel or voxel intensities in medical images; or irregular, such as disease rates over census divisions. Techniques for analyses may vary according to specific problems. If signal restoration is of interest, a statistical model, such as generalized linear mixed model, can be implemented to investigate the measurement error structure and to back-construct the signals. If the study purpose is classification or clustering, then we need methods of machine learning to find out data patterns. Sometimes, we may have very noisy lattice data, thus spatial smoothing approaches, such as spline approximation or kernel smoothing, are usually applied to reduce redundancies.

Since the location indices are discrete for lattice data, most techniques of time series can be directly applied. The only difference is that in time series, data is sequentially ordered in a natural way, whereas there is no such order for spatial data. By defining a neighborhood, one can use the correlation between a lattice random variable and its neighbors to define a spatial autocorrelation. For example, a temporal Markov chain is usually defined by

$$[Y(s)|Y(t-1),\ldots,Y(1)] = [Y(t)|Y(t-1)]$$

and $[Y(1)]$, while for a spatial version, we may use $[Y(s)|\partial Y(s)]$, where $\partial Y(s)$ are observations in the neighborhood of $Y(s)$. In addition, the autocorrelation can also be defined in a more flexible way:

$$[Y(2),\ldots,Y(\mathrm{s})|Y(1) = \Pi_{i=2}^{s} f_i(Y(i),Y(i-1)),$$

where $f_i(\cdot,\cdot)$ is some bivariate function.

7.10. Markov Random Field (MRF)[5,10]

For convenience, we consider a lattice process $\{Z(s_1),\ldots,Z(s_n)\}$ defined on infinite $D = \{s_1,\ldots,s_n\}$. The joint distribution $[Z(s_1),\ldots,Z(s_n)]$ then determines all conditional distributions $[Z(s_i)|Z_{-i}]$, where $Z_{-i} = \{Z(s_1),\ldots,Z(s_n)\}\backslash\{Z(s_i)\}$. The conditional distributions, however, cannot uniquely determine a joint distribution. This may cause problems in statistical analysis. For example in Bayesian analysis, when we use the Gibbs sampler to construct a MCMC, we need to make sure that the generated process converges to a random vector with a unique joint distribution. Similarly, to define a spatial Markov chain, the uniqueness of the joint distribution must be guaranteed.

For any $s_i \in D$, denote $\mathrm{N}(s_i) \subset D\backslash\{s_i\}$ as the neighborhood of $Z(s_i)$. We assume that for any $i = 1,\ldots,n$,

$$[Z(s_i)|Z_{-i}] = [Z(s_i)|Z(N(s_i))].$$

Moreover, we assume that all conditional distributions $[Z(s_i)|Z(N(s_i))]$ determine a unique joint distribution $[Z(s_1),\ldots,Z(s_n)]$. Then we call $\{Z(s_1),\ldots,Z(s_n)\}$ an MRF.

A special case of the MRF is the Conditional Autoregressive Model (CAR). For any $i = 1, \ldots, n$, a CAR assumes that all conditional distributions $[Z(s_i)|Z(N(s_i))]$ are Gaussian, and

$$E[Z(s_i)|Z(N(s_i))] = \mu(s_i) + \sum_{s_j \in N(s_i)} c_{ij}(Z(s_j) - \mu(s_j)),$$

where $\mu(s_i) := E[Z(s_i)]$ is the mean value. Denote the variance as τ_i^2, we have conditions

$$\frac{c_{ij}}{\tau_i^2} = \frac{c_{ji}}{\tau_j^2}.$$

Let $C = (c_{ij})|_{i,j=1,\ldots,n}$, $M = \text{diag}(\tau_1^2, \ldots, \tau_n^2)$, then the joint distribution $[Z(s_1), \ldots, Z(s_n)]$ is an n-dimensional multivariate Gaussian distribution with covariance matrix $(I - C)^{-1}M$. One can see that the weight matrix C characterizes the spatial correlation structure of the lattice data $\{Z(s_1), \ldots, Z(s_n)\}$.

Usually, in a CAR model, C and M are both unknown. But $(I - C)^{-1}M$ must be symmetric and non-negative definite so that it is a valid covariance matrix.

CAR models and Geostatistical models are tightly connected. Suppose a Gaussian random field $Z(s)$ with covariance function Σ_Z are sampled at points $\{s_1, \ldots, s_n\}$, then we can claim:

(1) If a CAR model on $\{s_1, \ldots, s_n\}$ has a covariance matrix $(I - C)^{-1}M$, then the covariance matrix of a random field $Z(s)$ on sample points $\{s_1, \ldots, s_n\}$ is $\Sigma_Z^s = (I - C)^{-1}M$.
(2) If the covariance matrix of a random field $Z(s)$ on $\{s_1, \ldots, s_n\}$ is Σ_Z^s, let $(\Sigma_Z^s)^{-1} = (\sigma^{(ij)})$, $M = \text{diag}(\sigma^{(11)}, \ldots, \sigma^{(nn)})^{-1}$, $C = I - M(\Sigma_Z^s)^{-1}$, then a CAR model defined on $\{s_1, \ldots, s_n\}$ has covariance $(I - C)^{-1}M$.

Since the CAR model has advantages in computing, it can be used to approximate Geostatistical models. In addition, the MRF or CAR model can also be constructed in a manner of BHMs, which can give us more computing conveniences.

7.11. Spatial Point Pattern (SPP)[11,12]

SPP is usually defined on random indices $\{s_1, \ldots, s_N\}$ in the sampling space $D \subset \mathbb{R}^d$. Each point is called an event. SPP has double randomness, meaning that the randomness is from both the location of s_i and the number N of events. The mechanism of generating such data is called a Spatial Point Process.

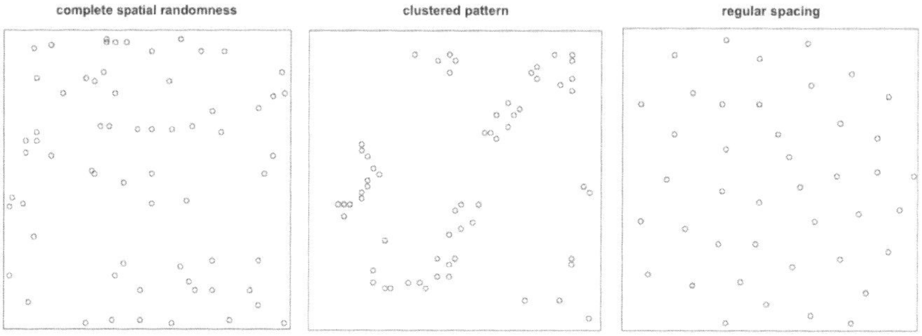

Fig. 7.11.1. Three SPPs: CSR (left), CP (middle) and RS (right)

Spatial point process N can be characterized by a probability model:

$$\{\Pr[N(D) = k];\ k \in \{0, 1, \ldots\},\ D \subset \mathbb{R}^d\},$$

where $N(D)$ denotes the number of events in D. If for any $s \in D$, we have $Pr[N(s) > 1] = 0$, i.e. there is at most one event at each location, we call N a simple spatial point process. By definition, an SPP pictures occurrence locations and the number of random events in a specific region. Therefore, it is very popular in the field of epidemiology, ecology and economics.

The simplest spatial point process is the homogeneous Poisson process. A homogeneous Poisson process N with Intensity λ is defined through the two aspects below:

(1) For any mutually disjoint areas $D_1, \ldots, D_k$ in $\mathbb{R}^d$, $N(D_1), \ldots, N(D_k)$ are independent.
(2) The volume of D is $|D|$, so we have $N(D) \sim \text{Poisson}(\lambda|D|)$.

The SPP generated by a homogeneous Poisson process is said to have the Complete Spatial Randomness (CSR). Event points $\{s_1, \ldots, s_N\}$ with CSR do not have spatial dependences. On the other hand, if a spatial point process is not homogeneous Poisson, the corresponding point patterns will be Cluster Pattern (CP), for which the event points are clustered, or Regular Spacing (RS), where there are some spaces between any two events. The three point patterns are illustrated in Figure 7.11.1.

7.12. CSR[11,13]

CSR is the simplest case of SPPs. The first step of analyzing point pattern data is to test if an SPP has the property of CSR. The goal is to determine whether we need to do subsequent statistical analysis or not, and whether there is a need to explore the dependence feature of the data.

To test the existence of CSR, we need to quantify the dependence structure of the SPP first. An approach to do this is to observe the distribution function of the distance between the observed event points and their neighboring events. If we denote W_i to be the distance between s_i and its nearest neighbor, then the probability distribution is

$$G(w) = \Pr[W_i \leq w].$$

Under the null hypothesis where CSR holds, it can be proved that $G(w) = 1 - \mathrm{Exp}(-\pi\lambda w^2)$. Through the empirical estimate of $G(w)$, $\hat{G}(w) = \frac{1}{N}\sum_{i=1}^{N} I(W_i \leq w)$, we can construct a Kolmogorov–Smirnov (KS) statistic

$$\mathrm{U}_{\mathrm{data}} = \sup_w |\hat{G}(w) - G(w)|.$$

Under the null hypothesis, one simulates K CSRs by Monte Carlo method and obtain $U_1, \ldots, U_k$, and compare $\mathrm{U}_{\mathrm{data}}$ with the quantiles of $U_1, \ldots, U_k$. By using this nearest neighbor method, we would roughly know if the CSR holds for current data. However, the G function is not correctly estimated if the CSR does not hold. Moreover, we do not make full use of all the data information of the events in the area D.

Another approach for testing CSR is to quantify both mean and dependence structures. If we define the first-order and second-order intensity function as

$$\lambda(s) = \lim_{(|ds| \to 0)} E\{N(ds)\}/|ds|$$

$$\lambda_2(s,u) = \lim_{\substack{|ds| \to 0 \\ |du| \to 0}} \frac{E\{\mathrm{N}(ds)N(\mathrm{du})\}}{|ds||\mathrm{du}|}.$$

Then $\lambda(s)$ and $\lambda_2(s,u)$ describe the mean and dependence structure of the point process N, respectively. Let $\rho(s,u) := \frac{\lambda_2(s,u)}{\lambda(s)\lambda(u)}$, then $\rho(s,u)$ is called Pair Correlation Function (PCF). If $\rho(s,u) = \rho(r)$, i.e. ρ only depends on the Euclidean distance r between location s and location u, and $\lambda(s) \equiv \lambda$, then N is said to be an isotropic second-order stationary spatial point process. It can be proved that in the case of CSR, CP and RS, we have $\rho(r) = 1$, $\rho(r) > 1$, and $\rho(r) < 1$, respectively. For isotropic second-order stationary spatial point process, another statistic for measuring the spatial dependence is K function. $K(r)$ is defined as a ratio between the expected number of all the event points located in a distance r from the the event point and the intensity λ. It can be proved that $K(r)$ is in an integral form of the second-order intensity function $\lambda_2(r)$. Moreover, under CSR, CP and RS, we have $K(r) = \pi r^2$, $K(r) > \pi r^2$, and $K(r) < \pi r^2$, respectively. Similar to the nearest neighbor distance function $G(w)$, through the empirical estimate of $K(r)$, $\hat{K}(r) = \frac{1}{\hat{\lambda} N} \sum_{i=1}^{N} \sum_{i \neq 1} I(\|s_i - s_j\| < r)$, we can construct a Cramér–von Mises test statistic $L = \int_0^{r_0} |\sqrt{\hat{K}(r)/\pi} - r|^2 dr$ and use Monte Carlo test method to test if CSR holds.

7.13. Spatial Point Process[11,14]

Fundamental properties of a homogeneous Poisson process N on region D include:

(1) $N(D)$ depends only on $|D|$, the area of D. It does not depend on the location or shape of D.
(2) Given $N(D) = n$, event points $s_1, \ldots, s_N$ are i.i.d as a uniform distribution with density $1/|D|$. In addition, according to the three kinds of SPPs, there are different point process models. We will introduce some commonly used models here.

The first one is the Inhomogeneous Poisson Process, where the first-order intensity function $\lambda(s)$ of Poisson process is changing w.r.t. s. This definition allows us to build regression models or Bayesian models. The SPP generated by an inhomogeneous Poisson process also has CSR. That is, the event points $\{s_1, \ldots, s_N\}$ do not have spatial dependence, but the probability model of the event points is no longer a uniform distribution. Instead, it is a distribution with density

$$f(s) = \lambda(s) / \left(\int_D \lambda(u) du \right).$$

By introducing covariates, the intensity function can usually be written as $\lambda(s; \beta) = g\{X'(s)\beta\}$, where β is the model parameter, $g(\cdot)$ is a known link function. This kind of model has extensive applications in the study of spatial epidemiology. Estimation of the model parameters can usually be made by optimizing Poisson likelihood functions, but explicit solutions usually do not exist. Therefore, we need iterative algorithm for calculations.

Cox Process is an extension of the inhomogeneous Poisson process. The intensity function $\lambda(s)$ of a Cox process is no longer deterministic, but a realization of a spatial random field $\Lambda(s)$. Since $\Lambda(s)$ characterizes the intensity of a point process, we assume that $\Lambda(s)$ is a non-negative random field. The first-order and second-order properties of Cox Process can be obtained in a way similar to the inhomogeneous Poisson process. The only difference lies in how to calculate the expectation in terms of $\Lambda(s)$. It can be verified that under the assumption of stationarity and isotropy, the first-order and second-order intensity of a Cox Process have the following relationship:

$$\lambda_2(r) = \lambda^2(r) + \mathrm{Cov}(\Lambda(s), \Lambda(u)),$$

where $r = \|s - u\|$. Therefore, the point pattern generated by a Cox Process is clustered. If we have $\Lambda(s) = \mathrm{Exp}(Z(s))$, where $Z(s)$ is a Gaussian random field, then the point process is called Log-Gaussian Cox Process (LGCP). LGCP is very popular in real applications. The first-order and second-order intensity functions of a LGCP are usually written in parametric forms. Parameter estimations can be obtained by a composite likelihood method.

RS usually occurs in the field of Biology and Ecology. For example, the gaps among trees are always further than some distance δ due to their "territories" of soil. Event points with this pattern must have an intensity function depending on spacing distance. As a simple illustration, we first consider an event point set X generated by a Poisson process with intensity ρ. By removing event pairs with a distance less than δ, we can get a new point pattern data $\tilde{X}$. The spatial point process generating $\tilde{X}$ is called the Simple Inhibition Process (SIP). The intensity function is $\lambda = \rho\mathrm{Exp}\{-\pi\rho\delta^2\}$. This intensity function has two characteristics: (1) The intensity of an event at any spatial location is only correlated with its nearest neighboring point. (2) This intensity is defined through the original Poisson process. Therefore, it is a conditional intensity. If we extend the SIP to a point process with some newly defined neighborhood, then we can construct a Markov point process, which is similar to the Markov random field for lattice data. However, the intensity function of this process is still a conditional intensity conditioning on Poisson processes. Therefore, it guarantees that the generated point pattern still has the RS feature.

7.14. Spatial Epidemiology[11,15]

A spatial epidemiology data set usually contains following information: (1) diseased individuals (cases) with their geocodes, for example, the latitude/longitude of family addresses; (2) incidence time; (3) risk factors, such as demographic info, exposure to pollutants, lifestyle variables, etc.; (4) control group sampled from the same region as the cases.

The analysis purpose of a spatial epidemiology data set usually focuses on the relationship between the risk of developing some disease and the risk factors. Denote N as the point process that generates the cases in region D, $f(s;\beta)$ the probability of an individual to get the disease, then a model of the risk intensity is in the form:

$$\lambda(s;\beta) = \lambda_0(s)f(X(s);\beta),$$

where $\lambda_0(s)$ is the population density in D, vector $X(s)$ are risk factors. Note that this model can be extended to a spatio-temporal version $\lambda(s,t;\beta) = \lambda_0(s)f(X(s,t);\beta)$, where s and t are space and time indices. If there is a control group, denote M as the underlying point process, then the risk of developing some disease for controls depends only on the sampling mechanism. To match the control group to cases, we usually stratified samples into some subgroups. For example, one can divide samples to males and females and use the gender proportions in cases to find matching controls. For simplicity, we use $\lambda_0(s)$ to denote the intensity of M, i.e. the controls are uniformly selected from the population.

For each sample, let $1-0$ indicate cases and controls, then we can use the logistic regression to estimate model parameters. Specifically, let $p(s;\beta) = \frac{f(s;\beta)}{1+f(s;\beta)}$ denote the probability that s comes from the case group, then an estimation of β can be obtained by maximizing the log likelihood function:

$$l(\beta) = \sum_{x\in N\cap D} \log\{p(x;\beta)\} + \sum_{y\in M\cap D} \log\{1-p(y;\beta)\}.$$

Once the estimator $\hat{\beta}$ is obtained, it can be plugged into the intensity function to predict the risk. In particular, we estimate $\hat{\lambda}_0(s)$ by using the control data, and plug $\hat{\lambda}_0(s)$ and $\hat{\beta}$ together into the risk model of cases. In this way we can calculate the disease risk $\hat{\lambda}(s;\beta)$ for any point s.

To better understand the spatial dependence of occurrences of certain diseases, we need to quantify the second order properties of case process N. A PCF $\rho(r)$ is usually derived and estimated. Existing methods include non-parametric and parametric models. The basic idea behind non-parametric methods is to use all the incidence pairs to empirically estimate $\hat{\rho}(r)$ by some smoothing techniques such as kernel estimation. In a parametric approach, the PCF is assumed to have a form $\rho(r) = \rho(r;\theta)$, where θ is the model parameter. By using all event pairs and a well defined likelihood, θ can be estimated efficiently.

7.15. Visualization[16–18]

Data in real life may have both spatial and temporal structures, its visualization is quite challenging due to the 3+1 data dimension. We introduce some widely used approaches of visualization below.

Animation is probably the most common way to illustrate spatio-temporal datasets. Usually one can use time points to sequence the data, and make a "movie" of the changing spatial maps. Marginal and Conditional plots, on the other hand, are used to illustrate wave-like features of data. One may pick an important space dimension (for example the North-South axis) and see how data progresses over time. This is called the 1-D Time Plot. Another way is blocking space maps to some small subregions, and draw time series over these blocks to show temporal changes. Sometimes multiple time series can be plotted in one figure for comparisons or other study purposes. The third way is to average spatial maps from the animation. One can take a weighted average over time, or just fix a time point and show the snap shot.

It would be very complicated to visualize correlation structures, which are of course more insightful for spatio-temporal data sets. Suppose the sample data is $Z_t = (Z(s_1;t), \ldots, Z(s_m;t))'$, we would like to see its correlation between two spatial point, or two time points, or the cross-correlation when both space and time are different. The empirical covariance matrix of time lag τ is:

$$\hat{C}_Z^{(\tau)} = \frac{1}{T-\tau} \sum_{t=\tau+1}^{T} (Z_t - \hat{\mu}_Z)(Z_{t-\tau} - \hat{\mu}_Z)',$$

where $\hat{\mu}_Z$ is the data average over time. By assuming stationarity, one can draw plots of $\hat{C}_Z^{(\tau)}$ against τ. There are many variations of $\hat{C}_Z^{(\tau)}$. For example, by dividing marginal variances, $\hat{C}_Z^{(\tau)}$ becomes a matrix of correlation coefficient; by replacing $Z_{t-\tau}$ with another random variable, say $Y_{t-\tau}$, $\hat{C}_Z^{(\tau)}$ is then $\hat{C}_{Z,Y}^{(\tau)}$, the cross-covariance between random fields Z and Y.

Another important method to better understand spatial and/or temporal correlations is to decompose the covariance matrix (function) into several components, and investigate features component by component. Local Indicators of Spatial Association (LISAs) is one of the approaches to check components of global statistics with spatio-temporal coordinates. Usually, the empirical covariance is decomposed by spatial principal component analysis (PCA), which in continuous case is called empirical orthogonal function (EOF). If the data has both space and time dimensions, spatial maps of leading components and their corresponding time courses should be combined. When one has a SPP data, LISAs are also used to illustrate empirical correlation functions.

7.16. EOF[10,12]

EOF is basically an application of the eigen decomposition on spatio-temporal processes. If the data are space and/or time discrete, EOF is the famous PCA; if the data are space and/or time continuous, EOF is the Karhunen–Leove Expansion. The purpose of EOF mainly includes: (1) looking for the most important variation mode of data; (2) reducing data dimension and noise in space and/or time.

Considering a time-discrete and space-continuous process $\{Z_t(s): s \in D, t = 1, 2, \ldots\}$ with zero mean surface, the goal of conventional EOF analysis is to look for an optimal and space–time separable decomposition:

$$Z_t(s) = \sum_{k=1}^{\infty} \alpha_t(k)\phi_k(s),$$

where $\alpha_t(k)$ can be treated as a time-varying random effect, whose variance decays to zero as k increases. For different k, $\alpha_t(k)$ are mutually uncorrelated, while functions $\phi_k(s)$ must satisfy some constraints, for instance orthonormality, to be identifiable. The role played by $\phi_k(s)$ can be seen as projection bases. In particular, let $C_Z^{(0)}(s,r)$ be the covariance between $Z_t(s)$ and $Z_t(r)$ for any arbitrary pair of spatial points s and r, then we have the Karhunen–Loeve expansion:

$$C_Z^{(0)}(s,r) = \sum_{k=1}^{\infty} \lambda_k \phi_k(s)\phi_k(r),$$

where $\{\phi_k(\cdot), k = 1, 2, \ldots\}$ are eigenfunctions of $C_Z^{(0)}(s,r)$, λ_k are eigenvalues in a decreasing order with k. In this way, $\alpha_t(k)$ is called the time series corresponding to the kth principal component. In fact, $\alpha_t(k)$ is the projection of $Z_t(s)$ on the kth function $\phi_k(s)$.

In real life, we may not have enough data to estimate the infinitely many parameters in a Karhunen–Leove Expansion, thus we usually pick a cut-off point and dispose all the eigen functions beyond this point. In particular, the Karhunen–Loeve Expansion can be approximately written as

$$Z_t(s) = \sum_{k=1}^{P} \alpha_t(k)\phi_k(s),$$

where the summation of up-to-Pth eigen values explains most of the data variation.

The EOF analysis depends on decompositions of the covariance surface (function), thus we need to obtain an empirical covariance first:

$$\hat{C}_z = \frac{1}{T}\sum_{t=1}^{T}(Z_t - \hat{\mu}_Z)(Z_t - \hat{\mu}_Z)'.$$

But real data can be collapsed with noise. Hence, to make $\hat{C}_z$ valid, we need to guarantee that $\hat{C}_z$ is non-negative definite. A commonly used approach is eigen decomposing $\hat{C}_z$ and throwing away all zero and negative eigenvalues, then back-construct the estimate of the covariance.

When the number of time points are more than spatial points, the empirical covariance is always singular. One solution is building a full-rank matrix by $A = \tilde{Z}'\tilde{Z}$ where $\tilde{Z} = (\tilde{Z}_1, \ldots, \tilde{Z}_T)$ and $\tilde{Z}_t$ is a centered vector. By eigen-decomposing A, we obtain eigen vectors ξ_i, then the eigen vectors of $C = \tilde{Z}\tilde{Z}'$ is

$$\psi_i = \tilde{Z}\xi_i \Big/ \sqrt{\xi_i'\tilde{Z}'\tilde{Z}\xi_i}.$$

7.17. Spatio-Temporal Kriging[19,20]

For a spatio-temporal data set, we can use methods similar to the spatial kriging to make predictions on both space and time. We first look at a general model for the corresponding process

$$Z(s;t) = \mu(s;t) + \delta(s;t) + \epsilon(s;t),$$

where $\mu(s;t)$ is the mean surface, $\delta(s;t)$ is the spatio-temporal random effect, $\epsilon(s;t)$ is white noise. Similar to geostatistics model, if $\mu(s;t) \equiv \mu$ and

$$\mathrm{Cov}[Z(s+h;t+\tau), Z(s;t)] = \mathrm{Cov}[Z(h;\tau), Z(0;0)] := C(h;\tau),$$

then we can define the stationarity of a spatio-temporal process. Here, h and τ are space and time lags, respectively. Moreover, we can define a spatio-temporal variogram $2\gamma(h;\tau) = C(0;0) - C(h;\tau)$.

Suppose we have observations on a $n \times T$ grid, then for any new point $(s_0;t_0)$, the kriged value can be written as

$$Z(s_0;t_0) = \mu(s_0;t_0) + c'\Sigma^{-1}(Z_{nT} - \mu_{nT}),$$

where $Z_{nT} = (Z_1', \ldots, Z_T')'$ is a $nT \times 1$ data matrix, $c = \mathrm{Cov}(Z(s_0;t_0), Z_{nT})$, Σ is the covariance matrix of Z_{nT}. For ordinary Kriging, $\mu(s;t)$ is unknown but can be estimated by generalized least square method $\hat{\mu} = (1'\Sigma^{-1}1)^{-1}1'\Sigma^{-1}Z_{nT}$.

To estimate the covariance or variogram, we first make an empirical estimate. For example

$$\hat{C}(h;\tau) = \frac{\sum_{N(h;\tau)} [Z(s_i;t_i) - \bar{Z}][Z(s_j;t_j) - \bar{Z}]}{N(h;\tau)},$$

then we use a parametric model $C(h;\tau) = C(h;\tau;\theta)$ to approximate. Note that the correlation in a spatio-temporal process includes spatial structure, temporal structure, and the interaction between space and time. Therefore, the covariance $C(h;\tau)$ is much more complicated than $C(h)$ or $C(\tau)$ alone. To propose a parametric correlation model, one needs to guarantee the validity, i.e. non-negative definiteness of the covariance matrix or conditional negative definiteness of the variogram. In addition, one should note that the covariance $C(h;\tau)$ is not necessarily symmetric, i.e. $C(h;\tau) = C(-h;\tau)$ or $C(h;\tau) = C(h;-\tau)$ does not hold in general. If $C(h;\tau)$ is symmetric, then we say that the covariance is fully symmetric. For a fully symmetric covariance function, if it can be written as

$$C(h;\tau) = C^{(s)}(h;0)C^{(t)}(0;\tau),$$

then this covariance is said to be separable. The separability assumption largely simplifies the estimation procedure and thus it is a key assumption in early spatio-temporal data analysis back in 1990s. For real world data, however, the cross-correlation between space and time may not be neglected. One needs more general models for the covariance $C(h;\tau)$. There have been increasing research interests on non-separable and not fully symmetric spatio-temporal covariances in recent years.

7.18. Functional Data[14,21]

Functional data is different from time series data or longitudinal data. For functional data, we assume the underlying process is space and/or time continuous and smooth in some sense. The basic unit of a functional data is not one or several random variables, but a stochastic trajectory or surface. There are in general three types of Functional data: (1) curve, i.e. the whole curve is observable, which is too ideal in most applications; (2) densely observed but noisy data, where the sample points of each curve are regularly spaced; (3) sparsely observed but noisy data, where observations are irregularly spaced and the frequency of sample points are very low.

For dense observations, usually we can smooth individual curves to reduce noises, and perform analysis accordingly. For sparse observations, however, it is hard to smooth curves individually. Thus, we need to assume similarities in the structure of curves so that we can pool all the curves to investigate the common feature.

The only important assumption for functional data is the smoothness. For simplicity, we only focus on data with time index. Suppose that the i-th individual $Y_i(t)$ can then be expressed as

$$Y_i(t) = X_i(t) + \varepsilon_i(t) = \mu(t) + \tau_i(t) + \varepsilon_i(t),$$

where $X_i(t)$ is a unobserved process trajectory, $\mu(t) = E[X_i(t)]$ is the common mean curve of all individuals, $\tau_i(t)$ the stochastic deviation of $X_i(t)$ from $\mu(t), \varepsilon_i(t)$ is a noise with variance σ^2. For model fitting, we can use spline approximations. Suppose $\mu(t) = \sum_{k=1}^{K} \beta_k B_k(t)$, $\tau_i(t) = \sum_{k=1}^{K} \alpha_{ik} B_k(t)$, where $B_k(t)$ are some basis functions defined in time interval T, K is the number of knots, β_k and α_{ik} are respectively coefficients of the mean and the random effect. In this way, a reduced rank model represents the functional data. If we further assume that the random effect α_{ik} is distributed with mean 0 and variance Γ, then the within-curve dependence can be expressed by:

$$\mathrm{Cov}(Y_i(t_p), Y_i(t_q)) = \sum_{l,m=1}^{K} \Gamma_{lm} B_l(t_p) B_m(t_q) + \sigma^2 \delta(p,q),$$

where $\delta(p,q) = 1$ if $p = q$, 0 otherwise.

Spline approximations are often combined with PCA. Let $G(s,t) = \mathrm{Cov}(X(s), X(t))$, it can be proved that $X_i(t)$ has a K-L expansion:

$$X_i(t) = \mu(t) + \sum_{k=1}^{\infty} \xi_{ik} \phi_k(t),$$

where $\phi_k(t)$ is an eigen function of $G(s,t)$ s.t. $G(s,t) = \sum_{k=1}^{\infty} \lambda_k \phi_k(t) \phi_k(t)'$, λ_k is the kth eigen value. If eigen values are in descending order $\lambda_1 \geq \lambda_2 \geq \ldots$, then $\phi_1(t)$ is called the first principal component, and the first several components account for the major variation of $X(t)$. Similar to EOF, we can just truncate the components to leading ones and make inferences accordingly. Furthermore, we can use splines to express $\mu(t)$ and $\phi_k(t)$ to make estimations easier. This model is known as the Reduced Rank Model, which not only enhances the model interpretability by dimension reduction, but also is applicable to sparse data analysis.

7.19. Functional Kriging[22,23]

Consider $\{Z(s;t)s \in D \subseteq R^d, t \in [0,T]\}$ as a functional spatial random field, where $Z(s;t)$ is a spatial random field when time t is given, and when

s is fixed, it is a squared integrable function on $[0, T]$ with inner product $\langle f, g\rangle = \int_0^T f(t)g(t)dt$ defined on the functional space. Assume that $Z(s;t)$ has the spatial second-order stationarity, but not necessarily stationary in time. A functional Kriging aims to predict a smooth curve $Z(s_0;t)$ at any non-sampled point s_0.

Suppose the prediction $\hat{Z}(s_0;t)$ has an expression,

$$\hat{Z}(s_0;t) = \sum_{i=1}^{n} \lambda_i Z(s_i;t),$$

where n is the sample size, then $\{\lambda_i, i = 1, \ldots, n\}$ can be obtained by minimizing $E[\int_0^T (\hat{Z}(s_0;t) - Z(s_0;t))^2 dt]$ subject to $\sum_{i=1}^n \lambda_i = 1$. The constraint guarantees unbiasedness of $\hat{Z}(s_0;t)$.

For $\forall t_1, t_2 \in [0, T]$, a variogram can be defined as

$$2\gamma_{t_1,t_2}(h) = \mathrm{Var}(Z(s+h;t_1) - Z(s;t_2)),$$

where we denote $2\gamma_{t,t}(h) = 2\gamma_t(h)$. Similar to the spatial kriging, we can obtain $\tilde{\lambda} = \Gamma^{-1}\tilde{\gamma}$, where $\tilde{\lambda} = (\hat{\lambda}_1, \ldots, \hat{\lambda}_n \hat{\rho})'$, by

$$\tilde{\gamma} = \begin{pmatrix} \int \gamma_t(s_1 - s_0)dt \\ \vdots \\ \int \gamma_t(s_n - s_0)dt \\ 1 \end{pmatrix}$$

$$\Gamma = \begin{cases} \int \gamma_t(s_i - s_j)dt & i = 1, \ldots, n; \quad j = 1, \ldots, n \\ 1 & i = n+1; \quad j = 1, \ldots, n \ , \\ 0 & i = n+1; \quad j = n+1 \end{cases}$$

where ρ is a Laplace operator. By using a Trace Variogram $2\gamma(h) = \int_0^T 2\gamma_t(h)dt$, the variance of the predicted curve is $\sigma_{s_0}^2 = \int_0^T \mathrm{Var}[\hat{Z}(s_0;t)]dt = \sum_{i=1}^n \lambda_i \gamma(s_i - s_0) + \rho$, which describes the overall variation of $\hat{Z}(s_0;t)$.

To estimate $\gamma(h)$, we can follow steps of the spatial kriging, i.e. we calculate an empirical variogram function and look for a parametric form that is close to it. An integral $\int (Z(s_i;t) - Z(s_j;t))^2 dt$ is needed to calculate the empirical variogram, which may cost a lot of computing, especially when the time interval $[0, T]$ is long. Therefore, the method of spline basis approximation to data curve $Z(s_i;t)$ will greatly reduce complexities. To control the degree of smoothness, we can use some penalties to regularize the shape of the approximated curves. Specifically, suppose

$$\tilde{Z}(s;t) = \sum_{k=1}^{K} \beta_k(s) B_k(t)$$

is an approximation to $Z(s;t)$, we estimate parameters $\beta_k(s)$ by minimizing

$$\sum_{j=1}^{M} [Z(s;t_j) - \tilde{Z}(s;t_j)]^2 + \alpha \int_0^T \tilde{Z}''(s;t)dt,$$

where M is the number of time points and α is a smoothing parameter. The smoothing parameter can be obtained by functional cross-validations.

References

1. Calhoun, V, Pekar, J, McGinty, V, Adali, T, Watson, T, Pearlson, G. Different activation dynamics in multiple neural systems during simulated driving. *Hum. Brain Mapping* (2002), 16: 158–167.
2. Cressie, N. *Statistics for Spatio Data.* New York: John Wiley & Sons INC., 1993.
3. Cressie, N, Davison, JL. Image analysis with partially ordered markov models. *Comput. Stat. Data Anal.* 1998, 29: 1–26.
4. Gaetan, C, Guyon, X. *Spatial Statistics and Modeling.* New York: Springer, 2010.
5. Banerjee, S, Carlin, BP, Gelfand, AE. *Hierarchical Modeling and Analysis for Spatial Data.* London: Chapman & Hall/CRC, 2004.
6. Diggle, PJ, Tawn, JA, Moyeed, RA. Model based geostatistics (with discussion). *Appl. Stat.*, 1998, 47: 299–350.
7. Stein, ML. *Interpolation of Spatial Data.* New York: Springer, 1999.
8. Davis, RC. On the theory of prediction of nonstationary stochastic processess. *J. Appl. Phys.*, 1952, 23: 1047–1053.
9. Matheron, G. *Traité de Geostatistique Apliquée, Tome II: le Krigeage. Memoires du Bureau de Recherches Geologiques et Minieres*, No. 24. Paris: Editions du Burean de Recherches geologques etmimieres.
10. Cressie, N, Wikle, CK. *Statistics for Spatio-Temporal Data.* Hoboken: John Wiley & Sons, 2011.
11. Diggle, PJ. *Statistical Analysis of Spatial and Spatio-Temporal Point Pattern.* UK: Chapman & Hall/CRC, London, 2014.
12. Sherman, M. *Spatial Statistics and Spatio-Temporal Data: Covariance Functions and Directional Properties.* Hoboken: John Wiley & Sons, 2011.
13. Moller, J, Waagepeterson, RP. *Statistical Inference and Simulation for Spatial Point Processes.* London, UK: Chapman & Hall/CRC, 2004.
14. Yao, F, Muller, HG, Wang, JL. Functional data analysis for sparse longitudinal data. *J. Amer. Stat. Assoc.*, 2005, 100: 577–590.
15. Waller, LA, Gotway, CA. *Applied Spatial Statistics for Public Health Data.* New Jersey: John Wiley & Sons, Inc., 2004.
16. Bivand, RS, Pebesma, E, Gomez-Rubio, V. *Applied Spatial Data Analysis with R,* (2nd Edn.). New York: Springer, 2013.
17. Carr, DB, Pickle, LW. *Visualizing Data Patterns with Micromaps.* London: Chapman & Hall/CRC, Boca Raton, Florida 2010.

18. Lloyd, CD. *Local Models for Spatial Analysis.* Boca Raton, Florida: Chapman & Hall/CRC, 2007.
19. Cressie, N, Huang, HC. Classes of nonseparable, spatiotemporal stationary covariance functions. *J. Amer. Stat. Assoc.*, 1999, 94: 1330–1340.
20. Gneiting, T. Nonseparable, stationary covariance functions for space-time data. *J. Amer. Stat. Assoc.*, 2002, 97: 590–600.
21. Ramsay, J, Silverman, B. Functional Data Analysis (2nd edn.). New York: Springer, 2005.
22. Delicado, P, Giraldo, R, Comas, C, Mateu, J. Statistics for spatial functional data: Some recent contributions. *Environmetrics*, 2010, 21: 224–239.
23. Giraldo, R, Delicado, P, Mateu, J. Ordinary kriging for function-valued spatial data. *Environ. Ecol. Stat.*, 2011, 18: 411–426.

About the Author

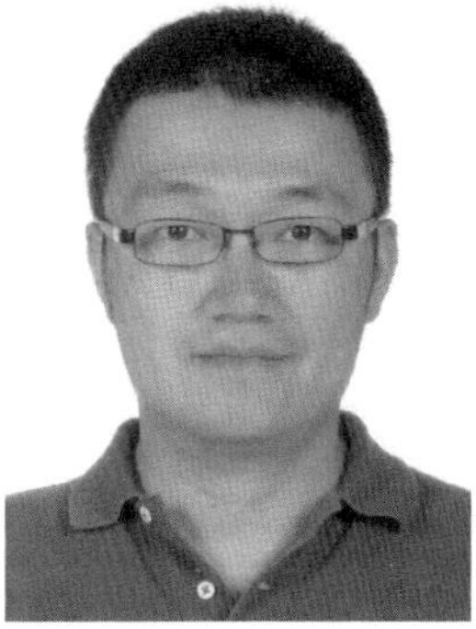

Dr. Hui Huang is an Assistant Professor of statistics at the Center for Statistical Science, Peking University. After receiving his PhD from the University of Maryland, Baltimore County in year 2010, he had worked for Yale University and the University of Miami as a post-doc associate for three years. In June 2013, he joined Peking University. In 2015, he received support from the "Thousand Youth Talents Plan" initiated by China's government. Dr. Huang's research interests include Spatial Point Pattern Analysis, Functional Data Analysis, Spatio-temporal Analysis, Spatial Epidemiology and Environmental Statistics.

CHAPTER 8

STOCHASTIC PROCESSES

Caixia Li*

8.1. Stochastic Process[1,2]

For any given $t \in T, X(t, \omega)$ is a random variable defined on a probability space (Ω, Σ, P). Then the t-indexed collection of random variables $X_T = \{X(t, \omega);\ t \in T\}$ is called a stochastic process on the probability space (Ω, Σ, P), where the parameter set $T \subset R$, and R is a real number set. For any specified $\omega \in \Omega, X(\cdot, \omega)$ is a function on the parameter $t \in T$, and it is often called a sample path or sample trajectory.

We often interpret the parameter t as time. If the set T is a countable set, we call the process a discrete-time stochastic process, usually denoted by $\{X_n, n = 1, 2, \ldots\}$. And if T is continuum, we call it a continuous-time stochastic process, usually denoted by $\{X(t), t \geq 0\}$. The collection of possible values of $X(t)$ is called state space. If the state space is a countable set, we call the process a discrete-state process, and if the space is a continuum, we call the process a continuous-state process.

8.1.1. *Family of finite-dimensional distributions*

The statistical properties of the stochastic process are determined by a family of finite-dimensional distributions $\{F_X(x_1, \ldots, x_n; t_1, \ldots, t_n), t_1, \ldots, t_n \in T, n \geq 1\}$, where

$$F_X(x_1, \ldots, x_n; t_1, \ldots, t_n) = P\{X(t_1) \leq x_1, \ldots, X(t_n) \leq x_n\}.$$

*Corresponding author: licx@mail.sysu.edu.cn

8.1.2. *Numerical characteristics*

Moments are usually to describe the numerical characteristics of a distribution, including mathematical expectation, variance and covariance, etc. The expectation and variance functions of stochastic process $\{X(t);\ t \in T\}$ are defined as

$$\mu_X(t) \hat{=} m(t) = E\{X(t)\}, \quad \sigma_X^2(t) \hat{=} E\{[X(t) - \mu_X(t)]^2\},$$

respectively. Autocovariance and correlation functions are given as

$$C_X(s,t) \hat{=} E\{[X(s) - \mu_X(s)][X(t) - \mu_X(t)]\}, \quad R_X(s,t) \hat{=} \frac{C_X(s,t)}{\sigma_X(s)\sigma_X(t)},$$

respectively. The crosscovariance function of two stochastic processes $\{X(t); t \in T\}$ and $\{Y(t); t \in T\}$ is defined as

$$C_{XY}(s,t) \hat{=} E\{[X(s) - \mu_X(s)][Y(t) - \mu_Y(t)]\}.$$

If $C_{XY}(s,t) = 0$, for any $s, t \in T$, then the two processes are said to be uncorrelated.

Stochastic process theory is a powerful tool to study the evolution of some system of random values over time. It has been applied in many fields, including astrophysics, economics, population theory and the computer science.

8.2. Random Walk[1,3]

A simple random walk is generalization of Bernoulli trials, which can be described by the movement of a particle makes a walk on the integer points. Wherever it is, the particle will either go up one step with probability p, or down one step with probability $1 - p$. $\{X_n\}$ is called a random walk, where X_n denote the site of the particle after n steps. In particular, when $p = 0.5$, the random walk is called symmetric.

Let $Z_i = 1$ (or -1) denote moving up (or down, respectively) one step. Then $Z_1, Z_2, \ldots$ are independent and identically distributed (i.i.d.), and $P(Z_i = 1) = p, P(Z_i = -1) = 1 - p$. Suppose the particle starts from the origin, then

$$X_0 = 0, \quad X_n = \sum_{i=1}^{n} Z_i, \quad n = 1, 2, \ldots.$$

It is easy to see that the simple random walk is a Markov chain. Its transition probability

$$p_{ij} = \begin{cases} p & j = i+1, \\ 1-p & j = i-1, \\ 0 & \text{else}. \end{cases}$$

8.2.1. *Distribution of simple random walk*

$\forall k = 0, \pm 1, \ldots$, the event $\{X_n = k\}$ means there are $x = (n+k)/2$ upward movements and $y = (n-k)/2$ downward movements. Therefore, $P\{X_n = k\} = 0$ if $n + k$ is odd, and

$$P\{X_n = k\} = \binom{n}{\frac{n+k}{2}} p^{\frac{n+k}{2}} (1-p)^{\frac{n-k}{2}},$$

otherwise. Then

$$E(X_n) = \sum_{i=1}^{n} E(Z_i) = 0, \quad \mathrm{var}(X_n) = E(X_n^2) = \sum_{i=1}^{n} \mathrm{var}(Z_i) = n.$$

A simple random walk is a one-dimensional discrete-state process. It can be extended to high dimensional or continuous-state type, such as Gaussian random walk with

$$X_n = \sum_{i=1}^{n} Z_i, \quad n = 1, 2, \ldots,$$

where $Z_i, i = 1, 2, \ldots$, are i.i.d. Gaussian distributed.

Definition: Let $\{Z_k, k = 1, 2, \ldots\}$ be a sequence of i.i.d. random variables. For each positive integer n, we let $X_n = \sum_{i=1}^{n} Z_i$, the sequence $\{X_n, n = 1, 2, \ldots\}$ is called a random walk. If the support of the Z_ks is $\mathbf{R}^m$, then we say $\{X_n\}$ is a random walk in $\mathbf{R}^m$.

Random walks have been to model the gambler's ruin and the volatility of the stock price patterns, etc. Maurice Kendall in 1953 found that stock price fluctuations are independent of each other and have the same probability distribution. In short, random walk says that stocks take a random and unpredictable path.

8.3. Stochastic Process with Stationary and Independent Increments[2,4]

Consider a continuous-time stochastic process $\{X(t), t \in T\}$. The increments of such a process are the differences $X_t - X_s$ between its values at different times $s < t$.

The process has independent increments

If for $t_1, t_2, \ldots, t_n \in T$ with $0 < t_1 < t_2 < \cdots < t_n$, the increments $X(t_1) - X(t_0)$, $X(t_2) - X(t_1), \ldots, X(t_n) - X(t_{n-1})$ are independent.

The process has stationary increments

If for $s, t \in T$ with $s < t$, the increments $X(t) - X(s)$ have the same distribution as $X(t - s)$.

In discrete time when $T = N = \{1, 2, \ldots\}$, the process $\{X(t),\ t \in T\}$ has stationary, independent increments if and only if it is the partial sum process associated with a sequence of i.i.d. variables.

8.3.1. *Distributions and moments*

Suppose that $\{X(t),\ t \in T\}$ has stationary, independent increments, and $X(t)$ has probability density (continuous case) or mass (discrete cases) function $f_t(x)$. If $t_1, t_2, \ldots, t_n \in T$ with $0 < t_1 < t_2 < \cdots < t_n$, then $(X(t_1), X(t_2), \ldots, X(t_n))$ has joint probability density or mass function

$f_{t_1}(x_1) f_{t_2 - t_1}(x_2 - x_1) \cdots f_{t_n - t_{n-1}}(x_n - x_{n-1})$. Suppose that $\{X(t), t \in T\}$ is a second-order process with stationary, independent increments. Then $E[X(t)] = \mu t$ and

$$\operatorname{cov}[X(s), X(t)] = \sigma^2 \min(s, t),$$

where μ and σ^2 are constants. For example, $\mathbf{X} = (X_1, X_2, \ldots)$ is a sequence of Bernoulli trials with success parameter $p \in (0, 1)$. Let $Y_n = \sum_{i=1}^{n} X_i$ be the number of successes in the first n trials. Then, the sequence $\mathbf{Y} = (Y_1, Y_2, \ldots)$ is a second-order process with stationary independent increments. The mean and covariance functions are given by $E[Y_n] = np$ and

$$\operatorname{cov}(Y_m, Y_n) = p(1 - p) \min(m, n).$$

A process $\{X(t),\ t \in T\}$ with stationary, independent increments is a Markov process. Suppose $X(t)$ has probability density or mass function $f_t(x)$. As a time homogeneous Markov process, the transition probability density function is $p_t(x, y) = f_t(y - x)$.

A Lévy process is a process with independent, stationary increments, $X(0) = 0$ and

$$\lim_{h \to 0} P\{|X(t + h) - X(t)| > \varepsilon\} = 0.$$

A Lévy process may be viewed as the continuous-time analog of a random walk. It represents the motion of a point whose successive displacements are random and independent, and statistically identical over different time intervals of the same length. The most well-known examples of Lévy processes are Brownian motion and Poisson process.

8.4. Markov processes[1,2]

Markov property refers to the memoryless property of a stochastic process. A stochastic process has the Markov property if its future and past states are conditional independent, conditional on the present state. A process with Markov property is called a Markov process.

Definition: A stochastic process $\{X(t) : t \in T\}$ is called a Markov process if

$$P(X(t_n) \leq x_n | X(t_{n-1}) = x_{n-1}, \ldots, X(t_1) = x_1)$$
$$= P(X(t_n) \leq x_n | X(t_{n-1}) = x_{n-1})$$

for any $t_1 < t_2 < \cdots < t_n, t_1, t_2, \ldots, t_n \in T$ and $n \geq 3$.

There are four kinds of Markov processes corresponding to two levels of state space and two levels of time indices: continuous-time and continuous-state, continuous-time and discrete-state, discrete-time and continuous-state, discrete-time and discrete-state Markov processes. Markov chain is used to indicate a Markov process which has a discrete (finite or countable) state space.

The finite-dimensional distribution of a Markov process is determined by conditional distribution and its initial state. The conditional cumulative distribution function (cdf) is given by

$$F(x; t|x_s; s) = P(X(t) \leq x | X(s) = x_s),$$

where $s, t \in T$ and $s < t$. We say the process is time-homogeneous, if $F(x; t|x_s; s)$, as a function of s and t, only depends on $t - s$.

For a time-homogeneous Markov chain, the conditional probability mass function (pmf)

$$p_{ij}(t) \hat{=} P(X(t + t_i) = x_j | X(t_i) = x_i), \quad \forall t > 0$$

describes the transition probability from state x_i to x_j, after time t.

For a time-homogeneous discrete-time Markov chain with $T = \{0, 1, 2, \ldots\}, p_{ij}(n)$ is called n-step transition probability, and $p_{ij}(1)$ (or p_{ij} in short) is one-step transition probability.

In real life, there are many random systems which change states according to a Markov transition rule, such as the number of animals in the forest changes, the number of people waiting for the bus, the Brownian movement of particles in the liquid, etc. In medical science, we usually divide a specified disease into several states. According to the transition probability between states under Markov assumption, we can evaluate the evolution of the disease.

A Markov process of order k is a generalization of a classic Markov process, where k is finite positive number. It is a process satisfying

$$P(X(t_n) \leq x_n | X(t_{n-1}) = x_{n-1}, \ldots, X(t_1) = x_1) = P(X(t_n) \leq x_n | X(t_{n-1}) = x_{n-1}, \ldots, X(t_{n-k}) = x_{n-k}), \quad \text{for any integer } n > k.$$

8.5. Chapman–Kolmogorov Equations[25]

For a homogeneous discrete-time Markov chain with $T = \{0, 1, 2, \ldots\}$, the k-step transition probability is defined as

$$p_{ij}(k) \hat{=} P(X(i+k) = x_j | X(i) = x_i).$$

The one-step transitions $p_{ij}(1)$(or p_{ij} in short) can be put together in a matrix form

$$P = \begin{pmatrix} p_{11} & p_{12} & \cdots \\ p_{21} & p_{22} & \cdots \\ \vdots & \vdots & \ddots \end{pmatrix}.$$

It is called (one-step) transition probability matrix. Note that

$$\sum_j p_{ij} = \sum_j P(X(t+1) = x_j | X(t) = x_i) = 1.$$

The k-step transition probability

$$p_{ij}(k) = \sum_l p_{il}(k-1) p_{lj}(1), i, l = 1, 2, \ldots,$$

and k-step transition probability matrix

$$P(k) \hat{=} \begin{pmatrix} p_{11}(k) & p_{12}(k) & \cdots \\ p_{21}(k) & p_{22}(k) & \cdots \\ \vdots & \vdots & \ddots \end{pmatrix} = P^k.$$

In general, as shown in Figure 8.5.1, for any m, n,

$$p_{ij}(m+n) = \sum_r p_{ir}(m) p_{rj}(n), i, r = 1, 2, \ldots.$$

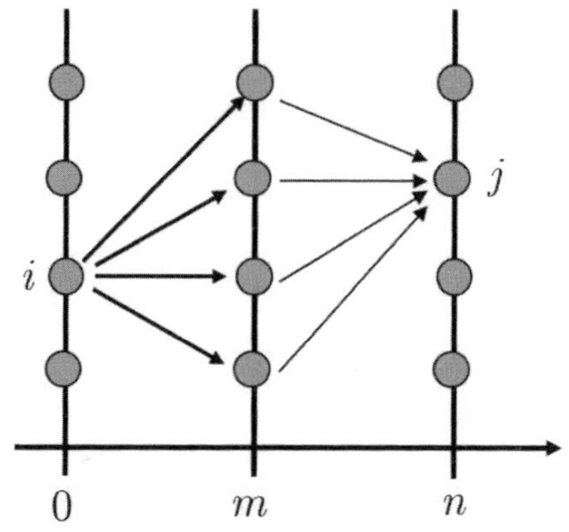

Fig. 8.5.1. The transition from state i to j.

Above equations are called Chapman–Kolmogorov equations. In terms of the transition probability matrices, $P(m+n) = P(m)P(n)$, and $P^{(n)} = P^n$, especially.

For a homogeneous continuous time discrete state Markov process, the state is transited into j from i after time Δt with the probability

$$p_{ij}(\Delta t) = P\{X(t+\Delta t) = j | X(t) = i\}.$$

Let $\delta_{ij} = 1$ if $i = j$, and $\delta_{ij} = 0$, otherwise.

$$q_{ij} \hat{=} \lim_{\Delta t \to 0+} \frac{p_{ij}(\Delta t) - \delta_{ij}}{\Delta t}$$

is said to be transition intensity. The matrix $Q \hat{=} (q_{ij})$ is called transition intensity matrix. It is easy to show that $\sum_j q_{ij} = 0$.

For the continuous-time Markov process with intensity matrix $Q = (q_{ij})$, the sojourn time of state i have exponential distribution with the mean $-q_{ii}$, and it steps into state j ($j \neq i$) with the probability $p_{ij} = -q_{ij}/q_{ii}$ after leaving state i. The transition probabilities satisfy Chapman–Kolmogorov equations

$$p_{ij}(t+s) = \sum_k p_{ik}(t) p_{kj}(s)$$

and two kinds of Chapman–Kolmogorov differential equations, i.e. Chapman–Kolmogorov forward equations

$$p'_{ij}(t) = \sum_k p_{ik}(t) q_{kj}, \text{ i.e. } P'(t) = P(t)Q$$

and Chapman–Kolmogorov backward equations

$$p'_{ij}(t) = \sum_k q_{ik}p_{kj}(t), \text{ i.e. } P'(t) = QP(t)$$

for all i, j and $t \geq 0$.

8.6. Limiting Distribution[1,2]

State j is said to be accessible from state i if for some $n \geq 0, p_{ij}^{(n)} > 0$. Two states accessible to each other are said to be communicative. We say that the Markov chain is irreducible if all states communicate with each other. For example, simple random walk is irreducible.

State i is said to have period d if $p_{ii}^{(n)} = 0$ whenever n is not divisible by d and d is the greatest integer with the property. A state with period 1 is called aperiodic.

A probability distribution $\{\pi_j\}$ related to a Markov chain is called stationary distribution if it satisfies $\pi_j = \sum_i \pi_i p_{ij}$.

A Markov chain is called finite if the state space is finite. If a Markov chain is finite and irreducible, there exists unique stationary distribution. Markov chain started according to a stationary distribution will follow this distribution at all points of time. Formally, if $P\{X_0 = j\} = \pi_j$ then $P\{X_n = j\} = \pi_j$ for all $n = 1, 2, \ldots$.

If there is a distribution $\{\pi_j\}$ such that

$$\lim_{n\to\infty} \sum_i \pi_i p_{ij}^{(n)} = \pi_j \quad \text{for any } i, j,$$

$\{\pi_j\}$ is called limiting distribution (or long-run distribution). A limiting distribution is such a distribution π that no matter what the initial distribution is, the distribution over states converges to π. If a finite Markov chain is aperiodic, its stationary distribution is limiting distribution.

8.6.1. *Hardy–Weinberg equilibrium in genetics*

Consider a biological population. Each individual in the population is assumed to have a genotype AA or Aa or aa, where A and a are two alleles. Suppose that the initial genotype frequency composition (AA, Aa, aa) equals $(d, 2h, r)$, where $d + 2h + r = 1$, then the gene frequencies of A and a are p and q, where $p = d + h, q = r + h$ and $p + q = 1$. We can use Markov chain to describe the heredity process. We number the three genotypes AA, Aa and aa by 1, 2, 3, and denote by p_{ij} the probability that an offspring has genotype j given that a specified parent has genotype i. The one-step transition probability matrix is

$$P = (p_{ij}) = \begin{pmatrix} p & q & 0 \\ \frac{1}{2}p & \frac{1}{2} & \frac{1}{2}q \\ 0 & p & q \end{pmatrix}.$$

The initial genotype distribution of the 0th generation is $(d, 2h, r)$. Then the genotype distribution of the nth generation $(n \geq 1)$

$$(d, 2h, r)P^n = (p^2, 2pq, q^2).$$

This is Hardy–Weinberg law of equilibrium. In this example, the stationary or limiting distribution is $(p^2, 2pq, q^2)$.

8.7. Poisson Process[6,1,8,9]

Let $N(t)$ be the total number of events that occur within the time interval $(0, t]$, and τ_i denote the time when the ith event occurs, $0 < \tau_1 < \tau_2 < \cdots$. Let $\{T_i, i = 1, 2, \ldots\}$ with $T_1 = \tau_1, T_2 = \tau_2 - \tau_1, \ldots$, be time intervals between successive occurrences.

$\{N(t), t \geq 0\}$ is called a Poisson process if $\{T_i, i = 1, 2, \ldots\}$ are identically independently exponential distributed. A Poisson process satisfies: (1) For any $t \geq 0$, the probability that an event will occur during $(t, t+\delta)$ is $\lambda\delta + o(\delta)$, where λ is constant and time-independent, and (2) the probability that more than one event will occur during $(t, t+\delta)$ is $o(\delta)$, and therefore the probability that no event will occur during $(t, t+\delta)$ is $1 - \lambda\delta - o(\delta)$. λ is called the intensity of occurrence.

A Poisson process can also be defined in terms of Poisson distribution. $\{N(t), t \geq 0\}$ is called an Poisson process if (1) it is a independent increment process, (2) $P(N(0) = 0) = 1$, and (3) $N(t) - N(s)(t > s)$ is Poisson distributed.

For a Poisson process $\{N(t), t \geq 0\}$ with intensity λ, we have $N(t) \sim P(\lambda t)$, and

$$P\{N(t) = k\} = \frac{\exp(-\lambda t)(\lambda t)^k}{k!}.$$

The occurrence time intervals $T_i \sim \exp(\lambda)$. To identify whether a process $\{N(t), t \geq 0\}$ is a Poisson process, we can check whether $\{T_i, i = 1, 2, \ldots\}$ are exponentially distributed. The maximum likelihood estimate (MLE) of λ

can be derived based on the n observed occurrence time $\{t_i, i = 1, 2, \ldots, n\}$. The likelihood

$$L(t_1, \ldots, t_n) = \lambda^n e^{-\lambda \sum_{i=0}^{n} (t_{i+1} - t_i)} = \lambda^n e^{-\lambda t_n}.$$

Let $d \ln L / d\lambda = 0$, and we get the MLE of $\lambda, \hat{\lambda} = n/t_n$.

Generalization of the Poisson process can be done in many ways. If we replace the constant intensity λ by a function of time $\lambda(t), \{N(t), t \geq 0\}$ is called time-dependent Poisson process. The probability

$$P\{N(t) = k\} = \frac{\exp(-\Lambda(t))\Lambda^k(t)}{k!},$$

where $\Lambda(t) = \int_0^t \lambda(s)ds$. If intensity λ of event is individual dependent, and it varies throughout the population according to a density function $f(\lambda)$, then the process is called a weighted Poisson process.

8.8. Branching Process[7,10]

Branching processes were studied by Galton and Watson in 1874. Suppose that each individual in a population can produce k offspring with probability $p_k, k = 0, 1, 2, \ldots$, and the production from each other is independent. Let X_0 denote the numbers of initial individuals, which is called the size of the 0th generation. The size of the first generation, which is constituted by all offspring of the 0th generation, is denoted by $X_1, \ldots$. Let $Z_j^{(n)}$ denote the number of offsprings produced by the jth individual in the nth Generation. Then

$$X_n = Z_1^{(n-1)} + Z_2^{(n-1)} + \cdots + Z_{X_{n-1}}^{(n-1)} = \sum_{j=1}^{X_{n-1}} Z_j^{(n-1)}.$$

It shows that X_n is a sum of X_{n-1} random variables with i.i.d. $\{p_k, k = 0, 1, 2, \ldots\}$. The process $\{X_n\}$ is called Branching Process.

The Branching Process is a Markov chain, and its transition probability is

$$p_{ij} = P\{X_{n+1} = j | X_n = i\} = P\left(\sum_{k=1}^{i} Z_k^{(n)} = j\right).$$

Suppose that there are x_0 individuals in the 0th generation, i.e. $X_0 = x_0$. Let

$$E(Z_j^{(n)}) = \sum_{k=0}^{\infty} kp_k = \mu \quad \text{and} \quad \mathrm{Var}(Z_j^{(n)}) = \sum_{k=0}^{\infty} (k - \mu)^2 p_k = \sigma^2.$$

Then it is easy to see

$$E(X_n) = x_0\mu^n, \quad \text{Var}(X_n) = \begin{cases} x_0^2\mu^{n-1}\sigma^2\frac{\mu^{n-1}}{\mu-1} & \mu \neq 1 \\ nx_0^2\sigma^2 & \mu = 1 \end{cases}.$$

Now we can see that the expectation and variance of the size will increase when $\mu > 1$ and will decrease when $\mu < 1$.

In Branching Processes, the probability π_0 that the population dies out is shown in the following theorem.

Theorem: *Suppose that $p_0 > 0$ and $p_0 + p_1 < 1$. Then $\pi_0 = 1$ if $\mu \leq 1$, and $\pi_0 = q^{x_0}$, otherwise, where q is the smallest positive number satisfying the equation $x = \sum_{k=0}^{\infty} p_k x^k$.*

Suppose that the life spans of the individuals are i.i.d. Let $F(x)$ denote the CDF, and $N(t)$ be the surviving individuals at time t. Then

$$E(N(t)) \approx \frac{(\mu - 1)e^{\alpha t}}{\mu^2\alpha\int_0^{\infty} xe^{-\alpha x}dF(x)},$$

when t is large enough, $\mu = \sum_{k=0}^{\infty} kp_k$ is the expected number of offspring of each individual, and $\alpha(> 0)$ is determined by

$$\int_0^{\infty} e^{-\alpha x}dF(x) = \frac{1}{\mu}.$$

8.9. Birth-and-death Process[1,7]

Birth–death processes represent population growth and decline. Let $N(t)$ denote the size of a population at time t. We say that 1 birth (or 1 death) occurs when the size increases by 1 (decreases by 1, respectively).

Birth–death processes are Markov chains with transition intensities satisfying $q_{ij} = 0$ if $|i - j| \geq 2$, and

$$q_{i,i+1} = \lambda_i, \quad q_{i,i-1} = \mu_i.$$

λ_i and μ_i are called birth rate and death rate, respectively.

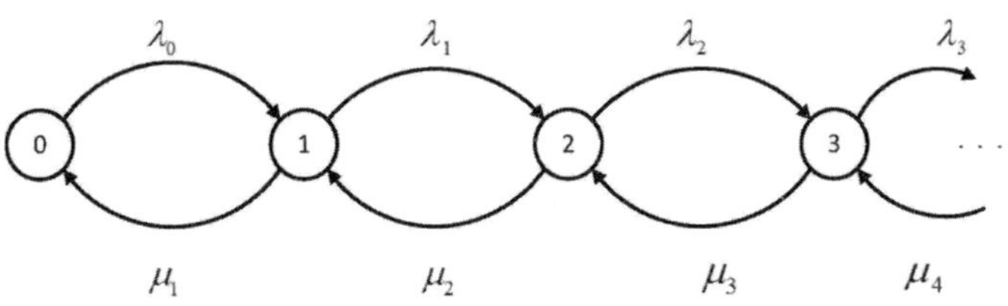

Fig. 8.9.1. Transitions in birth–death process.

The transition intensity matrix for birth–death processes is

$$Q = \begin{pmatrix} -\lambda_0 & \lambda_0 & 0 & 0 & \cdots \\ \mu_1 & -(\lambda_1+\mu_1) & \lambda_1 & 0 & \cdots \\ 0 & \mu_2 & -(\lambda_2+\mu_2) & \lambda_2 & \cdots \\ \vdots & \vdots & \vdots & \vdots & \vdots \end{pmatrix}.$$

According to the C–K forward equation, the distribution $p_k(t)$ $\hat{=}P\{N(t)=k\}$ satisfies the equations

$$p_0'(t) = -\lambda_0 p_0(t) + \mu_1 p_1(t),$$
$$p_k'(t) = -(\lambda_k+\mu_k)p_k(t) + \lambda_{k-1}p_{k-1}(t) + \mu_{k+1}p_{k+1}(t), \quad k \geq 1.$$

A birth–death process is called pure birth process if $\mu_i = 0$ for all i. Poisson process and Yule process are special cases of pure birth process with $\lambda_i = \lambda$ and $\lambda_i = i\lambda$, respectively.

8.9.1. *Mckendrick model*

There is one population which is constituted by 1 infected and $N-1$ susceptible individuals. The infected state is an absorbing state. Suppose that any given infected individual will cause, with probability $\beta h + O(h)$, any given susceptible individual infected in time interval $(t, t+h)$, where β is called infection rate. Let $X(t)$ denote the number of the infected individuals at time t. Then $\{X(t)\}$ is a pure birth process with birth rate

$$\lambda_n(t) = (N-n)n\beta.$$

This epidemic model was proposed by AM Mckendrick in 1926.

Let T denote the time until all individuals in the population are infected and T_i denote the time from i infective to $i+1$ infective. Then T_i has exponential distribution with mean

$$\frac{1}{\lambda_i} = \frac{1}{(N-i)i\beta}, \quad \text{and}$$

$$ET = E\left(\sum_{i=1}^{N-1} T_i\right) = \frac{1}{\beta}\sum_{i=1}^{N-1}\frac{1}{i(N-i)}$$
$$= \frac{1}{\beta N}\left[\sum_{i=1}^{N-1}\frac{1}{i} + \sum_{i=1}^{N-1}\frac{1}{N-i}\right] = \frac{2}{\beta N}\sum_{i=1}^{N-1}\frac{1}{i}.$$

8.10. Fix–Neyman Process[7]

Fix–Neyman process is Markov process with two transient states and one or more absorbing states. Fix–Neyman[1951] introduced the stochastic model of two transient states. A general illness–death stochastic model that can accommodate any finite number of transient states was presented by Chiang[1964]. In this general model, there are a finite number of health states and death states. An individual can be in a particular health state, or stay a death state if he dies of a particular cause. The health states are transient. An individual may leave a health state at any time through death, or by contracting diseases. Death states are absorbing states. If an individual enters a death state once, he will remain there forever.

Consider an illness–death process with two health states S_1 and S_2, and r death states $R_1, \ldots, R_r$, where r is a finite positive integer. Transitions are possible between S_1 and S_2, or from either S_1 or S_2 to any death state.

Let (τ, t) be a time interval with $0 \leq \tau < t < \infty$. Suppose an individual is in state S_α at time τ. During (τ, t), the individual may travel between S_α and S_β, for $\alpha, \beta = 1, 2$, or reach a death state. The transition is determined by the intensities of illness ($\nu_{\alpha\beta}$) and intensities of death ($\mu_{\alpha\delta}$). The health transition probability

$$P_{\alpha\beta}(\tau, t) = \Pr\{\text{state } S_\beta \text{ at } t | \text{ state } S_\alpha \text{ at } \tau\}, \quad \alpha, \beta = 1, 2,$$

and the death transition probability

$$Q_{\alpha\beta}(\tau, t) = \Pr\{\text{state } R_\delta \text{ at } t | \text{ state } S_\alpha \text{ at } \tau\}, \quad \alpha = 1, 2; \quad \delta = 1, \ldots, r.$$

The health transition probabilities satisfy

$$\begin{aligned} P_{\alpha\alpha}(\tau, \tau) &= 1, \quad \alpha = 1, 2 \\ P_{\alpha\beta}(\tau, \tau) &= 0, \quad \alpha \neq \beta; \ \alpha, \beta = 1, 2 \\ Q_{\alpha\delta}(\tau, \tau) &= 0, \quad \alpha = 1, 2; \ \delta = 1, \ldots, r. \end{aligned}$$

Based on Chapman–Kolmogorov equations,

$$\begin{aligned} \frac{\partial}{\partial t} P_{\alpha\alpha}(\tau, t) &= P_{\alpha\alpha}(\tau, t)\nu_{\alpha\alpha} + P_{\alpha\beta}(\tau, t)\nu_{\beta\alpha}, \\ \frac{\partial}{\partial t} P_{\alpha\beta}(\tau, t) &= P_{\alpha\alpha}(\tau, t)\nu_{\alpha\beta} + P_{\alpha\beta}(\tau, t)\nu_{\beta\beta}, \\ &\alpha \neq \beta; \ \alpha, \beta = 1, 2. \end{aligned}$$

The solutions from Chiang were given by

$$P_{\alpha\alpha}(\tau,t)=\sum_{i=1}^{2}\frac{\rho_i-\nu_{\beta\beta}}{\rho_i-\rho_j}e^{\rho_i(t-\tau)}$$

$$P_{\alpha\beta}(\tau,t)=\sum_{i=1}^{2}\frac{\nu_{\alpha\beta}}{\rho_i-\rho_j}e^{\rho_i(t-\tau)},\quad j\neq i,\ \alpha\neq\beta;\ \alpha,\beta=1,2.$$

Similarly, the death transition probability

$$Q_{\alpha\delta}(\tau,t)=\sum_{i=1}^{2}\frac{e^{\rho_i(t-t)}-1}{\rho_i(\rho_i-\rho_j)}[(\rho_i-\nu_{\beta\beta})\mu_{\alpha\delta}+\nu_{\alpha\beta}\mu_{\beta\delta}],$$

$$i\neq j;\ \alpha\neq\beta;\ j,\alpha,\beta=1,2;\ \delta=1,\cdots,r,$$

where

$$\rho_1=\frac{1}{2}\left[\nu_{11}+\nu_{22}+\sqrt{(\nu_{11}-\nu_{22})^2+4\nu_{12}\nu_{21}}\right],$$

$$\rho_2=\frac{1}{2}\left[\nu_{11}+\nu_{22}-\sqrt{(\nu_{11}-\nu_{22})^2+4\nu_{12}\nu_{21}}\right].$$

8.11. Stochastic Epidemic Models[11,12]

An epidemic model is a tool used to study the mechanisms by which diseases spread to predict the future course of an outbreak and to evaluate strategies to control an epidemic.

8.11.1. *SIS model*

The simplest epidemic model is SIS model. The SIS epidemic model has been applied to sexually transmitted diseases. In SIS epidemic model, the population is divided into two compartments, those who are susceptible to the disease (denoted by S), those who are infected (denoted by I). After a successful contact with an infectious individual, a susceptible individual becomes infected, but does not confer any long-lasting immunity. Therefore, the infected individual becomes susceptible again after recovery. The flow of this model is shown in Figure 8.11.1.

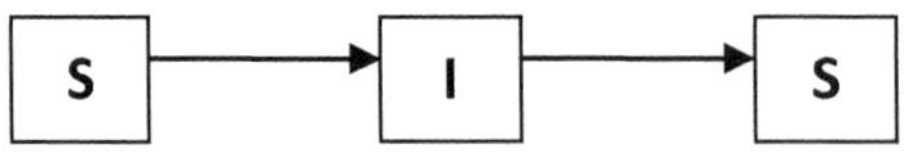

Fig. 8.11.1. SIS model.

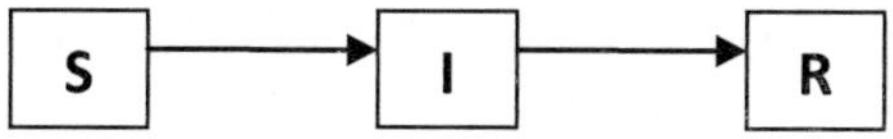

Fig. 8.11.2. SIR model.

Let $S(t)$ and $I(t)$ indicate the number of susceptible individuals and the number of infected individuals, respectively, at time t. Like previous Mckendrick model, suppose that any given infected individual will cause, with probability $\beta h + o(h)$, any given susceptible individual infected in time interval $(t, t+h)$, where β is called infection rate. In addition, any given infected individual will be recovery and be susceptible again with probability $\gamma h + o(h)$, where γ is called recovery rate. For a fixed population, $N = S(t) + I(t)$, The transition probabilities

$$P\{I(t+h) = i+1 | I(t) = i\} = \beta i(N-i)h + o(h),$$
$$P\{I(t+h) = i-1 | I(t) = i\} = i\gamma h + o(h),$$
$$P\{I(t+h) = i | I(t) = i\} = 1 - \beta i(N-i)h - i\gamma h + o(h),$$
$$P\{I(t+h) = j | I(t) = i\} = o(h), \quad |j-i| \geq 2.$$

8.11.2. *SIR model*

For most common diseases that confer long-lasting immunity, the population is divided into three compartments: susceptible$S(t)$, infected $I(t)$, and recovered $R(t)$. The recovered individuals are no longer spreading the disease when they are removed from the infection process. So, the population in SIR model is broken into three compartments: susceptible, infectious and recovered (Figure 8.11.2).

Similarly for a fixed population, the transition probabilities

$$P\{S(t+h) = k, I(t+h) = j | S(t) = s, I(t) = i\}$$
$$= \begin{cases} \beta i(N-i)h + o(h), & (k,j) = (s-1, i+1) \\ i\gamma h + o(h), & (k,j) = (s, i-1) \\ 1 - \beta i(N-i)h - i\gamma h + o(h), & (k,j) = (s,i) \\ o(h), & \text{otherwise} \end{cases}.$$

8.11.3. *SEIR model*

Many diseases have what is termed a latent or exposed phase, during which the individual is said to be infected but not infectious. The SEIR model takes into consideration the exposed or latent period of the disease. Hence, in this model, the population is broken into four compartments: susceptible (S), exposed (E), infectious (I) and recovered (R).

Maximum likelihood method can be used to estimate parameter values for the basic SIS, SIR, and SEIR model by using fully observed epidemic data.

8.12. Migration Process[7]

A population's growth is subject to immigration and emigration. The size of the population with various states changes through birth, death and migration. Migration processes are useful models for predicting population sizes, and forecasting future demographic composition.

Let $S_1, \ldots, S_s$ be s states. For each $\tau, 0 \leq \tau < t$, a change in the population size of state S_α during the time interval is assumed to take place according to

$$\begin{aligned}
\lambda_\alpha^*(\tau)\Delta + o(\Delta) &= \Pr\{\text{the size of } S_\alpha \text{ increase by 1 during } (\tau, \tau+\Delta)\},\\
\lambda_{\alpha\beta}^*(\tau)\Delta + o(\Delta) &= \Pr\{\text{one indivisidual move from } S_\alpha \text{ to } S_\beta\\
&\qquad \text{during } (\tau, \tau+\Delta)\},\\
\mu_\alpha^*(\tau)\Delta + o(\Delta) &= \Pr\{\text{the size of } S_\alpha \text{ will decrease by 1 during } (\tau, \tau+\Delta)\}.
\end{aligned}$$

Based on Chapman–Kolmogorov equations,

$$\begin{aligned}
\frac{d}{dt}P_{ij}(0,t) &= -P_{ij}(0,t)\sum_{\alpha=1}^{s}[\lambda_\alpha^*(t) - \lambda_{\alpha\alpha}^*(t)]\\
&\quad + \sum_{\alpha=1}^{s} P_{i,i-\delta_\alpha}(0,t)\lambda_\alpha^*(t) + \sum_{\alpha=1}^{s} P_{i,j+\delta_\alpha}(0,t)\mu_\alpha^*(t)\\
&\quad + \sum_{\substack{\alpha=1\\ \alpha\neq\beta}}^{s}\sum_{\beta=1}^{s} P_{i,j+\delta_\alpha-\delta_\beta}(0,t)v_{\alpha\beta}^*(t).
\end{aligned}$$

At $t = 0$, the initial condition $P_{i,j}(0,0) = 1$. The above equations describe the growth of a population in general.

8.12.1. *Immigration–emigration process*

Consider a migration process where an increase in population during a time interval $(t, t+\Delta)$ is independent of the existing population size. Then for state $S_\alpha, \lambda_\alpha^*(t) = \lambda_\alpha(t), a = 1, \ldots, s$, where $\lambda_\alpha(t)$ is known as immigration rate. The transition of an individual from one state to another is assumed to be independent of transitions made by other individuals, the corresponding intensity

$$v^*_{\alpha\beta}(t) = j_\alpha \mu_{\alpha\beta}, \quad \alpha \neq \beta; \beta = 1, \ldots, s,$$

where j_α is the population size of state S_α at time t, and $\lambda_\alpha(t)$ is known as immigration rate. A decrease in the population size of state S_α through death or emigration is measured by the intensity

$$\mu^*_\alpha(t) = j_\alpha \mu_\alpha, \quad \alpha = 1, \ldots, s,$$

where μ_α is known as emigration rate. Let

$$v_{\alpha\alpha} = -\left[\sum_{\substack{\beta=1\\ \beta\neq\alpha}}^{s} v_{\alpha\beta} + \mu_\alpha\right], \quad \alpha \neq \beta;\ \beta = 1, \ldots, s,$$

where $v_{\alpha\beta}$ is called internal migration rate (from S_α state to S_β).

In immigration–emigration process, $\lambda^*_\alpha(t) = \lambda(t)$. When $\lambda^*_\alpha(t)$ is a function of population size of j_α state S_α at time t, such as $\lambda^*_\alpha(t) = j_\alpha\lambda_\alpha$, we have a birth–illness–death process.

8.13. Renewal Process[7,3]

In the failure and renewal problem, for example, as soon as a component fails, it is replaced by a new one. The length of life of first, second, ... components, denoted by $\tau_1, \tau_2, \ldots$. Let $N(t)$ be the total number renewal events that occur within the time interval $(0, t]$, and T_i denote the time when the ith renewal event occurs, $0 < T_1 < T_2 < \cdots$. The renewal time intervals between two successive occurrences are

$$\tau_1 = T_1, \quad \tau_2 = T_2 - T_1, \ldots.$$

$\{N(t), t \geq 0\}$ is called a renewal process if $\tau_1, \tau_2, \ldots$ are i.i.d.

Renewal processes are counting processes with i.i.d. renewal time intervals. A Poisson process is a special renewal process with exponential distributed time intervals. Suppose the cumulative distribution function (CDF) of τ_i is $F(t)$, then the CDF $F_n(t)$ of the nth recurrence time $T_n = \sum_{i=1}^{n} \tau_i$

is n-fold convolution of $F(t)$, i.e.

$$F_n(t) = \int_0^t F_{n-1}(t-x)dF(x), \quad P\{N(t)=n\} = F_n(t) - F_{n-1}(t).$$

$m(t) = E\{N(t)\}$ is called renewal function, and it satisfies

$$m(t) = \sum_{n=1}^{\infty} nP\{N(t)=n\} = \sum_{n=1}^{\infty} P\{N(t) \geq n\} = \sum_{n=1}^{\infty} P\{S_n \leq t\} = \sum_{n=1}^{\infty} F_n(t).$$

In classical renewal process, the lengths of life of the components are i.i.d random variables. If the first component is not new but has been in use for a period and τ_1 is the residual of life of the first component, we have a delayed renewal process. Let the CDF of τ_1 is $F_0(x)$, then

$$m(t) = F_0(t) + \int_0^t m(t-x)dF(x), t \geq 0.$$

Theorem: If $\mu = E(\tau_n)$ and $\sigma^2 = \text{var}(\tau_n)$ are finite, then

$$\lim_{t\to\infty} \frac{m(t)}{t} = \frac{1}{\mu} \quad \text{and} \quad \lim_{t\to\infty} \frac{\text{var}[N(t)]}{t} = \frac{\sigma^2}{\mu^3}.$$

The theorem implies that the rate is about $1/\mu$ after a long run.

8.13.1. *Cramér–Lundberg ruin model*

The theoretical foundation of ruin theory is known as the Cramér–Lundberg model. The model describes an insurance company who experiences two opposing cash flows: incoming cash premiums and outgoing claims. Premiums arrive a constant rate $c > 0$ from customers and claims arrive according to a Poisson process or renewal process. So for an insurer who starts with initial surplus u, the balance at time $\boldsymbol{t}$ is

$$U(t) = u + ct - \sum_{n=1}^{N(t)} X_n,$$

where $N(t)$ is the number of claims during (0,t], X_n is the nth claim amount, and $\{X_1, X_2, \ldots\}$ are i.i.d non-negative random variables.

8.14. Queuing Process[7,14]

Queuing phenomenal can be observed in business transaction, in communications, medicine, transportation, industry, etc. For example, customers queue in banks and theaters. The purposes of queuing are to resolve congestion, to optimize efficiency, to minimize waiting time and to speed production. The queuing concept was originally formulated by Erlang in his study of telephone network congestion problems.

In a queuing system, a facility has s stations or servers for serving customers. The service discipline is first come, first served. If all stations are occupied, newly arriving customers must wait in line and form a queue. Generally, a queuing system includes: (1) Input process with random, planned or patterned arrivals, (2) service time, and (3) number of stations. It is simply represented by

Input distribution/service time/number of stations.

For example, in a queuing system with s stations, customers arrive according to a Poisson process, the service times are identically independently exponential distributed. The system is denoted by M/M/s, where M stands for Poisson arrivals or exponential service times. A queue with arbitrary arrivals, a constant service time and one station will be denoted by G/D/1.

8.14.1. *Differential equations for M/M/s queue*

In the system M/M/s, the arrivals follow a Poisson process with parameter λ, and the service times follow exponential distribution with parameter μ. When all the s stations are occupied at time t, one of the stations will be free for service within with probability $s\mu\Delta + o(\Delta)$. Let $X(t)$ be the number of customers in the system at time t, including those being served and those in the waiting line. $\{X(t), t > 0\}$ is time homogeneous Markov chain. Suppose $X(0) = i$, for $k = 0, 1, \ldots$, the transition probabilities,

$$p_{i,k}(0,t) = \Pr\{X(t) = k | X(0) = i\}$$

satisfy

$$\frac{d}{dt} p_{i,0}(0,t) = -\lambda p_{i,0}(0,t) + \mu p_{i,1}(0,t),$$

$$\frac{d}{dt} p_{i,0}(0,t) = -(\lambda + k\mu) p_{i,k}(0,t) + \lambda p_{i,k-1}(0,t) + (k+1)\mu p_{i,k+1}(0,t) \qquad k = 1, \ldots, s-1,$$

$$\frac{d}{dt} p_{i,k}(0,t) = -(\lambda + s\mu) p_{i,k}(0,t) + \lambda p_{i,k-1}(0,t) + s\mu p_{i,k+1}(0,t) \qquad k = s, s+1, \ldots.$$

If all states in M/M/s are communicative, there exists limiting distribution $\{\pi_k\}$ with $\pi_k = \lim_{t\to\infty} p_{i,k}(0,t)$ that satisfy

$$\lambda\pi_0 = \mu\pi_1,$$
$$(\lambda + k\mu)\pi_k = \lambda\pi_{k-1} + (k+1)\mu\pi_{k+1}, \quad k = 1,\ldots,s-1,$$
$$(\lambda + s\mu)\pi_k = \lambda\pi_{k-1} + s\mu\pi_{k+1}, \quad k = s, s+1, \ldots.$$

8.14.2. *M/M/1 queue*

When there is a single station in a system, the equations for limiting distribution become

$$0 = -\lambda\pi_0 + \mu\pi_1, \quad \text{and} \quad 0 = -(\lambda+\mu)\pi_k + \lambda\pi_{k-1} + \mu\pi_{k+1}, \quad k = 1,2,\ldots.$$

The solution $\pi_k = \rho\pi_0$, $k = 0,1,\ldots$, where $\rho = \lambda/\mu$ is the traffic intensity of the system.

8.15. Diffusion Process[15,16]

A sample path of a diffusion process models the trajectory of a particle embedded in a flowing fluid and subjected to random displacements due to collisions with molecules. A diffusion process is a Markov process with continuous paths. Brownian motion and Ornstein–Uhlenbeck processes are examples of diffusion processes.

In a simple discrete random walk, a particle hops at discrete times. At each step, the random the particle moves a unit distance to the right with probability p or to the left with probability $q = 1 - p$. Let $X(n)$ be the displacement after n steps. Then $\{X(n), n = 0,1,2,\ldots\}$ is a time-homogeneous Markov chain with transition probability

$$p_{i\,i+1} = p, p_{i\,i-1} = q, p_{ij} = 0, j \neq \pm 1.$$

Let

$$Z_i = \begin{cases} 1, & \text{move to the right at step } i \\ -1, & \text{move to the left at step } i \end{cases}.$$

Then $X(n) = \sum_{i=1}^{n} Z_i$, and $EX(n) = n(p-q), \mathrm{var}(X(n)) = 4npq$.

An appropriate continuum limit will be taken to obtain a diffusion equation in continuous space and time. Suppose that the particle moves an infinitesimal step length Δx during infinitesimal time interval Δt. Then there are $t/\Delta t$ moves during (0,t], and the expectation and variance of the displacement are given by

$$\frac{t}{\Delta t}(p-q)\Delta x = t(p-q)\frac{\Delta x}{\Delta t}, \quad \text{and} \quad 4\frac{t}{\Delta t}pq(\Delta x)^2 = 4tpq\frac{(\Delta x)^2}{\Delta t},$$

respectively. Taking the limit $\Delta x \to 0, \Delta t \to 0$ such that the quantities $(p-q)\Delta x/\Delta t$ and $(\Delta x)^2/\Delta t$ are finite, we let

$$\frac{(\Delta x)^2}{\Delta t} = 2D, \quad p = \frac{1}{2} + \frac{C}{2D}\Delta x, \quad q = \frac{1}{2} - \frac{C}{2D}\Delta x,$$

where C and $D(>0)$ are constants. Then, the expectation and variance of the displacement during (0,t] are given by

$$m(t) = 2Ct, \quad \sigma^2(t) = 2Dt.$$

Definition: Let $X(t)$ be the location of a particle at time t. The transition probability distribution during $(t, t+\Delta t]$ from location

$$F(t,x;t+\Delta t,y) = P\{X(t+\Delta t) \le y | X(t) = x\}.$$

If F satisfies

$$\lim_{\Delta t \to 0} \int_{|y-x|>\delta} d_y F(t,x;t+\Delta t,y) = 0$$

for any $\delta > 0$, and

$$\lim_{\Delta t \to 0} \frac{1}{\Delta t} \int_{-\infty}^{\infty} (y-x) d_y F(t,x;t+\Delta t,y) = a(t,x),$$

$$\lim_{\Delta t \to 0} \frac{1}{\Delta t} \int_{|x-y|>\delta}^{(y-x)^2 d_y} F(t,x;t+\Delta t,y) = b(t,x),$$

then $\{X(t), t > 0\}$ is called a diffusion process, where $a(t,x)$ and $b(t,x)$ are called drift parameter and diffusion parameter, respectively.

8.16. Brownian Motion[2,16]

Brownian motion was named after English physicist Brown Robert. He observed that a small particle suspended in a liquid (or a gas) moves randomly resulting in their collision with the molecules in the liquid or gas. In 1923, control theory founder Wiener gave a rigorous mathematical definition of Brownian motion. The Wiener process is often called standard Brownian motion. The Brownian motion $\{B_t: t \geq 0\}$ is characterized by the following properties:

(1) $\{B_t: t \geq 0\}$ has stationary independent increments.
(2) $\forall t > 0$, $B_t \sim N(0, t\sigma^2)$.

$\{B_t: t \geq 0\}$ with $B_0 = 0$ is called standard Brownian motion or Wiener process. Let $\tilde{B}_t = B_t - B_0$ if $B_0 = x$, then $\tilde{B}_t = \{\tilde{B}_{t,t} \geq 0\}$ is standard Brownian motion. The covariance and correlation functions of a standard Brownian motion

$$\mathrm{cov}(B_s, B_t) = \sigma^2 \min(s,t), \quad \mathrm{cor}(B_s, B_t) = \sqrt{\frac{\min(s,t)}{\max(s,t)}}.$$

Brownian motion $\{B_t: t \geq 0\}$ is a Markov process, and the transition probability density function

$$f(t-s, y-x) = \frac{\partial}{\partial y} P\{B_t \leq y | B_s = x\} = [2\pi\sigma^2(t-s)]^{-1/2} \exp\left[-\frac{(y-x)^2}{2\sigma^2(t-s)}\right].$$

The distribution of B_t depends on the initial distribution of B_0. Since B_0 is independent with $B_t - B_0$, the distribution of B_t is convolution of the distributions of B_0 and $B_t - B_0$.

The properties of a Brownian motion (BM) on R^d:

(1) If H is an orthogonal transformation on R^d, then $\{HB_t, t \geq 0\}$ is BM;
(2) $\{a + B_t, t \geq 0\}$ is BM, where a constant $a \in R^d$;
(3) $\{B(ct)/\sqrt{c}, t \geq 0\}$ is BM, where c is a positive constant.

Related processes: If $\{B_t: t \geq 0\}$ is Brownian motion, then

(1) $\{B_t - tB_1: t \in [0, 1]\}$ is a Brownian bridge.
(2) The stochastic process defined by $\{B_t + \mu t: t \geq 0\}$ is called a Wiener process with drift μ.

The mathematical model of Brownian motion has numerous real-world applications. For instance, the Brownian motion can be used to model the stock market fluctuations.

8.17. Martingale[2,19]

Originally, martingale referred to a class of betting strategies that was popular in 18th-century France. The concept of martingale in probability theory was introduced by Paul Lévy in 1934. A martingale is a stochastic process to model a fair game. The gambler's past events never help predict the mean of the future winnings. Let X_n denote the fortune after n bets, then

$$E(X_n|X_1,\ldots,X_{n-1}) = X_{n-1}.$$

Definition: Let T be a set of real numbers or integers, $(\mathcal{F})_{t\in T}$ be a sub σ-algebra of $\mathcal{F}$, and $X_T = \{X^t, t \in T\}$ is a stochastic process on the probability space $(\Omega, \mathcal{F}, P)$. If

$$E|X_t| < \infty, \quad \text{and} \quad E(X_t|\mathcal{F}_s) = X_s, \quad a.s., \ s < t, s, t \in T,$$

then X_T is called a martingale on $(\mathcal{F}_{\mathrm{t}})$. If

$$EX_t^+ < \infty, \quad [EX_t^- < \infty], \quad \text{and} \quad E(X_t|\mathcal{F}_s) \leq [\geq] X_s, \quad a.s., \ s < t, s, t \in T,$$

then X_T is called a supermartingale (submartingale, respectively) on $(\mathcal{F}_t)$.

Consider the gambler who wins \$1 when a coin comes up heads and loses \$1 when the coin comes up tails. Suppose that the coin comes up heads with probability p. If $p = 1/2$, the gambler's fortune over time is a martingale. If $p < 1/2$, the gambler loses money on average, and the gambler's fortune over time is a supermartingale. If $p > 1/2$, the gambler's fortune over time is a submartingale.

8.17.1. *Properties of martingales*

(1) If X_T is a martingale [supermartingale, submartingale], and a random variable $\eta > 0$ and measurable with regard to $\mathcal{F}_s$, then for $\forall t > s$

$$E(X_t\eta) = [\geq\leq] E(X_t\eta).$$

(2) If X_T is a martingale, then EX_t is constant, and $E|X_t| \uparrow$. If X_T is a submartingale, then $EX_t \uparrow$.

(3) If X_T is a submartingale [supermartingale], then $-X_T$ is a supermartingale [submartingale, respectively].

(4) If X_T is a martingale, and f is a continuous convex function with $Ef(X_t) < \infty, t \in T$, then $f(X_t)$ is a submartingale. If X_T is a submartingale [supermartingale], and f is a monotone non-decreasing continuous convex (concave) function with $Ef(X_t) < \infty, t \in T$, then $f(X_T) = \{f(X_t), t \in T\}$ is a submartingale [supermartingale].

(5) If X_T is a submartingale, then $\{(X_t - c)^+, t \in T\}$ is also a submartingale.

(6) If X_T and X_T, Y_T are both martingale [supermartingale], then $X_T + Y_T$ is martingale [supermartingale], and $(X \wedge Y)_T$ is supermartingale.

8.18. Markov Decision Process (MDP)[16,17]

An MDP is a discrete time stochastic control process. MDPs are a mathematical framework for modeling sequential decision problems under uncertainty. MDPs are useful for studying a wide range of optimization problems, including robotics, automated control, economics and manufacturing.

8.18.1. *Discrete-time MDP*

The basic definition of a discrete-time MDP contains five components, described using a standard notation $\langle S, A, q, r, V \rangle$. S is the state space, a finite set of all possible values relevant to the decision process, such as $S = \{1, 2, \ldots, m\}$. A is a finite set of actions. For any state $s \in S$, As is the action space, the set of possible actions that the decision maker can take at state s. $q = (q_{ij})$ denotes transition probabilities, where $q_{ij}(a)$ is the transition probability that determines the state of the system at time $t+1$, which are conditional on the state i and action a at time $t(t = 0, 1, 2, \ldots)$, and $q_{ij}(a)$ satisfies

$$q_{ij}(a) \geq 0, \quad \sum_{j \in s} q_{ij}(a) = 1, \quad i, j \in s, a \in A,$$

r is a reward function. Let $\Gamma = \{(i, a) : a \in A, i \in s\}$, $r{:}\Gamma \to R$, and R is the set of all real numbers. $r(i, a)$ is the immediate reward of taking action a at state s. The goal of solving an MDP is to find a policy $\pi \in \Pi$ for the decision maker that maximizes an objective function $V{:}\Pi \times S \to R$, such as cumulative function of the random rewards, where Π is the set of all policies. $V(\pi, i)$ measures the quality of a specified policy $\pi \in \Pi$ and an intial state $i \in S$. $\langle S, A, q, r, V \rangle$ collectively define an MDP.

8.18.2. *Continuous-time MDP*

For a continuous-time MDP with finite state space S and action space A, the components S, A, r, and V are similar to a discrete-time MDP, whereas $q = (q_{ij})$ denotes transition rates. $q_{ij}(a)$: $S \times A \to \Delta S$ is the transition rate that determine the state at time $t + \Delta t$, which are conditional on the state i and action a at time t, and $q_{ij}(a)$ satisfies

$$q_{ij}(a) \geq 0, \quad \sum_{j \in s} q_{ij}(a) = 0, \quad i, j \in s, a \in A.$$

In a discrete-time MDP, decisions can be made only at discrete-time intervals, whereas in a continuous-time MDP, the decisions can occur anytime.

Continuous time MDPs generalize discrete-time MDPs by allowing the decision maker to choose actions whenever the system state changes and/or by allowing the time spent in a particular state to follow an arbitrary probability distribution.

8.19. Stochastic Simulations[18,19]

A stochastic simulation is a simulation that traces the evolution of a stochastic process with certain probabilities.

8.19.1. *Simulation for discrete-time Markov chains*

Let $\{Y_n, n \geq 0\}$ be a Markov with state space $S = \{0, 1, 2, \ldots\}$ and one-step transition probability matrix $P = (p_{ij})$. Suppose the initial distribution $\pi = (\pi_0, \pi_1, \ldots)$.

Step 1. Initialize the state $y_0 = s_0$ by drawing s_0 from initial distribution π.

Generate a random number x_0 from a uniform distribution on [0,1] and take s_0 if $\sum_{i=0}^{s_0-1} \pi_i < x_0 \leq \sum_{i=0}^{s_0} \pi_i$.

Step 2. For the given state s, simulate the transition type by drawing from the discrete distribution with probability

$$P(\text{transition} = k) = p_{sk}.$$

Generate a random number x from a uniform distribution on [0,1] and choose the transition k if

$$\sum_{j=0}^{k-1} p_{sj} < x \leq \sum_{j=0}^{k} p_{sj}.$$

Step 3. Update the new system state.

Step 4. Iterate steps 2–3 until $n \geq n_{\text{stop}}$.

8.19.2. *Simulation for contiguous-time Markov chains*

Let $\{Y_t, t \geq 0\}$ be a Markov with state space $S = \{0, 1, 2, \ldots\}$ and intensity matrix $Q = (q_{ij})$. Suppose the initial distribution $\pi = (\pi_0, \pi_1, \ldots)$. Let

$$q_i = -q_{ii}, \quad p_{ii} = 0, \quad p_{ij} = q_{ij}/q_i, \quad i \neq j.$$

Step 1. Initialize the state $y_0 = s_0$ by drawing s_0 from initial distribution π.

Step 2. Simulate the sojourn time τ of current state s, until the next transition by drawing from an exponential distribution with mean $1/q_i$.

Step 3. For the given state s of the chain, simulate the transition type by drawing from the discrete distribution with probability $P(\text{transition} = k) = p_{sk}$.

Step 4. Update the new time $t = t + \tau$ and the new system state.

Step 5. Iterate steps 2–4 until $t \geq t_{\text{stop}}$.

Especially, if $p_{i,i+1} = 1, p_{ij} = 0, j \neq i+1$, then $\{Y_t, t \geq 0\}$ is a sample path of a Poisson process.

8.19.3. *Simulation for Wiener process (Brownian motion)*

Let $\{X(t), t \geq 0\}$ be a Wiener process with $X(t) \sim N(0, t\sigma^2)$. Let $X_n = X(n\Delta t)$ with a length of step Δt.

Step 1. Generate an independent random variable $\{W_n, n \geq 1\}$ from normal distribution $N(0,1)$.

Step 2. Let $X_0 = 0$ and

$$X_n = X_{n-1} + \sigma\sqrt{\Delta t}W_n.$$

Then $\{X_n, n = 0, 1, \ldots\}$ is a sample path of the Wiener process $\{X(t), t \geq 0\}$.

References

1. Lu, Y, Fang, JQ. *Advanced Medical Statistics.* Singapore: World Scientific Publishing Co., 2015.
2. Ross, SM. *Introduction to Probability Models* (10th edn). Singapore: Elsevier, 2010.
3. Lundberg, O. *On Random Processes and their Applications to Sickness and Accident Statistics.* Uppsala: Almqvist & Wiksells boktryckeri, 1964.
4. Wong, E. *Stochastic Processes in Information and Dynamical System.* Pennsylvania: McGraw-Hill, 1971.
5. Karlin, S, Taylor, HM. *A Second Course in Stochastic Processes.* New York: Academic Press, 1981.
6. Anderson, PK, Ørnulf Borgan, Gill, RD, *et al. Statistical Models Based on Counting Processes.* New York: Springer-Verlag, 1993.
7. Chiang, CL. *An Introduction to Stochastic Processes and their Application.* New York: Robert E. Krieger Publishing Company, 1980.
8. Chiang, CL. *The Life Table and its Application.* (1983) (The Chinese version is translated by Fang, JQ Shanghai Translation Press). Malabar, FL: Krieger Publishing, 1984.
9. Faddy, MJ, Fenlon, JS. Stochastic modeling of the invasion process of nematodes in fly larvae. *Appl. Statist.*, 1999, 48(1): 31–37.
10. Lucas, WF. *Modules in Applied Mathematics Vol. 4: Life Science Models.* New York: Springer-Verlag, 1983.

11. Daley, DJ, Gani, J. *Epidemic Modeling: An Introduction.* New York: Cambridge University Press, 2005.
12. Linda, JSA. *An Introduction to Stochastic Processes with Biology Applications.* Upper Saddle river: Prentice Hall. 2003.
13. Capasso, V. *An Introduction to Continuous-Time Stochastic Processes: Theory, Models, and Applications to Finance, Biology, and Medicine.* Cambridge: Birkhäuser, 2012.
14. Parzen, E. *Stochastic Processes.* San Francisco: Holden-Day, 1962 (the Chinese version is translated by Deng YL, Yang ZM, 1987).
15. Oliver, CI. *Elements of Random Walk and Diffusion Processes.* Wiley, 2013.
16. Editorial committee of Handbook of Modern Applied Mathematics. *Handbook of Modern Applied Mathematics — Volume of Probability Statistics and Staochatic Processes.* Beijing: Tsinghua University Press, 2000 (in Chinese).
17. Alagoz, O, Hsu, H, Schaefer, AJ, Roberts, MS. Markov decision processes: A tool for sequential decision making under uncertainty. *Medi. Decis. Making.* 2010, 30: 474–483.
18. Fishman, GS. *Principles of Discrete Event Simulation.* New York: Wiley, 1978.
19. Fix E. and Neyman J. A simple stochastic model of recovery, relapse, death and loss of patients. *Human Biology.* 1951, 23: 205–241.
20. Chiang C.L. *A Stochastic Model of Competing Risks of Illness and Competing Risks of Death. Stochastic Models in Medicine and Biology.* University of Wisconsin Press, Madison. 1964. pp. 323–354.

About the Author

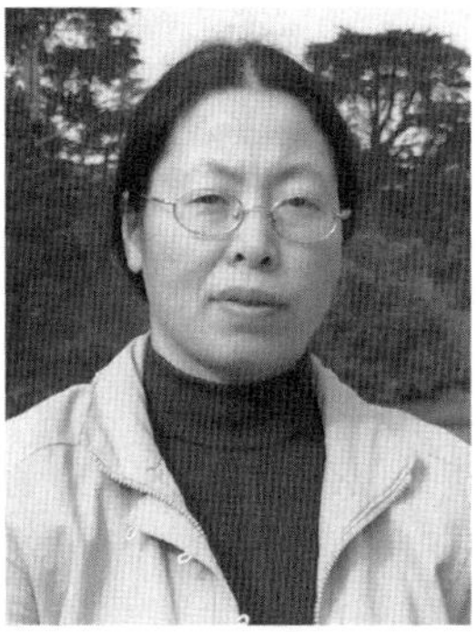

Dr. Caixia Li is presently employed as an Associate Professor at Sun Yat-Sen University. She received her Master's degree in Probability and Mathematical Statistics in 1996 and a PhD in Medical Statistics and Epidemiology from Sun Yat-Sen University in 2005. In 2006, she joined the postdoctoral program in Biostatistics at the University of California at San Francisco. In 2009, she returned to the Department of Statistics in Sun Yat-Sen University. Her research interests include biostatistics, statistical genetics and statistical modeling.

CHAPTER 9

TIME SERIES ANALYSIS

Jinxin Zhang*, Zhi Zhao, Yunlian Xue, Zicong Chen, Xinghua Ma and Qian Zhou

9.1. Time Series[1,2]

In the biomedical research, a random sequence $X_1, X_2, X_3, \ldots, X_T$ denoting the dynamic observations from the time point 1 to T is called a time series. The intervals to obtain the series may either be equal or unequal. Time series analysis method is a powerful tool to handle many issues in biomedicine. For examples, epidemiologists might be interested in the epidemical path of the influenza cases over time, so that the future prevalence will be predicted with some models and the seasonality of the epidemic can be discussed; the biologists focus on some important patterns in gene expression profiles which are associated with epigenetics or diseases; and in medicine, the blood pressure measurements traced over time could be useful for evaluating drugs used in treating hypertension.

Time series is a kind of discrete stochastic process, and stationary is the basic assumption to affect its estimation to structural parameters, i.e. the statistical properties characterizing the process are time-invariant. Specifically, a process $\{X_t\}$ is a strictly stationary process if the random sequences $X_{t_1}, X_{t_2}, \ldots, X_{t_n}$ and $X_{t_1-k}, X_{t_2-k}, \ldots, X_{t_n-k}$ have the same joint distribution for any delay k at time points $t_1, t_2, \ldots, t_n$. It will be more practical to weaken this condition to constrain a constant mean, finite and time-invariant second moments, which is called weakly stationary process. In this situation, the series can be treated roughly as stationary if the process

*Corresponding author: zhjinx@mail.sysu.edu.cn

of time series seems like random. More accurately, the unit root test can give a strictly statistical inference on stationary. Another prerequisite of time series analysis is invertibility, i.e. the current observation of series is the linear combination of the past observations and the current random noise.

Generally, the approaches to time series analysis are identified as the time domain approach and the frequency domain approach. The time domain approach is generally motivated by the assumption that the correlation between the adjacent points in series is explained well in terms of a dependence of the current value on the previous values, like the autoregressive moving average model, the conditional heteroscedasticity model and the state space model. In contrast, the frequency domain approach assumes the primary characteristics of interest in time series analysis related to the periodic or systematic sinusoidal variations found naturally in most data. The periodic variations are often caused by the biological, physical, or environmental phenomena of interest. The corresponding basic tool of a frequency domain approach is the Fourier transformation.

Currently, most researches focus on the multivariate time series, including (i) extending from the univariate nonlinear time series models to the multivariate nonlinear time series models; (ii) integrating some locally adaptive tools to the non-stationary multivariate time series, like wavelet analysis; (iii) reducing dimensions in the high-dimensional time series and (iv) combining the time series analysis and the statistical process control in syndromic surveillance to detect a disease outbreak.

9.2. ARIMA Model[1]

The autoregressive integrated moving average (ARIMA model) was first raised by Box and Jenkins in 1976, which was also called the Box–Jenkins model. Modeling and foresting can be done based on the analysis of the linear combination of past records and error values.

Identification of ARIMA model is based on the comparison of the Sample Autocorrelation Function (SACF) and the Sample Partial Autocorrelation Function (SPACF) of the time series data with those of known families of models. These families of models are autoregressives (AR) of the order $p = 1, 2, \ldots$, moving averages (MA) of the order $q = 1, 2, \ldots$, mixed autoregressive-moving averages of the orders (p, q), and autoregressive integrated moving averages of the orders (p, d, q), $d = 0, 1, 2, \ldots$, where d is the degree of differencing to reach stationary.

The ARIMA(p, d, q) model is defined as

$$(1 - \varphi_1 B - \varphi_2 B^2 - \cdots - \varphi_p B^p)\nabla^d X_t = (1 - \theta_1 B - \theta_2 B^2 - \cdots - \theta_q B^q)\varepsilon_t,$$

short for $\Phi(B)\nabla^d X_t = \Theta(B)\varepsilon_t$,

where $\Phi(B) = 1 - \varphi_1 B - \varphi_2 B^2 - \cdots - \varphi_p B^p$, $\Theta(B) = 1 - \theta_1 B - \theta_2 B^2 - \cdots - \theta_q B^q$ are AR(p) and MA (q), respectively. In ARIMA model, ∇ is the difference operator; p, d, q are non-negative integers, p is the order of an AR model, d is the difference order, q is the order of an MA model, and B is the backward shift operator, $B^j X_t = X_{t-j}$.

There are three steps in identification of ARIMA model: (1) Smooth of time series, which is a basic step. Many methods can be used to do the stationary test, such as data graph, SACF and SPACF, unit-root test, parameter test, inverted test, random walk test and so on. The simplest and mostly used methods are data graph test and autocorrelation (partial autocorrelation) function graph test. If n values do not fluctuate around a constant mean or do not fluctuate with constant variation, or SACF and SPACF decay extremely slowly then the series should be considered as non-stationary. If the series is not stationary, differencing or taking logarithmic transformation is recommended. (2) SACF and SPACF can also be used to recognize the parameters p and q of ARIMA model. If the SACF (or ACF) of the time series values cuts off at a lag of p(or q) observational intervals, then this series should be considered as AR(p) (or MA(q)). As for a mixture model with autoregressive coefficient of p and moving average coefficient of q, autocorrelation function may exhibit exponential decay, damped sine-wave or as a mixture of them at a lag of $p-q$ observational intervals; partial autocorrelation function is controlled by exponential decay, damped sine-wave or as a mixture of them at a lag of $p-q$ observational intervals. (3) Parameter test and residual test. Use the parameters p and q that are recognized before to do model fitting. If all parameters are significant and residual is white noise, then this model should be considered as adaptive. Otherwise, p and q are needed to be modified.

ARIMA model can be used to forecast. At present, the commonly used forecasting methods are linear minimum variance prediction and conditional expectation prediction. The lead time of prediction is expressed by L. The bigger the L, the bigger the error variance, that is, the worse the prediction accuracy.

9.3. Transfer Function Models[1,3]

The transfer function models are used to study the dynamic characteristics and forecasting of processes. In a study about the amount of fish and Nino phenomena, South Oscillation Index (SOI) is an important variable to predict the scale of recruitment (amounts of new fish). The dynamic relationship is

$$Y_t = \sum_{j=0}^{p_1} \alpha_j Y_{t-j} + \sum_{j=0}^{p_2} c_j X_{t-j} + \eta_t = A(L)Y_t + C(L)X_t + \eta_t, \tag{9.3.1}$$

where X_t denotes SOI, Y_t is the amount of new fish and $\sum_j |\alpha_j| < \infty$. That is, using past SOI and past amounts of new fish to predict current amount of new fish. The polynomial $C(L)$ is called transfer function, which reveals the time path of the influence from exogenous variable SOI to endogenous variable number of new fish. η_t is the stochastic impact to amounts of new fish, such as petroleum pollution in seawater or measurement error.

While building a transfer function model, it is necessary to differentiate each variable to stationary if the series $\{X_t\}$ and $\{Y_t\}$ are non-stationary. The interpretation of transfer function depends on the differences, for instance, in following three equations

$$Y_t = \alpha_1 Y_{t-1} + c_0 X_t + \varepsilon_t, \tag{9.3.2}$$

$$\Delta Y_t = \alpha_1 \Delta Y_{t-1} + c_0 X_t + \varepsilon_t, \tag{9.3.3}$$

$$\Delta Y_t = \alpha_1 \Delta Y_{t-1} + c_0 \Delta X_t + \varepsilon_t, \tag{9.3.4}$$

where $|\alpha_1| < 1$. In (9.3.2), a one-unit shock in X_t has the initial effect of increasing Y_t by c_0 units. This initial effect decays at the rate α_1. In (9.3.3), a one-unit shock in X_t has the initial effect of increasing the change in Y_t by c_0 units. The effect on the change decays at the rate α_1, but the effect on the level of $\{Y_t\}$ sequence never decays. In (9.3.4), only the change in X_t affects Y_t. Here, a pulse in the $\{X_t\}$ sequence will have a temporary effect on the level of $\{Y_t\}$.

A vector AR model can transfer to a MA model, like such a binary system

$$\begin{cases} Y_t = b_{10} - b_{12} Z_t + \gamma_{11} Y_{t-1} + \gamma_{12} Z_{t-1} + \varepsilon_{ty} \\ Z_t = b_{20} - b_{22} Y_t + \gamma_{21} Y_{t-1} + \gamma_{22} Z_{t-1} + \varepsilon_{tz} \end{cases}$$

that can be rewritten as VAR(2) or VMA(∞) models

$$\begin{pmatrix} Y_t \\ Z_t \end{pmatrix} = \begin{pmatrix} a_{10} \\ a_{20} \end{pmatrix} + \begin{pmatrix} a_{11} & a_{12} \\ a_{21} & a_{22} \end{pmatrix} \begin{pmatrix} Y_{t-1} \\ Z_{t-1} \end{pmatrix} + \begin{pmatrix} e_{t1} \\ e_{t2} \end{pmatrix}$$

$$\Leftrightarrow \begin{pmatrix} Y_t \\ Z_t \end{pmatrix} = \begin{pmatrix} \bar{Y}_t \\ \bar{Z}_t \end{pmatrix} + \sum_{i=0}^{\infty} \begin{pmatrix} a_{11} & a_{12} \\ a_{21} & a_{22} \end{pmatrix}^i \begin{pmatrix} e_{t-i,1} \\ e_{t-i,2} \end{pmatrix}$$

$$= \begin{pmatrix} \bar{Y}_t \\ \bar{Z}_t \end{pmatrix} + \sum_{i=0}^{\infty} \begin{pmatrix} \phi_{11}(i) & \phi_{12}(i) \\ \phi_{21}(i) & \phi_{22}(i) \end{pmatrix}^i \begin{pmatrix} \varepsilon_{t-i,y} \\ \varepsilon_{t-i,z} \end{pmatrix},$$

where the coefficients $\phi_{11}(i), \phi_{12}(i), \phi_{21}(i), \phi_{22}(i)$ are called impulse response functions. The coefficients $\phi(i)$ can be used to generate the effects of ε_{ty} and ε_{tz} shocks on the entire time paths of the $\{Y_t\}$ and $\{Z_t\}$ sequences. The accumulated effects of unit impulse in ε_{ty} and ε_{tz} can be obtained by the summation of the impulse response functions connected with appropriate coefficients. For example, after n periods, the effect of ε_{tz} on the value of Y_{t+n} is $\phi_{12}(n)$. Thus, after n periods, the cumulated effects of ε_{tz} on $\{Y_t\}$ sequence is $\sum_{i=0}^{n} \phi_{12}(i)$.

9.4. Trend Test[4,5]

If the time series $\{x_t\}$ satisfies $x_t = f(t) + \varepsilon_t$, where $f(t)$ is a deterministic function of time t and ε_t is a random variable, we can carry out the following hypothesis test:

H_0: $f(t)$ is a constant (not depending on time).

H_1: $f(t)$ is not a constant (a gradual monotonic change).

Constructing a test statistic to distinguish between the above H_0 and H_1, in presence of ε_t, is the general concept of the trend test. They can be divided into parametric tests and non-parametric tests.

For parametric tests, $\{x_t\}$ is generally expressed as the sum of a linear trend and a white noise term, written as

$$x_t = \alpha + \beta t + \varepsilon_t,$$

where α is a constant, β is the coefficient of time t, and $\varepsilon_t \sim N(0, \sigma^2)$. The estimate of α and β can be obtained by the least square estimation. Then we can construct the T statistic to test the hypothesis, of which the process is consistent with the general linear regression model. For special data, we need to make a proper transformation. For example, the logistic regression model can be applied to time series with qualitative data.

For non-parametric tests, a Mann–Kendall trend test can be used. It does not rely on an estimate of the trend itself, and is based on relative ranking of data instead of original values. Commonly, it is used in a combination with the Theil–Sen trend estimate.

The test statistic is

$$S = \sum_{i<k} \operatorname{sign}(x_k - x_i),$$

where

$$\operatorname{sign}(x) = \begin{cases} 1 & x > 0 \\ 0 & x = 0 \\ -1 & x < 0 \end{cases}.$$

The residuals are assumed to be mutually independent. For large samples (about $n > 8$) S is normally distributed with

$$E(S) = 0, \quad \operatorname{Var}(S) = \frac{n(n-1)(2n+5)}{18}.$$

In practice, the statistic Z is used and it follows a standard normal distribution

$$Z = \begin{cases} (S-1)/\sqrt{\operatorname{Var}(S)} & S > 0 \\ 0 & S = 0 \\ (S+1)/\sqrt{\operatorname{Var}(S)} & S < 0 \end{cases}.$$

A correction of $\operatorname{Var}(S)$ is necessary if there are any ties. In addition, since the correlation exists in time series, conducting a trend test directly will reject the null-hypothesis too often. Pre-whitening can be used to "wash-out" the serial correlation. For example, if $\{x_t\}$ is a combination of a trend and AR(1), it can be pre-whitened as

$$x'_t = (x_t - r_1 x_{t-1})/(1 - r_1),$$

where r_1 is the first-order autocorrelation coefficient. The new series $\{x'_t\}$ has the same trend as $\{x_t\}$, but its residuals are serially uncorrelated.

9.5. Autocorrelation Function & Partial Autocorrelation Function[1,6]

The definitions of autocorrelation function in different areas are not completely equivalent. In some areas, the autocorrelation function is equivalent to the self-covariance (autocovariance). We know that a stationary time series contains assumptions that data is obtained by equal intervals and the joint probability distribution keeps the same along with the series. Under the assumption of stationary, with the corresponding time interval k, the self-covariances are the same for any t, and called the autocovariance with lag k. It is defined as

$$\gamma_k = \mathrm{Cov}(z_t, z_{t+k}) = \mathrm{E}[(z_t - \mu)(z_{t+k} - \mu)].$$

Similarly, the autocorrelation function for the lag k is

$$\rho_k = \frac{\mathrm{E}[(z_t - \mu)(z_{t+k} - \mu)]}{\sqrt{\mathrm{E}[(z_t - \mu)^2]\mathrm{E}[(z_{t+k} - \mu)^2]}} = \frac{\mathrm{E}[(z_t - \mu)(z_{t+k} - \mu)]}{\sigma_z^2}.$$

The autocorrelation function reveals correlation between any pieces of the time series with specific time intervals. In a stationary autoregressive process, the autocorrelation function is exponential and sinusoidal oscillation damping. To achieve the minimal residual variance from the first-order coefficient $\hat{\phi}_{kk}$ regression model for a time-series $\{x_t\}$ is called the partial autocorrelation function with lag k. Using the Yule–Walker equation, we can get the formula of the partial autocorrelation function

$$\hat{\phi}_{kk} = \frac{\begin{vmatrix} \rho_0 & \rho_1 & \cdots & \rho_{k-2} & \rho_1 \\ \rho_1 & \rho_0 & \cdots & \rho_{k-3} & \rho_2 \\ \cdots & \cdots & \cdots & \cdots & \cdots \\ \rho_{k-1} & \rho_{k-2} & \cdots & \rho_1 & \rho_k \end{vmatrix}}{\begin{vmatrix} \rho_0 & \rho_1 & \cdots & \rho_{k-1} \\ \rho_1 & \rho_0 & \cdots & \rho_{k-2} \\ \cdots & \cdots & \cdots & \cdots \\ \rho_{k-1} & \rho_{k-2} & \cdots & \rho_0 \end{vmatrix}}.$$

It can be seen that the partial autocorrelation function is a function of the autocorrelation function. If the autocorrelation function is trailing and the partial autocorrelation function is truncated, then the data are suitable to an AR(p) model; if the autocorrelation function is truncated and partial autocorrelation function is trailing, the data are suitable to an MA(q) model; if the autocorrelation function and partial autocorrelation function are both trailing, the data are suitable to an ARMA (p, q) model.

9.6. Unit Root Test[1,3,7,8]

In practice, most time series are usually not stationary, in which the unit root series is a popular case. For instance, a random walk process is

$$Y_t = \alpha_1 Y_{t-1} + \varepsilon_t,$$

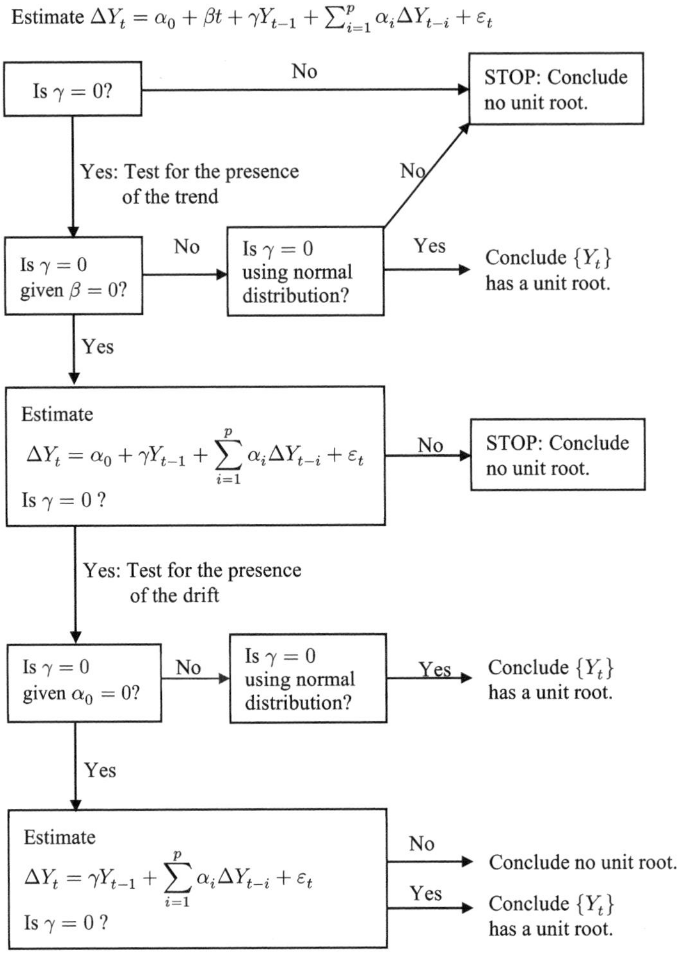

Fig. 9.6.1. A procedure to test for unit roots.

where $\alpha_1 = 1$ and $\varepsilon_t \sim IID(0, \sigma^2)$. The variance of the random walk process is $\mathrm{Var}(Y_t) = t\sigma^2$. It will be infinite if $t \to \infty$, which reveals the process is non-stationary. After the first-order difference, $\Delta Y_t = (\alpha_1 - 1)Y_{t-1} + \varepsilon_t$ becomes stationary, that is, the random walk process contains one unit root. Thus, the unit root test is to test the hypothesis $\gamma = \alpha_1 - 1 = 0$. Dickey and Fuller propose three different regression equations that can be used to test for the presence of a unit root:

$$\Delta Y_t = \gamma Y_{t-1} + \varepsilon_t,$$

$$\Delta Y_t = \alpha_0 + \gamma Y_{t-1} + \varepsilon_t,$$

$$\Delta Y_t = \alpha_0 + \gamma Y_{t-1} + \alpha_2 t + \varepsilon_t.$$

The testing statistic is

$$t = \frac{\hat{\gamma} - 1}{\hat{\sigma}_{\hat{\gamma}}},$$

where $\hat{\gamma}$ is the OLS estimator, $\hat{\sigma}_{\hat{\gamma}}$ is the standard deviation of $\hat{\gamma}$. The distribution of t-statistic is functional of the Brown motion, and the critical values can be found in DF tables. If the random terms in the three equations are still correlated, augment Dickey–Fuller (ADF) test transforms them into

$$\Delta Y_t = \gamma Y_{t-1} + \sum_{i=1}^{p} \alpha_i \Delta Y_{t-i} + \varepsilon_t,$$

$$\Delta Y_t = \alpha_0 + \gamma Y_{t-1} + \sum_{i=1}^{p} \alpha_i \Delta Y_{t-i} + \varepsilon_t,$$

$$\Delta Y_t = \alpha_0 + \beta t + \gamma Y_{t-1} + \sum_{i=1}^{p} \alpha_i \Delta Y_{t-i} + \varepsilon_t.$$

As for an intercept, a drift or a time trend term contained in the equation, the null hypothesis for unit root testing and corresponding t-statistic will be different. Doldado *et al.* suggest the procedure shown in Figure 9.6.1 to test for a unit root when the form of data-generating process is unknown.

The ADF test can also be modified to account for seasonal or multiple unit roots. In another extension, Perron and Vogelsang show how to test for a unit root when there are unknown structural breaks.

9.7. White Noise[9–11]

After building an ARIMA model, it is necessary to test whether any possible correlations still exist in the error series, that is, the residuals are white noise process or not.

Definition: A sequence $\{\varepsilon_t\}$ is a white noise process if each element has the zero mean, equal variances and is uncorrelated with others, i.e.

(i) $E(\varepsilon_t) = 0$,
(ii) $\mathrm{Var}(\varepsilon_t) = \sigma^2$,
(iii) $\mathrm{Cov}(\varepsilon_t, \varepsilon_{t-j}) = \gamma_j = 0$, for all $j > 0$.

From perspective of the frequency domain, white noise ε_t has spectrum density

$$f(\omega) = \frac{S(\omega)}{\gamma_0} = \frac{\gamma_0 + 2\sum_{j=1}^{\infty} \gamma_j \cos(j\omega)}{\gamma_0} = 1.$$

That is, the spectrum density of white noise series is a constant for different frequencies, which is analogous to the identical power of white light over all frequencies. This is why the series $\{\varepsilon_t\}$ is called white noise.

There are two main methods to test whether a series is a white noise process or not.

(1) Portmanteau test

The Portmanteau test checks the null hypothesis that there is no remaining residual autocorrelation at lags 1 to h against the alternative that at least one of the autocorrelations is non-zero. In other words, the pair of hypothesis

$$H_0\colon \rho_1 = \cdots = \rho_h = 0$$

versus

$$H_1\colon \rho_i \neq 0 \text{ for at least one } i = 1, \ldots, h$$

is tested. Here, $\rho_i = \mathrm{Corr}(\varepsilon_t, \varepsilon_{t-i})$ denotes an autocorrelation coefficient of the residual series. If the $\hat{\varepsilon}_t$'s are residuals from an estimated ARMA(p, q) model, the test statistic is

$$Q^*(h) = T \sum_{l=1}^{h} \hat{\rho}_l^2.$$

Ljung and Box have proposed a modified version of the Portmanteau statistic for which the statistic distributed as an approximate χ^2 was found to be more suitable with a small sample size

$$Q(h) = T(T+2) \sum_{l=1}^{h} \frac{\hat{\rho}_l^2}{T-l}.$$

If $Q(m) < \chi^2_\alpha$, residuals will be regarded as a white noise process.

(2) Breusch–Godfrey test

Another test for the residual autocorrelation, Breusch–Godfrey test, is based on considering an AR(h) model for the residuals

$$\varepsilon_t = \beta_1 \varepsilon_{t-1} + \cdots + \beta_h \varepsilon_{t-h} + \mathrm{error}_t$$

and checking the pair of hypothesis

$$H_0\colon \beta_1 = \cdots = \beta_h = 0 \quad \text{versus } H_0\colon \beta_i \neq 0 \quad \text{for one } 1 \leq i \leq h.$$

If the original model is an AR(p), then the auxiliary model

$$\hat{\varepsilon}_t = v + \alpha_1 X_{t-1} + \cdots + \alpha_p X_{t-p} + \beta_1 \hat{\varepsilon}_{t-1} + \cdots + \beta_h \hat{\varepsilon}_{t-h} + e_t$$

is fitted. Here, $\hat{\varepsilon}_t$ are the OLS residuals from the original AR(p) model. The LM statistic for the null hypothesis of interest can be obtained easily from the coefficient of determination R^2 of the auxiliary regression model as

$$LM_h = TR^2.$$

In the absence of any residual autocorrelations, it will be an asymptotic $\chi^2(h)$ distribution. An F version of the statistic with potentially better properties to data with a small sample may also be considered. It has the form

$$FLM_h = \frac{R^2}{1-R^2} \cdot \frac{T-p-h-1}{h} \sim F(h, T-p-h-1).$$

9.8. Exponential Smoothing Model[12,13]

Exponential smoothing model can make irregular time series data to be smoothed, meanwhile fluctuations and trends are decomposed. Thus, the future of time series can be inferred and predicted. Exponential smoothing model is developed from moving average model. Both exponential smoothing model and moving average model are popularly used for forecasting. The principle of exponential smoothing model is that the parameter in the model is a weight, which summarizes the contributions from previous observations. In the exponential smoothing model, the prediction of the next new value will be the weighted average of the previous and current values. A proper choice of weight is supposed to offset the impact of random fluctuations inherent in the time series. Exponential smoothing model does not discard the more previous data, but to older values, smaller weights will be assigned.

The basic formula for exponential smoothing is $S_t = \alpha y_t + (1-\alpha)S_{t-1}$, where S_t refers to the smoothed value at time t, y_t the actual value at time t, S_{t-1} the smoothed value at time $t-1$, and α the smoothing parameter, which ranges [0,1]. According to smooth different lags of historical values, exponential smoothing methods include at least the following patterns: exponential smoothing, secondary exponential smoothing and cubic exponential smoothing. In practice, exponential smoothing model has the following properties: (1) The series will be smoothed after the fitting by an exponential smoothing model. The smaller the smoothing parameter α used, the stronger the smoothing effect is. This α will make the prediction and will not respond rapidly to a new fluctuation. (2) In the linear part with the previously smoothed value, the impact from an older historical value will decease if a larger α is applied. One exception is when the time series consists of a linear trend while the exponential smoothing method is applied. In this case, we need to deal with the deviations which do not cease rapidly. The basic theory of correction is to perform a quadratic exponential smoothing.

The first step is to identify the patterns and directions of the impact from deviations. The second step is to set a linear part in the equation and create a trend forecasting model. This is the so-called secondary exponential smoothing method. The primary consideration whether a model is a successful one should be based on the effectiveness of prediction, while the parameter α level is the critical core to the model. The parameter α determines the proportions of information, comes from either the new values or previous values when constructing the prediction to the future. The larger the α, the higher the proportion of information from new data included in the prediction value while the lower proportion of information from historical data included, and vice versa.

Disadvantages of the exponential smoothing model are as follows: (1) Its lack of ability to identify the sudden turning points, but this can be made up by extra surveys or empirical knowledge. (2) The effect of long-term forecasting is poor. Advantages of the exponential smoothing model are as follows: (1) Gradually decreased weights are well in accordance with the real world circumstance. (2) There is only one parameter in the model. This will help enhance the feasibility of the method. (3) It is an adaptive method, since the prediction model can automatically measure the new information and take the information into consideration when realizing further predictions.

9.9. Heteroscedastic Time Series Model[14,15]

For traditional linear models, it is assumed that the error term is zero mean, homoscedastic and serially uncorrelated. However, a large number of empirical studies have shown that the error term of many series, in which high frequency is included, is obviously serially correlated. This will lead to the problem of heteroscedasticity. It means that the variance of the error term depends on the historical error levels, and changes over time and the series show volatility clustering. In this case, the variance cannot be assumed as a constant, but rather depends on the error of the historical data. So the model for such objective fact must have the characteristics of time variation. The traditional models cannot describe the fact of volatility clustering and time-varying variances. The first model that provides a systematic framework for volatility modeling, proposed by Engle[14], is the autoregressive conditional heteroscedastic (ARCH) model. This is a nonlinear time series model, which is widely applied to the analysis of heteroscedastic time series in economics because of its good statistical properties and accurate description of volatility phenomenon.

Generally, assuming that a stationary series $\{x_t\}$ can be expressed as

$$x_t = \beta_0 + \beta_1 x_{t-1} + \cdots + \beta_p x_{t-p} + a_t \tag{9.9.1}$$

and its error sequence $\{a_t\}$ can be expressed as

$$a_t = \sigma_t \varepsilon_t, \quad \sigma_t^2 = \alpha_0 + \alpha_1 a_{t-1}^2 + \cdots + \alpha_m a_{t-m}^2, \tag{9.9.2}$$

where $\{\varepsilon_t\}$ is a sequence of independent and identically distributed (i.i.d.) random variables with the mean zero and the variance 1. In practice, $\{\varepsilon_t\}$ is often assumed to follow the standard normal or a standardized Student-t or a generalized error distribution. Meanwhile, $\alpha_0 > 0$ and $\alpha_i \geq 0$ for $i > 0$. Then we can say that $\{a_t\}$ follows an ARCH(m) process and is denoted as $a_t \sim$ ARCH(m). Here, the model for x_t in Eq. (9.9.1) is referred to as the mean equation and the model for σ_t^2 in Eq. (9.9.2) is the volatility equation.

Characteristics of ARCH model: First, it characterizes the positive impact of the fluctuations of the past disturbance on the current disturbance to simulate the volatility clustering phenomenon, which means that large fluctuations generally are followed by large fluctuations and small fluctuations followed by small fluctuations. Second, it improves the adaptive ability of the model, which can improve the prediction accuracy. Third, the starting point of the ARCH model is that the apparent change in time series is predictable, and that the change follows a certain type of nonlinear dependence. Since Engle proposed the ARCH model, the scholars from various countries have developed a series of new models through the improvement and expansion of the ARCH model, including the Generalized ARCH, log ARCH, nonlinear ARCH, Asymmetric GARCH, Exponential ARCH, etc.

9.10. Threshold Autoregression (TAR) Model[15,16]

In practice, nonlinear characteristics are commonly observed. For example, the declining and rising patterns of a process are asymmetric, in which case piecewise linear models can obtain a better approximation to the conditional mean equation. However, changes of the traditional piecewise linear model occur in the "time" space, while the threshold autoregression (TAR) model utilizes threshold space to improve linear approximation.

Generally, a time series $\{x_t\}$ is said to follow a k-regime self-exciting threshold autoregression model (SETAR) model, if it satisfies

$$x_t = \varphi_0^{(j)} + \varphi_1^{(j)} x_{t-1} + \cdots + \varphi_p^{(j)} x_{t-p} + a_t^{(j)}$$

and $\gamma_{j-1} \leq x_{t-d} < \gamma_j$, where $j = 1, \ldots, k$, k and d are positive integers, and γ_j are real numbers such that $-\infty = \gamma_0 < \gamma_1 < \cdots < \gamma_{k-1} < \gamma_k = \infty$. The

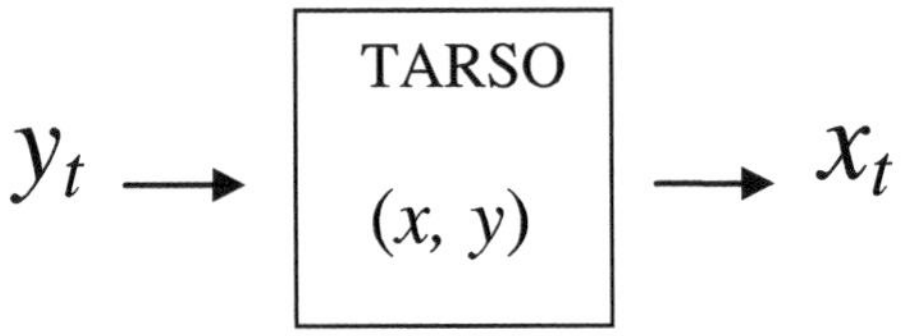

Fig. 9.10.1. TARSO flow diagram.

superscript (j) is used to signify the regime, $\{a_t^{(j)}\}$ are i.i.d. sequences with the mean 0 and the variance σ_j^2 and are mutually independent for different j. The parameter d is referred to as delay parameter and γ_j is the threshold. For different regimes, the AR models are different. In fact, a SETAR model is a piecewise linear AR model in the threshold space. It is similar in logic to the usual piecewise linear models in regression analysis, where the model changes occur in "time" space. If $k > 1$, the SETAR model is nonlinear. Furthermore, TAR model has some generalized forms like close-loop TAR model and open-loop TAR model.

$\{x_t, y_t\}$ is called an open-loop TAR system if

$$x_t = \phi_0^{(j)} + \sum_{i=1}^{m} \phi_i^{(j)} x_{t-i} + \sum_{i=0}^{n} \varphi_i^{(j)} y_{t-i} + a_t^{(j)},$$

and $\gamma_{j-1} \le x_{t-d} < \gamma_j$, where $j = 1, \ldots, k$, k and d are positive integers. $\{x_t\}$ is observable output, $\{y_t\}$ is observable input, and $\{a_t^{(j)}\}$ are white noise sequences with the mean 0 and the variance σ_j^2 being independent of $\{y_t\}$. The system is generally referred to as threshold autoregressive self-exciting open-loop (TARSO), denoted by

$$\text{TARSO}\ [d, k; (m_1, n_1), (m_2, n_2), \ldots, (m_k, n_k)].$$

The flow diagram of TARSO model is shown in Figure 9.10.1.

9.11. State Space Model[17–19]

State space model is a flexible method that can simplify maximum likelihood estimation and handle with missing data in time series analysis. It consists of vector autoregression of unobserved state vector $\boldsymbol{X}_t$ and observed equation of observed vector $\boldsymbol{Y}_t$, i.e.

$$\mathbf{X}_t = \Phi \mathbf{X}_{t-1} + \boldsymbol{e}_t,$$

$$\mathbf{Y}_t = A_t \mathbf{X}_t + \varepsilon_t,$$

where i.i.d. error matrices $\{\varepsilon_t\}$ and $\{\boldsymbol{e}_t\}$ are uncorrelated white noise processes, Φ is state transition matrix, A_t is measurement or observation matrix. The state error vector $\boldsymbol{e}_t$ has zero-mean vector and covariance matrix $\text{Var}(\boldsymbol{e}_t) = Q$. The additive observation noise $\boldsymbol{\varepsilon}_t$ is assumed to be Gaussian with covariance matrix $\text{Var}(\boldsymbol{\varepsilon}_t) = R$.

For example, we consider the issue of monitoring the levels of log(white blood cell count), log(platelet) and hematocrit after a cancer patient undergoes a bone marrow transplant, denoted Y_{t1}, Y_{t2}, and Y_{t3}, respectively, which are measurements made for 91 days. We model the three variables in terms of the state equation

$$\begin{pmatrix} X_{t1} \\ X_{t2} \\ X_{t3} \end{pmatrix} = \begin{pmatrix} \phi_{11} & \phi_{12} & \phi_{13} \\ \phi_{21} & \phi_{22} & \phi_{23} \\ \phi_{31} & \phi_{32} & \phi_{33} \end{pmatrix} \begin{pmatrix} X_{t-1,1} \\ X_{t-3,2} \\ X_{t-3,3} \end{pmatrix} + \begin{pmatrix} e_{t1} \\ e_{t2} \\ e_{t3} \end{pmatrix},$$

$$\begin{pmatrix} Y_{t1} \\ Y_{t2} \\ Y_{t3} \end{pmatrix} = \begin{pmatrix} A_{11} & A_{12} & A_{13} \\ A_{21} & A_{22} & A_{23} \\ A_{31} & A_{32} & A_{33} \end{pmatrix} \begin{pmatrix} X_{t,1} \\ X_{t,2} \\ X_{t,3} \end{pmatrix} + \begin{pmatrix} \varepsilon_{t1} \\ \varepsilon_{t2} \\ \varepsilon_{t3} \end{pmatrix}.$$

The maximum likelihood procedure yielded the estimators

$$\hat{\Phi} = \begin{pmatrix} 1.02 & -0.09 & 0.01 \\ 0.08 & 0.90 & 0.01 \\ -0.90 & 1.42 & 0.87 \end{pmatrix}, \quad \hat{Q} = \begin{pmatrix} 1.02 & -0.09 & 0.01 \\ 0.08 & 0.90 & 0.01 \\ -0.90 & 1.42 & 0.87 \end{pmatrix},$$

$$\hat{R} = \begin{pmatrix} 0.004 & 0 & 0 \\ 0 & 0.022 & 0 \\ 0 & 0 & 1.69 \end{pmatrix}.$$

The coupling between the first and second series is relatively weak, whereas the third series hematocrit is strongly related to the first two; that is,

$$\hat{X}_{t3} = -0.90X_{t-1,1} + 1.42X_{t-1,2} + 0.87X_{t-1,3}.$$

Hence, the hematocrit is negatively correlated with the white blood cell count and positively correlated with the platelet count. The procedure also provides estimated trajectories for all the three longitudinal series and their respective prediction intervals.

In practice, under the observed series $\{Y_t\}$, the choice of state pace model or ARIMA may depend on the experience of the analyst and oriented by the substantive purpose of the study.

9.12. Time Series Spectral Analysis[20,21]

Spectral analysis began with the search for "hidden periodicities" in time series data. The analysis of stationary processes by means of their spectral representations is often referred to as the frequency domain analysis of time series. For instance, in the design of a structure subject to a randomly fluctuating load, it is important to be aware of the presence in the loading force of a large harmonic with a particular frequency to ensure that the possible frequency does not overlap with a resonant frequency of the structure.

For the series $\{X_t\}$, defining its Fourier transform as

$$X(\omega) = \sum_{t=-\infty}^{\infty} e^{-i\omega t} X_t.$$

Further, the spectral density is defined as the Fourier transform of the autocovariance function

$$S(\omega) = \sum_{j=-\infty}^{\infty} e^{-i\omega j} \gamma_j.$$

Since γ_j is symmetric, the spectral density $S(\omega)$ is real

$$S(\omega) = \gamma_0 + 2\sum_{j=1}^{\infty} \gamma_j \cos(j\omega).$$

Equivalently, taking the Fourier transform of the autocorrelation function,

$$f(\omega) = \frac{S(\omega)}{\gamma_0} = \sum_{j=-\infty}^{\infty} e^{-i\omega j} \rho_j,$$

so that

$$\int_{-\pi}^{\pi} \frac{f(\omega)}{2\pi} d\omega = 1.$$

The integrated function $f(\omega)/2\pi$ looks just like a probability density. Hence, the terminology "spectral density" is used. In the analysis of multivariate time series, spectral density matrix and cross-spectral density are corresponding to autocovariance matrix and cross-covariance matrix, respectively.

For a MA(1) model $X_t = \varepsilon_t + \theta\varepsilon_{t-1}$, its spectral density is

$$f(\omega) = \frac{S(\omega)}{\gamma_0} = 1 + \frac{2\theta}{1+\theta^2} \cos\omega$$

that is demonstrated in Figure 9.12.1. We can see that "smooth" MA(1) with $\theta > 0$ have spectral densities that emphasize low frequencies, while "choppy" MA(1) with $\theta < 0$ have spectral densities that emphasize high frequencies.

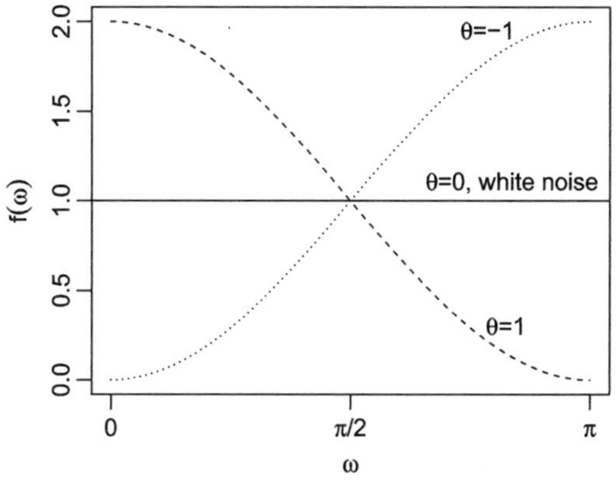

Fig. 9.12.1. MA(1) spectral density.

We can construct spectral density estimates by Fourier transforming these

$$\hat{S}(\omega) = \hat{\gamma}_0 + 2\sum_{j=1}^{N} \hat{\gamma}_j \cos(j\omega).$$

However, it is not consistent with the theoretical spectral density so that smoothed sample spectral density can be explored. The basic idea is that most spectral densities will change very little over small intervals of frequencies. As such, we should be able to average the values of the sample spectral density over small intervals of frequencies to gain reduced variability. Consider taking a simple average of the neighboring sample spectral density values centered on frequency ω and extending N Fourier frequencies on either side of ω. After averaging $2N+1$ values of the sample spectral, the smoothed sample spectral density is given by

$$\bar{S}(\omega) = \frac{1}{2N+1}\sum_{j=-N}^{N} \hat{S}\left(\omega + \frac{j}{T}\right).$$

More generally, a weight function or spectral window $W_m(\omega)$ may be used to smooth the sample spectrum.

9.13. Periodicity Detection[1,6,22]

As for the time series analysis, this is a main method in the frequency domain. Time series data often consist of rich information, such as trend variations, periodic or seasonal variations, random variations, etc. Periodicity is one of the most common characteristics in a time series, which exists in a large number of biomedical data, such as electrocardiogram (ECG) and electroencephalogram (EEG), monthly outpatient data, etc,. Accurately detecting the characteristics of periodicity in a time series is of great significance. One can use the periods obtained by periodicity detection methods to do sequence analysis of characteristics of information, such as life cycle analysis, DNA sequence analysis, etc. and also to use it as a prerequisite for modeling, forecasting and prediction, detection of irregular wave and to find sequence similarities or differences, such as differences in the levels of patients and normal people in a certain gene expression analysis and comparison of different subjects' sleeping structures, etc.

Frequency domain analysis methods of time series are mainly used to identify the periodic variations in time series data. Discrete Fourier Spectral Analysis is the basic in frequency domain, which is used to detect the dominant periods in a time series. For any time series samples $X_t, t = 1, 2, \ldots, N$, Discrete Fourier Transformation is defined as

$$\mathrm{dft}(\omega_j) = N^{-1/2} \sum_{t=1}^{N} x_t e^{-2\pi i \omega_j t},$$

where $\omega_j = j/N$, which is named as Fourier frequency, $j = 1, 2, \ldots, N$, and then periodogram is obtained,

$$I(\omega_j) = |\mathrm{dft}(\omega_j)|^2,$$

where $j = 1, 2, \ldots, N$. Based on periodogram, Fisher g statistics is promoted according to the formula:

$$g_1 = \max_{1 \le j \le k} (I(\omega_j)) \Big/ \sum_{j=1}^{k} I(\omega_j),$$

where $I(\omega_j)$ is the periodogram at each $\omega_j, j = 1, 2, \ldots, k$. Fisher g statistic is used to identify the highest peak of a periodogram, and to judge whether there is a significant periodicity component in a time series or not. Since then, several improved methods based on Fisher g test were proposed by researchers, which were developed in order to be applied under different situations, such as the short or long sequence length, the strength of the background noise, etc.

In recent years, periodicity test in qualitative time series or categorical time series achieved many improvements. Stoffer *et al.* promoted a method called spectral envelope analysis to detect periods of categorical time series which made dummy transformation first to a categorical time series, and then doing Discrete Fourier transformation, which proves to be suitable to be applied in real data. In addition, Walsh transformation is an alternative method to detect periodicity in the categorical time series.

9.14. Moving Holiday Effects of Time Series[13,23]

The moving holiday effect of time series is also called the calendar effect, that is, date of the same holiday determined by lunar calendar are different in solar calendar years. In China, important moving holidays are New Year, Lantern Festival, Mid-Autumn Festival, and Dragon-Boat Festival.

There are two important elements to describe moving holidays. First, time series around moving holiday shows up and down trend. Second, effect of moving holidays depends on the different date that appeared in solar calendar.

When the date of a holiday shifts from year to year, it can affect the time series in an interval of two or more months. This will violate the comparability for the same month among different years.

First, the calendar effect in monthly time series could sometimes cause considerable distortions in analytical tools such as the correlogram, which makes it more difficult in model identification. Second, it will distort important characters of time series (such as turning point and turning direction) and further on affect comparability of observations in different months. Third, the calendar effect can reduce the forecasting ability of a model for time series. Especially, in the construct of a regression equation, if such seasonal fluctuations affect the dependent and independent variables differently, the precision of estimation to coefficients will decrease. Fourth, the calendar effect caused by determined seasonality factors cannot be correctly extracted, which is called "over seasonal adjustment".

This means characteristic peak on spectrum of December is weakened. Furthermore, the calendar effect may easily cover up the significant periodicity. In medicine, once the changing levels of pathogen are distorted, it will mislead etiological explanation.

Identification of moving holiday effect: first, draw a day-by-day sequence chart using daily observations around the moving holidays (Figure 9.14.1) to see clearly whether there is a drift or not; Then, draw a day-by-day sequence chart by taking moving holiday (e.g. Chinese New Year) as the midpoint (Figure 9.14.2), from which we can determine the pattern of the moving holiday effect on the outpatient capacity sequence. According to Figure 9.14.2 and paired t-test, we can determine the interval of moving holiday effect (see Ref. [1]).

Nowadays, the adjustment method of moving holiday effect is embedded in the seasonal adjustment methods, such as TRAMO/SEATS, X-11-ARIMA, X-12-ARIMA , X-13A-S, and NBS-SA (developed by Chinese Statistical Bureau in 2009). All these softwares are based on days in moving

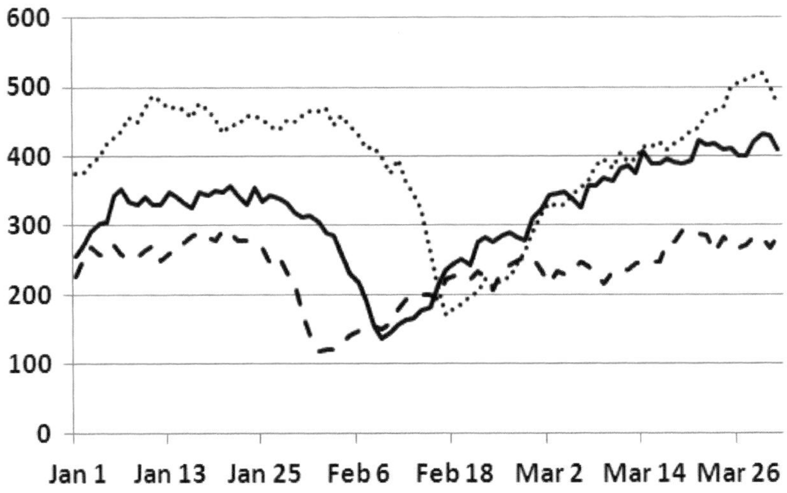

Fig. 9.14.1. Day-by-day sequence.

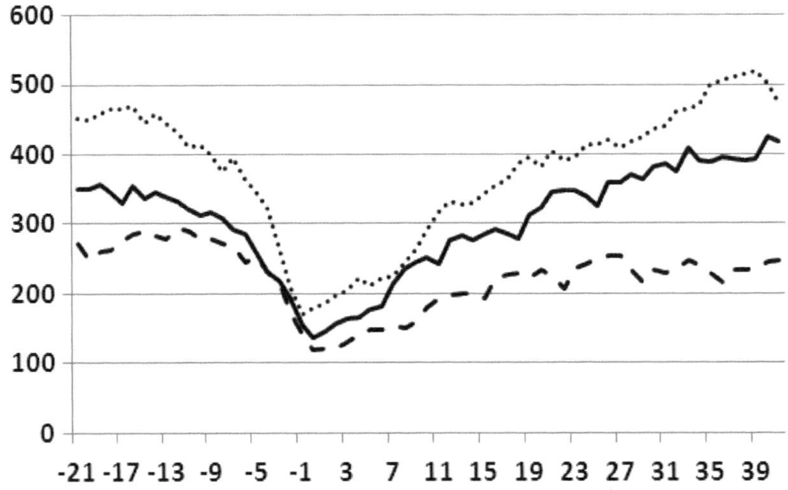

Fig. 9.14.2. Day-by-day sequence with Chinese New Year as the midpoint.

holiday effect interval, which are not so accurate. It is recommended to use observation-based proportional model instead of days-based proportional model when performing adjustment of moving holiday effects.

9.15. Vector Autoregressive Model (VAR)[1,2,19]

Most theories and methodologies in univariate time series analysis can be extended to multivariate time series analysis, especially the VAR. For many time series arising in practice, a more effective analysis may be obtained by considering individual series as components of a vector time series and analyzing the series jointly. Multivariate processes arise when several related time series are observed simultaneously over time, instead of observing just a single series as is the case in univariate time series analysis.

For instance, Shumway *et al.* study the possible effects of temperature and pollution on weekly mortality in Los Angeles County. By common knowledge, cardiovascular mortality will decrease under warmer temperatures and in lower particulate densities, while temperatures are possibly associated with pollutant particulates. For the three-dimensional series, cardiovascular mortality X_{t1}, temperature X_{t2}, and pollutant particulate levels X_{t3}, taking $\boldsymbol{X}_t = (X_{t1}, X_{t2}, X_{t3})'$ as a vector, the VAR(p) model is

$$\boldsymbol{X}_t = A_0 + \sum_{i=1}^{p} \boldsymbol{A}_i \boldsymbol{X}_{t-i} + \varepsilon_t, \tag{9.15.1}$$

where A_0 is a three-dimensional constant column vector, $\boldsymbol{A}_i$ are 3×3 transition matrix for $i > 0$, and ε_t is three-dimensional white noise process with covariance matrix $E(\varepsilon_t \varepsilon_t') = \Sigma_\varepsilon$. If $p = 1$, the dynamic relations among the three series are defined as the first-order relation,

$$X_{t1} = a_{10} + a_{11}X_{t-1,1} + a_{12}X_{t-1,3} + a_{13}X_{t-1,3} + \varepsilon_{t1},$$

which expresses the current value of mortality as a linear combination of the trend and its immediate past value and the past values of temperature and the particulate levels. Similarly,

$$X_{t2} = a_{20} + a_{21}X_{t-1,1} + a_{22}X_{t-1,3} + a_{23}X_{t-1,3} + \varepsilon_{t2}$$

and

$$X_{t3} = a_{30} + a_{31}X_{t-1,1} + a_{32}X_{t-1,3} + a_{33}X_{t-1,3} + \varepsilon_{t3}$$

express the dependence of temperature and particulate levels on the other series. If the series are stationary and its parameters are identifiable, $\hat{A}_0$, $\hat{\boldsymbol{A}}_1$, and $\hat{\Sigma}_\varepsilon$ can be estimated by Yule–Walker estimation. The selection criteria on lag order is based on BIC

$$\text{BIC} = \ln \left| \hat{\sum}_\varepsilon \right| + (k^2 p \ln n)/n,$$

where $k = 3$. The optimal model is VAR(2) given in Table 9.15.1.

Table 9.15.1. Lag order selection of VAR model.

Order (p)	$\lvert\hat{\Sigma}_\varepsilon\rvert$	BIC
1	118520	11.79
2	74708	11.44
3	70146	11.49
4	65268	11.53
5	59684	11.55

Analog to univariate time series, VMA(q) and VARMA(p, q) models are defined as

$$\boldsymbol{X}_t = \mu + \boldsymbol{B}_0 \varepsilon_t + \sum_{i=1}^{q} \boldsymbol{B}_i \varepsilon_{t-i} \tag{9.15.2}$$

and

$$\boldsymbol{X}_t = \boldsymbol{\mu} + \sum_{i=1}^{p} \boldsymbol{A}_i \boldsymbol{X}_{t-i} + \sum_{i=0}^{q} \boldsymbol{B}_i \boldsymbol{\varepsilon}_{t-i}. \tag{9.15.3}$$

Compared to VAR model, it is more complex in VMA model. However, VMA model is highly related to impulse response function which can explore the effects of random shocks. As for VARMA(p, q), there are too many parameters to estimate and they are hardly identifiable so that only VARMA(1,1) and VARMA(2,1) can be useful in practice.

9.16. Granger Causality[3,11,24]

Granger causality measures whether current and past values of one variable help to forecast future values of another variable. For instance, a VAR(p) model

$$\boldsymbol{X}_t = A_0 + \boldsymbol{A}_1(L)\boldsymbol{X}_{t-1} + \varepsilon_t$$

can be written as

$$\begin{pmatrix} Y_t \\ Z_t \end{pmatrix} = \begin{pmatrix} A_{10} \\ A_{20} \end{pmatrix} + \begin{pmatrix} A_{11}(L) & A_{12}(L) \\ A_{21}(L) & A_{22}(L) \end{pmatrix} \begin{pmatrix} Y_{t-1} \\ Z_{t-1} \end{pmatrix} + \begin{pmatrix} \varepsilon_{t1} \\ \varepsilon_{t2} \end{pmatrix},$$

Table 9.16.1. Granger causality test base on a VAR(4) model.

Causality hypothesis	Statistic	Distribution	P value
$Y_t \xrightarrow{\text{Gr}} Z_t$	2.24	$F(4, 152)$	0.07
$Z_t \xrightarrow{\text{Gr}} Y_t$	0.31	$F(4, 152)$	0.87
$Y_t \xrightarrow{\text{inst}} Z_t$	0.61	$\chi^2(1)$	0.44

Note: "Gr" denotes the Granger cause and "inst" denotes the instantaneous cause.

where $\boldsymbol{X}_t = (Y_t, Z_t)$, $A_{ij}(L)$ is the polynomial of the lag operator L, and its coefficients are $a_{ij}(1), a_{ij}(2), \ldots, a_{ij}(p)$. If and only if

$$a_{ij}(1) = a_{ij}(2) = \cdots = a_{ij}(p) = 0,$$

then $\{Y_t\}$ is not the Granger causality to $\{Z_t\}$. The bivariate example can be extended to any multivariate VAR(p) model:

$$\text{Non-Granger causality } X_{tj} \Leftrightarrow \text{All the coefficients of } A_{ij}(L) \text{ equal zero.}$$

Here, Granger causality is different from instantaneous causality that measures whether the current values of one variable are affected by the contemporaneous values of another variable.

If all variables in the VAR model are stationary, conducting a standard F-test of the restriction

$$H_0\colon a_{ij}(1) = a_{ij}(2) = \cdots = a_{ij}(p) = 0$$

and the testing statistic is

$$F = \frac{(\text{RSS}_R - \text{RSS}_{\text{UR}})/p}{\text{RSS}_{\text{UR}}/(n-k)},$$

where RSS_R and RSS_{UR} are the restricted and unrestricted residuals sum of squares, respectively, and k is the number of parameters needed to be estimated in the unrestricted model. For example, Table 9.16.1 depicts the Granger causality tests in a bivariate VAR(4) model.

Before testing Granger causality, there are three points to be noted: (i) Variables need to be differentiated until every variable is stationary; (ii) The lags in the model are determined by AIC or BIC; (iii) The variables will be transformed until the error terms are uncorrelated.

9.17. Cointegration Test[3,25]

In univariate models, the series can become stationary by difference so that ARMA model will be built. However, spurious regression will appear, though every variable is stationary after differentiating. For a bivariate system example,

$$X_{t1} = \gamma X_{t2} + \varepsilon_{t1}, \quad (9.17.1)$$

$$X_{t2} = X_{t-1,2} + \varepsilon_{t2} \quad (9.17.2)$$

with ε_{t1} and ε_{t2} uncorrelated white noise processes, both X_{t1} and X_{t2} are cointegrated of order 1 (i.e. $I(1)$ processes). But differenced VMA(1) model

$$\Delta \boldsymbol{X}_t = \begin{pmatrix} \Delta X_{t1} \\ \Delta X_{t2} \end{pmatrix} = \begin{pmatrix} 1-L & \gamma L \\ 0 & 1 \end{pmatrix} \begin{pmatrix} \varepsilon_{t1} \\ \varepsilon_{t2} \end{pmatrix},$$

still exists a unit root. Nevertheless, the linear combination $(X_{t1} - \gamma X_{t2})$ is stationary since it eliminates the random trends in two series. We say $\boldsymbol{X}_t \equiv (X_{t1}, X_{t2})'$ is cointegrated with a vector $(1, -\gamma)'$. More formally, the component of vector $\boldsymbol{X}_t$ is said to be cointegrated of order d, b, denoted $\boldsymbol{X}_t \sim CI(d, b)$ if

(i) all components of $\boldsymbol{X}_t = (X_{t1}, \cdots, X_{tn})'$ are $I(d)$;
(ii) $\exists$ a vector $\beta = (\beta_1, \ldots, \beta_n)' \neq 0$ such that the linear combination $\beta' X_t = \beta_1 X_{t1} + \cdots + \beta_n X_{tn} \sim I(d-b)$, where $b > 0$.

The vector β is called the cointegrating vector, which eliminates all the random trends among variables.

Engle–Granger method and Johansen–Stock–Watson method are used to test cointegrating usually. As for Engle–Granger method, two variables are cointegrated if the regression residuals of the two integrated variables are stationary by ADF test. One shortcoming in the procedure is the variable is defined as the dependent variable for the regression. Hence, the following Johansen–Stock–Watson method is applied to test cointegration by analyzing the relationship between rank of coefficient matrix and eigenvalues. Essentially, it is the multivariate form of ADF test

$$\Delta \boldsymbol{X}_t = \boldsymbol{\pi} \boldsymbol{X}_{t-1} + \sum_{i=1}^{p-1} \boldsymbol{\pi}_i \Delta \boldsymbol{X}_{t-i} + \boldsymbol{e}_t,$$

where the rank of matrices $\boldsymbol{\pi}$ is the dimension of integrating vector. For $1 \leq \text{rank}(\boldsymbol{\pi}) < n$, $\boldsymbol{\pi}$ can be decomposed as

$$\boldsymbol{\pi} = \alpha \beta',$$

where α and β are two $n \times r$ matrices with $\text{rank}(\beta) = \text{rank}(\boldsymbol{\pi}) = r$. Then β is the integrating vector.

Further, error correction model will be made for the bivariate systems (9.17.1) and (9.17.2), that is,

$$\Delta X_{t1} = \alpha_1(X_{t1} - \gamma X_{t2}) + \sum a_{11}(i)\Delta X_{t-i,1} + \sum a_{12}(i)\Delta X_{t-i,2} + \varepsilon_{t1},$$

$$\Delta X_{t2} = \alpha_2(X_{t1} - \gamma X_{t2}) + \sum a_{21}(i)\Delta X_{t-i,1} + \sum a_{22}(i)\Delta X_{t-i,2} + \varepsilon_{t2},$$

where $\alpha_1(X_{t1} - \gamma X_{t2})$ is the error correction term to correct the VAR model of $\Delta \boldsymbol{X}_t$. Generally, the error correction model corresponding to vector $\boldsymbol{X}_t = (X_{t1}, \ldots, X_{tn})'$ is

$$\Delta \boldsymbol{X}_t = \pi \boldsymbol{X}_t + \sum_{i=1}^{p} \pi_i \Delta \boldsymbol{X}_{t-i} + \boldsymbol{\varepsilon}_t,$$

where $\pi = (\pi_{jk})_{n\times n} \neq 0$, $\pi_i = (\pi_{jk}(i))_{n\times n}$, and the error vector $\boldsymbol{\varepsilon}_t = (\varepsilon_{ti})_{n\times 1}$ is stationary and uncorrelated.

9.18. Categorical or Qualitative Time Series[12,29–31]

Categorical or qualitative time series also named as categorical time series is defined as an ordered sequence of categorical values of a variable at equally spaced time intervals. The values are gathered in terms of states (or categories) at discrete time points in a categorical time series.

Categorical time series exists in a variety of fields, such as biomedicine, behavior research, epidemiology, genetics, etc. Figure 9.18.1 depicts a categorical time series of the sleep pattern of a normal infant when sleeping ($n = 525$ minutes as a total). Six sleep states are recorded including quiet sleep — trace alternate, quiet sleep — high voltage, indeterminate sleep, active sleep — low voltage, active sleep — mixed, and awake. The states were coded using the numbers 1–6, respectively. There is another way to depict categorical time series data (see Figure 9.18.2). Without coding each

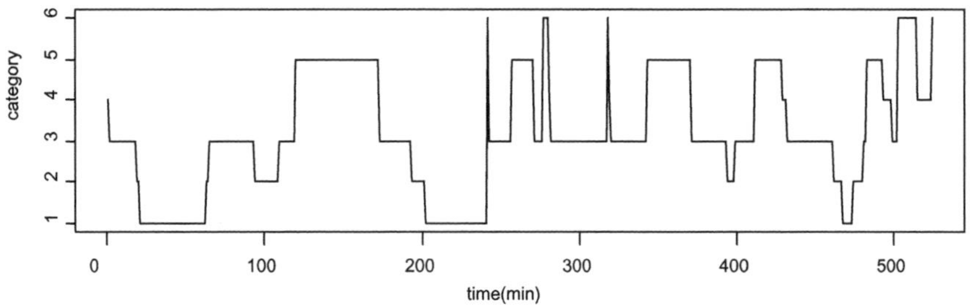

Fig. 9.18.1. Realization of sleep state data for one infant.

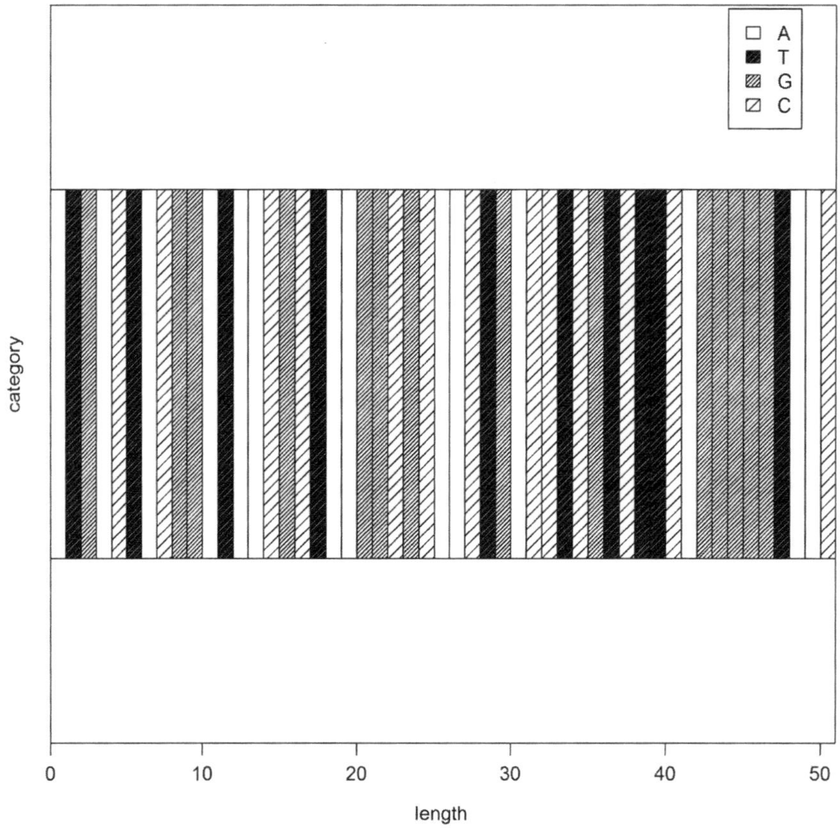

Fig. 9.18.2. First 50 SNPs plot in trehalose synthase gene of Saccharomyces cerevisiae.

state as a number, rectangle with different style instead is used to represent each category of a gene sequence.

There are numerous statistical techniques for analyzing continuous-valued time series in both the time and frequency domains. If a time series is discrete-valued, there are a number of available techniques, for example, DARMA models, INAR models, and truncated models in the time domain, Fourier and Walsh–Fourier analysis in the spectral domain. If the time series is categorical-valued, then there is the theory of Markov chains, and the link function approach for the time domain analysis, the spectral envelop method for the frequency domain analysis. Stoffer *et al.* created the spectral envelope analysis to detect periodicity of categorical time series, in which dummy transformation was first made for a categorical time series to a multivariate time series, and then Discrete Fourier Transformation was applied. The spectral envelope method was used in real long DNA sequence periodicity detection and achieved good results. Walsh Transformation Spectral Analysis is an alternative method to process categorical time series in the spectral domain. Tests for stationary in a categorical time series is one concern of researchers in recent years.

9.19. Non-parametric Time Series[12,29–31]

The GARCH model builds a deterministic nonlinear relationship between time series and error terms, whereas non-parametric models can handle unknown relationship between them. For instance, series $\{X_t\}$ has the model

$$X_t = f_1(X_{t-1}) + \cdots + f_p(X_{t-p}) + \varepsilon_t, \tag{9.19.1}$$

where $f_i(X_{t-i})$, $i = 1, 2, \ldots, p$, are unknown smoothing functions. It is a natural extension of the AR(p) model, which is called additive autoregressive (AAR) model, denoted as $\{X_t\} \sim \mathrm{AAP}(p)$. If the functions $f_i(\cdot)$ are linear forms, i.e. $f_i(X_{t-i}) = \phi_i X_{t-i}$, AAR($p$) model will degenerate into AR(p) model. For moderately large p, the functions in such a "saturated" non-parametric form are difficult to estimate unless the sample size is astronomically large. The difficulty is intrinsic and is often referred to as the "curse of dimensionality".

An extension of the threshold model is the so-called functional/varying-coefficient autoregressive (FAR) model

$$X_t = f_1(X_{t-d})X_{t-i} + \cdots + f_p(X_{t-d})X_{t-p} + \sigma(X_{t-d})\varepsilon_t, \tag{9.19.2}$$

where $d > 1$ and $f_1(\cdot), \ldots, f_p(\cdot)$ are unknown coefficient functions, denoted as $\{X_t\} \sim \mathrm{FAR}(p, d)$. It allows the coefficient functions to change gradually, rather than abruptly as in the TAR model, as the value of X_{t-d} varies continuously. This can be appealing in many applications such as in understanding the population dynamics in ecological studies. As the population density X_{t-d} changes continuously, it is reasonable to expect that its effects on the current population size X_t will be continuous as well.

The FAR model depends critically on the choice of the model dependent variable X_{t-d}. The model-dependent variable is one of the lagged variables. This limits the scope of its applications. The adaptive functional/varying-coefficient autoregressive (AFAR) model is a generalization of FAR model

$$X_t = g_0(\boldsymbol{X}'_{t-1}\beta) + g_1(\boldsymbol{X}'_{t-1}\beta)X_{t-1} + \cdots + g_p(\boldsymbol{X}'_{t-1}\beta)X_{t-p} + \varepsilon_t, \tag{9.19.3}$$

where ε_t is independent of $X_{t-1}, \ldots, X_{t-p}, \ldots, \boldsymbol{X}_{t-1} = (X_{t-1}, \ldots, X_{t-p})'$ and $\beta = (\beta_1, \ldots, \beta_p)'$. The model is denoted by AFAR(p). It allows a linear combination of past values as a model dependent variable. This is also a generalization of single index models and threshold models with unknown threshold directions.

Another useful non-parametric model, which is a natural extension of the ARCH model, is the following functional stochastic conditional variance model:

$$X_t = f(X_{t-1}, \dots, X_{t-p}) + \sigma(X_{t-1}, \dots, X_{t-p})\varepsilon_t, \tag{9.19.4}$$

where ε_t is white noise independent of $\{X_{t-1}, \dots, X_{t-p}\}$, $\sigma^2(\cdot)$ is the conditional variance function, $f(\cdot)$ is an autoregressive function. It can be derived that the variance of residuals is

$$\mathrm{Var}(r_t|X_{t-1}, \dots, X_{t-p}) \approx \sigma^2(X_{t-1}, \dots, X_{t-p}).$$

Generally, the estimation of non-parametric time series model is fulfilled by local linear kernel estimation. A simple and quick method to select the bandwidth proposed in Cai *et al.* (2000) is regarded as a modified multifold cross-validation criterion that is attentive to the structure of stationary time series data. The variable selection is to use a stepwise deletion technique for each given linear component together with a modified AIC and t-statistic.

9.20. Time Series Forecasting[1,32]

By summarizing the historical time series data, we may find a model which is proper to fit the series. With observed values at time t and before, it will be possible to forecast values in the future time of $(t + l)$, where l is the lead time for time series prediction.

The components of a time series are trend, cycle, seasonal variations, and irregular fluctuations, which are important to identify and forecast the historical characteristics of time series. Time series modeling is the procedure of identifying and recognizing these four components. The time series components already discussed above, do not always appear alone. They can appear in any combination or can appear altogether. Therefore, the so-called proper forecasting models are generally not unique. A selected forecasting model that successfully includes a certain component may fail to include another essential component.

One of the most important problems in forecasting is matching the appropriate forecasting model to the pattern of the available time series data. The key issues in time series modeling are assuming that a data pattern can be recognized by historical time series data and the influence of external factors on time series is constant. Thus, time series forecasting is suitable for objective factors or those that cannot be controlled, such as macroeconomic situation, the employment level, medical income and expenditure and outpatient capacity, rather than subjective factors, such as commodity prices.

There are five steps in time series forecast: (1) draw time series graph to ensure stationary, (2) model identification and modeling, (3) estimation and assessment, (4) forecast and (5) analysis of predictive validity. The key issue is proper model identification according to the characters of time series.

If a time series is linear, then AR, MA, ARMA or ARIMA model is available. VAR model which is extended from these models is multitime series model based on vector data.

If a time series is nonlinear, chaotic time series model can be chosen. Empirical studies point out that the forecast effect of nonlinear model (nonlinear autoregressive exogenous model) is better than that of linear model. Some other nonlinear time series models can describe various changes of the sequence along with time, such as conditional heteroscedasticity models: ARCH, GARCH, TARCH, EGARCH, FIGARCH and CGARCH. This variation is related with recent historical values, and can be forecasted by the time series.

Nowadays, model-free analyses, the methods based on wavelet transform (locally stationary wavelet and neural network based on wavelet decomposition) are focused by researchers. The multiscale (or multiresolution) technology can be used for time series decomposition, attempts to elucidate the time dependence in multiscale. The Markov Switching Model (MSMF) is used for modeling volatility changes of time series. We can use the latent Markov model to fulfill the modeling when the Markov process cannot be observed, and considering as simple dynamic Bayesian networks which can be widely used in speech recognition, converting the time series of speech to text.

Acknowledgment

Dr. Madafeitom Meheza Abide Bodombossou Djobo reviewed the whole chapter and helped us express the ideas in a proper way. We really appreciate her support.

References

1. Box, GEP, Jenkins, GM, Reinsel, GC. *Time Series Analysis: Forecasting and Control*. New York: Wiley & Sons, 2008.

2. Shumway, RH, Azari, RS, Pawitan, Y. Modeling mortality fluctuations in Los Angeles as functions of pollution and weather effects. *Environ. Res.*, 1988, 45(2): 224–241.
3. Enders, W. *Applied Econometric Time Series*, (4th edn.). New York: Wiley & Sons, 2015.
4. Kendall, MG. *Rank Correlation Methods.* London: Charler Griffin, 1975.
5. Wang, XL, Swail, VR. Changes of extreme wave heights in northern hemisphere oceans and related atmospheric circulation regimes. *Amer. Meteorol. Soc.* 2001, 14(10): 2204–2221.
6. Jonathan, D. Cryer, Kung-Sik Chan. *Time Series Analysis with Applications in R*, (2nd edn.). Berlin: Springer, 2008.
7. Doldado, J, Jenkinso, T, Sosvilla-Rivero, S. Cointegration and unit roots. *J. Econ. Surv.*, 1990, 4: 249–273.
8. Perron, P, Vogelsang, TJ. Nonstationary and level shifts with an application to purchasing power parity. *J. Bus. Eco. Stat.*, 1992, 10: 301–320.
9. Hong, Y. *Advanced Econometrics.* Beijing: High Education Press, 2011.
10. Ljung, G, Box, GEP. On a measure of lack of fit in time series models. *Biometrika*, 1978, 66: 67–72.
11. Lutkepohl, H, Kratzig, M. *Applied Time Series Econometrics.* New York: Cambridge University Press, 2004.
12. An, Z, Chen, M. *Nonlinear Time Series Analysis.* Shanghai: Shanghai Science and Technique Press, (in Chinese) 1998.
13. Findley, DF, Monsell, BC, Bell, WR, *et al.* New capabilities and methods of the X-12-ARIMA seasonal adjustment program. *J. Bus. Econ. Stat.*, 1998, 16(2): 1–64.
14. Engle, RF. Autoregressive Conditional Heteroscedasticity with Estimates of the Variance of United Kingdom Inflation. *Econometrica*, 1982, 50(4): 987–1007.
15. Tsay, RS. *Analysis of Financial Time Series*, (3rd edn.). New Jersey: John Wiley & Sons, 2010.
16. Shi, J, Zhou, Q, Xiang, J. An application of the threshold autoregression procedure to climate analysis and forecasting. *Adv. Atmos. Sci.* 1986, 3(1): 134–138.
17. Davis, MHA, Vinter, RB. *Stochastic Modeling and Control.* London: Chapman and Hall, 1985.
18. Hannan, EJ, Deistler, M. *The Statistical Theory of Linear Systems.* New York: Wiley & Sons, 1988.
19. Shumway, RH, Stoffer, DS. *Time Series Analysis and Its Application With R Example*, (3rd edn.). New York: Springer, 2011.
20. Brockwell, PJ, Davis, RA. *Time Series: Theory and Methods*, (2nd edn.). New York: Springer, 2006.
21. Cryer, JD, Chan, KS. *Time Series Analysis with Applications in R*, (2nd edn.). New York: Springer, 2008.
22. Fisher, RA. Tests of significance in harmonic analysis. *Proc. Ro. Soc. A*, 1929, 125(796): 54–59.
23. Xue, Y. *Identification and Handling of Moving Holiday Effect in Time Series.* Guangzhou: Sun Yat-sen University, Master's Thesis, 2009.
24. Gujarati, D. *Basic Econometrics*, (4th edn.). New York: McGraw-Hill, 2003.
25. Brockwell, PJ, Davis, RA. *Introduction to Time Series and Forecasting.* New York: Springer, 2002.
26. McGee, M, Harris, I. Coping with nonstationarity in categorical time series. *J. Prob. Stat.* 2012, 2012: 9.
27. Stoffer, DS, Tyler, DE, McDougall, AJ. Spectral analysis for categorical time series: Scaling and the spectral envelope. *Biometrika.* 1993, 80(3): 611–622.

28. WeiB, *CH. Categorical Time Series Analysis and Applications in Statistical Quality Control.* Dissertation. de-Verlag im Internet GmbH, 2009.
29. Cai, Z, Fan, J, Yao, Q. Functional-coefficient regression for nonlinear time series. *J. Amer. Statist. Assoc.*, 2000, 95(451): 888–902.
30. Fan, J, Yao, Q. *Nonlinear Time Series: Parametric and Nonparametric Methods.* New York: Springer, 2005.
31. Gao, J. *Nonlinear Time Series: Semiparametric and Nonparametric Methods.* London: Chapman and Hall, 2007.
32. Kantz, H, Thomas, S. *Nonlinear Time Series Analysis.* London: Cambridge University Press, 2004.
33. Xu, GX. *Statistical Prediction and Decision.* Shanghai University of Finance and Economic Press, Shanghai: 2011 (In Chinese).

About the Author

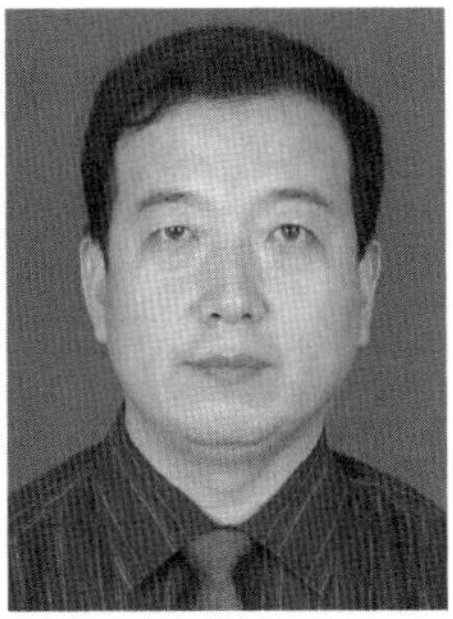

Jinxin Zhang is an Associate Professor and Director in the Department of Medical Statistics and Epidemiology, School of Public Health, Sun Yat-sen University, China. He got his PhD degree from the Fourth Military Medical University, China in 2000. He is the editor of more than 20 text or academic books and has published more than 200 papers, of which more than 20 has been included by Science Citation Index. He has taken part in more than 40 projects funded by governments. He is one of the main teaching members for the Chinese National Excellent Course, Chinese National Bilingual Teaching Model Course, Chinese Brand Course for International Students, Chinese National Brand Course of MOOCs. He has a written or reviewed the *Chinese Health Statistics*, *Chinese Preventive Medicine* and 10 other academic journals. He is a member of the core leaders of the Center for Guiding Clinical Trials in Sun Yat-sen University. His research interests include dynamic data analysis and research design for medical research.

CHAPTER 10

BAYESIAN STATISTICS

Xizhi Wu*, Zhi Geng and Qiang Zhao

10.1. Bayesian Statistics[1,2]

Bayesian statistical method is developed based on Bayesian Theorem which is used to expound and solve statistical problems systematically. Logically, the content of Bayesian statistics is to add data to the initial probability, and then get one new initial probability by Bayesian theory. Bayesian statistics uses probability to measure the degree of trust to the fidelity of an uncertain event based on the existing knowledge. If H is an event or a hypothesis, and K is the knowledge before the test, then we use $p(H|K)$ as the probability or trust after giving K. If there is a data named D in the test, then you should revise the probability to $p(H|D \cap K)$. Such a kind of revision will be included in uncertain data when giving the judgment of H to be right or not. There are three formal rules of probability theory, but other properties can be derived from them as well.

1. Convexity. For every event A and $B, 0 \leq p(A|B) \leq 1$ and $p(A|A) = 1$.
2. Additivity. For the incompatible event A and B and the random event C, there is

$$p(A \cup B|C) = p(A|C) + p(B|C).$$

   (This rule is usually extended to a countable infinite collection of mutually exclusive events.)
3. Multiplication. For every three random events, there is

$$p(A \cap B|C) = p(B|C)p(A|B \cap C).$$

*Corresponding author: xizhi_wu@163.com

It is to be noted that the probability is always a function which has two variables: one is the event which you are interested in its uncertainty, and the other is the knowledge you hold when you study its uncertainty, as mentioned like $p(H|K)$. The second variable is often forgotten, causing the neglect of the information known before, which could lead to serious error. When revising the uncertainty of H according to D, only the conditional event changes from K to $D \cap K$ and H is not changed.

When we say that uncertainty should be described by probability, we mean that your belief obeys the presentation of operational rules. For example, we can prove Bayesian Theorem, and then, from these rules, we can get $p(H|D \cap K)$ from $p(H|K)$. Because K is one part of the conditional event, and it can be elliptical from the mark, thus the Bayesian Theorem is

$$p(H|D) = p(D|H)p(H)/p(D),$$

where $p(D) = p(D|H)p(H) + p(D|H^C)p(H^C)$. H^C is the complementary event to H, which means when H is not true, H^C is true and vice versa. Thus, how to combine $p(D|H), p(D|H^C)$ and $p(H)$ to get $p(H|D)$ can be observed. Because it is the most usual task for statisticians to use the data to change the trust of H, Bayesian Theorem plays an important role, and becomes the name of this method.

In Bayesian theory, probability is interpreted as a degree of trust, so $p(x|\theta)$ is the trust to x when it has parameter value θ, and then it causes trust to $p(\theta|x)$ by $p(\theta)$ when x is given. It differs from the usual method where the probability and frequency are associated with each other. Bayesian theory is not involved in the subjective individual — "you". Although these two interpretations are completely different, there is also connection within them that all come from particular forms of trust which are often used.

Frequency school argues that parameters are constant, but Bayesian school thinks that if a parameter is unknown, it is very reasonable to give a probability distribution to describe its possible values and the likelihood. Bayesian method allows us to use the objective data and subjective viewpoint to confirm the prior distribution. Frequency school states that it reflects different people producing different results with lack of objectivity.

10.2. Prior Distribution[2]

Let us assume that the sampling distribution of the density of the random variable X is $p(x|\theta)$, and the prior distribution of parameter θ is $p(\theta)$, then the posterior distribution is the conditional distribution

$$p(\theta|x) = p(x|\theta)p(\theta)/p(x)$$

after giving sample x. Here, the denominator,

$$p(x) = \int p(x|\theta)p(\theta)d\theta,$$

is the marginal distribution of x, which is called the forecast distribution or marginal distribution of x, and the numerator is the joint distribution of sample x and parameter θ, which is $p(x|\theta)p(\theta) = p(x, \theta)$. So, the posterior distribution can be considered to be proportional to the product of the likelihood function $p(x|\theta)$ and the prior distribution $p(\theta)$, i.e.

$$p(\theta|x) \propto p(x|\theta)p(\theta).$$

Posterior distribution can be viewed as the future prior distribution. In practices, such as life tests, when researchers observe a life sequence $x = (x_1, \dots, x_n)$, they also need to predict the future life $y = (y_1, \dots, y_m)$. At this moment, the posterior expectation of $p(x|\theta)$, i.e.

$$h(y|x) \propto \int p(y|\theta)p(\theta|x)d\theta,$$

is regarded as a distribution, which is called the predictive distribution. In this case, $p(\theta)$ is just replaced by $p(\theta|x)$, the posterior distribution (the future prior distribution). From that, a $(1 - \alpha)$ equal-tailed prediction interval (L, U) can be defined for the future observation Y, which meets

$$1 - \alpha = P(L < Y < U) = \int_L^U h(y|x)dy,$$

where

$$\frac{1}{\alpha} = \int_{-\infty}^L h(y|x) \int_U^\infty h(y|x)dy.$$

Usually, the steps of Bayesian inference based on posterior distributions are to consider a family of distributions of a random variable with parameter θ at first. Then according to past experience or other information, a prior distribution of parameter θ is determined. Finally, the posterior distribution is calculated by using the formula above, based on which necessary deductions can be obtained. Usually, the posterior mean value is used to estimate parameters, such as applying $\int \theta p(\theta|x)d\theta$ to estimate θ.

The confidence interval for θ can yet be obtained by its posterior distribution. For example, for a given sample x, probability $1 - \alpha$, and the posterior distribution $p(\theta|x)$ of parameter θ, if there is an interval $[a, b]$ such that $P(\theta \in [a, b]|x) \geq 1 - \alpha$, then the interval is called as the Bayesian credible interval (BCI) of θ with coverage probability $1 - \alpha$, which is briefly called the confidence interval. The confidence interval is a special case for the more general confidence set. What is worth mentioning is the highest posterior density (HPD) confidence interval, which is the shortest one in all the confidence intervals with the same coverage probability. Certainly, it is generally applied in the case of single-peaked continuous distribution (in this case, the confidence set must be a confidence interval). Of course, there is also similarly one-sided confidence interval, that is, one of the endpoints is infinite. If the probability of θ in the left and right of the interval is both $\alpha/2$, then it is named as an equal-tailed confidence interval. The HPD confidence interval is a set C, such that $P(\theta \in C|x) = 1 - \alpha$, and $p(\theta_1|x) > p(\theta_2|x)$ for $\theta_1 \in C$ and $\theta_2 \notin C$.

The parameters in the prior distribution are called hyper-parameters. The II method of maximum likelihood (ML-II) method can be used to estimate hyper-parameters. In this method, the likelihood is equal to the last hyper-parameter after integrating middle parameters.

Conjugate distribution family is the most convenient prior distribution family. Assume $F = \{f(x|\theta)\}$, $(x \in X)$ is the distribution family which is identified by parameter θ. A family of prior distribution Π is conjugate to F, if all the posterior distributions belong to Π for all $f \in F$, all prior distributions in Π and all $x \in X$.

For an exponential family distribution with density,

$$f(x|\theta) = h(x)e^{\theta x - \psi(\theta)},$$

its conjugate distribution about θ is

$$\pi(\theta|\mu, \lambda) = K(\mu, \lambda)e^{\theta\mu - \lambda\psi(\theta)},$$

and the corresponding posterior distribution is $\pi(\theta|\mu + x, \lambda + 1)$.

10.3. Bayesian Decision[2]

Bayesian statistical decision is the decision which minimizes the following Bayesian risk. Consider a statistical model, the distribution of observations $x = (x_1, \ldots, x_n)$ depends on the parameter $\theta \in \Theta$, where Θ refers to state space, θ refers to "the natural state". Making A as the possible action space, for act $a \in A$ and the parameter $\theta \in \Theta$, a loss function $l(\theta, a)$ is needed (can also use the utility functions which is opposite to the loss function). For example, act a represents the estimator for some $q(\theta)$. At that time, the common loss function involves the quadratic loss function $l(\theta,a)=(q(\theta)-a)^2$ or the absolute loss function $l(\theta,a)=|q(\theta)-a|$ and so on. In testing $H_0\colon\theta\in\Theta_0 \Leftrightarrow H_1\colon\theta\in\Theta_1$, the $0-1$ loss function can be useful, where $l(\theta,a)=0$ if $\theta\in\Theta_a$ (i.e. the judgment is right), otherwise $l(\theta,a)=1$.

Let $\delta(x)$ be the decision made based on data x, the risk function is defined as

$$R(\theta,\delta)=E\{l(\theta,\delta(x))|\theta\}=\int l(\theta,\delta(x))p(x|\theta)dx.$$

For the prior distribution $p(\theta)$, Bayesian risk is defined as the

$$r(\delta)=E\{R(\theta,\delta)\}=\int R(\theta,\delta)p(\theta)d(\theta).$$

The decision minimizing the Bayesian decision is called the Bayesian decision (the Bayesian estimation in estimation problems). For posterior distribution $P(\theta|x)$, the posterior risk is

$$r(\delta|x)=E\{l(\theta,\delta(X))|X=x\}=\int l(\theta,\delta(X))p(\theta|x)dx.$$

To estimate $q(\theta)$, the Bayesian estimation is the posterior mean $E(q(\theta)|x)$ while using quadratic loss function, and the Bayesian estimation is the posterior medium $med(q(\theta)|x)$ while using absolute loss function.

Then, we will study the posterior risk for $0-1$ loss function. Considering the estimation problem ($\delta(x)$ is the estimator.),

$$l(\theta,\delta(x))=\begin{cases}1, & \delta(x)\neq\theta\\ 0, & \delta(x)=\theta,\end{cases}$$

then

$$r(d|x)=\int_{\delta(x)\neq\theta} P(q|x)dq=1-P(q|x).$$

It means that the decision maximizing the posterior probability is a good decision. To be more intuitive, let us consider the binary classification problem, which contains two parameters θ_1,θ_2, and two risks $1-P(\theta_1|x)$ and $1-P(\theta_2|x)$ can be obtained. Obviously, the θ which maximizes the posterior probability $P(\theta|x)$ is our decision, i.e.

$$\delta(x)=\begin{cases}\theta_1, & P(\theta_1|x)>P(\theta_2|x)\\ \theta_2, & P(\theta_2|x)>P(\theta_1|x)\end{cases}$$

or

$$\delta(x) = \begin{cases} \theta_1, & \frac{P(x|\theta_1)}{P(x|\theta_2)} > \frac{P(\theta_2)}{P(\theta_1)} \\ \theta_2, & \frac{P(x|\theta_2)}{P(x|\theta_1)} > \frac{P(\theta_1)}{P(\theta_2)} \end{cases}.$$

In this case, the decision error is

$$P(\text{error}|x) = \begin{cases} P(\theta_1|x), & \delta(x) = \theta_2 \\ P(\theta_2|x), & \delta(x) = \theta_1 \end{cases}$$

and the average error is

$$P(\text{error}) = \int P(\text{error}|x)d(x)d(x).$$

Bayesian decision minimizes that error because

$$P(\text{error}|x) = \min(P(\theta_1|x), P(\theta_2|x)).$$

10.4. Bayesian Estimation[2]

To assume that X is a random variable depending on the parameter λ, we need to make a decision about λ and use $\delta(x)$ to represent the decision dependent on data x. According to the pure Bayesian concepts, λ is an implementation of a random variable (written as Λ, whose distribution is $G(\lambda)$. For a fixed λ, the expected loss (also known as the risk) is $R_\delta(\lambda) = \int L(\delta(x), \lambda) f(\theta|x))dx$, where $L(\delta(x), \lambda) \geq 0$ is the loss function, and $f(x|\lambda)$ is density function of X. And the total expected loss (or expected risk) is

$$r(\delta) = \iint L(\delta(x), \lambda) f(x|\lambda) dx dG(\lambda).$$

Let $\delta_G(x)$ denote the Bayesian decision function d, which minimizes $r(\delta)$. In order to get the Bayesian decision function, we choose d which can minimize the "expected loss"

$$E(L|x) = \frac{\int L(\delta(x), \lambda) f(x|\theta) dG(\lambda))}{\int f(x|\lambda) dG(\lambda)}$$

for each x. And $r(\delta_G)$ is called the Bayesian risk or the Bayesian envelope function. Considering the quadratic loss function for point estimation,

$$\begin{aligned} r(\delta) &= \iint [\delta(x) - \lambda]^2 dF(x|\lambda) dG(\lambda) \\ &= r(d_G) + \iint [\delta(x) - \delta_G(x)]^2 dF(x|\lambda) dG(\lambda) \\ &\quad +2 \iint [\delta(x) - \delta_G(x)][\delta(x) - \lambda] dF(x|\lambda) dG(\lambda). \end{aligned}$$

The third item above is 0 because $r(\delta) \geq r(\delta_G)$, i.e. for each x, we have

$$\int [\delta_G(x) - \lambda] dF(x|\lambda) dG(\lambda) = 0$$

or

$$\delta_G(x) = \frac{\int \lambda dF(x|\lambda) dG(\lambda)}{\int dF(x|x) dG(\lambda)}.$$

That means after given $x, \delta_G(x)$ is the posterior mean of Λ. Let $F_G(x) = \int dF(x|x)dG(\lambda)$ be a mixed distribution, and X_G denotes the random variable with this distribution. From that, we can deduce many results for some important special distributions, for example,

(1) If $F(x|\lambda) = N(\lambda, \delta^2)$, and $G(\lambda) = N(u_G, \delta_G^2)$, then $X_G \sim N(u_G, \delta + \delta_G^2)$, and the joint distribution of Λ and X_c is bivariate normal distribution with correlation coefficient ρ, and $\delta_G(x) = \{x/s^2 + u_G/s_G^2\}/\{1/s^2 + 1/s_G^2\}, r(\delta_G) = (1/s^2 + 1/s_G^2)^{-1}$.

(2) If $p(x|\lambda) = e^{-\lambda}\lambda^x/x!, x = 0, 1, \ldots, \infty$, and $dG(\lambda) = (\Gamma(\beta))^{-1}\alpha^\beta\lambda^{\beta-1} e^{-\alpha\lambda}d\lambda$, then $\delta_G(x) = \frac{\beta+x}{\alpha+1}$, and $r(\delta_G) = \frac{\beta}{\alpha(\alpha+1)}$. The posterior medium is

$$\delta_G(x) = \frac{1x! \int \lambda^{x+1}e^{-\lambda}dG(\lambda)}{1x! \int \lambda^x e^{-\lambda}dG(\lambda)} = \frac{(x+1)p_G(x+1)}{p_G(x)},$$

where the marginal distribution is $p_G(x) = \int p(x|\lambda)dG(\lambda)$.

(3) If the likelihood function is $L(r|m) = \frac{(m-1)!}{(r-1)!(m-r)!}, r = 1, \ldots, m$ and the prior distribution is $\phi(r) \propto 1/r, r = 1, \ldots, m^*$, then

$$p(r|m) = \frac{j(r)}{(r-1)!(m-r)!} = \frac{m!}{r!(m-r)!}, \quad r = 1, \ldots, \min(m^*, m)$$

and $E(r|m) = m/2, \mathrm{Var}(r|m) = \sqrt{m}/2$.

(4) If $p(x|\lambda) = (1-\lambda)\lambda^x, x = 0, 1, \ldots, 0 < \lambda < 1$, then

$$\delta_G(x) = \frac{\int (1-\lambda)\lambda^{x+1}dG(\lambda)}{\int (1-\lambda)\lambda^x dG(x)} = \frac{p_G(x+1)}{p_G(x)}.$$

(5) For random variable Y with distribution $\exp[A(\theta) + B(\theta)W(y) + U(y)]$, let $x = W(y)$ and $\lambda = \exp[c(\lambda) + V(x)]$. If G is the prior distribution of λ, then in order to estimate λ,

$$\delta_G(x) = \exp[V(x) - V(x+1)]\frac{f_G(x+1)}{f_G(x)}.$$

10.5. Bayes Factor (BF)[1–3]

To test hypotheses, Jeffreys[3] introduced a category of statistics which is known as BF. BF of hypothesis H versus A is defined as the rate of posterior odds α_H/α_A to prior odds π_H/π_A. Suppose that Ω_H and Ω_A, which are in parameter space Ω, represent the two normal subsets corresponding to the two hypotheses, μ is the probability measure on Ω, and for given θ, $f_{X|\theta}(\cdot|\theta)$ is the density (or discrete distribution) of random variable X. Then we have the following expressions:

$$\alpha_H = \frac{\int_{\Omega_H} f_{X|\theta}(\theta|x)d\mu(\theta)}{\int_{\Omega} f_{X|\theta}(\theta|x)d\mu(\theta)}; \quad \alpha_A = \frac{\int_{\Omega_A} f_{X|\theta}(\theta|x)d\mu(\theta)}{\int_{\Omega} f_{X|\theta}(\theta|x)d\mu(\theta)};$$

$$\pi_H = \mu(\Omega_H); \quad \pi_A = \mu(\Omega_A).$$

Thus, the BF is

$$\frac{\alpha_H/\alpha_A}{\pi_H/\pi_A} = \frac{\int_{\Omega_H} f_{X|\theta}(\theta|x)d\mu(\theta)/\mu(\Omega_H)}{\int_{\Omega_A} f_{X|\theta}(\theta|x)d\mu(\theta)/\mu(\Omega_A)} = \frac{f_H(x)}{f_A(x)},$$

where the numerator $f_H(x)$ and denominator $f_A(x)$ represent predictive distribution when $H{:}\,\theta \in \Omega_H$ and $A{:}\,\theta \in \Omega_A$, respectively. So BF can also be defined as the ratio of predictive distributions, i.e. $f_H(x)/f_A(x)$. Obviously, the posterior odds for H is $\frac{\mu(\Omega_H)f_H(x)}{\mu(\Omega_A)f_A(x)}$.

Usually, Bayesian statisticians will not appoint prior odds. BFs can be interpreted as "tendency to model based on the evidence of data" or "the odds of H_0 versus H_1 provided by data". If the BF is less than some constant k, then it rejects certain hypothesis. Compared with the posterior odds, one advantage of calculating BF is that it does not need prior odds, and the BF is able to measure the degree of support for hypotheses from data. All these explanations are not established on strict meaning. Although the BF does not depend on prior odds, it does depend on how the prior distribution distributes on the two hypotheses. Sometimes, BF is relatively insensitive for reasonable choices, so we say that "these explanations are plausible".[1]

However, some people believe that BF intuitively provides a fact on whether the data x increases or reduces the odds of one hypothesis to another. If we consider the log-odds, the posterior log-odds equals prior log-odds plus the logarithm of the BF. Therefore, from the view of log-odds, the logarithm of BF will measure how the data changes the support for hypotheses.

The data increase their support to some hypothesis H, but it does not make H more possible than its opposite, and just makes H more possible than in prior cases.

The distributions of two models $M_i i = 1, 2$, are $f_i(x|\theta_i) i = 1, 2$, and the prior distribution of θ_i is represented by μ_i^0. In order to compare these two models, we usually use the BF of M_1 to M_2:

$$BF_{12}(x, \mu_1^0, \mu_2^0) \equiv \frac{\int f_1(x|\theta)\mu_1^0(d\theta_1)}{\int f_2(x|\theta)\mu_2^0(d\theta_2)}.$$

When lacking of prior information, some people suggest using fractional BF, which divides data x with size n into two parts $x = (y, z)$, with size m and $n - m(0 < m < n)$ respectively. Firstly, we use y as the training sample to get a posterior distribution $\mu_i^0(\theta_i|y)$, and then we apply $\mu_i^0(\theta_i|y)$ as the prior distribution to get the BF based on z:

$$\begin{aligned} BF_{12}(z, \mu_1^0, \mu_2^0|y) &= \frac{\int f_1(z|\theta_1)\mu_1^0(d\theta_1|y)}{\int f_2(z|\theta_2)\mu_2^0(d\theta_2|y)} \\ &= \frac{\int f_1(x|\theta_1)\mu_1^0(d\theta_1)}{\int f_1(y|\theta_2)\mu_1^0(d\theta_1)} \Big/ \frac{\int f_2(x|\theta_1)\mu_2^0(d\theta_2)}{\int f_2(y|\theta_2)\mu_2^0(d\theta_2)}. \end{aligned}$$

The fractional BF is not as sensitive as the BF, and it does not rely on any constant which appears in abnormal prior cases. Its disadvantage is that it is difficult to select the training sample.

10.6. Non-Subjective Prior[2,3]

According to the Bayesian, any result of inference is the posterior distribution of the variable that we are interested in. Many people believe that it is necessary to study non-subjective priors or non-informative prior. All kinds of non-subjective prior distribution should more or less meet some basic properties. Otherwise, there will be paradox. For instance, the most commonly used non-subjective priors is the local uniform distribution. However, the uniforms distribution generally is not invariant to parameter transformation, that is, the parameter after transformation is not uniformly distributed. For example, the uniform prior distribution of standard deviation σ would not be transformed into a uniform distribution of σ^2, which causes inconsistencies in the posterior distributions.

In general, the following properties are taken into account while seeking non-subjective priors:

(1) Invariance: For one-to-one function $\theta(\phi)$ of ϕ, the posterior distribution $\pi(\phi|x)$ obtained from the model $p(x|\phi, \lambda)$ must be consistent with the posterior distributions $\pi(\phi|x)$ obtained from the model $p(x|\theta, \lambda)$ which

is derived from parameter transformation. That is, for all data x,

$$\pi(\phi|x) = \pi(\theta|x)\left|\frac{d\theta}{d\phi}\right|.$$

And if the model $p(x|\phi, \lambda)$ has sufficient statistic $t = t(x)$, then the posterior distribution $\pi(\phi|x)$ should be the same as the posterior distribution $\pi(\phi|t)$ obtained from $p(t|\phi, \lambda)$.

(2) Consistent Marginalization: If the posterior distribution $\pi_1(\phi|x)$ of ϕ obtained by the model $p(x|\phi, \lambda)$ which of the form $\pi_1(\phi|x) = \pi_1(\phi|t)$ for some statistic $t = t(x)$, and if the sample distribution of t, $p(t|\phi, \lambda) = p(t|\phi)$ only depends on ϕ, then the posterior distributions $\pi_2(\phi|t)$ derived from the marginal model $p(t|\phi)$ must be the same as the posterior distribution $\pi_1(\phi|t)$ obtained from the complete model $p(x|\phi, \lambda)$.

(3) Consistency of Sample Property: The properties of the posterior distribution acquired from repeated sampling should be consistent with the model. In particular, for any large sample and $p(0 < p < 1)$, the coverage probability of confidence interval of the non-subjective posterior probability p should be close to p for most of the parameter values.

(4) Universal: Recommended method which results in non-subjective posterior distribution should be universal. In other words, it can be applied to any reasonably defined inference.

(5) Admissibility: Recommended method which results in non-subjective posterior distribution should not hold untenable results. In particular, in every known case, there is no better posterior distribution in the sense of general acceptability.

Jeffreys[3] proposed the Jeffreys' rule for selection of prior distribution. For the likelihood function $L(\theta)$, Jeffreys' prior distribution is proportional to $\sqrt{|I(\theta)|}$, where $I(\theta)$ is Fisher information matrix, that is to say that Jeffreys' prior distribution is

$$p(\theta) \propto \sqrt{|I(\theta)|} = \left\{E\left[\left(\frac{\partial L(\theta)}{\partial\theta}\right)^2\right]\right\}^{\frac{1}{2}}.$$

Jeffreys' distribution can remain the same in the one-to-one parameter transformation (such prior distribution is called as a constant prior distribution). If $p(\theta)$ is a Jeffreys' prior distribution, and $\xi = f(\theta)$ is a one-to-one parameter transformation, then the Jeffreys' prior distribution of ξ is $p \circ f^{-1}(\xi)|df^{-1}(\xi)/d\xi|$. Box and Tiao (1973) introduced the concept of the likelihood function based on the data transformation. For different data, the posterior distribution deduced from the prior distribution can ensure that the position is different, but the shape is the same. So Jeffreys' prior distribution can approximately maintain the shape of posterior distribution.

Sometimes, Jeffreys' prior distributions and some other certain non-subjective priors of uniform distribution $p(x)$ may be an irregular distribution, that is $\int p(\theta)d\theta = \infty$. However, the posterior distributions may be regular.

In multiparameter cases, we are often interested in some parameters or their functions, and ignore the rest of the parameters. In this situation, the Jeffreys' prior method seems to have difficulties. For example, the estimator produced by Jeffreys' prior method may inconsistent in the sense of frequency, and we cannot find the marginal distributions for nuisance parameters.

10.7. Probability Matching Prior[2,4]

Probability matching priors were first proposed by Welch and Peers (1963), and later received wide attention because of Stein (1985) and Tibshirani (1989). The basic idea is to make Bayesian probability match the corresponding frequency probability when the sample size approaches infinity. So, $x_1, \ldots, x_n$ are independent, identically distributed with density $f(x|\theta, w)$, where θ is the parameter we are interested in, and w is the nuisance parameter. A prior density $p(\theta, \omega)$ is called to satisfy the first-order probabilisty matching criteria if

$$p\{\theta > \theta_{1-\alpha}(p(\cdot), x_1, \ldots, x_n|\theta, w)\} = \alpha + o(n^{-\frac{1}{2}}),$$

where $\theta_{1-\alpha}(p(\cdot), x_1, \ldots, x_n)$ is the $100 \times a$ percentile of the posterior distribution $p^n(\cdot|x)$ derived from the prior distribution $p(\cdot)$.

Peers (1965) showed that the first-order probability matching prior distribution is the solution of a differential equation. Datta and Ghosh (1995) gave a more rigorous and general statement. But there is a lot of first-order probability matching priors, and it is hard to decide which one to choose. So, Mukerjee and Dey (1993) introduced the second-order probability matching priors. The difference between the second-order and first-order is that $o(n^{-\frac{1}{2}})$ is replaced by $o(n^{-1})$. As long as a first-order probability matching prior distribution is the solution of a second-order differential equation, it is also the second-order probability matching prior distribution. The second-order probability matching prior distribution is often unique.

Example of deviation models: Jorgenson (1992) defined the deviation model as an arbitrary class with the following probability density:

$$f(x|u, \lambda) = c(\lambda, x)\exp\{\lambda t(x, u)\},$$

where $c(\cdot)$ and $t(\cdot)$ are two functions. A common case is that $c(\lambda, x)$ is the multiplication of functions containing λ and x, respectively (for example, $c(\lambda, x) = a(\lambda)b(x)$), and it is called a normal deviation model. A normal deviation model with position parameters has density form

$$f(x|u, \lambda) = \frac{\exp\{\lambda t(x-u)\}}{\int \exp\{\lambda t(x)\}dx}$$

and one of its special classes is generalized linear models with density

$$f(x|\theta, \lambda) = c(\lambda, x)\exp[\lambda\{\theta x - k(\theta)\}]$$

which is widely well known (McCullagh and Nelder, 1983). When μ is the interested parameter and λ is the nuisance parameter, $p_\mu^{(1)}(u, \lambda)$ and $p_\mu^{(2)}(u, \lambda)$ represent the prior density of first-order and second-order matching probability prior distribution, respectively. But when λ is the interested parameter, and μ is a nuisance, $p_\lambda^{(1)}(u, \lambda)$ and $p_\lambda^{(2)}(u, \lambda)$ represent the prior density of first-order and second-order matching probability prior distribution. The related information matrix is

$$I(u, \lambda) = \text{diag}\{I_{11}, I_{22}\},$$

where

$$I_{11} = \lambda E\left\{-\frac{\partial^2 t(x, \mu)}{\partial^2 \mu^2}\bigg|\mu, \lambda\right\}; \quad I_{22} = \lambda E\left\{-\frac{\partial^2 \log c(\lambda, x)}{\partial^2 \lambda^2}\bigg|\mu, \lambda\right\}.$$

Garvan and Ghosh (1997) got the following results for deviation models:

$$p_\mu^{(1)}(\mu, \lambda) = I_{11}^{\frac{1}{2}} g(\lambda); \quad p_\lambda^{(1)}(\mu, \lambda) = I_{22}^{\frac{1}{2}} g(\mu),$$

where $g(\cdot)$ is any arbitrary function. From that, we can get that, it has an infinite number of first-order probability matching prior distributions. For a normal deviation model, the above formulas can be turned into

$$p_u^{(1)}(u, \lambda) = E^{\frac{1}{2}}\{-t''(x)|u, \lambda\}g(\lambda);$$

$$p_\lambda^{(1)}(u, \lambda) = \left\{-\frac{d^2 \log\{1/(\int \exp\{\lambda t(x)\}dx)\}dx)\}}{d\lambda^2}\right\}^{-\frac{1}{2}} g(u),$$

In order to get the unique matching probability distribution, we need to choose the second-order probability matching prior distributions.

10.8. Empirical Bayes (EB) Methods[2]

EB originated from von Mises (1942) and later the EB introduced by Robbins[4] is known as the non-parametric EB, which is distinguished from parametric empirical Bayes method put forward by Efron and Morris (1972, 1973, 1975). The difference between these two EB methods is that: Non-parametric EB does not require the prior distribution any more, and it uses data to estimate the related distribution. However, parametric EB methods need indicate a prior distribution family. Because at each level, the prior distribution has to be determined by parameters, parametric EB method uses observed data to estimate the parameters at each level.

(1) Non-parametric Empirical Bayes Estimation: Suppose that parameter $\theta \in \Theta$, the action $a \in A$, the loss $L(a, \theta)$ is a function from $A \times \Theta$ to $[0, \infty)$, G is prior distribution on Θ, and for given θ (its distribution is G), random variable $X \in \chi$ has probability density $f_\theta(\cdot)$ (corresponding to the measure μ on σ-field of χ). For a decision function t, the average loss on $\chi \times \Theta$ is $R(t, \theta) = \int L(t(x), \theta) f_\theta(x) d\mu(x)$, $R(t, G) = \int R(t, \theta) G(\theta)$ is the Bayesian risk based on prior distribution, and t_G is regarded as the Bayesian decision minimizing the Bayesian risk.

In reality, we are unable to get t_G because G is often unknown. Assume that our decision problems are repeated independently, and have the same unknown prior distribution G, which means that $(\theta_1, x_1), \ldots, (\theta_n, x_n)$ are independent and identically distributed random pairs, where θ_i is i.i.d. and obeys distribution G and X_i obeys the distribution density $f_{\theta_i}(\cdot)$. For given $G, X_1, \ldots, X_n, \ldots$ are observable while $\theta_1, \ldots, \theta_n, \ldots$ are unobservable. Assume that we have observed $x_1, \ldots, x_n$ and x_{n+1}, we want to make decision about loss L for θ_{n+1}. Because $x_1, \ldots, x_n$ come from population $f_G(x) = \int f_\theta(x) dG(\theta)$, we can judge that they contain information about G. Thus we can extract information about G from these observations, and determining the decision, $t_n(\cdot) = t_n(x_1, \ldots, x_n)$, about θ_{n+1} based on the information above. The $(n+1)$-th step of the Bayesian loss is

$$R_n(T, G) = E[R(t_n(\cdot), G)] = \iint E[L(t_n(\cdot), \theta)] f_\theta(x) d\mu(x) dG(\theta).$$

According to Robbins (1964), if $\lim_{n\to\infty} R_n(T, G) = R(G)$, $T = \{t_n\}$ is called asymptotically optimal to G (denoted as a.o.). If $\lim_{n\to\infty} R_n(T, G) - R(G) = O(\alpha_n) \cdot (\alpha_n \to 0)$, then $T = \{t_n\}$ is known as α_n-order asymptotically optimal to G. In application, the second definition is more practical.

(2) Parametric Empirical Bayes Estimation: In order to illustrate, the normal population is considered. Suppose that p random variables are observed, and they come from normal populations, which may have different average values but always have the same known variance: $X_i \sim N(\theta_i, \sigma^2), i = 1, \ldots, p$. In the sense of frequency, the classical estimator of θ_i is X_i, which is the best linear unbiased estimator (BLUE), the maximum likelihood estimator (MLE) and minimum maximum risk estimator (MINIMAX estimator), etc. Bayesian methods assume that the prior distribution of θ_i is $\theta_i \sim N(\mu, \tau^2)(i = 1, \ldots, p)$. Thus, Bayesian estimation of θ_i (the posterior mean of θ_i) is $\tilde{\theta}_i = \frac{\sigma^2}{\sigma^2+\tau^2}\mu + \frac{\tau^2}{\tau^2+\sigma^2}X_i$, which is a weighted average of μ and X_i, and the posterior distribution of θ_i is $N[\tilde{\theta}_i, \sigma^2\tau^2/(\sigma^2+\tau^2)]$. What different is that empirical Bayes approach does not specify the values of hyper-parameters μ and τ^2, and thinks that all information about these two parameters are involved in marginal distribution $p(X_i) \sim N(\mu, \sigma^2 + \tau^2), (i = 1, \ldots, p)$. Because of the assumption that all θ_i have the same prior distribution, this unconditional assumption is reasonable, just as in the single-factor analysis of variance, there is similarity among each level.

10.9. Improper Prior Distributions[5,6]

Usually, the uniform distribution on an interval and even the real axis is used as the prior distribution. But this prior distribution is clearly an improper prior because its cumulative probability may be infinite. In articles about Bayesian, the improper prior distributions are often explained as the "limit" of proper prior distributions. The meaning of the limit is that the posterior distribution derived by an improper prior is the limit of the posterior distribution derived by a proper prior, while the paradox of marginalization discussed by Dawid *et al.*[6] shows that the improper prior distribution does not have Bayesian properties. Since there is no paradox appearing in the case of the proper prior distribution, the improper prior distribution may not be the limit of a sequence of proper prior distributions sometimes. According to Akaike,[5] it is more reasonable to interpret improper prior distribution as the limit of some proper prior distribution related to the data.

To explain this problem, let us look at a simple example. Assume that the data obey distribution

$$p(x|m) = (2\pi)^{-1/2} \exp\{-(x - m)^2/2\},$$

and we use a non-informative prior distribution (also called as improper uniform prior distribution) as the prior of mean m. Clearly, the posterior distribution is

$$p(m|x) = (2\pi)^{-1/2} \exp\{-(m-x)^2/2\}.$$

In addition, assume that proper prior distribution of m is

$$ps(m) = (2\pi S^2)^{-1/2} \exp\{-(m-M)^2/(2S^2)\},$$

such that the corresponding posterior distribution is

$$p_s(m|x) = \left(\frac{1+S^2}{2\pi S^2}\right)^{1/2} \exp\left\{-\frac{1}{2}\left(\frac{1+S^2}{S^2}\right)\left(m - \frac{M+S^2x}{1+S^2}\right)^2\right\}.$$

Obviously, for each x,

$$\lim_{S\to\infty} p_S(m|x) = p(m|x),$$

which makes the interpretation of "limit" seem reasonable. But the trouble appears in the measurement. We often use entropy, which is defined as

$$B[f\colon g] = -\int \frac{f(y)}{g(y)} \log \frac{f(y)}{g(y)} g(y)dy$$

to measure the goodness of fit between the hypothetical distribution $g(y)$ and the true distribution $f(y)$. Suppose that $f(m) = p(m|x), g(m) = ps(m|x)$, we find that $B[p(\cdot|x); ps(\cdot|x)]$ is negative and tends to 0 as S tends to be infinite. However, only when the prior distribution $p_s(m)$s mean $M = x$, it can be guaranteed that $p_s(m|x)$ converges uniformly to $p(m|x)$ for any x. Otherwise, for fixed $M, p_s(m|x)$ may not approximate $p(m|x)$ well when x is far away from M. This means that the more appropriate name for posterior distribution $p(m|x)$ is the limit of the posterior distribution $p(m|x)$ which is determined by the prior distribution $p_s(m)$ (where $M = x$) adjusted by data.

Since Dawid has shown that there will not be paradox for proper prior distribution, the culprit of the paradox is the property that the improper prior distribution relies on data. There is another example in the following.

Jaynes (1978) also discussed this paradox. If the prior distribution is $\pi(\eta|I_1) \propto \eta^{k-1}e^{-t\eta}, t > 0$, the related posterior distribution is

$$p(\varsigma|y, z, I_1) \propto \pi(\varsigma)c^{-\varsigma}\{\frac{y}{t + yQ(\varsigma, z)}\}^{n+k},$$

where I_1 is prior information, and

$$Q(\varsigma, z) = \sum_1^{\varsigma} z_i + c\sum_{\varsigma+1}^{n} z_i, y = x_1.$$

Jaynes believed that it was reasonable to directly make $t = 0$ when $t \ll yQ$. It suggests that the result is obtained when $t = 0$ is also reasonable and

$t \ll yQ$. Thus, we can conclude that the improper prior distribution is another form of the prior distribution depending on the data.

10.10. Nuisance Parameters[7]

In estimation, suppose that the parameter is composed of two parts $\theta = (\gamma, \delta)$, we are interested in parameter γ and regard δ as a nuisance parameter. We can get the joint posterior distribution $p(\theta|x) = p(\theta, \delta|x)$ based on the prior distribution $p(\theta) = p(\gamma, \delta)$ at first, and calculate γ's posterior distribution $p(\gamma|x) = \int_\Delta p(\theta, \delta|x)d\delta$ (assume that Γ and Δ are the range of γ and δ, respectively). At last, we use the posterior expectation $\int \gamma p(\gamma|x)d\gamma$ as the estimation of γ. However, in practice, especially when there are many parameters, it may be difficult to determine the prior distribution $p(\gamma, \delta)$. In addition to using reference prior distributions, there are also many other ways to deal with nuisance parameters (refer to Dawid, 1980; Willing, 1988). Here, we will introduce a method which fixes the value of δ. Assume that the ranges Γ and Δ are open intervals. According to de la Horra (1992), this method can be divided into the following steps:

(1) Determine the prior distribution of γ: $p(\gamma)$;
(2) Select a sensitive value of nuisance parameter δ: β;
(3) Calculate $p_\beta(\gamma|x) \propto p(\gamma)f(x|\gamma, \beta)$;
(4) Calculate $T_\beta(x) \equiv \int_\Gamma \gamma p_\beta(\gamma|x)d\gamma$ and use it as the estimate of γ.

It should be noted that $p(\gamma)$ should be calculated by the joint prior distribution, i.e. $p(\gamma) = \int_\Delta dp(\gamma, \delta)$. But because of the difficulties in detemining $p(\gamma, \delta)$, we directly determine $p(\gamma)$. The selected sensitive value should make the estimator of $T_\beta(x)$ have good properties. De la Horra (1992) showed that if the prior mean of δ was selected as the sensitive value, $T_\beta(x)$ was optimal in the sense of mean squared error (MSE). Denoting as the range of observations, the optimal property of $T_\beta(x)$ minimizes MSE,

$$\int_{\Gamma\times\Delta}\int_{\chi}(\gamma - T_\beta(x))^2 f(x|\gamma, \beta)dxdp(\gamma, \delta),$$

when β equals the prior mean (β_0). Although the prior mean $\beta_0 = \int_{\Gamma\times\Delta}\delta dp(\gamma, \delta)$, we can determine β_0 directly without through $p(\gamma, \delta)$. MSE does not belong to Bayesian statistical concept, so it can be used to compare various estimates. For example, assume that the observations $x_1, \ldots, x_n$ come from distribution $N(\gamma, \delta)$, whose parameters are unknown, and assume that prior distribution of γ is $N(\mu, 1/\tau)$. The above estimator

$$T_\beta(x) = \{\tau\mu + (n/\beta)\bar{x}\}/\{\tau + (n/\beta)\}$$

has the minimum MSE.

Then we use approximation methods to deal with nuisance parameters. The distribution of random variables $X_1, \ldots, X_n$ has two parameters θ and v. We are only interested in parameter θ and regard v as a nuisance parameter. Assume that the joint prior distribution is $p(\theta, v)$, what we care about is the marginal posterior distribution

$$p(\theta|x) \propto \int p(\theta, v)L(\theta, v)dv,$$

where $L(\theta, v) = \prod_{i=1}^{n} f(x_i|\theta, v)$ is the likelihood function. If $p(\theta, v)$ is the uniform distribution, that is just the integral of the likelihood function. In addition, we can also remove nuisance parameters through maximizing the method. Suppose that $\hat{v}(\theta)$ is the v which maximizes the joint posterior distribution $p(\theta, v|x)(\propto p(\theta, v)L(\theta, v))$, then we get profile posterior

$$p^p(\theta|x) \propto p(\theta, \hat{v}(\theta)|x),$$

which is the profile likelihood for uniform prior distribution. Of course, from the strict Bayesian point of view, $p(\theta|x)$ is a more appropriate way to remove a nuisance parameter. However, because it is much easier to calculate the maximum value than to calculate the integral, it is easier to deal with profile posterior. In fact, profile posterior can be regarded as an approximation of the marginal posterior distribution. For fixed θ, we give the Taylor expansion of $p(\theta, v|x) = \exp\{\log p(\theta, v|x)\}$ to the second item at $\hat{v}(\theta)$, which is also called the Laplace approximation:

$$p(\theta, v|x) \approx Kp(\theta, \hat{v}(\theta)|x)|j(\theta, \hat{v}(\theta))|^{-\frac{1}{2}},$$

where $j(\theta, \hat{v}(\theta)) = -\frac{\partial^2}{\partial v^2}\log p(\theta, v|x)|_{v=\hat{v}(\theta)}$ and K is a proportionality constant. If $j(\cdot)$ is independent of θ, or if the posterior distribution of θ and v is independent, then the profile posterior is equal to the marginal posterior distribution.

10.11. Bayesian Interval Estimates[8]

When looking for a confidence region for an unknown parameter θ, which comes from the density of i.i.d. random variables $Y_1, \ldots, Y_n$, we often consider the likelihood-based confidence regions and the HPD regions. The LB confidence region can be represented as

$$L(c) = \{\theta \in \Theta: 2\{l(\hat{\theta}) - l(\theta)\} \leq c^2\},$$

where c can control the convergence probability of this interval to achieve the expected value, i.e. $P_\theta\{L(c)\} = \alpha$ The HPD region can be represented as

$$H(b) = \{\theta \in \Theta: 2\{l(\hat{\theta}) - l(\theta) + h(\hat{\theta}) - h(\theta)\} \leq b^2\},$$

where b aims to make this region have a suitable posterior probability $\pi\{H(b)\} = \alpha$ and $\exp h(\theta)$ is the prior distribution of θ in Θ.

About these two approaches, we have three questions naturally:

(1) In what case does the posterior probability of the LB confidence region with convergence probability is α equal to α yet?
(2) In what cases does the convergence probability of the HPD region with posterior probability is α equal to α?
(3) In what cases does the LB confidence region with convergence probability α and the HPD region with posterior probability α coincide or at least coincide asymptotically?

Severini[8] answered these three questions:

(1) If c_α leads to $P_\theta\{L(c)\} = \alpha$, the posterior probability $\pi\{L(c_\alpha)\}$ of the LB confidence regions $L(c_\alpha)$ is

$$\pi\{L(c_\alpha)\} = \alpha + \{2\hat{i}_{01}\hat{i}_{11} - \hat{i}_{11}\hat{i}_{01} + \hat{i}_{001}\hat{i}_{01}\hat{h}' - \hat{h}''\hat{i}_{01}^2 - (\hat{h}')^2\hat{i}_{01}^2\} \\ \times \hat{i}_{20}^{-3} q_{\alpha/2}\phi(q_{\alpha/2})/n + O_p(n^{-3/2}).$$

(2) If b_α leads to $\pi\{H(b_\alpha)\} = \alpha$ the convergence probability $P_\theta\{H(b_\alpha)\}$ of the HPD region $H(b_\alpha)$ is

$$P_\theta\{H(b_\alpha)\} = \alpha + \{i'_{11}i_{01} - 2i'_{01}i_{11} - i_{001}i_{01}h' + 2i'_{01}i_{01}h' \\ -h''i_{01}^2 - (h')^2 i_{01}^2\} i_{20}^{-3} q_{\alpha/2}\phi(q_{\alpha/2})/n + O_p(n^{-3/2}).$$

(3) If $h' = 0$ and $i'_{11}i_{01} - 2i'_{01}i_{11} = 0$, then we have $P_\theta\{\Delta_\alpha\} = O(n^{-3/2}), \pi(\Delta_\alpha) = O(n^{-3/2})$,

where Δ_α is the symmetric difference between $H(b_\alpha)$ and $L(c_\alpha)$. Denote $\phi(\cdot)$ and $\Phi(\cdot)$. ql as the density and the distribution function of the standard normal distribution, respectively, and ql meets $\phi(ql) = 0.5+l$. For any k, l, m, we define

$$i_{klm} = i_{klm}(\theta) = E\{U^k W^l V^m; \theta\},$$

where $U = \partial\{\log p(Y;\theta)\}/\partial\theta, V = \partial^2\{\log p(Y;\theta)\}/\partial\theta^2$ and $W = \partial^3\{\log p(Y;\theta)\}/\partial\theta^3$. i_{kl0} is abbreviated as i_{kl}, $i_{klm}(\hat{\theta})$ is denoted as $\hat{i}_{klm}$, and $\hat{h}$ is used to refer to $h(\hat{\theta})$.

Using the above conclusions, we can effectively answer the three questions mentioned ahead. Clearly, when $h' = i_{11}/i_{20}$, the posterior probability of the LB confidence region with convergence probability α is $\alpha + O(n^{-3/2})$. In addition, as long as h' meets

$$(h')^2 i_{01}^2 + h'' i_{01}^2 + (i_{001} i_{01} - 2i'_{01} i_{01})/h' + 2i'_{01} i_{11} - i'_{11} i_{01} = 0,$$

the convergence probability of the HPD region with posterior probability α is $\alpha + O(n^{-3/2})$. However, since the equation above does not have general solution, we pay special attention to two important cases, where the Fisher information i'_{01} equals 0 and i_{11}/i_{01}^2 has no connection with θ. In the case of the Fisher information equals 0, $h' = i_{11}/i_{01}$ is the solution of the equation. In the latter case, $h' = 0$ is the solution. Therefore, in these cases, as long as the prior distribution is selected properly, the convergence probability of the HPD region, with posterior probability α, is $\alpha + O(n^{-3/2})$.

Now, let us consider some examples meeting those conditions. If the density comes from the exponential family $p(y;\theta) = \exp\{y\theta + D(\theta) + W(y)\}$, and the natural parameter θ is unknown, we have $i_{11} = 0$. Thus, when the prior density is constant, the LB confidence region with convergence probability α and the HPD region with posterior probability α coincide asymptotically.

When the density function is like

$$p(y;\theta) = \exp\{yT(\theta) + D(\theta) + W(y)\}$$

and the parameter θ is unknown, we get $i_{11}/i_{20} = T''/T'$. Then just selecting $h = \log T'$, that is, the prior density is proportional to $T'(\theta)$, the posterior probability of the LB confidence region, with convergence probability α, will be $\alpha + O(n^{-3/2})$.

If the distribution is like $g(y - \theta)$ where g is a density function on the real axis and $\Theta = (-\infty, +\infty)$, i_{ii} and i_{01} are independent on θ. Therefore, when the prior density is uniform distribution, the HPD region equals the LB confidence region asymptotically.

10.12. Stochastic Dominance[10]

SD is a widely applied branch in decision theory. Suppose that F and G are cumulative distribution functions of X and Y, respectively. The following definitions are the first- or second-order control, $Y(G)$ (represented by $\succeq_1$ and $\succeq_2$), of $X(F)$

$$X \succeq_1 Y \Leftrightarrow F \succeq_1 G \Leftrightarrow (F(x) \leq G(x), \forall X \in R),$$

$$X \succeq_2 Y \Leftrightarrow F \succeq_2 G \Leftrightarrow \left(\int_{-\infty}^{x} |G(t) - F(t)| dt \geq 0, \forall X \in R \right).$$

If the inequalities in the definitions are strict, SD can be represented by $\succ_1$ and $\succ_2$ separately. According to the usual Bayesian estimation theory, to compare a decision d with a decision d'', we need to compare the posterior expected values of their corresponding loss function $L(\theta, d)$ and $L(\theta, d'')$. According to SD concept, Giron[9] proposed to compare the whole distribution instead of a feature. Because what we are concerned about is the loss function, it does not matter if we change the direction of inequality in the SD definition, i.e.

$$X \succeq_1 Y \Leftrightarrow F \succeq_1 G \Leftrightarrow (F(x) \geq G(x), \forall x \in R),$$

$$X \succeq_2 Y \Leftrightarrow F \succeq_2 G \Leftrightarrow \left(\int_{x}^{\infty} |G(t) - F(t)| dt \geq 0, \forall x \in R \right).$$

According to this definition and the related theorems of SD, we can infer that if $\mathcal{U}_1 = \{u: R \to R; u \uparrow\}$ and $\mathcal{U}_2 = \{u \in \mathcal{U}_1; u: \text{convex}\}$, then (as long as the expectation exists)

$$F \succeq_1 G \Leftrightarrow \left(\int u dF \leq \int u dG, \forall u \in \mathcal{U}_1 \right),$$

$$F \succeq_2 G \Leftrightarrow \left(\int u dF \leq \int u dG, \forall u \in \mathcal{U}_2 \right).$$

So, we can define SD of estimations d, d'' (according to the posterior distribution): for $i = 1, 2$,

$$d \succeq_i d' \Leftrightarrow L(\theta, d) \succeq_i L(\theta, d').$$

For example, if $\theta | x \sim N(m_n, \sigma_n^2), L(\theta, d) = |\theta - d|$, then for any $r > 0, d \in R, d \neq m_n$, it is easy to verify that

$$P(|\theta - m_n| \leq r) > P(|\theta - d| \leq r);$$

which means that for each loss function: $L(\theta, d) = \omega(|\theta - d|)$ (here, $\omega: R^+ \to R$ is a non-decreasing function), such that the first-order SD m_n stochastically dominates any other estimator $d \neq m_n$. This result is still valid for many other distributions.

Giron[9] presented some general results on SD:

$$Y \succeq_{cs} X \Leftrightarrow f(Y) \succeq_1 f(X) \quad \forall f \in \mathcal{F},$$

where $\mathcal{F}$ represents a unimodal symmetric family

$$Y \succeq_{cs} X \Leftrightarrow P(X \in A) \leq P(Y \in A) \quad \forall A \in \mathcal{A}_{cs},$$

where $\mathcal{A}_{cs}$ is the lower convex symmetric set in R^n, and $Y \succeq_{cs} X$ indicates that Y is more concentrated than X.

For an n-dimensional random vector X which has a symmetric unimodal density, if $\forall y \neq 0 \in R^n$, then $X \succeq_{cs} X - y$.

For an n-dimensional random vector X who has a symmetric unimodal density, and any function g which is symmetric and unimodal, if $\forall y \neq 0 \in R^n$, then $g(X) \succeq_1 g(X - y)$.

For an n-dimensional random vector X who has a non-degenerate and symmetric density, and g: $R^n \to R$ which is a strictly lower convex function, if $\forall y \neq 0 \in R^2$, then $g(X) \succ_2 g(X - y)$.

According to Fang *et al.* (1990) and Fang and Zhang (1990), the n-dimensional random vector X is said to have a spherical distribution if

$$\forall O \in O(n), X \stackrel{d}{=} OX,$$

where $O(n)$ is the set containing all the $n \times n$ orthogonal matrices. X is spherical, if and only if the eigenfunction of X has the form $\phi(\|t\|^2)$ which is noted as $X \sim S_n(\phi)$. The n-dimensional random vector X is said to have an ellipsoidal distribution: $X \sim EC_n(\mu, \Sigma; \phi)$, if $x = \mu + A'y$, where $y \sim S_n(\phi), A'A = \Sigma$. μ is called as the position vector and Σ is the spread for ECD.

10.13. Partial BF[2,10]

Suppose that s models $M_i (i = 1, \ldots, s)$ need to be compared based on the data $y = (y_1, \ldots, y_n)$. The density of y_i and the prior density of unknown parameter $\theta_i \in \Theta_i$ are $p_i(y|\theta_i)$ and $p_i(\theta_i)$, respectively. For each model and prior probability $p_1, \ldots, p_s$, the posterior probability

$$P(M_i|y) = \frac{p_i f_i(y)}{\sum_{j=1}^{s} p_j f_j(y)},$$

where $f_i(y) = \int_{\Theta_i} p(y|\theta_i)p_i(\theta_i)$. We can make choices by the ratio of the posterior probabilities

$$\frac{P(M_j|y)}{P(M_k|y)} = \frac{p_j}{p_k} \mathrm{BF}_{jk}(y),$$

where $BF_{jk}(y) = f_j(y)/f_k(y)$ is the BF. If the two models are nested, that is, $\theta_j = (\xi, \eta), \theta_k = \xi$ and $p_k(y|\xi) = p_j(y|\eta_0, \xi)$, where η_0 is a special value for the parameter η, and ξ is a common parameter, the BF is

$$\mathrm{BF}_{jk}(y) = \frac{\iint p_j(y|\eta,\xi)p_j(\xi,\eta)d\xi d\eta}{\int p_j(y|\eta_0,\xi)p_k(\xi)d\xi}.$$

Such models are consistent, that is, when $n \to \infty, BF_{jk}(y) \to \infty$ (under model M_j) or $BF_{jk}(y) \to 0$ (under model M_k).

BFs play a key role in the selection of models, but they are very sensitive to the prior distribution. BF are instable when dealing with non-subjective (non-informative or weak-informative) prior distributions, and they are uncertain for improper prior distributions. The improper prior can be written as $p_i^N(\theta_i) = c_i g_i(\theta)$, where $g_i(\theta_i)$ is a divergence function for the integral in Θ_i, and c_i is an arbitrary constant. At this time, the BF depending on the ratio c_j/c_k is

$$\mathrm{BF}_{jk}^N(y) = \frac{c_j}{c_k}\frac{\int_{\Theta_j} p_j(y|\theta_j)g_j(\theta_j)d\theta_j}{\int_{\Theta_k} p_k(y|\theta_k)g_k(\theta_k)d\theta_k}.$$

Considering the method of partial BFs, we divide the sample y with size n into the training sample $y(l)$ and testing sample $y(n-l)$ with sizes l and $n-l$, respectively. Using the BF of $y(l)$,

$$\begin{aligned}\mathrm{BF}_{jk}(l) &= \frac{f_j(y(n-l)|y(l))}{f_k(y(n-l)|y(l))}\\ &= \frac{\int_{\Theta_j} f_j(y(n-l)|\theta_j)p_j^N(\theta_j|y(l))d\theta_j}{\int_{\Theta_k} f_k(y(n-l)|\theta_k)p_k^N(\theta_k|y(l))d\theta_k} = \frac{\mathrm{BF}_{jk}^N(y)}{\mathrm{BF}_{jk}^N(y(l))}\end{aligned}$$

is called the partial Bayes factor (PBF), where $\mathrm{BF}_{jk}^N(y)$ and $\mathrm{BF}_{jk}^N(y(l))$ are the complete BFs to y and $y(l)$, respectively. The basic idea of the PBF introduced by O'Hagan[10] is that when n and l are large enough, different training samples give basically the same information, that is, $p_i(y(l)|\theta_i)$ does not vary with $y(l)$ approximately. So,

$$p_i^{\frac{1}{l}}(y(l)|\theta_i) \approx p_i^{\frac{1}{n}}(y|\theta_i); \quad p_i(y(l)|\theta_i) \approx p_i^b(y|\theta_i), \quad \left(b = \frac{1}{n}\right).$$

O'Hagan[10] replaced the denominator of the PBF $\mathrm{BF}_{jk}^N(y(l))$ above by

$$\mathrm{BF}_{jk}^b(y) = \frac{f_j^b(y)}{f_k^b(y)} = \frac{\int_{\Theta_j} f_j^b(y|\theta_j)p_j^N(\theta_j)d\theta_j}{\int_{\Theta_k} f_k^b(y|\theta_k)p_k^N(\theta_k)d\theta_k},$$

and defined

$$\text{FBF}_{jk} = \frac{\text{BF}_{jk}^N(y)}{\text{BF}_{jk}^b(y)}.$$

Through that transformation, if the prior distribution is improper, they would cancel each other out in the numerator and the denominator, so the BF is determined. But there is one problem: how to choose b, about which there are a lot of discussions in the literatures on different purposes.

10.14. ANOVA Under Heteroscedasticity[10,11]

Consider k normal distributions $N(y_i|\mu_i, \sigma_i^2), i = 1, \ldots, k$; with samples $y_i = (y_{i1}, \ldots, y_{in_i})$ with size n_i, sample mean $\bar{y}_i$, and sample variance s_i^2/n_i. Classic method (frequency or Bayesian) to test equality of μ_i usually assumes homoscedasticity. For heteroscedasticity, Bertolio and Racugno[11] proposed that the problem of analysis of variance can be regarded as a model selection problem to solve. Consider the nested sampling model:

$$p_1(z|\theta_1) = N(y_1\mu, \tau_1^2) \cdots N(y_k\mu, \tau_k^2),$$
$$p_2(z|\theta_2) = N(y_1\mu, \sigma_1^2) \cdots N(y_k\mu, \sigma_k^2),$$

where $z = (y_1, \ldots, y_k), \theta_1 = (\mu, \tau_1, \ldots, \tau_k), \theta_2 = (\mu_1, \ldots, \mu_k, \sigma_1, \ldots, \sigma_k)$. Assume that μ is prior independent of τ_i. Usually, the prior distribution of μ and $\log(\tau_i)$ is uniform distribution $p_1^N(\theta_1) = c_1/\prod_{i=1}^k \tau_i$. Assume that μ and σ_i are prior independent yet, and their prior distribution is $p_2^N(\theta_2) = c_2/\prod_{i=1}^k \sigma_i$. None of the two prior distributions above is integrable. Let M_1 and M_2 denote these two models, whose probabilities are $P(M_1)$ and $P(M_2)$. The posterior probability of the model M_1 is

$$P(M_1|z) = \left\{1 + \text{BF}_{21}^N(z)\frac{P(M_2)}{P(M_1)}\right\}^{-1},$$

where

$$\text{BF}_{21}^N(z) = \frac{p_2(z|\theta_2)p_2^N(\theta_2)d\theta_2}{p_1(z|\theta_1)p_1^N(\theta_1)d\theta_1}$$

is the BF. For an improper prior, BF depends on c_2/c_1. Bertolio and Racugno[11] pointed out that neither the PBF nor the intrinsic BF is a true BF, and they are consistent asymptotically. This makes it possible under a very weak condition to deduce the rational prior distribution, that is, the intrinsic and fractional prior distribution to calculate the true BF. The features of this method are: the selection of Bayesian model can be completed automatically, these BFs depend on samples through sufficient statistics rather than individual training samples, and $\mathrm{BF}_{21}(z) = 1/\mathrm{BF}_{12}(z)$ such that $P(M_2|z) = 1 - P(M_1|z)$. Suppose that the sample y with size n is divided into $y(l)$ and testing sample $y(n-l)$ with sizes l and $n-l$, respectively. The testing sample is used to convert the improper prior distribution $p_i^N(\theta_i)$ to the proper distribution

$$p_i(\theta_i|y(l)) = \frac{p_i(y(l)|\theta_i)p_i^N(\theta_i)}{f_i^N(y(l))},$$

where

$$f_i^N(y(l)) = \int p_i(y(l)|\theta_i)p_i^N(\theta_i)d\theta_i, \quad i = 1, 2.$$

The BF is

$$\mathrm{BF}_{21}(y(n-l)|y(l)) = \mathrm{BF}_{21}^N(y)\mathrm{BF}_{12}^N(y(l)),$$

where $\mathrm{BF}_{12}^N(y(l)) = f_1^N(y(l))/f_2^N(y(l))$. As long as $0 < f_i^N(y(l)) < \infty$, $i = 1, 2$, we can define $\mathrm{BF}_{21}(y(n-l)|y(l))$. If it is not true for any subset of $y(l)$, $y(l)$ is called a minimum training sample. Berger and Pericchi (1996) recommended calculation of $\mathrm{BF}_{21}(y(n-l)|y(l))$ with the minimum training samples, and averaged all (L) the minimum training samples included in y. Then we get the arithmetic intrinsic BF of M_2 to M_1:

$$\mathrm{BF}_{21}^{AI}(y) = BF_{21}^N(y)\frac{1}{L}\sum BF_{12}^N(y(l)),$$

which does not rely on any constant in the improper priors.

The PBF introduced by O'Hagan[10] is

$$\mathrm{FBF}_{21}(b_n, y) = \mathrm{BF}_{21}^N(y)\frac{\int p_1(y|\theta_1)^{b_n}p_1^N(\theta_1)d\theta_1}{\int p_2(y|\theta_2)^{b_n}p_2^N(\theta_2)d\theta_2},$$

where $b_n(b_n = m/n, n \geq 1)$ represents the ratio of the minimum training sample size to the total sample size. FBF_{21} does not rely on any constant in the improper priors either.

10.15. Correlation in a Bayesian Framework[12]

Given random variable $X \sim p(x|\theta)$ and its parameter $\theta \sim p(\theta)$, we consider the Pearson correlation between $g(x,\theta)$ and $h(x,\theta)$, particularly when $g(x,\theta) = \theta$ is the parameter and $h(x,\theta) = \delta(X)$ is the estimator of θ. At this time, (θ, X) is a pair of random variables with the joint distribution P, and π is the marginal distribution of θ. Denote $r(\pi,\delta) = E[\{\delta(X) - \theta\}^2]$ as the

Bayes risk under squared loss and $r(\pi)$ as the risk of the Bayesian estimator $\delta_\pi(X) = E(\theta|X)$.

Dasgupta *et al.*[12] gave the following result: if $\delta = \delta(X)$ is an estimator of θ with the deviation $b(\theta) = E\{\delta(X)|\theta\} - \theta$, the correlation coefficient under the joint distribution of θ and X is

$$\rho(\theta, \delta) = \frac{\mathrm{Var}(\theta) + \mathrm{Cov}\{\theta, b(\theta)\}}{\sqrt{\mathrm{Var}(\theta)}\sqrt{\mathrm{Var}\{\theta + b(\theta)\} + r(\pi, \delta) - E\{b^2(\theta)\}}}.$$

When δ is unbiased or the Bayesian estimator δ_π, correlation coefficients are

$$\rho(\theta, \delta) = \sqrt{\frac{\mathrm{Var}(\theta)}{\mathrm{Var}(\theta) + r(\pi, \delta)}}; \quad \rho(\theta, \delta_\pi) = \sqrt{1 - \frac{r(\pi)}{\mathrm{Var}(\theta)}},$$

respectively.

For example, $\bar{X}$ is the sample mean from the normal distribution $N(\theta, 1)$, and the prior distribution of θ belongs to a large distribution class $c = \{\pi: E(\theta) = 0, Var(\theta) = 1\}$. We can obtain

$$1 - \rho^2(\theta, \delta_\pi) = \frac{r(\pi)}{\mathrm{Var}(\theta)} = r(\pi) = \frac{1}{n} - \frac{1}{n^2} I(f_\pi),$$

where $f_\pi(x)$ is the marginal distribution of $\bar{X}$, and $I(f)$ is the Fisher information matrix:

$$f_\pi(x) = \sqrt{n/2\pi} \int e^{-n(x-\theta)^2} d\pi(\theta); \quad I(f) = \int \left\{\frac{f'(x)}{f(x)}\right\}^2 f(x)dx.$$

We can verify that $\inf_{\pi \in c}\{1 - \rho^2(\theta, \delta_\pi)\} = 0$, that is, $\sup_{\pi \in c} \rho(\theta, \delta_\pi) = 1$.

The following example is to estimate $\boldsymbol{F}$ by the empirical distribution $\boldsymbol{F_n}$. Assume that the prior information of $\boldsymbol{F}$ is described by a Dirichlet process, and the parameter is a measure γ on R. Thus, $\boldsymbol{F}(x)$ has a beta distribution π, and its parameter is $\alpha = \gamma(-\infty, x], \beta = \gamma(x, \infty)$.

Dasgupta *et al.*[12] also showed that

(1) The correlation coefficient between θ and any unbiased estimator is non-negative, and strictly positive if the prior distribution is non-degenerate.
(2) If δ_U is a UMVUE of θ, and δ is any other unbiased estimator, then $\rho(\theta, \delta_U) \geq \rho(\theta, \delta)$; If δ_U is the unique UMVUE and π supports the entire parameter space, the inequality above is strict.
(3) The correlation coefficient between θ and the Bayesian estimator $\delta_\pi(X)$ is non-negative. If the estimator is not a constant, the coefficient is strictly positive.

(4) If the experiment ξ_1 contains more information than ξ_2 in the Blackwell's framework, then $\rho_{\xi_2}(\theta, \delta) \geq \rho_{\xi_1}(\theta, \delta)$, for the prior distribution π.
(5) If the likelihood function is unimodal for every x, then the correlation coefficient is between θ and its MLE is non-negative.
(6) If the density $p(x|\theta)$ has a monotone likelihood ratio, the correlation coefficient between θ and its any permissible estimator is non-negative.
(7) If the distribution of X is $\boldsymbol{F}(x-\theta)$, and $\boldsymbol{F}$ and the prior distribution π of θ belong to the class of c_1, c_2, respectively, the criteria maximizing $\inf_{F\in c_1, \pi\in c_2} \rho(\theta, \delta)$, where δ is unbiased for all $F \in c_1$, is equivalent to the criteria minimizing $\sup_{F\in c_1} \operatorname{Var}\{\delta(X)|\theta\}$.
(8) If the likelihood function is unimodal for every x, then the correlation coefficient is between the Bayesian estimation δ_π of θ and the MLE of θ is non-negative for any prior distribution.

10.16. Generalized Bayes Rule for Density Estimation[2,13]

There is a generalized Bayes rule, which is related to all α divergence including the Kullback–Leibler divergence and the Hellinger distance. It is introduced to get the density estimation. Let $x^{(n)} = (x_1, \ldots, x_n)$ denote n independent observations, and assume that they have the same distributions which belong to the distribution class $\mathcal{P} = \{p(x; u), u \in U\}$, where $p(x; u)$ is the density of some α – finite referenced measure μ on R^n. We hope to get the predictive density $\hat{p}(x; x^{(n)})$ of future x based on $x^{(n)}$. Different from $\hat{p}(x; x^{(n)}) = p(x; \tilde{u})$, which is produced by putting the estimate $\tilde{u}$ of μ into the density family which we are interested in, the Bayesian predictive density is defined as

$$\hat{p}(x; x^{(n)}) = p(x|x^{(n)}) = \int_U p(x; u) p(u|x^{(n)}) du,$$

where

$$p(u|x^{(n)}) = \frac{p(x^{(n)}; u)p(u)}{\int_U p(x^{(n)}; u)p(u)du}$$

is the posterior distribution of u after given $x^{(n)}$. In repeated sampling, the quality of a predictive density can be measured by the average divergence of the real density. If we take the divergence $D(p, \hat{p})$ as a loss function, then the measurement is

$$E_{X^{(n)}}(D(p, \hat{p})) = \int D(p(x; u), \hat{p}(x; x^{(n)}))p(x^{(n)}; u)\mu(dx^{(n)}).$$

After integrating with the prior distribution, we can get the Bayes risk $\int_U E_{X^{(n)}}(D(p,\hat{p}))p(u)du$, which is used to measure the goodness-of-fit with the real distribution. When using the Kullback–Leibler divergence,

$$D(p(x;u),\hat{p}(x;x^{(n)})) = \int \log\left(\frac{p(x;u)}{\hat{p}(x;x^{(n)})}\right)p(x;u)\mu(dx).$$

Let us consider the α divergence introduced by Csiszar (1967) next:

$$D_\alpha(p(x;u),\hat{p}(x;x^{(n)})) = \int f_\alpha\left(\frac{\hat{p}(x;x^{(n)})}{p(x;u)}\right)p(x;u)\mu(dx),$$

where

$$f_\alpha(z) = \begin{cases} \frac{4}{1-\alpha^2}(1 - z^{(1+\alpha)/2}), & |\alpha| < 1, \\ z\log z, & \alpha = 1, \\ -\log z, & \alpha = -1. \end{cases}$$

The Hellinger distance is equivalent to $\alpha = 0$ and the Kullback–Leibler divergence is equivalent to $\alpha = -1$.

Given prior distributions $p(u)$, because $|\alpha| \leq 1$, the generalized Bayesian predictive density based on α divergence is defined as

$$\hat{p}_\alpha(x;x^{(n)}) \propto \begin{cases} [\int p^{(1-\alpha)/2}(x;u)p(u|x^{(n)})du]^{2/(1-\alpha)}, & \alpha \neq 1, \\ \exp\{\int \log p(x;u)p(u|x^{(n)})du\}, & \alpha = 1. \end{cases}$$

When $\alpha = -1$, this is the Bayesian predictive density mentioned above. Corcuera and Giummole[13] showed that this $\hat{p}_\alpha(x;x^{(n)})$ defined here is the Bayesian estimation of $p(x;u)$ when using α divergence as the loss function.

Through the following examples, let us study the property of the generalized Bayes predictive density under the assumption of non-Bayesian distribution. Let $x_1,\ldots,x_n$ and x be the variables with normal distribution $N(\mu,\sigma^2)$, where $\mu \in R, \sigma \in R^+$. When $\hat{\mu} = n^{-1}\sum_{i=1}^n x_i, \hat{\sigma}^2 = n^{-1}\sum_{i=1}^n (x_i - \hat{\mu})^2$, because $r = (x-\hat{\mu})/\hat{\sigma}$ is the largest invariant, the form of the optimal predictive density, which is sought for, is $\hat{p}(x;\hat{\sigma}) = \frac{1}{\hat{\sigma}}g(\frac{x-\hat{\mu}}{\hat{\sigma}})$. Corcuera and Giummole[13] concluded that the preferably invariant predictive density (for $|\alpha| < 1$ and $\alpha = -1$) is

$$\hat{p}(x;\hat{\sigma}) \propto \left[1 + \frac{1-\alpha}{2n+1-\alpha}\left(\frac{x-\hat{\mu}}{\hat{\sigma}}\right)^2\right]^{-[(2n-1-\alpha)/2(1-\alpha)]}.$$

When $\alpha = 1$, we only need to replace $\hat{\sigma}$ in the result above with $\sqrt{n/(n-1)}\hat{\sigma}$.

10.17. Maximal Data Information Prior[14]

The Maximal data information prior (MDIP) is proposed for constructing non-informative prior and informative prior. Considering the joint distribution $p(y, \theta)$ of the observation vector y and the parameter vector θ, where $\theta \subset R_\theta, y \subset R_y$, the negative entropy $-H(p)$, which measures the information in $p(y, \theta)$ related to the uniform distribution, is (note that p in the entropy $H(p)$ represents the distribution $p(y, \theta)$ rather than the prior distribution $p(\theta)$)

$$-H(p) = \int_{R_\theta} \int_{R_y} \log p(y, \theta) dy d\theta,$$

that is, $E \log p(y, \theta)$. This is the average of the logarithm of the joint distribution, and the larger it is, the more information it contains. For the prior distribution $p(\theta)$ of θ, $p(y, \theta) = f(y|\theta)p(\theta)$, and then (refer to Zellner,[20] and Soofi, 1994):

$$-H(p) = \int_{R_\theta} I(\theta)p(\theta)d\theta + \int_{R_\theta} p(\theta) \log p(\theta) d\theta,$$

where

$$I(\theta) = \int_{R_y} f(y|\theta) \log f(y|\theta) dy$$

is the information in $f(y|\theta)$. The $-H(p)$ above contains two parts: the first one is the average of the prior information in data density $f(y|\theta)$, and the second one is the information in the prior density $p(\theta)$.

If the prior distribution is optional, we want to view the information in the data. Under certain conditions, such as the prior distribution is proper and both its mean and variance are given, we can choose the prior distribution to maximize the discriminant function represented by $G(p)$:

$$G(p) = \int_{R_\theta} I(\theta)p(\theta)d\theta - \int_{R_\theta} p(\theta) \log p(\theta) d\theta.$$

The difference just happens between the two items on the right of $-H(p)$. So, $G(p)$ is a measure of the general information provided by an experiment. If $p(y, \theta) = g(\theta|y)h(y)$ and $g(\theta|y) = f(y|\theta)p(\theta)/h(y)$, from the formula above, we can get

$$G(p) = \int_{R_\theta} \left[\int_{R_\theta} g(\theta|y) \log \left\{ \frac{L(\theta|y)}{p(\theta)} \right\} \right] h(y) dy,$$

where $L(\theta|y) \equiv f(y|\theta)$ is the likelihood function. Therefore, we see that $p(\theta)$ is selected to maximize G such that it maximizes the average of the logarithm of the ratio between likelihood function and prior density. This is another explanation of $G(p)$.

It does not produce clear results when using the information offered by an experiment as a discriminant function to emerge prior distributions. So, it has been suggested that we approximate the discriminant function by large sample and select the prior distribution with maximal information of not included. However, this needs to contain the data that we do not have, and the increases of the sample are likely to change the model. Fortunately, $G(p)$ is an accurately discriminant functional with finite sample which can lead to the optimal prior distribution.

y is a scale or vector, $y_1, y_2, \ldots, y_n$ are independent identically distributed observations, it is easy to get

$$G_n(p) = \sum_{i=1}^{n} \left[\int I_i(\theta)p(\theta)d\theta - \int p(\theta)\log p(\theta)d\theta \right].$$

because $I_i(\theta) = I(\theta) = \int f(y_i|\theta)\log f(y_i|\theta)dy_i, i = 1, \ldots, n$, $G_n(p) = nG(p)$.

When the observations are independent but not identically distributed, the MDIP based on n observations derived from the above formula is the geometric average of the individual prior distributions.

About the derivation of the MDIP, under some conditions, the procedure to select $p(\theta)$ to maximize $G(p)$ is a standard variation problem. The prior distribution is proper if $\int_{R_\theta} p(\theta)d\theta = 1$, where R_θ is the region containing θ. R_θ is a compact region, may be very large or a bounded region such as (0,1). Under these conditions, the solution maximizing $G(p)$ is

$$p^*(\theta) = \begin{cases} ce^{I(\theta)} & \theta \subset \mathrm{R}_\theta \\ 0 & \theta \not\subset \mathrm{R}_\theta \end{cases}.$$

where c is a standardized constant meeting $c = 1/\int_{R_\theta} \exp\{I(\theta)\}d\theta$.

10.18. Conjugate Likelihood Distribution of the Exponential Family[15]

According to Bayes theorem, the posterior distribution is proportional to the product of the likelihood function and the prior distribution. Thus, the nature of the likelihood function, such as integrability, has received great attention, which relates to whether we can get the proper prior distribution from an improper prior distribution, and also relates to whether we can effectively use Gibbs sampling to generate random variables for inference. George *et al.* (1993) discussed the conjugate likelihood prior distribution of the exponential family. As for researches associated to the conjugate distribution of the exponential distribution family, we are supposed to refer to Arnold *et al.* (1993, 1996).

v is a fixed σ-finite measure on a Borel set in R^k. For $\theta \in R^k$, the natural parameter space is defined as $N = \{\theta | \int \exp(x\theta)dv(x) < \infty\}$. For $\Theta \subset N$, through the exponential family of v, probability measure $\{P_\theta | \theta \in \Theta\}$ is defined as

$$dP_\theta(x) = \exp[x\theta - \psi(\theta)]dv(x), \theta \in \Theta,$$

where $\psi(\theta) \equiv \ln \int \exp(x\theta)dv(x)$. What we have known is that N is a lower convex, and ψ is a lower convex function in N. The conjugate prior distribution measure of P_θ is defined as

$$d\Pi(\theta|x_0, n_0) \propto \exp[x_0\theta - n_0\psi(\theta)]I_\Theta(\theta)d\theta, \quad x_0 \in R^k, n_0 \geq 0.$$

Diaconis and Ylvisaker[15] put forward the sufficient and necessary conditions of proper conjugate prior distribution. Measure $\Pi(\theta|x_0, n_0)$ is finite, that is, $\int_\Theta \exp[x_0\theta - n_0\psi(\theta)]d\theta < \infty$ if and only if $x_0/n_0 \in K^0$ and $n_0 > 0$, where K^0 is the internal of the lower convex support of v. Π which meets the above condition can be expressed as a proper conjugate prior distributions on R^k, that is,

$$d\Pi(\theta|x_0, n_0) = \exp[x_0\theta - n_0\psi(\theta) - \phi(x_0, n_0)]I_\Theta(\theta)d\theta,$$

where $\phi(x_0, n_0) = \ln \int \exp[x_0\theta - n_0\psi(\theta)]d\theta$.

George *et al.* (1993) proved that $\phi(x_0, n_0)$ is lower convex. If $\theta_1, \ldots, \theta_p$ are samples coming from the conjugate prior distribution $d\Pi(\theta|x_0, n_0)$, then

$$d\Pi(\theta|x_0, n_0) = \exp\left[x_0 \sum_{i=1}^p \theta_i - n_0 \sum_{i=1}^p \psi(\theta_i) - p\phi(x_0, n_0)\right] \times \left[\prod_{i=1}^p I_\Theta(\theta_i)d\theta_i\right].$$

The conjugate likelihood distribution derived from this prior distribution is defined as

$$L(x_0, n_0|\theta_1, \ldots, \theta_p) \propto \exp\left[x_0 \sum_{i=1}^p \theta_i - n_0 \sum_{i=1}^p \psi(\theta_i) - p\phi(x_0, n_0)\right]$$
$$\times I_{K^0}(x_0/n_0)I_{(0,\infty)}(n_0).$$

George *et al.* proved the following result: if $\theta_i \in \Theta$ for $\theta_1, \ldots, \theta_p$, then $L(x_0, n_0|\theta_1, \ldots, \theta_p)$ is log-convex in (x_0, n_0). Moreover, if Θ is lower convex,

$\psi(\theta)$ is strictly lower convex, and dx_0 and n_0 are the Lebesgue measure on R^k and R, respectively, then for all p, $\int_{R^k} L(x_0, n_0|\theta_1, \ldots, \theta_p)dx_0 < \infty$ and

$$\int_{R^{k+1}} L(x_0, n_0|\theta_1, \ldots, \theta_p)dx_0 dn_0 < \infty \Leftrightarrow p \geq 2.$$

Thus, they showed that the likelihood function family $L^G(\alpha, \beta|\theta_1, \ldots, \theta_p)$ is log-upper convex, who comes from the gamma (α, β) distribution of $\theta_1, \ldots, \theta_p$. And for all p,

$$\int_0^\infty L^G(\alpha, \beta|\theta_1, \ldots, \theta_p)d\alpha < \infty$$

and $\int_0^\infty \int_0^\infty L^G(\alpha, \beta|\theta_1, \ldots, \theta_p)d\alpha d\beta < \infty \Leftrightarrow p \geq 2$.

Similarly, the likelihood function family $L^B(\alpha, \beta|\theta_1, \ldots, \theta_p)$ is log-upper convex, which comes from the distribution beta (α, β) of $\theta_1, \ldots, \theta_p$.

10.19. Subjective Prior Distributions Based on Expert Knowledge[16–18]

When estimating the hyperparameters (parameters of the prior distribution) of the subjective prior distribution, we can use the expert opinion to obtain some information about the parameters. These prior distributions we get above are called the subjective prior distributions based on the expert experience. Kadane and Wolfson[16] suggested that experts should provide a range for parameters of the prior distribution, which can be better than guessing unknown parameter information.

Assume that what we are interested in is X, and H is the background information. $P(X|H)$ represents uncertainty about X based on H if the analyzer has consulted an expert and the expert estimates X using two variables m and s, where m is the best guess for X from the expert, and S measures the uncertainty on m from experts. When $X = x, L(X = x; m, s, H)$ is the likelihood function of m and s, which is provided by the expert. According to Bayes Theorem,

$$P(X = x|m, s, H) \propto L(X = x; m, s, H)P(X = x|H).$$

For example, the analyzer could believe that m is actually $\alpha + \beta x$, and different values of α and β illustrate the analyzer's views about expert opinions. The analyzer can also use γs to adjust the value of s. α, β, γ are called the adjusted coefficients. Select the normal form:

$$L(X = x; m, s, H) \propto \exp\left[-\frac{1}{2}\left(\frac{m - (\alpha + \beta x)}{\gamma s}\right)^2\right].$$

If the analyzer's prior distribution $P(X = x|H)$ is non-subjective (flat), the posterior distribution $f(x|m, s, H)$ is proportional to $L(X = x; m, s, H)$. This model can be extended. When there are k experts, the analyzer has the expert opinions $(m_i, s_i), (i = 1, \ldots, k)$ corresponding to the adjusted coefficients $(\alpha_i, \beta_i, \gamma_i)$. The likelihood function is $L(X = x; (m_i, s_i), i = 1, \ldots, k, H)$. If it is not easy to determine the adjusted coefficient, the past expert opinions (m_i, s_i) and the corresponding value x_i can be used to get the posterior distribution of the adjusted coefficients. Their posterior distribution is

$$P(\alpha, \beta, \gamma|(m_i, s_i), x_i, i = 1, \ldots, k, H) \propto \gamma^{-n} \exp\left[-\frac{1}{2}\left(\frac{m - (\alpha + \beta x)}{\gamma s}\right)^2\right].$$

Singpurwalla and Wilson[18] considered the example of previously deduced probability of the software failure model. Suppose that the Poisson process is determined completely by its mean function $\Lambda(t)$, the logarithm of Poisson run time model is used to describe the failure time of a software, and Λ has the form of $\ln(\lambda\theta t + 1)\theta$. If $T_1 \le T_2$ are two time points selected by an expert about the location and the scale, the prior distribution of $\lambda, \theta > 0$ can be obtained from

$$\frac{e^{\Lambda(T_1)\theta} - 1}{e^{\Lambda(T_2)\theta} - 1} = \frac{T_1}{T_2}, \quad \lambda = \frac{e^{\Lambda(T_1)\theta} - 1}{\theta T_1}.$$

They also deduced the joint posterior distribution of $\Lambda(T_1)$ and $\Lambda(T_2)$.

Singpurwalla and Percy[17] did a lot of work about determining hyperparameters. For random variable X with density $f(x|\theta)$, θ is the unknown parameter with subjective prior density $f(\theta)$, which has unknown hyperparameters such that it can affect the prior information of θ. Thus, we can get the posterior density of X,

$$f(x) = \int_{-\infty}^{\infty} f(x|\theta) f(\theta) d\theta,$$

which contains unknown hyperparameters. Our expert will provide information about X rather than θ, that is, how big the value of $F(x) = \int_{-\infty}^{x} f(x)dx$ should be. It is equivalent to give values of the hyperparameters.

10.20. Bayes Networks[19,20]

A Bayes network is defined as $\boldsymbol{B} = (\boldsymbol{G}, \boldsymbol{\Theta})$ in form, where $\boldsymbol{G}$ is a directed acyclic graph (DAG) whose vertices correspond to random variables $X_1, X_2, \ldots, X_n$, and edges represent direct dependence between variables. A Bayes Network meets the causal Markov assumption, in other words, each variable in the Bayes network is independent of its ancestors given its parents. Thus, the figure $\boldsymbol{G}$ depicts the independence assumption, that is, each variable is independent of its non-descendants in $\boldsymbol{G}$ given its parents in $\boldsymbol{G}$. $\boldsymbol{\Theta}$ represents the set of network parameters, which includes the parameter $\theta_{x_i|\pi_i} = P_B(x_i|\pi_i)$ concerning the realization x_i of X_i on the condition of π_i, where π_i is the parent set of X_i in $\boldsymbol{G}$. Thus, a Bayes network defines the unique joint probability distribution of all the variables, and under the independence assumption:

$$P_B(X_1, X_2, \ldots, X_n) = \prod_{i=1}^{n} P_B(x_i|\pi_i).$$

If there is no independence assumption, according to the chain principle of the conditional distribution,

$$P_B(X_1 = x_1, \ldots, X_n = x_n) = \prod_{i=1}^{n} P_B(X_i = x_i|X_{i+1} = x_{i+1}, \ldots, X_n = x_n).$$

According to the independence assumption,

$$P_B(X_1 = x_1, X_2 = x_2, \ldots, X_n = x_n) = \prod_{i=1}^{n} P_B(X_i = x_i|X_j = x_j, \forall X_j \in \pi_i).$$

Obviously, the independence assumptions greatly simplify the joint distribution.

Given the factorization form of the joint probability distribution of a Bayes Network, we can deduce from the marginal distributions by summing all "irrelevant" variables. There are general two kinds of inferences:

(1) To forecast a vertex X_i through the evidence of its parents (top-down reasoning).
(2) To diagnose a vertex X_i through the evidence of its children (bottom-up reasoning).

From the perspective of algorithm, there are two main kinds of structural learning algorithms of Bayes networks: the first one is the constraint-based algorithms, which analyze the probability relationship by conditional independence testing that is used to analyze the Markov property of Bayes networks. For example, the search is limited to the Markov blanket of a vertex, and then the figure corresponding to d-separation is constructed statistically. We usually regard the edge (arc or arrow) in all directions as a part of a ternary v structure (such as $X_j \to X_i \to X_k, X_j \to X_i \leftarrow X_k, X_j \leftarrow X_i \to X_k$). For subjective experiences, or ensuring loop-free conditions, we may also add some constraints. Eventually, the model is often interpreted as a causal model, even if it is learned from observational data. The second one is score-based algorithms, which give a score to each candidate Bayes Network. These scores are defined variously, but they measure the network according to some criteria. Given the scoring criteria, we can use intuitive search algorithms, such as parsimony search algorithm, hill climbing or tabu search-based algorithm, to achieve the network structure which maximizes the score. The score functions are usually score equivalent, in other words, those networks with the same probability distribution have the same score. There are many different types of scores, such as the likelihood or log-likelihood score, AIC and BIC score, the Bayesian Dirichlet posterior density score for discrete variables, K2 score, the Wishart posterior density score for continuous normal distribution and so on.

A simple driving example is given below. Consider several dichotomous variables: Y (Young), D (Drink), A (Accident), V (Violation), C (Citation), G (Gear). The data of the variable is 0,1 dummy variables, "yes" corresponding to 1, and "no" corresponding to 0. The following chart is the corresponding DAG, which shows the independence and relevance of each vertex. The arrows indicate the presumed causal relationships. The variable Accident, Citation, and Violation have the same parents, Young and Drink.

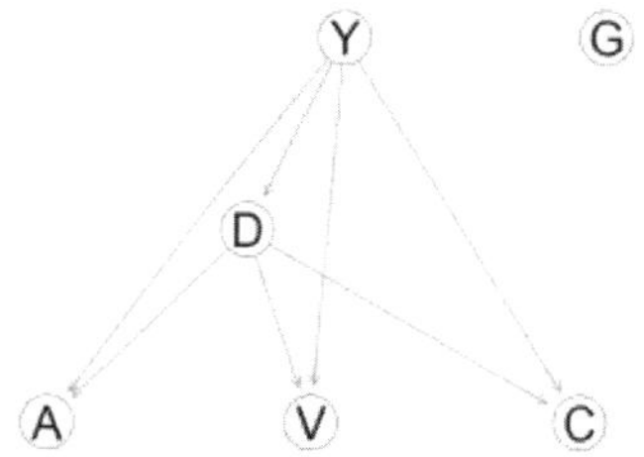

References

1. Berger, JO. *Statistical Decision Theory and Bayesian Analysis* (2nd edn.). New York: Springer-Verlag, 1985.
2. Kotz, S, Wu, X. *Modern Bayesian Statistics*, Beijing: China Statistics Press, 2000.
3. Jeffreys, H. *Theory of Probability* (3rd edn.). Oxford: Clarendon Press, 1961.
4. Robbins, H. An Empirical Bayes Approach to Statistics. *Proceedings of the Third Berkeley Symposium on Mathematical Statistics and Probability*, Volume 1: Contributions to the Theory of Statistics: 157–163, 1955.
5. Akaike, H. The interpretation of improper prior distributions as limits of data dependent proper prior distributions. *J. R. Statist. Soc. B*, 1980, 42: 46–52.
6. Dawid, AP, Stone, M, Zidek, JV. Marginalization paradoxes in Bayesian and structural inference (with discussion). *JRSS B*, 1973, 35: 189–233.

7. Albert, JH. Bayesian analysis in the case of two-dimentional parameter space. *Amer. Stat.* 1989, 43(4): 191–196.
8. Severini, TA. On the relationship between Bayesian and non-Bayesian interval estimates. *J. R. Statist. Soc. B*, 1991, 53: 611–618.
9. Giron, FJ. Stochastic dominance for elliptical distributions: Application in Bayesian inference. *Decision Theory and Decison Analysis.* 1998, 2: 177–192, Fang, KT, Kotz, S, Ng, KW. *Symmetric Multivariate and Related Distributions.* London: Chapman and Hall, 1990.
10. O'Hagan, A. Fractional Bayes factors for model comparison (with discussion). *J. R. Stat. Soc. Series B*, 1995, 56: 99–118.
11. Bertolio, F, Racugno, W. Bayesian model selection approach to analysis of variance under heteroscedasticity. *The Statistician*, 2000, 49(4): 503–517.
12. Dasgupta, A, Casella, G, Delampady, M, Genest, C, Rubin, H, Strawderman, E. Correlation in a bayesian framework. *Can. J. Stat.*, 2000, 28: 4.
13. Corcuera, JM, Giummole, F. A generalized Bayes rule for prediction. *Scand. J. Statist.* 1999, 26: 265–279.
14. Zellner, A. *Bayesian Methods and Entropy in Economics and Econometrics. Maximum Entropy and Bayesian Methods.* Dordrecht: Kluwer Acad. Publ., 1991.
15. Diaconis, P, Ylvisaker, D. Conjugate priors for exponential families, *Ann. Statist.* 1979, 7: 269–281.
16. Kadane, JB, Wolfson, LJ. Experiences in elicitation. *The Statistician*, 1998, 47: 3–19.
17. Singpurwalla, ND, Percy, DF. Bayesian calculations in maintenance modelling. University of Salford technical report, CMS-98-03, 1998.
18. Singpurwalla, ND, Wilson, SP. *Statistical Methods in Software Engineering, Reliability and Risk.* New York: Springer, 1999.
19. Ben-Gal, I. Bayesian networks, in Ruggeri, F, Faltin, F and Kenett, R, *Encyclopedia of Statistics in Quality & Reliability*, Hoboken: Wiley & Sons, 2007.
20. Wu, X. *Statistical Methods for Complex Data* (3rd edn.). Beijing: China Renmin University Press, 2015.

About the Author

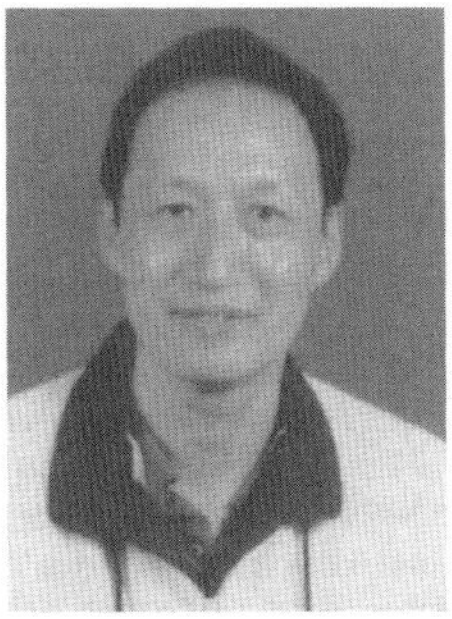

Xizhi Wu is a Professor at Renmin University of China and Nankai University. He taught at Nankai University, University of California and University of North Carolina at Chapel Hill. He graduated from Peking University in 1969 and got his Ph.D. degree at University of North Carolina at Chapel Hill in 1987. He has published 10 papers and more than 20 books so far. His research interests are statistical diagnosis, model selection, categorical data analysis, longitudinal data analysis, component data analysis, robust statistics, partial least square regression, path analysis, Bayesian statistics, data mining, and machine learning.

CHAPTER 11

SAMPLING METHOD

Mengxue Jia and Guohua Zou*

11.1. Survey Sampling[1,2]

Survey sampling is a branch of statistics which studies how to draw a part (sample) from all objects or units (population), and how to make inference about population target variable from the sample. Its basic characteristics are cost saving and strong timeliness. All advantages of survey sampling are based on investigating a part of population, and this part of population will directly affect the quality of the survey. In order to get a reliable estimate of the target variable of population and estimate its error, we must use the method of probability sampling by which a sample is randomly selected with given probability strictly. We mainly introduce this kind of sampling in this chapter.

The alternative to probability sampling is non-probability sampling by which a sample is not randomly selected with given probability but accidentally or purposively. There are several common non-probability sampling methods: (i) Haphazard sampling: sampling with no subjective purpose and casual way or based only on the principle of convenience, such as "street intercept" survey; (ii) Purposive sampling: select the required samples purposefully according to the needs of survey; (iii) Judgement sampling: select representative samples for population according to the experience and knowledge on population of the investigators; (iv) Volunteer sampling: all respondents are volunteers.

Non-probability sampling can provide some useful information, but population cannot be inferred based on such samples. In addition, the sampling

*Corresponding author: ghzou@amss.ac.cn

error cannot be calculated according to the samples from non-probability sampling, and so it cannot be controlled.

The following methods can be utilized to collect data after selecting the sample.

(1) Traditional data collection modes

(a) Mail survey: The respondents fill out and send back the questionnaires that the investigators send or fax to them.
(b) Interview survey: The investigators communicate with the respondents face to face. The investigators ask questions and the respondents give their answers.
(c) Telephone survey: The investigators ask the respondents questions and record their answers by telephone.

(2) Computer-assisted modes

Computer technology has had a great impact on the above three traditional data collection methods, and a variety of computer-assisted methods have been applied to mail survey, interview survey and telephone survey.

(a) Computer-Assisted Self-Interviewing (CASI): By using computer, the respondents complete the questionnaires sent by email by the investigators.
(b) Computer-Assisted Personal Interviewing (CAPI): The respondents read the questionnaire on the computer screen and answer the questions with the interviewer being present.
(c) Computer-Assisted Telephone Interviewing (CATI): Computer replaces the pattern of paper and pencil in telephone survey.

The development and application of computer have also produced some new ways of data collection, such as the Internet survey based on Internet which greatly reduces the survey cost. In addition, the pictures, dialogue and even video clip can be included in the Internet survey questionnaire.

11.2. Simple Random Sampling[1,3]

Simple random sampling is the most basic sampling method, and its way of selecting a sample is to draw a sample without replacement one by one or all at once from the population such that every possible sample has the same chance of being selected.

In practice, simple random sample can be obtained by taking the random number: An integer is randomly selected from 1 to N and denoted by r_1, then the r_1th unit is included in the sample. Similarly, the second integer is randomly selected from 1 to N and denoted by r_2, then the r_2th unit is included in the sample if $r_2 \neq r_1$, or the r_2th unit is omitted and another random number is selected as its replacement if $r_2 = r_1$. Repeat this process until n different units are selected. Random numbers can be generated by dices or tables of random number or computer programs.

Let $Y_1, \ldots, Y_N$ denote N values of the population units, $y_1, \ldots, y_n$ denote n values of the sample units, and $f = n/N$ be the sampling fraction. Then an unbiased estimator and its variance of the population mean $\bar{Y} = \sum_{i=1}^{N} Y_i/N$ are

$$\bar{y} = \frac{1}{n}\sum_{i=1}^{n} y_i, \quad V(\bar{y}) = \frac{1-f}{n}S^2,$$

respectively, where $S^2 = \frac{1}{N-1}\sum_{i=1}^{N}(Y_i - \bar{Y})^2$ is the population variance. An unbiased estimator of $V(\bar{y})$ is $v(\bar{y}) = \frac{1-f}{n}s^2$, where $s^2 = \frac{1}{n-1}\sum_{i=1}^{n}(y_i - \bar{y})^2$ is the sample variance.

The approximate $1-\alpha$ confidence interval for $\bar{Y}$ is given by

$$\left(\bar{y} - z_{\alpha/2}\sqrt{\frac{1-f}{n}} \cdot s, \bar{y} + z_{\alpha/2}\sqrt{\frac{1-f}{n}} \cdot s\right),$$

where $z_{\alpha/2}$ is the $\alpha/2$ quantile of the standard normal distribution.

In practical surveys, an important problem is how to determine the sample size. The determination of sample size requires a balance of accuracy and cost. For a fixed total cost C_T, the sample size can be directly determined by the formula $C_T = c_0 + cn$, where c_0 denotes the cost related to organization, etc., which is irrelevant to the sample size, and c denotes the average cost of investigating a unit. Considering sampling accuracy, a general formula of the required sample size is $n = \frac{n_0}{1+n_0/N}$ if one focuses on estimating the population mean, where n_0 is determined as follows:

(1) If the absolute error limit $\leq d$ is required, then $n_0 = (\frac{z_{\alpha/2}S}{d})^2$;
(2) If the relative error limit $\leq r$ is required, then $n_0 = (\frac{z_{\alpha/2}S}{r\bar{Y}})^2$;
(3) If the variance of $\bar{y} \leq V$ is required, then $n_0 = \frac{S^2}{V}$;
(4) If the coefficient of variation of $\bar{y} \leq C$ is required, then $n_0 = \frac{1}{C^2}(\frac{S}{\bar{Y}})^2$.

Note that in the above n_0, the population standard deviation S and population variation coefficient $S/\overline{Y}$ are unknown, so we need to estimate them by using historical data or pilot investigation in advance.

11.3. Stratified Random Sampling[1,3]

Stratified sampling is a sampling method that the population is divided into finite and non-overlapping groups (called strata) and then a sample is selected within each stratum independently. If simple random sampling is used in each stratum, then the stratified sampling is called the stratified random sampling.

If the stratified sample is obtained, the estimator of the population mean $\bar{Y}$ is the weighted mean of the estimator of each stratum $\hat{\bar{Y}}_h$ with the stratum weight $W_h = \frac{N_h}{N}$:

$$\hat{\bar{Y}}_{\text{st}} = \sum_{h=1}^{L} W_h \hat{\bar{Y}}_h,$$

where N_h denotes the number of units in stratum h, and L denotes the number of strata.

The variance of $\hat{\bar{Y}}_{\text{st}}$ is

$$\mathrm{V}(\hat{\bar{Y}}_{\text{st}}) = \sum_{h=1}^{L} W_h^2 \mathrm{V}(\hat{\bar{Y}}_h),$$

and the estimated variance of $\hat{\bar{Y}}_{\text{st}}$ is given by

$$v(\hat{\bar{Y}}_{\text{st}}) = \sum_{h=1}^{L} W_h^2 v(\hat{\bar{Y}}_h),$$

where $\mathrm{V}(\hat{\bar{Y}}_h)$ and $v(\hat{\bar{Y}}_h)$ are the variance and the estimated variance of $\hat{\bar{Y}}_h$ in stratum h, respectively.

For stratified sampling, how to determine the total sample size n and how to allocate it to the strata are important. For the fixed total sample size n, there are some common allocation methods: (1) Proportional allocation: The sample size of each stratum n_h is proportional to its size N_h, i.e. $n_h = \frac{n}{N} N_h = nW_h$. In practice, the allocation method that n_h is proportional to the square root of N_h is sometimes adopted when there is a great difference among stratum sizes. (2) Optimum allocation: This is an allocation method that minimizes the variance $\mathrm{V}(\hat{\bar{Y}}_{\text{st}})$ for a fixed cost or minimizes cost for a fixed value of $\mathrm{V}(\hat{\bar{Y}}_{\text{st}})$. If the cost function is linear: $C_T = c_0 + \sum_{h=1}^{L} c_h n_h$, where C_T denotes total cost, c_0 is the fixed cost which is unrelated to the sample size, and c_h is the average cost of investigating a unit in the h-th stratum, then the optimum allocation is given by $n_h = n \frac{W_h S_h / \sqrt{c_h}}{\sum_h W_h S_h / \sqrt{c_h}}$ for stratified random sampling. The optimum allocation is called Neyman allocation if $c_1 = c_2 = \cdots = c_L$. Further, Neyman allocation reduces to the proportional allocation if $S_1^2 = S_2^2 = \cdots = S_L^2$, where S_h^2 denotes the variance of the h-th stratum, $h = 1, 2, \ldots, L$.

In order to determine the total sample size of stratified random sampling, we still consider the estimation of the population mean. Suppose the form of sample size allocation is $n_h = nw_h$, which includes the proportional allocation and the optimum allocation above as special cases. If the variance of estimator $\leq V$ is required, then the required sample size is

$$n = \frac{\sum_h W_h^2 S_h^2 / w_h}{V + \frac{1}{N}\sum_h W_h S_h^2}.$$

If the absolute error limit $\leq d$ is required, then the required sample size is

$$n = \frac{\sum_h W_h^2 S_h^2 / w_h}{\frac{d^2}{u_\alpha^2} + \frac{1}{N}\sum_h W_h S_h^2}.$$

If the relative error limit $\leq r$ is required, then the required sample size can be obtained by substituting $d = r\bar{Y}$ into the above formula.

If there is no ready sampling frame (the list including all sampling units) on strata in practical surveys, or it is difficult to stratify population, the method of post-stratification can be used, that is, we can stratify the selected sample units according to stratified principle, and then estimate the target variable by using the method of stratified sampling introduced above.

11.4. Ratio Estimator[3,4]

In simple random sampling and stratified random sampling, the classical estimation method is to estimate the population mean by directly using the sample mean or its weighed mean, which does not make use of any auxiliary information. A common method using auxiliary information to improve estimation accuracy is the ratio estimation method which is applicable to the situation where the variable of interest is almost proportional to the auxiliary variable, or there is a linear relationship through the origin between the two variables.

Denote $\bar{y}$ and $\bar{x}$ as the sample means of the variable of interest and auxiliary variable, respectively, and assume that the population mean $\bar{X}$ is known. Then the ratio estimator of $\bar{Y}$ is defined as $\bar{y}_R = \frac{\bar{y}}{\bar{x}}\bar{X}$. $\bar{y}_R$ is nearly unbiased when the sample size is large, and its variance is

$$V(\bar{y}_R) \approx \frac{1-f}{n} \cdot \frac{1}{N-1}\sum_{i=1}^{N}(Y_i - RX_i)^2$$

$$= \frac{1-f}{n}(S_y^2 + R^2 S_x^2 - 2R\rho S_x S_y),$$

where $R = \frac{\bar{Y}}{\bar{X}}$ is the population ratio, S_y^2 and S_x^2 denote the population variances, and ρ denotes the population correlation coefficient of the two variables:

$$\rho = \frac{S_{yx}}{S_y S_x} = \frac{\sum_{i=1}^N (Y_i - \bar{Y})(X_i - \bar{X})}{\sqrt{\sum_{i=1}^N (Y_i - \bar{Y})^2 \cdot \sum_{i=1}^N (X_i - \bar{X})^2}}.$$

A nearly unbiased variance estimator of $\bar{y}_R$ is given by

$$v(\bar{y}_R) = \frac{1-f}{n} \cdot \frac{1}{n-1} \sum_{i=1}^{n} (y_i - \hat{R}x_i)^2,$$

where $\hat{R} = \frac{\bar{y}}{\bar{x}}$.

The condition that the ratio estimator is better than the sample mean is $\rho > \frac{RS_x}{2S_y} = \frac{1}{2}\frac{C_x}{C_y}$, where $C_x = S_x/\bar{X}$ and $C_y = S_y/\bar{Y}$ are the population variation coefficients.

The idea of ratio estimation can also be applied to stratified random sampling: Construct ratio estimator in each stratum, and then use the stratum weight W_h to average these ratio estimators–separate ratio estimator; or the estimators of population means of the variable of interest and auxiliary variable are obtained first, then construct ratio estimator–combined ratio estimator. The former requires large sample size in each stratum, while the latter requires only large total sample size. In general, the separate ratio estimator is more effective than the combined ratio estimator when the sample size is large in each stratum.

Specifically, the separate ratio estimator is defined as

$$\bar{y}_{RS} = \sum_h W_h \bar{y}_{Rh} = \sum_h W_h \frac{\bar{y}_h}{\bar{x}_h} \bar{X}_h.$$

It is nearly unbiased, and its variance is

$$\mathrm{V}(\bar{y}_{RS}) \approx \sum_h \frac{W_h^2(1-f_h)}{n_h} (S_{yh}^2 + R_h^2 S_{xh}^2 - 2R_h \rho_h S_{xh} S_{yh}),$$

where the subscript h denotes the h-th stratum.

The combined ratio estimator is defined as

$$\bar{y}_{RC} = \frac{\bar{y}_{\mathrm{st}}}{\bar{x}_{\mathrm{st}}} \bar{X} \hat{=} \hat{R}_C \bar{X},$$

where $\bar{y}_{\mathrm{st}} = \sum_h W_h \bar{y}_h$ and $\bar{x}_{\mathrm{st}} = \sum_h W_h \bar{x}_h$ are the stratified simple estimators of $\bar{Y}$ and $\bar{X}$, respectively, and $\hat{R}_C = \frac{\bar{y}_{\mathrm{st}}}{\bar{x}_{\mathrm{st}}}$. $\bar{y}_{RC}$ is also nearly unbiased, and its variance is

$$V(\bar{y}_{RC}) \approx \sum_h \frac{W_h^2(1-f_h)}{n_h}(S_{yh}^2 + R^2 S_{xh}^2 - 2R\rho_h S_{xh} S_{yh}).$$

As for the estimated variances, we can use the sample ratio, sample variance and sample correlation coefficient to replace the corresponding population values in the above variance formulas.

11.5. Regression Estimator[3,4]

The estimation accuracy can be improved by using regression estimator when the variable of interest approximately follows a general linear relationship (i.e. not through the origin) with the auxiliary variable. For simple random sampling, the regression estimator of the population mean $\bar{Y}$ is defined as

$$\bar{y}_{lr} = \bar{y} + b(\bar{X} - \bar{x}),$$

where

$$b = \frac{s_{yx}}{s_x^2} = \frac{\sum_{i=1}^n (x_i - \bar{x})(y_i - \bar{y})}{\sum_{i=1}^n (x_i - \bar{x})^2}$$

is the sample regression coefficient. It is nearly unbiased when the sample size n is large, and its variance is

$$V(\bar{y}_{lr}) \approx \frac{1-f}{n}(S_y^2 + B^2 S_x^2 - 2BS_{yx}),$$

where S_{yx} is the population covariance, and

$$B = \frac{S_{yx}}{S_x^2} = \frac{\sum_{i=1}^N (Y_i - \bar{Y})(X_i - \bar{X})}{\sum_{i=1}^N (X_i - \bar{X})^2}.$$

The estimated variance is

$$v(\bar{y}_{lr}) = \frac{1-f}{n}(s_y^2 + b^2 s_x^2 - 2bs_{yx}).$$

Similar to stratified ratio estimator, stratified regression estimator can also be defined: construct regression estimator in each stratum, and then use the stratum weight W_h to average all the regression estimators–separate regression estimator; or the estimators of $\bar{Y}$ and $\bar{X}$ are obtained first, then construct the regression estimator–combined regression estimator. Similarly, the former requires large sample size in each stratum, while the latter requires only large total sample size.

For stratified random sample, the separate regression estimator is defined as

$$\bar{y}_{lrs} = \sum_h W_h \bar{y}_{lrh} = \sum_h W_h[\bar{y}_h + b_h(\bar{X}_h - \bar{x}_h)],$$

where

$$b_h = \frac{s_{yxh}}{s_{xh}^2} = \frac{\sum_{i=1}^{n_h}(x_{hi} - \bar{x}_h)(y_{hi} - \bar{y}_h)}{\sum_{i=1}^{n_h}(x_{hi} - \bar{x}_h)^2}.$$

$\bar{y}_{lrs}$ is nearly unbiased, and its variance is

$$V(\bar{y}_{lrs}) \approx \sum_h \frac{W_h^2(1 - f_h)}{n_h}(S_{yh}^2 - 2B_h S_{yxh} + B_h^2 S_{xh}^2),$$

where $B_h = S_{yxh}/S_{xh}^2$.

For stratified random sample, the combined regression estimator is defined as

$$\bar{y}_{lrc} = \bar{y}_{\text{st}} + b_c(\bar{X} - \bar{x}_{\text{st}}),$$

where

$$b_c = \frac{\sum_h W_h^2(1 - f_h)s_{yxh}/n_h}{\sum_h W_h^2(1 - f_h)s_{xh}^2/n_h}.$$

$\bar{y}_{lrc}$ is also nearly unbiased, and its variance is

$$V(\bar{y}_{lrc}) \approx \sum_h \frac{W_h^2(1 - f_h)}{n_h}(S_{yh}^2 - 2B_c S_{yxh} + B_c^2 S_{xh}^2),$$

where

$$B_c = \frac{\sum_h W_h^2(1 - f_h)S_{yxh}/n_h}{\sum_h W_h^2(1 - f_h)S_{xh}^2/n_h}.$$

Similarly, the estimated variances can be obtained by replacing population values by the corresponding sample values.

11.6. Unequal Probability Sampling with Replacement[1,4]

Equal probability sampling is very convenient to implement and simple in data processing. Its significant characteristic is that each unit of population is treated equally. But this equal treatment is unreasonable when there are great differences among the population units. One solution is to use sampling with unequal probabilities. Unequal probability sampling with replacement is the easiest sampling with unequal probabilities, and it is defined as follows: n units are taken with replacement from the population of size N such that the probability of the ith unit being selected in each sampling is $Z_i, i = 1, \ldots, N, \sum_{i=1}^{N} Z_i = 1$.

The usual selection of the probability Z_i is such that it is proportional to the corresponding unit size, i.e. $Z_i = M_i/M_0$, where M_i is the size or scale of the ith unit, and $M_0 = \sum_{i=1}^{N} M_i$. Such an unequal probability sampling with replacement is called the sampling with probability proportional to size and with replacement, or PPS sampling with replacement for short.

In general, code method is used when implementing unequal probability sampling with replacement: For given sampling probability $Z_i(i = 1, 2, \ldots, N)$, select an integer M_0 such that all of $M_i = M_0 Z_i$ are integers, then give the ith unit M_i codes. Specifically, the first unit has codes $1 \sim M_1$, the second unit has codes $M_1 + 1 \sim M_1 + M_2, \ldots$, the ith unit has codes $\sum_{j=1}^{i-1} M_j + 1 \sim \sum_{j=1}^{i} M_j, \ldots$, and the last unit has codes $\sum_{j=1}^{N-1} M_j + 1 \sim M_0$ $(= \sum_{j=1}^{N} M_j)$. A random integer, say m, is generated from $[1, M_0]$ in each sampling, then the unit having code m is selected in this sampling. n sample units can be drawn by repeating this procedure n times.

We can also use the Lahiri method: Let M_i be the same as defined in code method, and $M^* = \max_{1 \le i \le N}\{M_i\}$. First, a pair of integers i and m are selected from $[1, N]$ and $[1, M^*]$, respectively. Then the ith unit is included in the sample if $M_i \ge m$; otherwise, a new pair (i, m) is selected. Repeat this process until n sample units are drawn.

Suppose $y_1, y_2, \ldots, y_n$ are n sample observations, then the following Hansen–Hurwitz estimator is the unbiased estimator of the population total Y: $\hat{Y}_{\mathrm{HH}} = \frac{1}{n}\sum_{i=1}^{n} \frac{y_i}{z_i}$. Its variance is

$$V(\hat{Y}_{\mathrm{HH}}) = \frac{1}{n}\sum_{i=1}^{N} Z_i \left(\frac{Y_i}{Z_i} - Y\right)^2.$$

The unbiased estimator of $V(\hat{Y}_{\mathrm{HH}})(n > 1)$ is given by

$$v(\hat{Y}_{\mathrm{HH}}) = \frac{1}{n(n-1)}\sum_{i=1}^{n} \left(\frac{y_i}{z_i} - \hat{Y}_{\mathrm{HH}}\right)^2.$$

11.7. Unequal Probability Sampling without Replacement[1,4]

The same unit is likely to be repeatedly selected when using unequal probability sampling with replacement, and it is intuitively unnecessary to repeatedly investigate the same units, so unequal probability sampling without replacement is more efficient and attractive in practice.

Similar to unequal probability sampling with replacement which needs to consider the sampling probability Z_i in each sampling, unequal probability sampling without replacement needs to consider the probability of each unit being included in the sample, say π_i. In addition, the probability of any two units being included in the sample, say π_{ij}, also needs to be considered. The most common situation is to let π_i be in proportion to the corresponding unit size, i.e. $\pi_i = nZ_i$, where $Z_i = M_i/M_0$ with M_i being the size of the ith unit and $M_0 = \sum_{i=1}^N M_i$. Such an unequal probability sampling without replacement is called the sampling with inclusion probabilities proportional to size, or πPS sampling for short.

It is not easy to implement πPS sampling or make $\pi_i = nZ_i$. For $n = 2$, we can use the following two methods:

(1) Brewer method: The first unit is selected with probability proportional to $\frac{Z_i(1-Z_i)}{1-2Z_i}$, and the second unit is selected from the remaining $N-1$ units with probability proportional to Z_j.
(2) Durbin method: The first unit is selected with probability Z_i, and let the selected unit be unit i; the second unit is selected with probability proportional to $Z_j(\frac{1}{1-2Z_i} + \frac{1}{1-2Z_j})$.
These two methods require $Z_i < \frac{1}{2}$ for each i.

If $n > 2$, the following three methods can be used:

(1) Brewer method: The first unit is selected with probability proportional to $\frac{Z_i(1-Z_i)}{1-nZ_i}$, and the rth ($r \geq 2$) unit is selected from the units not included in the sample with probability proportional to $\frac{Z_i(1-Z_i)}{1-(n-r+1)Z_i}$;
(2) Midzuno method: The first unit is selected with probability $Z_i^* = \frac{n(N-1)Z_i}{N-n} - \frac{n-1}{N-n}$, and then $n-1$ units are selected from the remaining $N-1$ units by using simple random sampling;
(3) Rao–Sampford method: The first unit is selected with probability Z_i, then $n-1$ units are selected with probability proportional to $\lambda_i = \frac{Z_i}{1-nZ_i}$ and with replacement. All of the units which have been selected would be omitted once there are units being repeatedly selected, and new units are drawn until n different units are selected.

For unequal probability sampling without replacement, we generally use the Horvitz–Thompson estimator to estimate the population total Y: $\hat{Y}_{\mathrm{HT}} = \sum_{i=1}^n \frac{y_i}{\pi_i}$. It is unbiased and its variance is

$$\mathrm{V}(\hat{Y}_{\mathrm{HT}}) = \sum_{i=1}^N \frac{1-\pi_i}{\pi_i} Y_i^2 + 2\sum_{i=1}^N \sum_{j>i}^N \frac{\pi_{ij} - \pi_i\pi_j}{\pi_i\pi_j} Y_i Y_j.$$

An unbiased variance estimator of $\hat{Y}_{\mathrm{HT}}$ is given by

$$v(\hat{Y}_{\mathrm{HT}}) = \sum_{i=1}^{n} \frac{1-\pi_i}{\pi_i^2} y_i^2 + 2\sum_{i=1}^{n}\sum_{j>i}^{n} \frac{\pi_{ij}-\pi_i\pi_j}{\pi_i\pi_j\pi_{ij}} y_i y_j.$$

In the above formulas, we naturally assume $\pi_i > 0, \pi_{ij} > 0, i \neq j$.

11.8. Double Sampling[1,3]

In practical surveys, we often require the auxiliary information of population to obtain samples and/or perform data processing. For example, the information of the size of each unit is needed when implementing unequal probability sampling, the stratum weight is required to know when implementing weighted estimation and so on. When there is lack of the required auxiliary information, we can select a large sample to obtain such information, and then select a small sample from the large sample to investigate the target variable of interest. This is the idea of double sampling.

(1) Double stratified sampling: A large sample of size n' (the first phase sample) is drawn from the population by using simple random sampling. Let n'_h denote the number of units in the hth stratum, then $w'_h = \frac{n'_h}{n'}$ is the unbiased estimator of the stratum weight $W_h = N_h/N$. A small sample of size n (the second phase sample) is then drawn from the large sample by using stratified random sampling to conduct main investigation.

Let y_{hj} denote the jth-unit observation from stratum h of the second phase sample, and $\bar{y}_h = \frac{1}{n_h}\sum_{j=1}^{n_h} y_{hj}$ be the sample mean of stratum h. Then the estimator of the population mean $\bar{Y}$ is $\bar{y}_{\mathrm{stD}} = \sum_{h=1}^{L} w'_h \bar{y}_h$. It is unbiased and its variance is

$$\mathrm{V}(\bar{y}_{\mathrm{stD}}) = \left(\frac{1}{n'} - \frac{1}{N}\right) S^2 + \sum_h \frac{W_h S_h^2}{n'}\left(\frac{1}{v_h} - 1\right),$$

where S^2 and S_h^2 are the population variance and the variance of stratum h, respectively, v_h denotes the sampling fraction of stratum h, and n_h is the sample size of stratum h.

A nearly unbiased variance estimator of $\bar{y}_{\mathrm{stD}}$ is given by

$$v(\bar{y}_{\mathrm{stD}}) = \sum_h \left(\frac{1}{n_h} - \frac{1}{n'_h}\right) w_h'^2 s_h^2 + \left(\frac{1}{n'} - \frac{1}{N}\right) \sum_h w'_h (\bar{y}_h - \bar{y}_{\mathrm{stD}})^2,$$

where s_h^2 is the variance of stratum h of the second phase sample.

(2) Ratio estimator and regression estimator for double sampling: We investigate only the auxiliary variable in the first phase sampling, and let $\bar{x}'$ denote

the sample mean; then we investigate the target variable of interest in the second phase sampling, and let $\bar{y}$ denote the sample mean. Accordingly, $\bar{x}$ denotes the mean of auxiliary variable of the second phase sample.

Double ratio estimator: $\bar{y}_{RD} = \frac{\bar{y}}{\bar{x}}\bar{x}' \hat{=} \hat{R}\bar{x}'$. It is nearly unbiased, and its variance is

$$\mathrm{V}(\bar{y}_{RD}) \approx \left(\frac{1}{n'} - \frac{1}{N}\right) S_y^2 + \left(\frac{1}{n} - \frac{1}{n'}\right)(S_y^2 + R^2 S_x^2 - 2RS_{yx}),$$

where $R = \bar{Y}/\bar{X}$. The estimated variance of $\bar{y}_{RD}$ is

$$v(\bar{y}_{RD}) = \frac{s_y^2}{n} + \left(\frac{1}{n} - \frac{1}{n'}\right)(\hat{R}^2 s_x^2 - 2\hat{R}s_{yx}),$$

where s_y^2, s_x^2, and s_{yx} are the variances and covariance of the second phase sample, respectively.

Double regression estimator: $\bar{y}_{lrD} = \bar{y} + b(\bar{x}' - \bar{x})$, where b is the regression coefficient based on the second phase sample. $\bar{y}_{lrD}$ is nearly unbiased, and its variance is

$$\mathrm{V}(\bar{y}_{lrD}) \approx \left(\frac{1}{n'} - \frac{1}{N}\right) S_y^2 + \left(\frac{1}{n} - \frac{1}{n'}\right) S_y^2(1 - \rho^2).$$

The estimated variance of $\bar{y}_{lrD}$ is

$$v(\bar{y}_{lrD}) \approx \left(\frac{1}{n'} - \frac{1}{N}\right) s_y^2 + \left(\frac{1}{n} - \frac{1}{n'}\right) s_y^2(1 - r^2),$$

where r is the correlation coefficient of the second phase sample.

11.9. Successive Sampling[1,3]

In practice, the successive sampling conducted at different time points is required in order to obtain current information and understand the trend of change of population. For convenience, a fixed sample is often utilized for the successive sampling, this is so-called panel survey. However, repeatedly investigating a fixed sample can lead to many problems differing from common surveys. A main problem is that repeated investigation is likely to make respondents bored and so unwilling to actively cooperate or offer untrue answers carelessly, in other words, it would produce the sample aging or the sample fatigue; on the other hand, the target population would change over time, so the long-term fixed sample could not represent the changed population very well.

Sample rotation is a method of overcoming the sample aging and retaining the advantage of panel surveys. With this method, a portion of sample units are replaced at regular intervals and the remaining units are retained.

Here, we consider the successive sampling on two occasions. Suppose simple random sampling is used on each occasion, and the sample size is n. m units which are drawn from the sample on the previous occasion are surveyed on the current occasion (such units are called the matched sample units), and $u = n - m$ new units drawn from $N - n$ units which are not selected on the previous occasion are surveyed on the current occasion (such units are called the rotation or unmatched sample units). Obviously, there are observations of the matched sample units on both occasions. We let $\bar{y}_{1m}$ and $\bar{y}_{2m}$ be the sample means on the previous and current occasions, respectively, $\bar{y}_{2u}$ be the mean of the u rotation sample units on the current occasion, and $\bar{y}_{1n}$ be the mean of the n units on the previous occasion.

For the m matched sample units, the previous observations can be considered as the auxiliary information, and so we can construct the double regression estimator of $\bar{Y}$: $\bar{y}'_{2m} = \bar{y}_{2m} + b(\bar{y}_{1n} - \bar{y}_{1m})$; for the rotation sample units, the estimator of $\bar{Y}$ is $\bar{y}'_{2u} = \bar{y}_{2u}$. A natural idea is to use their weighted mean: $\bar{y}'_2 = \varphi\bar{y}'_{2u} + (1-\varphi)\bar{y}'_{2m}$, where ϕ is weight. Clearly, the optimal weight is given by $\varphi = \frac{V_m}{V_u+V_m}$ with the finite population correction being ignored, where

$$V_m \triangleq \mathrm{V}(\bar{y}'_{2m}) = \frac{S_2^2(1-\rho^2)}{m} + \frac{\rho^2 S_2^2}{n},$$

$$V_u \triangleq \mathrm{V}(\bar{y}'_{2u}) = \frac{S_2^2}{u},$$

S_2^2 denotes the population variance on the current occasion, and ρ denotes the population correlation coefficient between the two occasions. The corresponding variance of $\bar{y}'_2$ is

$$V(\bar{y}'_2) = \frac{V_u V_m}{V_u + V_m} = \frac{n - u\rho^2}{n^2 - u^2\rho^2} S_2^2.$$

Therefore, the optimal rotation fraction is $\frac{u}{n} = \frac{1}{1+\sqrt{1-\rho^2}}$. Obviously, the bigger the ρ, the more the rotation units. With the optimal rotation fraction, the variance of $\bar{y}'_2$ is given by

$$\mathrm{V}_{\mathrm{opt}}(\bar{y}'_2) = \frac{1+\sqrt{1-\rho^2}}{2n} S_2^2.$$

11.10. Cluster Sampling[1,3]

Population is divided into a number of large units or groups of small units called clusters. Cluster sampling is the sampling method that some clusters are selected in a certain way and all the small units included in the selected clusters are surveyed. Compared with simple random sampling, cluster sampling is cheaper because the small sample units within a cluster are gathered relatively and so it is convenient to survey; also, the sampling frame of units within a cluster is not required. However, in general, the efficiency of cluster sampling is relatively low because the units in the same cluster are often similar to each other and it is unnecessary to investigate all the units in the same cluster intuitively. So, for cluster sampling, the division of clusters should make the within-cluster variance as large as possible and the between-cluster variance as small as possible.

Let $Y_{ij}(y_{ij})$ denote the j-th unit value from cluster i of population (sample), $i = 1, \ldots, N, j = 1, \ldots, M_i(m_i)$, where $M_i(m_i)$ denotes the size of cluster i of population (sample); and let $M_0 = \sum_{i=1}^{N} M_i$. In order to estimate the population total $Y = \sum_{i=1}^{N} \sum_{j=1}^{M_i} Y_{ij} \equiv \sum_{i=1}^{N} Y_i$, the clusters can be selected by using simple random sampling or directly using unequal probability sampling.

(1) Select clusters by using simple random sampling

In this case, we should use the ratio estimator: $\hat{Y}_R = M_0 \hat{\bar{\bar{Y}}}_R \equiv M_0 \frac{\sum_{i=1}^{n} y_i}{\sum_{i=1}^{n} m_i}$, where $y_i = \sum_{j=1}^{m_i} y_{ij}$. It is nearly unbiased and its variance is

$$V(\hat{Y}_R) \approx \frac{N^2(1-f)}{n} \frac{\sum_{i=1}^{N} M_i^2 (\bar{Y}_i - \bar{\bar{Y}})^2}{N-1},$$

where $\bar{Y}_i = \sum_{j=1}^{M_i} Y_{ij}/M_i, \bar{\bar{Y}} = \sum_{i=1}^{N} \sum_{j=1}^{M_i} Y_{ij}/M_0$.

The estimated variance of $\hat{Y}_R$ is

$$v(\hat{Y}_R) = \frac{N^2(1-f)}{n} \frac{1}{n-1} \left(\sum_{i=1}^{n} y_i^2 + \hat{\bar{\bar{Y}}}_R^2 \sum_{i=1}^{n} m_i^2 - 2\hat{\bar{\bar{Y}}}_R \sum_{i=1}^{n} m_i y_i \right).$$

When $M_1 = M_2 = \cdots = M_N = M$, the variance of $\hat{Y}_R$ reduces to

$$V(\hat{Y}_R) \approx \frac{N^2 M(1-f)}{n} S^2 [1 + (M-1)\rho_c],$$

where ρ_c is the intra-class correlation coefficient. Note that if nM small units are directly drawn from the population by using simple random sampling, the variance of the corresponding estimator $\hat{Y}$ of the population total is

$$V_{\text{ran}}(\hat{Y}) = \frac{N^2 M(1-f)}{n} S^2.$$

So the design effect of cluster sampling is

$$\text{deff} \equiv \frac{V(\hat{Y}_R)}{V_{\text{ran}}(\hat{Y})} \approx 1 + (M-1)\rho_c.$$

(2) Select clusters by using unequal probability sampling

A more effective way is to select clusters by using unequal probability sampling with probability proportional to cluster size, i.e. PPS sampling with replacement or πPS sampling without replacement, and the corresponding estimators are the Hansen–Hurwitz estimator and Horvitz–Thompson estimator, respectively.

11.11. Equal Probability Systematic Sampling[5,6]

Systematic sampling is a sampling technique to select random numbers from the specified range after placing the population units in order, and then determine the sample units by a certain rule. The most significant advantages of systematic sampling are its convenience in implementing, and its simplicity in the requirement for sampling frame. The disadvantage of systematic sampling is its difficulty in estimating the variance of estimator.

The simplest systematic sampling is the equal interval sampling, which is a kind of equal probability systematic sampling. When the N population units are ordered on a straight line, the equal interval sampling is conducted as follows: determine an integer k which is the integer closest to N/n with n being the sample size; select an integer r at random from the range of 1 to k; and then the units $r + (j-1)k, j = 1, 2, \ldots, n$ are selected. k is called the sampling interval.

Let $N = nk$, then the population can be arranged in the form of Table 11.11.1, where the top row denotes random starting points, and the leftmost column denotes sample units and mean. Obviously, a systematic sample is just constituted with a column in the table. It is also observed

Table 11.11.1. k systematic samples when $N = nk$.

	1	2	$\cdots$	r	$\cdots$	k
1	Y_1	Y_2	$\cdots$	Y_r	$\cdots$	Y_k
2	Y_{k+1}	Y_{k+2}	$\cdots$	Y_{k+r}	$\cdots$	Y_{2k}
$\vdots$	$\vdots$	$\vdots$	$\vdots$	$\vdots$	$\vdots$	$\vdots$
n	$Y_{(n-1)k+1}$	$Y_{(n-1)k+2}$	$\cdots$	$Y_{(n-1)k+r}$	$\cdots$	Y_{nk}
mean	$\bar{y}_1$	$\bar{y}_2$	$\cdots$	$\bar{y}_r$	$\cdots$	$\bar{y}_k$

that systematic sampling can be regarded as a kind of cluster sampling if we consider the column as the cluster, and a kind of stratified sampling if we take the row as the stratum.

Let $y_1, y_2, \ldots, y_n$ denote the systematic sample observations in the order they appear in the population, then the estimator of the population mean $\bar{Y}$ is $\bar{y}_{sy} = \frac{1}{n}\sum_{i=1}^{n} y_i$. It is unbiased and its variance is

$$V(\bar{y}_{sy}) = \frac{1}{k}\sum_{r=1}^{k}(\bar{y}_r - \bar{Y})^2.$$

It can also be expressed as

$$V(\bar{y}_{sy}) = \frac{S^2}{n}\left(\frac{N-1}{N}\right)[1 + (n-1)\rho_{\text{wsy}}],$$

where ρ_{wsy} denotes the intra-sample (cluster) correlation coefficient. We can use the following methods to estimate the variance of $\bar{y}_{sy}$:

$$v_1 = \frac{1-f}{n}s^2 = \frac{N-n}{Nn}\frac{1}{n-1}\sum_{i=1}^{n}(y_i - \bar{y}_{sy})^2.$$

This estimator is obtained by treating the systematic sample as the simple random sample;

$$v_2 = \frac{1-f}{n}\frac{1}{n}\sum_{i=1}^{n/2}(y_{2i} - y_{2i-1})^2,$$

where n is an even number. Let two sample observations y_{2i-1} and y_{2i} be a group and calculate their sample variance, then v_2 is obtained by averaging the sample variances of all groups and multiplying by $(1-f)/n$;

$$v_3 = \frac{1-f}{n}\frac{1}{2(n-1)}\sum_{i=2}^{n}(y_i - y_{i-1})^2.$$

Its construction method is similar to that of v_2, and the difference between them is that the group here is composed of each observation and the observation ahead of it.

Finally, for the population with periodic variation like department-store sales, we should be very careful in selecting the sampling interval, for example, the sampling interval should not be the integral multiple of the variation period.

11.12. Unequal Probability Systematic Sampling[5,6]

Let π_i denote the inclusion probability that satisfies $\sum_{i=1}^{N} \pi_i = n$. A random number is selected from the interval $[0,1]$, say r, then the i_0th, i_1th, $\ldots, i_{n-1}$th units of population are selected as the sample units when $\sum_{j=1}^{i_k-1} \pi_j < r+k, \sum_{j=1}^{i_k} \pi_j \geq r+k, k=0,1,\ldots,n-1$. Such sampling is called unequal probability systematic sampling. This sampling is a kind of sampling without replacement, and the randomness of sample is fully reflected in the selection of r. So it has the advantages of high accuracy of unequal probability sampling without replacement and convenience in implementing.

In practice, the most common unequal probability systematic sampling is systematic sampling with inclusion probabilities proportional to size, or πPS systematic sampling for short, i.e. π_i is proportional to the unit size M_i: $\pi_i = nM_i/M_0 \equiv nZ_i$, where $M_0 = \sum_{i=1}^{N} M_i$.

In general, unequal probability systematic sampling is conducted by using code method. For πPS systematic sampling, for example, the implementation method is as follows: accumulate M_i first, and select the codes every $k = \frac{M_0}{n}$ with the unit r selected randomly from $(0, \frac{M_0}{n}]$ as the starting unit, then the units corresponding to the codes $r, r+k, \ldots, r+(n-1)k$ are sample units (if k is an integer, then the random number r can be selected from the range of 1 to k).

Let $y_1, y_2, \ldots, y_n$ denote the systematic sample observations in the order they appear in the population, then the estimator of the population mean $\bar{Y}$ is $\hat{Y}_{\mathrm{HT}} = \sum_{i=1}^{n} \frac{y_i}{\pi_i}$. It is unbiased and its variance is

$$\mathrm{V}(\hat{Y}_{\mathrm{HT}}) = \sum_{i=1}^{N} \frac{1-\pi_i}{\pi_i} Y_i^2 + 2\sum_{i=1}^{N}\sum_{j>i}^{N} \frac{\pi_{ij}-\pi_i\pi_j}{\pi_i\pi_j} Y_i Y_j.$$

We can use the following methods to estimate the variance of $\hat{Y}_{\mathrm{HT}}$:

(1) $v_1' = \frac{1-\hat{f}}{n(n-1)} \sum_{i=1}^{n} \left(\frac{ny_i}{\pi_i} - \hat{Y}_{\mathrm{HT}}\right)^2$,
where $\hat{f} = \frac{1}{n}\sum_{i=1}^{n} \pi_i$, v_1' is obtained by treating the πPS systematic sample without replacement as the PPS sample with replacement and multiplying by the estimator of finite population correction $1-\hat{f}$;

(2) $v_2' = \frac{1-\hat{f}}{n}\frac{1}{n} \sum_{i=1}^{n/2} \left(\frac{ny_{2i}}{\pi_{2i}} - \frac{ny_{2i-1}}{\pi_{2i-1}}\right)^2$;

(3) $v_3' = \frac{1-\hat{f}}{n}\frac{1}{2(n-1)} \sum_{i=2}^{n} \left(\frac{ny_i}{\pi_i} - \frac{ny_{i-1}}{\pi_{i-1}}\right)^2$.

The ideas of constructing the two estimators are similar to those of constructing v_2 and v_3 in the equal probability systematic sampling (y_i is replaced by ny_i/π_i).

As regards the choice of estimated variances, generally speaking, for the population in a random order, $v_1'(v_1)$ is better; while $v_2'(v_2)$ and $v_3'(v_3)$ apply more broadly, especially to the population with linear trend.

11.13. Two-stage Sampling[3,5]

Suppose each unit of population (primary unit) includes several small units (secondary unit). For the selected primary units, not all but only part of the secondary units are surveyed, such sampling is called two-stage sampling. Two-stage sampling has the advantages of cluster sampling that the samples are relatively concentrated and so the investigation is convenient, and the sampling frames on the secondary units are needed only for those selected primary units. Also, two-stage sampling has high sampling efficiency because only part of the secondary units are surveyed.

For two-stage sampling, the estimator of target variable can be obtained stage by stage, i.e. the estimator constructed by the secondary units is treated as the "true value" of the corresponding primary unit, then the estimator of target variable of population is constructed by these "true values" of primary units.

(1) The first-stage sampling is the unequal probability sampling with replacement

Let Z_i denote the probability of selecting the primary units in the first-stage sampling. If the i-th primary unit is selected, then m_i secondary units are selected from this primary unit. Note that if a primary unit is repeatedly selected, those secondary units selected in the second-stage sampling need to be replaced, and then select m_i new secondary units.

In order to estimate the population total Y, we can estimate the total Y_i of each selected primary unit first, and treat the estimator $\hat{Y}_i$ (suppose it is unbiased and its variance is $\mathrm{V}_2(\hat{Y}_i)$) as the true value of the corresponding primary unit, then estimate Y based on the primary sample units: $\hat{Y}_{\mathrm{HH}} = \frac{1}{n}\sum_{i=1}^{n}\frac{\hat{Y}_i}{z_i}$. This estimator is unbiased and its variance is

$$\mathrm{V}(\hat{Y}_{\mathrm{HH}}) = \frac{1}{n}\left[\sum_{i=1}^{N} Z_i\left(\frac{Y_i}{Z_i} - Y\right)^2 + \sum_{i=1}^{N}\frac{\mathrm{V}_2(\hat{Y}_i)}{Z_i}\right].$$

The variance of $\hat{Y}_{\mathrm{HH}}$ consists of two parts, and in general, the first term from the first-stage sampling is the dominant term. An unbiased estimator of $V(\hat{Y}_{\mathrm{HH}})$ is

$$v(\hat{Y}_{\mathrm{HH}}) = \frac{1}{n(n-1)}\sum_{i=1}^{n}\left(\frac{\hat{Y}_i}{z_i} - \hat{Y}_{\mathrm{HH}}\right)^2.$$

We can observe that it has the same form as the estimator of single-stage sampling; in addition, the form of $v(\hat{Y}_{\mathrm{HH}})$ is irrelevant to the method used in the second-stage sampling.

(2) The first-stage sampling is the unequal probability sampling without replacement

Let π_i, π_{ij} denote the inclusion probabilities of the first-stage sampling. Similar to the sampling with replacement above, the estimator of the population total Y is $\hat{Y}_{\mathrm{HT}} = \sum_{i=1}^{n} \frac{\hat{Y}_i}{\pi_i}$. This estimator is unbiased and its variance is

$$V(\hat{Y}_{\mathrm{HT}}) = \sum_{i=1}^{N}\frac{1-\pi_i}{\pi_i}Y_i^2 + 2\sum_{i=1}^{N}\sum_{j\rangle i}^{N}\frac{\pi_{ij}-\pi_i\pi_j}{\pi_i\pi_j}Y_iY_j + \sum_{i=1}^{N}\frac{\mathrm{V}_2(\hat{Y}_i)}{\pi_i}.$$

Assuming that $v_2(\hat{Y}_i)$ is an unbiased estimator of $V_2(\hat{Y}_i)$, an unbiased estimator of $V(\hat{Y}_{\mathrm{HT}})$ is given by

$$v(\hat{Y}_{\mathrm{HT}}) = \sum_{i=1}^{n}\frac{1-\pi_i}{\pi_i^2}\hat{Y}_i^2 + 2\sum_{i=1}^{n}\sum_{j>i}^{n}\frac{\pi_{ij}-\pi_i\pi_j}{\pi_i\pi_j\pi_{ij}}\hat{Y}_i\hat{Y}_j + \sum_{i=1}^{n}\frac{v_2(\hat{Y}_i)}{\pi_i}.$$

11.14. Multi-stage Sampling[3,5]

Suppose population consists of N primary units, each primary unit consists of secondary units, and each secondary unit consists of third units. After the second-stage sampling, select the third units from the selected secondary units, and such sampling is called three-stage sampling; if we survey all the third units included in the selected secondary units, then such sampling is called two-stage cluster sampling. General multi-stage sampling or multi-stage cluster sampling can be defined similarly.

Like two-stage sampling, the estimator of target variable for multi-stage sampling can be obtained stage by stage, i.e. the estimator constructed by the next stage units is treated as the true value of their previous stage unit. In practical surveys, unequal probability sampling is often used in the first two or three stages sampling, and equal probability sampling or cluster sampling is used in the last stage sampling. On the other hand, when dealing with the data from unequal probability sampling without replacement, the formula of unequal probability sampling with replacement is often utilized to simplify the data processing. So here, we mainly discuss the situation where unequal probability sampling with replacement is used in the first two stages sampling. For the last stage sampling, we consider two cases:

(1) The third-stage sampling is the unequal probability sampling with replacement

Suppose the sample sizes of three-stage sampling are n, m_i and k_{ij}, respectively, and the probability of each unit being selected in each sampling is Z_i, Z_{ij} and Z_{iju} ($i = 1, \dots, N; j = 1, \dots, M_i; u = 1, \dots, K_{ij}$; and M_i denotes the size of primary unit, K_{ij} denotes the size of secondary unit), respectively. Let $Y_{iju}(y_{iju})$ denote the unit values of population (sample), then an unbiased estimator of the population total $Y = \sum_{i=1}^{N}\sum_{j=1}^{M_i}\sum_{u=1}^{K_{ij}} Y_{iju} \equiv \sum_{i=1}^{N} Y_i$ is

$$\hat{Y} = \frac{1}{n}\sum_{i=1}^{n}\frac{1}{z_i}\frac{1}{m_i}\sum_{j=1}^{m_i}\frac{1}{z_{ij}}\frac{1}{k_{ij}}\sum_{u=1}^{k_{ij}}\frac{y_{iju}}{z_{iju}}.$$

The variance of $\hat{Y}$ and its unbiased estimator are

$$\mathrm{V}(\hat{Y}) = \frac{1}{n}\left(\sum_{i=1}^{N}\frac{Y_i^2}{Z_i} - Y^2\right) + \frac{1}{n}\sum_{i=1}^{N}\frac{1}{Z_i}\frac{1}{m_i}\left(\sum_{j=1}^{M_i}\frac{Y_{ij}^2}{Z_{ij}} - Y_i^2\right)$$
$$+\frac{1}{n}\sum_{i=1}^{N}\frac{1}{Z_i}\left[\frac{1}{m_i}\sum_{j=1}^{M_i}\frac{1}{Z_{ij}}\frac{1}{k_{ij}}\left(\sum_{u=1}^{K_{ij}}\frac{Y_{iju}^2}{Z_{iju}} - Y_{ij}^2\right)\right]$$

and

$$v(\hat{Y}) = \frac{1}{n(n-1)}\sum_{i=1}^{n}(\hat{Y}_i - \hat{Y})^2,$$

respectively, where $Y_{ij} = \sum_{u=1}^{K_{ij}} Y_{iju}, \hat{Y}_i = \frac{1}{z_i m_i}\sum_{j=1}^{m_i}\frac{1}{z_{ij}}(\frac{1}{k_{ij}}\sum_{u=1}^{k_{ij}}\frac{y_{iju}}{z_{iju}})$.

(2) The third-stage sampling is the equal probability sampling

Suppose PPS sampling with replacement is used in the first two stages sampling, and simple random sampling with replacement is used in the last-stage sampling, then the estimator $\hat{Y}$ and its estimated variance are simplified as follows:

$$\hat{Y} = \frac{M_0}{n}\sum_{i=1}^{n}\frac{1}{m_i}\sum_{j=1}^{m_i}\frac{1}{k_{ij}}\sum_{u=1}^{k_{ij}} y_{iju} \equiv M_0\bar{\bar{y}},$$

$$v(\hat{Y}) = \frac{M_0^2}{n(n-1)}\sum_{i=1}^{n}(\bar{\bar{y}}_i - \bar{\bar{y}})^2,$$

where $M_0 = \sum_{i=1}^{N}\sum_{j=1}^{M_i} K_{ij}, \bar{\bar{y}}_i = \frac{1}{m_i}\sum_{j=1}^{m_i}\frac{1}{k_{ij}}\sum_{u=1}^{k_{ij}} y_{iju}$.

If simple random sampling without replacement is used in the last stage sampling, the above formulas on $\hat{Y}$ and $v(\hat{Y})$ still hold.

11.15. Variance Estimation for Complex Surveys[6]

In practical survey sampling, the sampling method adopted is generally a combination of various basic sampling methods, thus there is a difficulty in estimating variance due to the complex surveys, and the variance estimator is often complicated even if it can be given, especially when nonlinear estimator is adopted. The methods for dealing with the variance estimation of complex surveys mainly include random group method, balanced half-sample method, Jackknife method (bootstrap method), and Taylor series method. As random group method is the basis for balanced half-sample method and Jackknife method, and Taylor series method used for the linearization of nonlinear estimator cannot be applied by itself, we introduce only random group method.

The idea of random group method is to select two or more samples from population by using the same sampling method, and construct the estimator of target variable of population for each sample, then calculate the variance based on the difference between these estimators or between these estimators and the estimator using the whole sample. In practice, the selected sample is generally divided into several subsamples or groups, and the variance estimator can be constructed by the estimators based on these subsamples and the whole sample. We consider two cases:

(1) Independent random groups

If the selected sample is put back each time, then the random groups are independent. The implementation process is as follows: (a) Select the sample S_1 from the population using a certain sampling method; (b) After the first sample S_1 is selected, put it back to the population, and then select the sample S_2 using the same way as (a); (c) Repeat the process until k samples $S_1, \ldots, S_k$ are selected. The k samples are called random groups.

For each random group, an estimator of the population target variable θ is constructed in the same way and denoted by $\hat{\theta}_\alpha (\alpha = 1, \ldots, k)$. Then the random group estimator of θ is $\hat{\hat{\theta}} = \frac{1}{k}\sum_{\alpha=1}^{k}\hat{\theta}_\alpha$. If $\hat{\theta}_\alpha$ is assumed to be unbiased, then $\hat{\hat{\theta}}$ is also unbiased. An unbiased variance estimator of $\hat{\hat{\theta}}$ is $v(\hat{\hat{\theta}}) = \frac{1}{k(k-1)}\sum_{\alpha=1}^{k}(\hat{\theta}_\alpha - \hat{\hat{\theta}})^2$.

Based on the combined sample of k random groups, we can also construct an estimator $\hat{\theta}$ of θ in the same way as $\hat{\theta}_\alpha$. For the variance estimation of $\hat{\theta}$, the following two estimators can be used:

$$v_1(\hat{\theta}) = v(\hat{\hat{\theta}}), \quad v_2(\hat{\theta}) = \frac{1}{k(k-1)} \sum_{\alpha=1}^{k} (\hat{\theta}_\alpha - \hat{\theta})^2.$$

(2) Dependent random groups

In practical surveys, the sample is usually drawn from the population all at once. In this case, the random groups can be obtained only by dividing the sample into several groups randomly. Thus, random groups are not independent. In order to get a good random group estimator, the division of random groups must follow the following basic principle: Each random group is required to have the same sampling structure as the original sample in nature. After the random groups are obtained, the estimator can be constructed in the same way as independent random group situation.

11.16. Non-sampling Error[7]

In survey sampling, because only part of population units is investigated, an estimation error is unavoidable. The error caused by sampling is called sampling error. The error caused by other various reasons is called non-sampling error. Non-sampling error can occur in each stage of surveys, and it mainly includes the following three types:

(1) Frame error: The error is caused by the incomplete sampling frame (i.e. the list for sampling does not perfectly correspond to the target population) or the incorrect information from sampling frame. The causes of the error include: some units of target population are missing (zero to one, i.e. no units in the sampling frame correspond to these units in target population), some units of non-target population are included (one even many to zero), multiplicity problems (one to many, many to one or many to many), and data aging of sampling frame and so on.

It is generally difficult to find the error caused by the first reason (i.e. the missingness of the units of target population), while the influence of such an error is great. One solution is to find the missing units by linking these units and the units of sampling population in some way; another solution is to use multiple sampling frames, i.e. use two or more sampling frames such as list frame and region frame, thus the flaw that one sampling frame cannot cover the whole target population can be overcome.

(2) Non-response error: The error is caused by non-response or incomplete information of the selected units. Non-response often has serious impact on the results. Unfortunately, in practical surveys, the non-response rate is on

the rise in recent years. A variety of reasons lead to non-response, such as respondents not being contacted, refusing to cooperate, and not being able to answer questions.

In order to reduce the non-response error, we should do our best to increase the response rate. In this regard, the following suggestions can be provided: (a) Strengthen the management of survey, try to get support from the related departments, give more publicity to the survey, and provide appropriate material reward; (b) Choose the investigators with responsibility and strong communication ability, and strengthen the training of investigators; (c) Revisit the respondents who have not responded, i.e. follow up the unanswered units. In addition, it is also important to improve the design of questionnaire.

No matter how we work hard, it is in general impossible to avoid non-response completely, so how to treat the survey data containing non-response is important. Here are some common methods: (a) Replace the missing sample units by others. We need to be very careful when using this method, and the following basic principle should be followed: The two should have similar characteristics; and replacement procedure should be determined before the survey. (b) Bias adjustment: Estimate the possible bias through the difference between respondents and non-respondents (for instance, the difference of auxiliary variables), and then adjust the estimate. (c) Weighting adjustment: Weighting adjustment to the survey data can be employed to correct the bias caused by non-response. (d) Resampling: The data of non-response subsample is obtained by resampling the non-response units. (e) Imputation: Use the appropriate estimates to impute the non-response data.

(3) Measurement error: The error is caused by the difference between the survey data and their true values. The causes of error include: the design of survey is not scientific enough, and the measurement tool is not accurate enough; the investigators have no strong professional ability and responsibility; the respondents cannot understand questions or remember their answers correctly, or offer untruthful answers purposely. One solution is to use the method of resampling adjustment (i.e. adjust the estimate based on the more accurate information from a selected subsample) besides the total quality control of the whole survey.

11.17. Survey on Sensitive Question[3,8]

Sensitive question is the question related to highly private secret such as drug addiction and tax evasion. If we investigate such questions directly, the respondents often refuse to cooperate or offer untruthful answers due to their misgivings. A method of eliminating respondents' worries is to use the randomized response technique, with the characteristic that the survey questions are randomly answered, or the answers to other questions are used to interfere with the true answer in order to protect respondents' privacy.

(1) Warner randomized response model

Randomized response technique was first proposed by S. L. Warner in 1965. Two questions are shown to the respondents: Question I: "Do you have the character A?"; Question II: "Don't you have the character A?". The answers to these two questions are "yes" or "no". Its magic lies in the fact that the respondents answer the first question with probability P, and answer the second question with probability $1-P$, i.e. answer one of the two questions randomly. This can be achieved by designing randomized device, and the specific operation is as follows:

The respondents are given a closed container with two kinds of identical balls except the color (red and white), and the ratio of red balls to white balls is $P\colon(1-P)$. Let the respondents draw a ball randomly from the container and answer Question I if a red ball is selected, answer Question II if a white ball is selected. Note that only the respondent himself/herself knows which question he/she answers, thus his/her privacy is effectively protected.

Suppose simple random sample with replacement of size n is selected, and there are m persons of them answering "yes"; Let π denote the proportion of the persons with the character A in population, then an unbiased estimator of π is

$$\hat{\pi} = \frac{1}{2P-1}\left[\frac{m}{n} - (1-P)\right],$$

where $P \neq 1/2$. The variance of $\hat{\pi}$ and its unbiased estimator are given by

$$V(\hat{\pi}) = \frac{\pi(1-\pi)}{n} + \frac{P(1-P)}{n(2P-1)^2}$$

and

$$v(\hat{\pi}) = \frac{\hat{\pi}(1-\hat{\pi})}{n-1} + \frac{P(1-P)}{(n-1)(2P-1)^2},$$

respectively.

(2) Simmons randomized response model

To eliminate respondents' misgivings further, Warner model was improved by W. R. Simmons as follows: Change the second question in

Warner model to a non-sensitive question which is irrelevant to the sensitive question A, i.e. Question II′: "Do you have the character B?". The operation is similar to that of Warner method: The proportion π_B of persons with the character B needs to be known, and the ratio of the two questions (i.e. red balls and white balls) is still $P\colon(1-P)$.

An unbiased estimator of π is

$$\hat{\pi}_A = \frac{1}{P}\left[\frac{m}{n} - (1-P)\pi_B\right].$$

The variance of $\hat{\pi}_A$ is

$$V(\hat{\pi}_A) = \frac{\pi_A(1-\pi_A)}{n} + \frac{(1-P)^2\pi_B(1-\pi_B)}{nP^2} + \frac{P(1-P)(\pi_A+\pi_B-2\pi_A\pi_B)}{nP^2}$$

and an unbiased estimator of $V(\hat{\pi}_A)$ is

$$v(\hat{\pi}_A) = \frac{1}{(n-1)P^2}\left(\frac{m}{n}\right)\left(1-\frac{m}{n}\right).$$

11.18. Small Area Estimation[9]

The subpopulation that consists of the units with special characteristics in population is called area. The area with small size is called small area. The estimation methods of area and small area have been widely applied in medical and health statistics (such as the investigation of diseases and symptoms) and other fields. It is difficult to estimate the target variable for small area because the sample size of small area is usually small or even zero. Traditionally, small area estimation is based mainly on sampling design, with the advantage that it is unrelated to specific model assumption, and so is robust to models. For the estimation of the area total Y_d, there are three main methods:

(1) Direct estimation: Estimate Y_d by using the area sample directly, and this method is suitable to the large area sample cases.

The most common direct estimator of Y_d is the Horvitz–Thompson estimator: $\hat{Y}_{d;HT} = \sum_{k\in s_d} y_k/\pi_k$, where π_k is the inclusion probability of unit k, and s_d denotes the sample of the d-th area.

Assuming that the total auxiliary information X_d (say p-dimensional) is known, and the auxiliary information x_k of each selected unit is feasible, the generalized regression estimator of Y_d can be used: $\hat{Y}_{d;\mathrm{GR}} = \hat{Y}_{d,\mathrm{HT}}+$

$(X_d - \hat{X}_{d,\mathrm{HT}})' \hat{B}_d$, where

$$\hat{B}_d = \left(\sum_{k\in s_d} \mathbf{x}_k \mathbf{x}'_k/(\pi_k c_k)\right)^{-1} \left(\sum_{k\in s_d} \mathbf{x}_k y_k/(\pi_k c_k)\right)$$

with c_k being a given constant.

(2) Synthetic estimation: It is an indirect estimation method, and the idea is to obtain the small area estimator with the assistance of the big population estimator due to lots of sample information from the big population. Here, there is an implicit assumption that the big population shares its characteristics with all small areas covered by itself. A common synthetic estimator is the regression synthetic estimator.

Use the same notations as (1), and let s denote the collection of all samples, and

$$\hat{B} = \left(\sum_{k\in s} \mathbf{x}_k \mathbf{x}'_k/\pi_k c_k\right)^{-1} \left(\sum_{k\in s} \mathbf{x}_k y_k/\pi_k c_k\right),$$

then the regression synthetic estimator is defined as follows: $\hat{Y}_{d;s} = X'_d \hat{B}$. It is nearly unbiased when each area has the characteristics similar to population.

(3) Composite estimation: It is a weighted mean of the direct estimator and synthetic estimator: $\hat{Y}_{d;\mathrm{com}} = \varphi_d \hat{Y}_d + (1-\varphi_d)\hat{Y}_{d;s}$, where $\hat{Y}_d$ denotes a direct estimator, $\hat{Y}_{d;s}$ denotes a synthetic estimator, and φ_d is the weight satisfying $0 \le \varphi_d \le 1$. Clearly, the role of φ_d is to balance the bias from synthetic estimation (the implicit assumption may not hold) and the variance from direct estimation (the area sample size is small). The optimal φ_d can be obtained by minimizing $\mathrm{MSE}(\hat{Y}_{d;\mathrm{com}})$ with respect to φ_d.

If the sum of mean square errors of all small area estimators is minimized with respect to a common weight φ, then James–Stein composite estimator is obtained. This method can guarantee the overall estimation effect of all small areas.

Another method for estimating the target variable of small area is based on statistical models. Such models establish a bridge between survey sampling and other branches of Statistics, and so various models and estimation methods of traditional Statistics can be applied to small area estimation.

11.19. Sampling for Rare Population[10,11]

Conventional sampling methods are hardly suitable for surveys of the population with rare features (such as aids, a rare gene, and rare medicinal herbs) because the units with these features in population are rare and so the probabilities of such units being selected are close to 0, or it is difficult to determine the required sample size in advance. For the sampling for rare population, the following methods can be used:

(1) Inverse sampling: Determine an integer m greater than 1 in advance, then select the units with equal probability one by one until m units with features of interest are selected.

For the population proportion P, an unbiased estimator is $\hat{P} = (m-1)/(n-1)$, and the unbiased variance estimator of $\hat{P}$ is given by

$$v(\hat{P}) = \frac{m-1}{n-1}\left[\frac{m-1}{n-1} - \frac{(N-1)(m-2)}{N(n-2)} - \frac{1}{N}\right].$$

(2) Adaptive cluster sampling: Adaptive cluster sampling method can be used when the units with features of interest are sparse and present aggregated distribution in population. The implementation of this method includes two steps: (a) Selection of initial sample: Select a sample of size n_1 by using a certain sampling method such as simple random sampling considered in this section; (b) Expansion of initial sample: Check each unit in the initial sample, and include the neighboring units of the sample units that meet the expansion condition; then continue to enlarge the neighboring units until no new units can be included.

The neighbourhood of a unit can be defined in many ways, such as the collection of the units within a certain range of this unit. The expansion condition is often defined as that the unit value is not less than a given critical value. In the unit collection expanded by an initial unit u, the unit subcollection satisfying the expansion condition is called a network; the unit which does not satisfy the expansion condition is called an edge unit. If unit u cannot be expanded, the unit itself is considered as a network. Let Ψ_k denote the network that unit k belongs to, m_k denote the number of units in Ψ_k, and $\bar{y}_k^* = \frac{1}{m_k}\sum_{j\in\Psi_k} y_j \equiv \frac{1}{m_k} y_k^*$.

The following two methods can be used to estimate the population mean $\overline{Y}$:

(i) Modified Hansen–Hurwitz estimator: $t_{\mathrm{HH}^*} = \frac{1}{n_1}\sum_{k=1}^{n_1} \bar{y}_k^*$. An unbiased variance estimator of t_{HH*} is

$$v(t_{\mathrm{HH}^*}) = \frac{N-n_1}{Nn_1}\frac{1}{n_1-1}\sum_{k=1}^{n_1}(\bar{y}_k^* - t_{\mathrm{HH}*})^2.$$

(ii) Modified Horvitz–Thompson estimator: $t_{\mathrm{HT}^*} = \frac{1}{N}\sum_{k=1}^{r}\frac{y_k J_k}{\pi_k}$, where r denotes the number of distinct units in the sample, J_k equals to 0 if the kth unit is an edge unit, and 1 otherwise, and $\pi_k = 1 - \binom{N-m_k}{n_1} \Big/ \binom{N}{n_1}$. An unbiased variance estimator of $t_{\mathrm{HT}*}$ is

$$v(t_{HT*}) = \frac{1}{N^2} \sum_{k=1}^{\gamma} \sum_{l=1}^{\gamma} \frac{y_k^* y_l^* (\pi_{kl} - \pi_k \pi_l)}{\pi_k \pi_l \pi_{kl}},$$

where γ denotes the number of distinct networks formed by the initial sample, and

$$\pi_{kl} = 1 - \left[\binom{N-m_k}{n_1} + \binom{N-m_l}{n_1} - \binom{N-m_k-m_l}{n_1}\right] \Big/ \binom{N}{n_1}.$$

11.20. Model-based Inference[12,13]

There are essentially two forms of statistical inferences in survey sampling: design-based inference and model-based inference. The former argues that each unit value in population is fixed, and the randomness is only from sample selection; the evaluation of inference is based on repeated sampling. This is the traditional inference method, and the methods introduced in previous sections of this chapter are based on this kind of inference method. The latter argues that the finite population is a random sample from a superpopulation, and the evaluation of inference is based on the superpopulation model.

In the framework of model-based inference, the estimation problem of the target variable of finite population actually becomes the prediction problem of the unsampled unit values, thus traditional statistical models and estimation methods are naturally applied to the inference of finite population. In recent decades, the application of statistical models in survey sampling has received much attention. Here is an example of model-based estimation.

Consider the following superpopulation model:

$$y_k = \beta x_k + \varepsilon_k, \quad k \in U \equiv \{1, \ldots, N\},$$

where x_k is a fixed auxiliary variable, the disturbances ε_k are mutually independent, and $E(\varepsilon_k) = 0, V(\varepsilon_k) = v(x_k)\sigma^2$, with $v(x_k)$ being a known function of x_k, σ^2 being an unknown parameter, and $E(V)$ denoting expectation (variance) with respect to the model.

Note that the finite population total Y can be divided into two parts: $Y = \sum_{k\in s} y_k + \sum_{k\in U\backslash s} y_k$, where $U\backslash s$ denotes the collection of the unsampled units, so in order to estimate Y, we need only to estimate $\sum_{k\in U\backslash S} y_k$. The estimation of $\sum_{k\in U\backslash S} y_k$ can be made by predicting $y_k (k \in U\backslash s)$ with the above model. Thus, the following estimator of Y is obtained:

$$\hat{Y}_m = \sum_{k\in s} y_k + \hat{\beta} \sum_{k\in U\setminus s} x_k$$

where $\hat{\beta} = \frac{\sum_{k\in s} y_k x_k/v(x_k)}{\sum_{k\in s} x_k^2/v(x_k)}$. As a special case, when $v(x_k) = x_k$, $\hat{Y}_m$ becomes the ratio estimator $(\bar{y}/\bar{x})X$. The construction of the above estimator totally depends on the model and is unrelated to the sampling design. In the framework of model-based inference, the model mean square error $E(\hat{Y}_m - Y)^2$ is usually used to evaluate the performance of $\hat{Y}_m$.

Another method of using statistical model is as follows: Construct the estimator of target variable of finite population with the help of model, but the evaluation of estimator is based only on sampling design, and unrelated to the model once the estimator is obtained. Such a method is known as model-assisted inference, which is essentially an inference form based on sampling design. In the framework of this inference, a general process of constructing estimator is as follows: Model parameters are estimated by using the whole finite population first, and we write the "estimator" as B; then by virtue of the "estimator" B and the model, the "estimator" $\hat{Y}$ of target variable of finite population is derived; finally, B is estimated by combining sampling design (B is unknown in fact because it depends on the whole finite population) and the corresponding estimator is inserted into $\hat{Y}$.

References

1. Feng, SY, Ni, JX, Zou, GH. *Theory and Method of Sample Survey.* (2nd edn.). Beijing: China Statistics Press, 2012.
2. Survey Skills project team of Statistics Canada. *Survey Skills Tutorials.* Beijing: China Statistics Press, 2002.
3. Cochran, WG. *Sampling Techniques.* (3rd edn.). New York: John Wiley & Sons, 1977.
4. Brewer, KRW, Hanif, M. *Sampling with Unequal Probabilities.* New York: Springer-Verlag, 1983.
5. Feng, SY, Shi, XQ. *Survey Sampling — Theory, Method and Practice.* Shanghai: Shanghai Scientific and Technological Publisher, 1996.
6. Wolter, KM. *Introduction to Variance Estimation.* New York: Springer-Verlag, 1985.
7. Lessler, JT, Kalsbeek, WD. *Nonsampling Error in Surveys.* New York: John Wiley & Sons, 1992.
8. Warner, SL. Randomized response: A survey technique for eliminating evasive answer bias. *J. Amer. Statist. Assoc.*, 1965, 60: 63–69.
9. Rao, JNK. *Small Area Estimation.* New York: John Wiley & Sons, 2003.
10. Singh, S. *Advanced Sampling Theory with Applications.* Dordrecht: Kluwer Academic Publisher, 2003.
11. Thompson, SK. Adaptive cluster sampling. *J. Amer. Statist. Assoc.*, 1990, 85: 1050–1059.

12. Royall, RM. On finite population sampling theory under certain linear regression models. *Biometrika*, 1970, 57: 377–387.
13. Sarndal, CE, Swensson, B, Wretman, JH. *Model Assisted Survey Sampling*. New York: Springer-Verlag, 1992.

About the Author

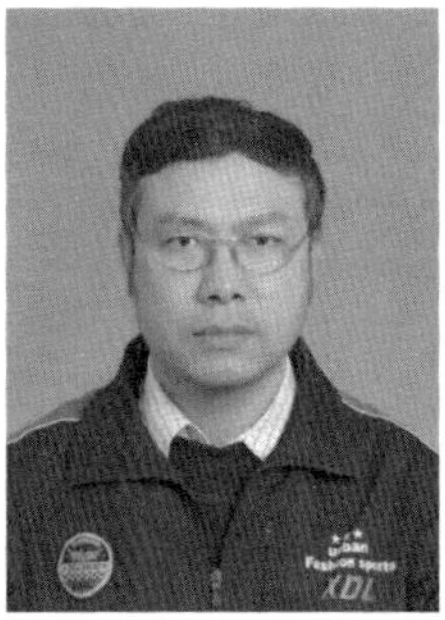

Guohua Zou is a Full Professor of School of Mathematical Sciences at the Capital Normal University, China. He got his Bachelor's degree in Mathematics from Jiangxi University in 1985, his Master's degree in Probability and Statistics from Jilin University in 1988, and PhD in Statistics from the Institute of Systems Science, Chinese Academy of Sciences in 1995.

Professor Zou is interested in developing statistical theory and methods to analyze practical economic, medical and genetic data. Special focuses are on design and data analysis in surveys, statistical model selection and averaging, and linkage and association studies between diseases and genes. He has published one book and more than 90 papers in leading international and national scholarly journals.

CHAPTER 12

CAUSAL INFERENCE

Zhi Geng*

12.1. Yule–Simpson paradox[1–2]

The association between two variables Y and T may be changed dramatically by the appearance of a third variable Z. Table 12.1.1 gives a numerical example.

In Table 12.1.1, we have the risk difference RD $= 80/200 - 100/200 = -0.10$, which means that "New drug" has no effect. But after we stratify the 400 patients by sex as shown in Table 12.1.2, we can see that RD $= 35/50 - 90/150 = +0.10$ for male and RD $= 45/150 - 10/50 = +0.10$ for female, which mean that "New drug" has effects for both male and female.

Table 12.1.1. "New drug" group and "Placebo" group.

	Recover	Unrecover	Total
New drug	80	120	200
Placebo	100	100	200

Table 12.1.2. Stratification by sex.

	Male		Female	
	Rec	Unrec	Rec	Unrec
New drug	35	15	45	105
Placebo	90	60	10	40

*Corresponding author: zhigeng@pku.edu.cn

Table 12.1.3. The number of UTI patients.

	Low UTI hospitals		High UTI hospitals		All hospitals	
AB-proph	UTI	No-UTI	UTI	No-UTI	UTI	No-UTI
Yes	20	1,093	22	144	42	1,237
No	5	715	99	1,421	104	2,136
	$RR_L = 2.6$		$RR_H = 2.0$		$RR = 0.7$	

The conclusions are reversed by omitting "sex". This is called Yule–Simpson paradox.[41,46] Such a factor "sex" which rises this phenomenon is called a confounder.

It makes an important issues: Is a statistical conclusion reliable? Are there any other factors (such as "age") which can change the conclusion? Is the conclusion more reliable if more factors are considered?

Reintjes *et al.*[38] gave an example from hospital epidemiology. A total of 3519 gynecology patients from eight hospitals in a non-experimental study were used to study the association between antibiotic prophylaxis (AB-proph.) and urinary tract infections (UTI). The eight hospitals were stratified into two groups with a low incidence percentage ($<2.5\%$) and a high percentage ($\geq 2.5\%$) of UTI. In Table 12.1.3, the relative risk (RR) was $(42/1279)/(104/2240) = 0.7$ for the overall eight hospitals, which means that AB-proph. had a protective effect on UTI. But the RRs were 2.6 and 2.0 for the low and the high incidence groups, respectively, which means that AB-proph. had a risk effect on UTI for both groups. The real effect of AB-proph. on UTI has been shown to be protective in randomized clinical trials, which is consistent with the crude analysis rather than the stratified analysis. This result explains that there were more unidentified confounders which canceled out their effects on each other in the crude analysis.

As pointed by Yule–Simpson paradox, we should select carefully which confounders need to be observed in observational and experimental studies. If some necessary confounders are omitted, the conclusion of data analysis may be unreliable.

12.2. Causal Models[3,4]

To define causal effects, Neyman[37] and Rubin[40] proposed the potential outcome model, also called the counterfactual model. They made the Stable Unit Treatment Value Assumption (SUTVA): for any unit i, its potential outcome is not affected by other units, and the potential outcome is unique for any treatment level. SUTVA assumption implies no interference, that is, any treatment accepted by a unit does not affect other units. Thus, the potential outcome of a unit i under an exposure level t can be denoted as $Y_t(i)$. Let Y denote the observed outcome. The observed variable $Y(i) = Y_t(i)$ if unit i was exposed to treatment t. Consider a binary treatment variable T (value 0 or 1). The individual causal effect of treatment T for individual i is defined as $\text{ICE}(i) = Y_1(i) - Y_0(i)$. For an individual i, we cannot usually obtain both $Y_1(i)$ and $Y_0(i)$, where the unobserved one is a counterfactual outcome. The average causal effect is defined as

$$\text{ACE}(T \to Y) = E[Y_1 - Y_0],$$

where $E[\,]$ denotes the expectation over the population. Without any other assumption, neither the individual causal effect nor the average causal effect is identifiable.

Fisher[33] proposed the randomized experiment that treatment T is randomly assigned. In a randomized experiment, treatment variable T is independent of any other covariate. Thus, T is independent of $Y_t(i)$, denoted as $T \perp Y_t(i)$. For a randomized trial, we have

$$\text{ACE}(T \to Y) = E[Y|T = 1] - E[Y|T = 0],$$

where $E[Y|T = t]$ denotes the expectation of observed variable Y in treatment group of $T = t$. This expectation is identifiable from observed data, that is, it can be expressed by distributions of observed variables. Thus, the average causal effect is identifiable for a randomized experiment.

In an observational study, the identifiability of causal effects requires other assumptions. Rosenbaum and Rubin[5] presented the assumption of the strongly ignorable treatment assignment. Let X denote an observed covariate vector. If the potential outcomes (Y_1, Y_0) are independent of treatment T conditionally on X (denoted as $(Y_1, Y_0) \perp T|X$) and $0 < P(T = 1|X = x) < 1$ for any x, then we say that given X, the assignment of treatment T is strongly ignorable. Under this assumption, the average causal effect can be represented as the expectation of observed variables: $\text{ACE}(T \to Y) = E\{E[Y|T = 1, X] - E[Y|T = 0, X]\}$, that is, the average causal effect is identifiable.

Pearl[4] made use of Bayesian networks and external intervention to explain causal relationships and causal effects, called causal networks. In a causal network, every node X_i denotes a variable, a directed arrow $X_i \to X_j$ denotes a causal relationship between cause X_i and effect X_j.

For the potential outcome model, the joint distribution of potential outcomes, say $f(y_1, y_0)$, is used to evaluate causal effects, and the causal relationships between all variables that are not considered. The causal network model describes the causal relationships among variables and makes use of intervention for breaking the paths between causes and effects to evaluate causal effects.

12.3. Confounders[6–7]

When evaluating the causal effect of an exposure or a treatment T on an outcome variable Y, a spurious statistical conclusion may be obtained due to omission of a third variable X, which is called a confounder (see Yule–Simpson paradox). There are two criteria for detecting whether a factor is a confounder or not: a collapsibility-based criterion and a comparability-based criterion.

Collapsibility-based criterion: A factor is not a confounder if the conditional association measure given by the factor equals the marginal association measure obtained by omitting the factor. For example, consider the RR of treatment T on outcome Y. The marginal relative risk RR by omitting sex X equals the conditional relative risk $\mathrm{RR}(x)$ given sex $X = x$, that is, $\mathrm{RR}(x) = \mathrm{RR}$. It means the RR is collapsible over sex X. But the collapsibility of the RR does not imply the collapsibility of the risk difference or odds ratio. Thus, the collapsibility-based criterion depends on what the association measure is used. On the other hand, an association measure is not a measure of causal effect, even if it is collapsible. It is because the conditional association measure given by X may not be used to measure a real cause effect.

Comparability-based criterion: A factor is not a confounder if the factor is identically distributed between the exposed and unexposed groups. For example, sex is not a confounder if the distribution of the sex in the smoking group is the same as that in non-smoking group.

In epidemiological studies, the following causal effect of the exposure on the exposed group is often interested:

$$\begin{aligned}\mathrm{ACE}(T \to Y|T = 1) &= E[Y_1 - Y_0|T = 1]\\ &= E(Y|T = 1) - E(Y_0|T = 1).\end{aligned}$$

The confounding bias is defined as the difference between the average causal effect and the risk difference:

$$\begin{aligned}B &= E[Y_1 - Y_0|T = 1] - [E(Y|T = 1) - E(Y|T = 0)]\\ &= E(Y|T = 0) - E(Y_0|T = 1).\end{aligned}$$

That is, it is the difference of the expectation of the observed outcome Y and that of potential outcome Y_0 in the exposed group. If the confounding bias $B \neq 0$ and the conditional confounding bias in every stratum $X = x$

$$B_x = E(Y_0|T = 1, x) - E(Y|T = 0, x) = 0,$$

then X is a confounder. That is, the confounding bias can be removed by the stratification with X. The strongly ignorable treatment assignment assumption $(Y_1, Y_0) \perp T|X$ and the weakly ignorable treatment assignment assumption $Y_0 \perp T|X$ mean that the variable set X is a sufficient confounder set.

In an observational study, it is critical to determine confounders. For a design of observational study, in order to avoid the results of spurious associations, we must determine which variables need to be observed and which need not. Greenland *et al.*[6] reviewed the criteria for confounders. Greenland *et al.*[7] described a causal network approach to detect confounders. Geng *et al.*[2] discussed the necessary and sufficient conditions for detecting confounders.

12.4. Collapsibility[6,8,9]

Let Y be a binary outcome, T be a binary exposure or treatment variable, and X a discrete variable with K values ($X = 1, \ldots, K$) denoting a background factor. Let $p_{\text{ijk}} = P(Y = i, T = j, X = k)$ denote a joint probability, $p_{\text{ij+}} = P(Y = i, T = j)$ denote a marginal probability and $p_{i|\text{jk}} = P(Y = i|T = j, X = k)$ denote a conditional probability. The RR of exposure T to outcome Y is denoted as

$$\text{RR}_+ = \frac{P(Y = 1|T = 1)}{P(Y = 1|T = 0)} = \frac{p_{1|1+}}{p_{1|0+}},$$

and the conditional RR given $X = k$ is denoted as

$$\text{RR}_k = \frac{p_{1|1k}}{p_{1|0k}}.$$

If all conditional RRs are the same (i.e. $\text{RR}_1 = \cdots = \text{RR}_K$), then we say that the RR is consistent. If all of them are equal to the marginal RR (i.e. $\text{RR}_+ = \text{RR}_k$), then we say that the RR is collapsible. If the RR,

$$\text{RR}_\omega = \frac{P(Y = 1|T = 1, X \in \omega)}{P(Y = 1|T = 0, X \in \omega)},$$

from any partial marginal table that is obtained by pooling any number of tables is equal to the marginal relative risk RR_+ (i.e. $\text{RR}_+ = \text{RR}_\omega$ for any subset ω of values of X), then we say that the RR is strongly collapsible. The necessary and sufficient condition for the strong collapsibility of the RR is that 1) Y and X are conditionally independent given T (denoted as

$Y \perp X|T$), or 2) T and X are independent ($T \perp X$) and the RRs are consistent. Similarly, we can define the collapsibilities of risk differences and odds ratios, although the conditions for their collapsibilities are different.

Now, consider the continuous outcome Y and T. For a discrete covariate X, let the model be

$$E(Y|t, x) = \alpha(x) + \beta(x)t.$$

When $\beta(x) = \beta(x')$ for all $x \neq x'$, the model is a parallel linear regression model. For a continuous covariate X, let the model be $E(Y|t, x) = \alpha + \beta t + \gamma x$. If the partial marginal regression model is

$$E(Y|t, x \in \omega) = \alpha(\omega) + \beta(\omega)t,$$

and $\beta(\omega) = \beta$ holds for any possible interval, then we say that the parameter β is uniformly collapsible over X. Particularly, we have $E(Y|t, x \in \omega) = E(Y|t) = \alpha' + \beta' t$ when ω is the full domain of X. If the marginal model holds and $\beta' = \beta$, then we say that the parameter β is simply collapsible over X. The necessary and sufficient condition for the uniform collapsibility of parameter β is (a) $\alpha(x) = \alpha(x')$ for the case of discrete $X, \gamma = 0$ for the case of continuous X or (b) the independence $T \perp X$ and $\beta(x) = \beta(x')$ for the case of discrete X.

For the logistic regression model, let Y be a binary outcome with value 0 or 1. The logistic regression model is

$$\log \frac{P(Y = 1|T = t, X = x)}{1 - P(Y = 1|T = t, X = x)} = \alpha(x) + \beta(x)t.$$

For a continuous X, let model be

$$\log \frac{P(Y = 1|T = t, X = x)}{1 - P(Y = 1|T = t, X = x)} = \alpha + \beta t + \gamma x.$$

If the partially marginal logistic regression model,

$$\log \frac{P(Y = 1|T = t, X \in \omega)}{1 - P(Y = 1|T = t, X \in \omega)} = \alpha(\omega) + \beta(\omega)t$$

holds and $\beta(\omega) = \beta$ for any ω, then we say that the parameter β is uniformly collapsible over X. The necessary and sufficient condition for the uniform collapsibility of β is (a) $Y \perp X|T$ or (b) $Y \perp T|X$.

12.5. Propensity Score[5]

The observed data in each stratum may be too sparse if they are stratified by a multi-value covariate or by a high-dimensional covariate vector. It reduces the efficiency of statistical inference. By use of the propensity score, the observed data can be stratified as crudely as possible such that there are as many data as possible in each stratum. Let T be a binary exposure variable and X be a discrete or continuous covariate. Let $b(X)$ be a function of X. If the conditional independence $T \perp X | b(X)$ holds, then $b(X)$ is defined as a balance score. It means that given the score $b(X) = c$, the treatment group and the control group have the same distribution of covariate X. According to the condition of confounders, we can know that omitting X cannot induce confounding bias conditionally on $b(X)$ if X is a sufficient confounder set. Thus, we only need to control for $b(X)$. The propensity score is defined as the conditional probability $f(X) = P(T = 1|X)$ which is a function of variable X. The propensity score is a balance score, that is, $T \perp X | f(X)$. The necessity and sufficient condition for that $b(X)$ is a balance score is $f(X) = g[b(X)]$. It means that $f(X)$ is the crudest balance score.

If the treatment assignment T is strongly ignorable conditionally on X, then it is also strongly ignorable conditionally on $b(X)$.

Let $b(X)$ be a balance score. Given $b(X) = b(x)$, the difference between the expectations of observed outcome for two groups is the average treatment effect conditionally on $b(X) = b(x)$, that is,

$$E(Y|b(x), T = 1] - E(Y|b(x), T = 0] = E[Y_1 - Y_0|b(x)].$$

The total average treatment effect $E(Y_1 - Y_0)$ can be obtained by finding the expectation over $b(X)$.

By use of balance scores, we can match the treated individuals and the control individuals or make pairs of them. First, we randomly draw x and calculate a balance score $b(x)$, and then randomly draw a treated individual ($T = 1$) and a control individual ($T = 0$) from the groups with the score value $b(x)$. Note that the expectation of the difference of the outcomes for the drawn pair is the average treatment effect conditioning on $b(x)$. Repeating the process, we can obtain the unbiased estimate of the total average treatment effect $E(Y_1 - Y_0)$.

Because the propensity score $f(X)$ is a function of X and is the crudest balance score, the strata obtained by the propensity score are the densest for all by other balance scores. For a continuous X, we can use a logistic regression model as the model of propensity score. The propensity scores are estimated by the observed data, and the estimated scores are used to stratify the sample. The estimated scores may be categorized into several levels (say five levels). To balance these strata, the levels of the categorization can be determined such that the numbers of individuals in all levels are almost the same.

12.6. Instrumental Variable[10–12]

The instrumental variable (IV) approach was presented by Durbin[11] for the parameter estimation of simple linear models with measurement errors. Now, it is being applied widely to econometrics (Heckman,[34]; Angrist *et al.*,[10]), epidemiology (Robins *et al.*,[39]) and so on. The IV approach is also applied to causal inference.

If there is an unobserved confounder which relates to both treatment T and outcome Y, then the causal effect of treatment T on outcome Y is not identifiable without any other assumption. Another way of evaluating the causal effect is the IV approach, in which it is crucial to find an IV Z. Assume that there is an unobserved confounder U and the assumption of the latent treatment assignment ignorability $(Y_1, Y_0) \perp T | U$ holds. We say that Z is an IV if Z relates to treatment T and is independent of $U (Z \perp U)$. By the independency of the IV Z and the confounder U, the causal effect of treatment T on outcome Y may be identifiable or partially identifiable.

In a randomized trial with non-compliance, the randomized treatment assignment Z is strongly associated to the really accepted treatment T, and it is independent of all covariates U, including all confounders. Further assume that the outcome Y depends only on the really accepted treatment T, but not on treatment assignment Z. For example, for a double blind trial, there is no psychological effect of treatment assignment Z on outcome Y. The causal network in Figure 12.6.1 describes the relationships among variables in randomized clinical trials with non-compliance. In such a network, treatment assignment Z satisfies the conditions of IV.

Generally, it is difficult to verify experimentally whether a covariate is an IV.

Consider a linear model $Y = \beta t + \gamma u + \varepsilon_Y$, where ε_Y is independent of other variables and $E(\varepsilon_Y) = 0$. Parameter β can be presented as $\beta = \mathrm{Cov}(Z, Y)/\mathrm{Cov}(Z, T)$, and thus its IV estimator is $\mathrm{Cov}'(Z, Y)/\mathrm{Cov}'(Z, T)$, where $\mathrm{Cov}(\cdot, \cdot)$ denotes covariance, and $\mathrm{Cov}'(\cdot, \cdot)$ denotes its estimator.

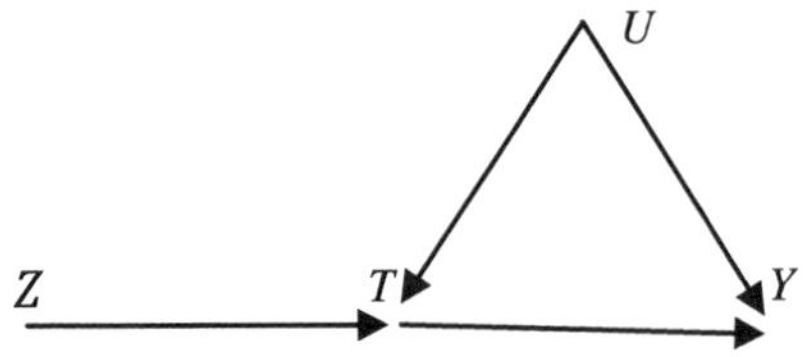

Fig. 12.6.1. Randomized trial with non-compliance.

Especially for the case of a binary IV Z, we have

$$\beta = \frac{E(Y|Z=1) - E(Y|Z=0)}{E(T|Z=1) - E(T|Z=0)}.$$

When the treatment assignment Z is randomized, the average causal effect of the treatment assignment Z on outcome Y is $E(Y|Z=1)-E(Y|Z=0)$, and the average causal effect of Z on T is $E(T|Z=1)-E(T|Z=0)$. Dividing the former by the latter, we obtain the average causal effect of the treatment T on the outcome Y: $E(Y|T=1) - E(Y|T=0)$.

12.7. Principal Stratification[13]

For a commonly used stratification, the covariates which are not affected by treatment are used to stratify the population. For example, the covariate "sex" is used to stratify the population to subpopulations "male" and "female". If a post-treatment variate which is affected by treatment is used for stratification, it may induce the confounding bias of the causal effect of treatment on outcome. For example, consider a binary treatment T (1 for treated, 0 for control), a post-treatment variable S denotes the heartbeat (1 for regular, 0 for irregular) and the outcome Y denotes the sudden death (1 for no, 0 yes). If the heartbeat S is used to stratify the patients, it may induce the confounding bias of treatment effect on outcome. It is because the heartbeat S is an intermediate variable between the path from treatment T to outcome Y. For a subpopulation (say $S = 1$ "regular"), some patients are treated and the others are untreated, and thus, they are not comparable. Similarly, a model of outcome Y including an intermediate variable S may also induce confounding bias. For example, consider a linear model $Y = \alpha+\beta t+\gamma s+\varepsilon$, where S denotes an intermediate variable. Even if there is no confounder affecting both treatment T and outcome Y, β cannot present the causal effect of treatment T on outcome Y. Frangakis and Rubin[13] proposed the principal stratification approach, in which the potential outcomes of the intermediate variable, i.e. (S_1, S_0), are used to stratify the population. Although $S_1(i)$ and $S_0(i)$ may be different, the values of $(S_1(i), S_0(0))$ are not affected by treatment T. The principal stratification does not induce confounding bias.

For the basic principal stratification, a basic stratum is a set of all individuals in which each individual i has $(S_1(i), S_0(i)) = (s', s'')$. For a principal stratification, each stratum Ω is a union of some basic principal strata. A causal effect for a principal stratum Ω is defined as a comparison between the potential outcomes $\{Y_1(i): i \in \Omega\}$ and $\{Y_0(i): i \in \Omega\}$.

The challenging issue for using the principal stratification is the identifiability because the principal stratum for any individual is not observed. For a treated individual, only S_1 is observed, but S_0 is unobserved. To identify the causal effects for the principal stratification, we require some assumptions or an IV.

Below, we introduce some applications of the principal stratification with an intermediate variable. The later sections in this chapter discuss the identifiability of causal effects in the principal strata.

For the non-compliance problem in clinical trials, let T denote the treatment assignment, S denote the accepted treatment. Let the principal strata (S_1, S_0) denote the compliance groups: $(S_1, S_0) = (0, 0)$ denotes the never-treated group no matter what the treatment assignment is, $(S_1, S_0) = (1, 1)$ denotes the always treated group no matter what the treatment assignment, is $(S_1, S_0) = (1, 0)$ denotes the complier group, and $(S_1, S_0) = (0, 1)$ denotes the defier group.

For the problem of evaluating quality of life with censoring by death, there is confounding bias of treatment effects on quality of life if only survival patients are used for the evaluation. It is because the survival patients are not comparable, some of whom are treated and some of whom are untreated. Let (S_1, S_0) denote the survival, and $(S_1, S_0) = (1, 1)$ denote the always survival principal stratum no matter what the treatment assignment is. The effect of treatment on the quality of life is meaningful only for the always survival principal stratum because there is no suitable definition of quality of life for death.

12.8. Non-compliance[14,15]

For clinical trials, non-compliance often occurs when patients do not comply with the treatment assignment. The patients assigned to the treatment group do not accept the treatment and change to the control group, while the patients assigned to the control group change to the treatment group. The comparability of the treatment group and the control group in the randomized clinical trials is destroyed by the non-compliance.

Let Z denote the randomized treatment assignment, $Z = 1$ denote the assignment to a treatment group, and $Z = 0$ denote the assignment to a control group (e.g. placebo). Let a binary variable D denote the accepted treatment of a patient, $D = 1$ denotes that the patient accepts the treatment, and $D = 0$ denote that the patient accepts the placebo. Let Y be a binary outcome, $Y = 0$ denote unrecovered, and $Y = 1$ denote recovered. The causal effect of accepted treatment D on outcome Y is not identifiable because there may be an unobserved confounder U between D and Y.

Since the treatment assignment Z is randomized, the causal effect of the treatment assignment Z on outcome Y can be evaluated by the association measure between Z and Y. The intention-to-treat (ITT) analysis uses the causal effect of Z on Y to evaluate the treatment effect. The reason for using the ITT analysis is that the effect value obtained by the ITT analysis is between 0 and the value of causal effect of accepted treatment D on Y for a randomized trial. Therefore, the ITT analysis does not overevaluate the causal effect of D on outcome. Particularly, no causal effect of D on Y implies no causal effect of Z on Y. Thus, the ITT analysis is a conservative approach for evaluating the causal effect of treatment D on outcome Y. There are two problems for the ITT approach. One is that it may underestimate the drug toxicity when evaluating the drug safety. The other is that when the two treatments with equivalent effects have different compliances in their trials, the spurious difference between them is obtained by the ITT analysis.

There are several approaches for non-compliance analysis, such as the inverse probability weighting and G-estimation. But they require some assumption, such as $D \perp Y_d | X$ where X is observed or the IV assumption. Some investigators prefer to use the ITT analysis, and they think that the effect obtained by the ITT analysis includes the effect of patients' non-compliance in practice. But the non-compliance in clinical trials may be different from that in practice.

Let T denote treatment assignment, and S denote the accepted treatment. The principal stratum (S_1, S_0) denotes the compliance, and then $(S_1, S_0) = (1, 0)$ denotes the complier group. Imbens and Rubin[15] discussed the complier average treatment effect (CACE), which equals the causal effect of treatment assignment on outcome divided by the proportion of the compliers in all patients.

12.9. Surrogate Endpoint[13,16–17]

In a clinical trial, a surrogate endpoint may be used for assessing the treatment effect on a true endpoint when the measurement of the true endpoint may be expensive or infeasible. For example, CD4 count is often used as a surrogate for survival time in clinical trials of AIDS, and bone mass is often used as a surrogate for fracture in osteoporosis studies.

Let T denote a binary treatment, Y denote a true endpoint, and S denote a surrogate. Suppose that the treatment T is randomized. Since the surrogate

S cannot be randomized, there may be an unobserved confounder U which affects both the surrogate S and the endpoint Y.

There have been several criteria of surrogates. The most intuitive one requires that there is a strong correlation between the surrogate and the true endpoint. But even when the correlation of the surrogate and the endpoint is 1, the treatment effect on the surrogate cannot be used to predict the treatment effect on the endpoint. For example, the size of children's shoes is strongly correlated to the number of words remembered by the children, but the causal effect of a treatment on the shoes' size cannot predict the causal effect of the treatment on the number of remembered words. Prentice[17] proposed the criteria for a statistical surrogate S, which further requires the conditional independence of the treatment T and the endpoint Y given the statistical surrogate S. It means that the surrogate S breaks the dependency of treatment T on the endpoint Y. Frangakis and Rubin[13] pointed out that a statistical surrogate does not satisfy the property of causal necessity, and they proposed the criterion for the principal surrogate to satisfy the causal necessity. Lauritzen[36] used a causal diagram to depict a strong surrogate criterion which requires that the surrogate S breaks the causal path from the treatment T to the endpoint Y. Thus, a strong surrogate S also satisfies the property of causal necessity.

Chen *et al.*[16] presented the surrogate paradox for all these criteria, which means that a treatment has a positive effect on a surrogate and the surrogate has a positive effect on or a positive association with the endpoint, but the treatment has a negative effect on the endpoint. This means that the sign of causal effect of the treatment on the surrogate and the sign of causal effect of the surrogate on the endpoint cannot be used to predict the sign of causal effect of the treatment on the endpoint.

To avoid the surrogate paradox, Chen *et al.*[16] proposed the causation-based criteria, and Wu *et al.*[44] presented the association-based criteria. VanderWeele[43] discussed whether various criteria cannot avoid the surrogate paradox. Several other criteria require that the endpoint is observed, and the observed data of surrogate and endpoint are used to assess the surrogacy (Burzykowski *et al.*,[32]).

12.10. Interaction[18–19]

"Interaction" is a term for multiple factor analysis. But it is used for different concepts. Rothman *et al.*[19] described three kinds of interactions: statistical interaction, biological interaction and public health interaction. Various concepts of interactions are separated as two classes. The first class is a quantity assessment based on statistical models with multiple risk factors and parameters, called the statistical interaction. Let A and B denote two binary risk factors with values 0 and 1 representing unexposed and exposed, respectively. Let Y denote a binary response variable with values 0 and 1 representing undiseased and diseased, respectively. Let $\pi_{\mathrm{ij}} = P(Y = 1|A = i, B = j)$ denote the probability of diseased under the exposure $A = i$ and $B = j$. No additive interaction is defined as follows:

$$\pi_{11} - \pi_{00} = (\pi_{10} - \pi_{00}) + (\pi_{01} - \pi_{00}).$$

It means that the joint risk difference of two risk factors A and B on the disease Y is equal to the sum of the risk differences of a single risk factor A on Y and a single risk factor B on Y. No multiplicative interaction is defined as follows:

$$\pi_{11}/\pi_{00} = (\pi_{10}/\pi_{00})(\pi_{01}/\pi_{00}).$$

It means that the RR of risk factors A and B on the disease Y is equal to the multiplicativity of the RRs of a single factor A on Y and a single factor B on Y. When both A and B have single effects (that is, $\pi_{10} \neq \pi_{00}$ and $\pi_{01} \neq \pi_{00}$), there must be the multiplicative interaction if there is no additive interaction, and there must be the additive interaction if there is no multiplicative interaction. When both A and B have only weak effects (that is, both π_{01} and π_{10} are small), no additive interaction is approximatively equivalent to the following no multiplicative interaction:

$$\frac{1 - \pi_{11}}{1 - \pi_{00}} = \left(\frac{1 - \pi_{10}}{1 - \pi_{00}}\right)\left(\frac{1 - \pi_{01}}{1 - \pi_{00}}\right).$$

The existence of interaction depends on the association measurements used. The parameters of interaction in a model are often used to represent statistical interactions. When a term "interaction" is used, we should explain what association measurement is used.

The second class is a quality assessment based on biologic mechanisms, called biologic interaction (or synergism). Let $Y_{A=i,B=j}$ denote the potential outcome of a binary response under exposures $A = i$ and $B = j$. According to four binary potential outcomes $(Y_{00}, Y_{01}, Y_{10}, Y_{11})$ of each individual, all individuals can be partitioned into $2^4 = 16$ classes. The class with $(0, 0, 0, 1)$ denotes the individuals each of which has the disease if and only if both the exposures are present. The proportion of this class in the whole population is used to measure the synergism effect. For example, such a biologic interaction is the synergism effect of a gene A and smoking B on cancer Y. For the persons in the class $(0, 0, 0, 1)$, they should avoid smoking $(B = 1)$ if they have the gene exposure ($A = 1$). For the persons in class $(0, 0, 1, 0)$, they have the disease only if they are exposed to a single exposure ($B = 1$), but they do not have the disease if they are exposed to both ($A = 1, B = 1$). We say that there is an antagonism between A and B.

12.11. Mediation Analysis[13,20]

The path analysis, structural equations, mediation analysis and direct and indirect effects are used to investigate the mechanisms among multiple variables. For example, treatment T reduces sudden deaths Y through correcting irregular heartbeat S (Treatment $T \to$ Heartbeat $S \to$ Sudden death Y), and the treatment reduces sudden death through another path (Treatment $T \to$ Sudden death Y). The path analysis and the mediation analysis make use of the structural equations: $Y = \alpha + \beta S + \gamma T + \varepsilon_Y$ and $S = \lambda + \eta T + \varepsilon_S$. The parameter γ denotes the direct effect of T on Y, and $\beta\eta$ denotes the indirect effect of T on Y. The conditional independency of Y and T given S implies $\gamma = 0$, which means no direct effect. The conclusion requires the assumption of no confounders which affect both S and Y. But in many real applications, this assumption may not hold because the intermediate variable S (e.g. heartbeat) cannot be randomized. For this case, the direct effect of treatment on sudden death cannot be evaluated by comparing the treatment group ($T = 1$) and the control group ($T = 0$) conditionally on heartbeat S. It is because conditionally on regular (or irregular) heartbeat, the treatment group is not comparable with the control group. The stratification by the intermediate variable S may induce the confounding bias of the direct effect of treatment T on the endpoint Y.

Frangakis and Rubin[13] proposed the principal stratification approach. The potential outcomes $(S_{T=1}, S_{T=0})$ of the intermediate variable are used for stratification. In terms of the principal stratification, the direct effect is assessed by comparing the distributions of $Y_{T=1}$ and $Y_{T=0}$ in the principal stratum of $S_{T=1} = S_{T=0}$. If there is the causal effect of T on Y in the stratum, then there is the direct effect of treatment T on Y, called the principal direct effect. But there is no clear definition of the principal indirect effect. The total effect of treatment T on response Y is assessed by comparing the distributions of $Y_{T=1}$ and $Y_{T=0}$. If the indirect effect is assessed by the difference of the total effect and the principal direct effect, it also contains the direct effect except for the principal direct effect.

Let Y_{ts} denote the potential outcome of response under the external intervention of the treatment $T = t$ and the intermediate variable $S = s$. Pearl[20] defined the control direct effect of treatment T on response Y for individual i

as $\text{CDE}_s(i) = Y_{1s}(i) - Y_{0s}(i)$. It describes the effect of treatment on response under the external intervention on the intermediate variable $S = s$. The average control direct effect $ACDE_s$ is the expectation of $\text{CDE}_s(i)$. The control direct effect depends on the value s of the intermediate variable. To identify $ACDE_s$, we need the conditional independencies: (1) $Y_{\text{ts}} \perp T|X$ and (2) $Y_{\text{ts}} \perp S|(T, X)$, where X is an observed covariate. Because it is impossible to remove the direct effect by controlling for some variables, there is no definition of the control indirect effect. The natural direct effect for individual i is defined as $\text{NDE}(i) = Y_{1s_0}(i) - Y_{0s_0}(i)$. It describes the causal effect of treatment T on response Y if the intermediate variable was s_0. Different individuals may have different values of s_0. The average natural direct effect (ANDE) is the expectation of $\text{NDE}(i)$. To identify ANDE, we need an additional conditional independency: (3) $Y_{ts} \perp S_{t'}|X$.

12.12. Missing Not at Random[21,22]

If data missing depends neither on values of missing data nor on observed data, we say that data are missing completely at random. If data missing depends on observed data but is conditionally independent of missing data given the observed data, we say that data is missing at random (MAR). Otherwise, we say that data are missing not at random (MNAR). When values of confounders are MAR, it does not affect the evaluation of causal effects. But if they are MNAR, it may induce confounding bias so that causal effects cannot be identified.

Consider the case of discrete variables. Let response Y have K levels, treatment T be binary and covariate or confounder X have J values. Suppose that confounder X is subject to missing. Let M be an indicator of X missing, $M_i = 1$ denote that the value x_i is missing for individual i and $M_i = 0$ denote that x_i is observed. The goal is to identify the conditional causal effect for the strarum $x.\text{CE}_x = D[E(Y_{T=1}|x), E(Y_{T=0}|x)]$ and the marginal causal effect $\text{CE}_+ = D[E(Y_{T=1}), E(Y_{T=0})]$, where $D[\cdot,\cdot]$ denotes a function for comparing two parameters. For example, the conditional average causal effect $\text{ACE}(x) = E(Y_{T=1}|x) - E(Y_{T=0}|x)$, and the marginal average causal RR $\text{CRR} = E(Y_{T=1})/E(Y_{T=0})$.

Assume that X is a sufficient confounder set so that $Y_{\text{t}} \perp T|X$ holds. Ding and Geng[21] discussed the identifiability of causal effects under the following mechanisms of missing data:

M1: Given T and Y, X missing does not depend on its values (MAR). The probability of X missing is $P(M = 1|x, t, y) = P(M = 1|t, y)$, but M depends on (T, Y), denoted as $M \perp X|(T, Y)$ and $M \uparrow (T, Y)$.

For this mechanism of data missing, the joint distribution $p(m, x, t, y)$ is identifiable, and thus, the causal effects of treatment T on response Y (CE_x and CE_+) are identifiable.

M2: X missing depends on values of X (i.e. MNAR). But given T and X, X missing is independent of Y, that is, $P(M = 1|x, t, y) = P(M = 1|t, x)$, and the indicator M depends on (T, X), denoted as $M \perp Y|(T, X)$ and $M \uparrow (T, X)$.
For this mechanism of data missing, the causal effect CE_x is identifiable.

M3: Given X and Y, X missing is independent of T: $P(M = 1|x, t, y) = P(M = 1|x, y)$, and depends on (X, Y) (i.e. MNAR), denoted as $M \perp T|(X, Y)$ and $M \uparrow (X, Y)$.
For this mechanism of data missing, the causal odds ratio OR_x of treatment T and a binary Y is identifiable, and thus, other causal measurements can be evaluated qualitatively, that is, positive, negative or null.

M4: X missing depends on (T, X, Y) by the logistic regression model,

$$\log \frac{P(M = 1|x, t, y)}{1 - P(M = 1|x, t, y)} = \beta_0 + \beta_T t + \beta_X x + \beta_Y y.$$

For this mechanism of data missing, the joint distribution $p(m, x, t, y)$ is identifiable and the causal effects of T on Y (CE_x and CE_+) are identifiable if Y is binary and the conditional odd ratios $\mathrm{OR}_{\mathrm{TY}|M=1}$ is between $OR_{\mathrm{TY}|M=0,X=1}$ and $\mathrm{OR}_{TY|M=0,X=0}$, where

$$\mathrm{OR}_{\mathrm{TY}|C} = \frac{P(T = 1, Y = 1|C)P(T = 0, Y = 0|C)}{P(T = 1, Y = 0|C)P(T = 0, Y = 1|C)}.$$

M5: X missing depends on (T, X, Y), and there is no model assumption.

For this case, causal effects are not identifiable but are partially identifiable, that is, their bounds can be found.

Zhang and Rubin[22] discussed the causal effect of treatment T on death Y for the case where confounder X may be censored by death ($Y = 1$).

12.13. Causal Network[4,23]

Causal networks are used to describe the causal relationships among multiple variables. A causal network is represented by a directed acyclic graph (DAG) or a Bayesian network $G = (V, E)$, where $V = \{X_1, \ldots, X_p\}$ is a set of nodes denoting p variables, $E = \{e_1, \ldots, e_K\}$ is a set of directed edges, and each directed edge $e_k = <X_i, X_j>$ denotes an arrow $X_i \to X_j$, and where X_i is a cause or a parent node of X_j, and X_j is an effect or a child node of X_i. Let pa_i denote the parent set of node X_i. In Figure 12.13.1, $\mathrm{pa}_4 = \{X_2, X_3\}$, X_2 and X_3 are the causes of X_4, and X_4 is the effect of X_2 and X_3. Each node in a causal network is a function of its parents, i.e. $x_i = f_i(\mathrm{pa}_i, \varepsilon_i)$, where ε_i is an external variable which affects only X_i in the network. The joint probability or density is represented as

$$p(x_1, \ldots, x_p) = \prod_{i=1}^{p} p(x_i|\mathrm{pa}_i),$$

where $p(x_i|pa_i)$ is the conditional probability or density of X_i given pa_i.

An external intervention $\mathrm{set}(x_i)$ sets a variable X_i to a constant x_i so that it is not affected by its parents pa_i. For example, $\mathrm{set}(x_2)$ breaks $X_1 \to X_2$ in Figure 12.13.1, and the joint distribution after the intervention becomes

$$p(x_1, x_3, x_4, x_5|\mathrm{set}(x_2)) = p(x_1)p(x_3|x_1)p(x_4|x_2, x_3)p(x_5|x_4)$$

and $p(x_1, x_3, x_4, x_5|\mathrm{set}(x_2)) = 0$ for $X_2 \neq x_2$. Particularly, $p(x_1, x_3|\mathrm{set}(x_2)) = p(x_1, x_3) \neq p(x_1, x_3|x_2)$, that is, the intervention does not affect the distribution of non-descendants. The distribution after the intervention $\mathrm{set}(x_2)$ is not equal to the conditional distribution given $X_2 = x_2$.

A causal network represents a set of conditional independencies. Given pa_i, X_i is conditionally independent of non-descendants of X_i. For example, in Figure 12.13.1, X_2 and X_3 are conditionally independent given X_1. Let C be an arbitrary subset of V. We say that a path between node X_i and node X_j is not blocked by C if each node X_k on the path satisfies the two following conditions:

(1) If X_k is a collider (i.e. $\to X_k \leftarrow$), then X_k or its descendant is in C;
(2) If X_k is not a collider, then X_k is not in C.

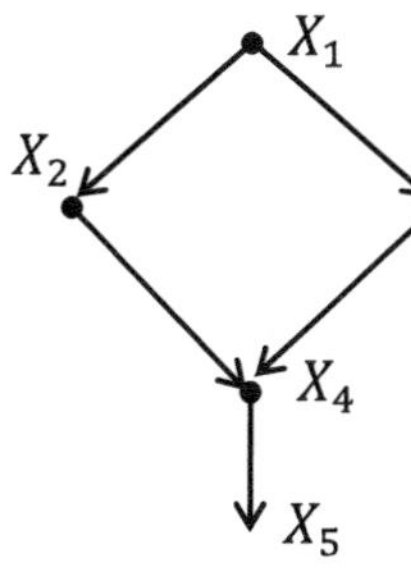

Fig. 12.13.1. DAG for a causal network.

Otherwise, we say that the path is blocked by C. Let A, B and C be three disjoint sets of nodes. We say that C d-separates A and B (denoted as $d(A, B, C)$) if and only if C blocks every path from a node in A to a node in B. By the concept of d-separation, we can read the conditional independencies from a causal network. $d(A, B, C)$ implies the conditional independency of A and B given C. From the network in Figure 12.13.1, we can read $d(X_2, X_3, X_1)$, and thus, we know that X_2 and X_3 are conditionally independent given X_1. Since $d(X_2, X_3, \{X_1, X_4\})$ does not hold, generally X_2 and X_3 are not conditionally independent given $\{X_1, X_4\}$, although the conditional independency may coincidentally hold, which is called unfaithfulness.

12.14. Identifiability of Causal Effects[7,24,25]

Various causal effects are used to evaluate effects of a treatment on a response or outcome, which are different from association and correlation measurements. For example, the results would be produced if a drug intervention or a policy was implemented. By observational studies, we can obtain the distribution $p(x_1, \ldots, x_p)$ of observed variables experimentally. If the causal effects of interest can be represented by this distribution of observed variables, then we say that the causal effects are identifiable. Otherwise, this distribution may be produced by two different values of a causal effect, and we say that the causal effect is not identifiable. For example, when a correlation between smoking and cancer may be interpreted no matter whether smoking is a cause of cancer, the causal effect is not identifiable. Let $X = X_O \cup X_U$ denote the set of all variables, where X_O denotes observed variables and X_U denotes unobserved ones. The goal is to identify the post-intervention distribution of X_j after the intervention of X_i, that is, $p(x_j|\text{set}(x_i))$ using the distribution of observed variables, $p(x_O)$. If there is a unique $p(x_j|\text{set}(x_i))$ which can be interpreted by $p(x_O)$, then the causal distribution $p(x_j|\text{set}(x_i))$ is identifiable. When both X_i and X_j are observed, no confounding bias is equivalent to $p(x_j|\text{set}(x_i)) = p(x_j|x_i)$. Pearl gave the following properties:

(1) An intervention $\text{set}(x_i)$ affects only the descendants of X_i;
(2) $P_{x'_i}(S|\text{pa}_i) = P(S|x'_i, \text{pa}_i)$ holds for any set S of variables;
(3) $X_j \perp \text{Pa}_i | X_i$ is a sufficient condition for no confounding.

Property (1) implies that $P_{x'_i}(S) = P(S)$ if S is not the descendants of X_i. Property (2) implies no confounding, which means that the causal effect of X_i on any set S is equal to the distribution conditional on the parent set of

X_i. Geng and Li (2002) proved that the conditional independence in property (3) is a necessary and sufficient condition for uniform non-confounding.

To check whether there are other confounders outside a set S, we delete all directed edges emanating from exposure E in a given causal diagram, that is, remove all effects of exposure. If there still exists a path between E and response D which is not blocked by S, then there may exist some association between E and D conditional on S. The association cannot be interpreted by the causal effect of E on D, and thus there are some confounders outside S. Greenland *et al.* (1999) presented the following algorithm. Given a set of variables $S = \{S_1, \ldots, S_n\}$ which does not include descendants of E and D,

(1) Delete the arrows emanating from E (i.e. remove all exposure effects).
(2) In the new DAG without exposure effects, check whether there is any unblocked path between E and D which is not blocked by S.
(3) If yes, then there are some other confounders outside S; otherwise S is a sufficient set of confounders, but there may be some redundant non-confounders in S.

Wang *et al.*[25] proposed an algorithm for deleting non-confounders from a sufficient confounder set.

12.15. Network Structural Learning[8,26–27]

There are two kinds of learning for Bayesian networks, DAGs and causal networks: one is the parameter learning and the other is the structural learning.

The parameter learning is to estimate the parameters or the distributions for the case of a known structure of the networks. For the case of discrete variables, it is to estimate the conditional probabilities $p(x_i|\text{pa}_i)$. For the case of normal distributions, it is to estimate the parameters of conditional normal distributions of X_i given pa_i.

There have been two primary approaches for learning the structures of DAGs from data. One is the search-and-score approach. It defines a score for each possible structure, and then it tries to search the best structure over all possible structures heuristically. Heckerman[34] proposed a Bayesian approach for learning Bayesian networks. The other is the constraint-based approach. It evaluates the presence or absence of an edge by testing conditional independencies among variables from data. Verma and Pearl[26] resented the inductive causation (IC) algorithm which searches for a separator S_{ab} of two variables (say a and b) from all possible variable subsets such that a and b are independent conditionally on S_{ab}. For two non-adjacent variables a and b, we determine a v-structure ($a \to c \leftarrow b$) if their common neighbor c is not contained in the separator S_{ab}. After finding all edges and v-structures, we determine the directions of other undirected edges such that no new v-structures and cycles are generated. A systematic way of searching for separators in increasing order of cardinality was proposed by Spirtes and Glymour.[42] The PC algorithm limits possible separators to variables that are adjacent to a or b.

Xie *et al.*[27] proposed a structural learning approach for multiple incomplete databases. With the knowledge of conditional independencies among variables, the structure can be learnt correctly from the incomplete data. At first, the local structures are discovered from each incomplete database, which may have spurious edges. Then the local structures are combined together to a global network. Xie and Geng[45] presented a recursive learning algorithm, which recursively separates a large structural learning to two small ones.

From observational data, we can discover a class of networks which have the same conditional independencies, called a Markov equivalence class. In such a Markov class, the directions of some edges cannot be oriented. For example, two DAGS $a \to b \leftarrow c \to d$ and $a \to b \leftarrow c \leftarrow d$ belong to an equivalence class, denoted by a partially directed graph $a \to b \leftarrow c - d$, but the DAG $a \to b \to c \to d$ does not belong to this class. To determine which one is true in the class, we have to use other prior knowledge or experimental data. To orient all undirected edges in an equivalence class, He and Geng[28] presented an active learning approach which tried to manipulate as few variables as possible.

12.16. Local Causal Relationship[29–31]

Consider a causal network of lung cancer in Figure 12.16.1. We try to find the causes of lung cancer and then make a public health policy for lung cancer. Using the ordinary regression model based on correlation, we shall select four variables (Smoking, Genetics, Coughing, Fatigue, Allergy), called Markov blanket. Given the Markov blanket, the response variable (Lung Cancer) is conditionally independent of other six variables, that is, the parameters of the six variables in the regression model are zero. Although these variables in the blanket can be used to diagnose lung cancer, the intervention of Coughing and Fatigue in the blanket may not reduce the risk of lung cancer. The ordinary variable selection cannot distinguish the causes from the effects.

If the goal is to discover the local causal relationships of a given target variable and to find out what its causes and effects are or if the goal is to make an intervention policy, then we only need to discover the local causal

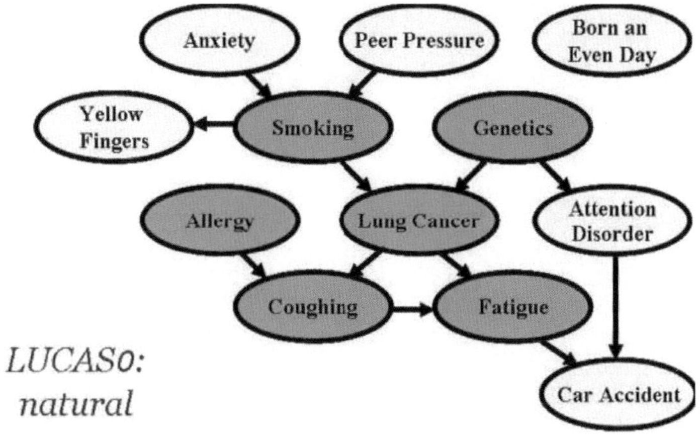

Fig. 12.16.1. Causal network of lung cancer.[29]

relationships between the target variable and its neighbors without having to find the global network structure.

Tsamardinos *et al.*[30] presented a local structural learning algorithm for finding the nodes of parents–children–descendants of the target node. But their algorithm does not distinguish between the parent nodes and the children nodes. Wang *et al.*[28] presented a stepwise local structural learning approach, called the MB-by-MB algorithm. This algorithm starts from the target node Y and finds the neighbors and then the neighbors of neighbors stepwise. At first, it finds the Markov blanket MB(Y) of the target Y, and discovers the local network over the MB(Y). Next, it finds the neighbor MB(X_i) of each node X_i in MB(Y). Then the process is repeated until we can determine the causes and effects of the target Y. If the conditional independencies are checked correctly, the MB-by-MB algorithm can discover the correct local structure of the global network.

References

1. Geng, Z. Collapsibility of relative risks in contingency tables with a response variable. *J. Royal Statist. Soc. B*, 1992, 54: 585–593.
2. Geng, Z, Guo, J, Fung, WK. Criteria for confounders in epidemiological studies. *J. Royal Statist. Soc. B*, 2002, 64: 3–15.
3. Imbens, GW, Rubin, DB. *Causal Inference for Statistics, Social and Biomedical Sciences: An Introduction.* Cambridge: Cambridge University Press, 2015.
4. Pearl, J. *Causality: Models, Reasoning, and Inference.* (2nd edn.). Cambridge: Cambridge University Press, 2009.
5. Rosenbaum, PR, Rubin, DB. The central role of the propensity score in observational studies for causal effects. *Biometrika*, 1983, 70: 41–55.

6. Greenland, S, Robins, J, Pearl, J. Confounding and collapsibility in causal inference. *Statist. Sci.* 1999, 14: 29–46.
7. Greenland, S, Pearl, J, Robins, JM. Causal diagrams for epidemiologic research. *Epidemiology* 1999, 10: 37–48.
8. Guo, JH, Geng, Z. Collapsibility of logistic regression coefficients. *J. Royal Statist. Soc. B*, 1995, 57: 263–267.
9. Ma, ZM, Xie, XC, Geng, Z. Collapsibility of distribution dependence. *J. Royal Statist. Soc. Ser. B*, 2006, 68: 127–133.
10. Angrist, J, Imbens, G, Rubin, D. Identification of causal effects using instrumental variables. *J. Amer. Statist. Assoc.* 1996, 91: 444–472.
11. Durbin, J. Errors in Variables. *Inter. Stat. Rev.*, 1954, 22: 23–32.
12. Greenland, S. An introduction to instrumental variables for epidemiologists. *Int. J. Epidemiol.* 2000, 29: 722–729.
13. Frangakis, CE, Rubin, DB. Principal stratification in causal inference. *Biometrics*, 2002, 58: 21–29.
14. Chen, H, Geng, Z, Zhou, X. Identifiability and estimation of causal effects in randomized trials with noncompliance and completely non-ignorable missing-data (with discussion). *Biometrics*, 2009, 65: 675–691.
15. Imbens, GW, Rubin, DB. Bayesian inference for causal effects in randomized experiments with noncompliance. *Ann. Stat.* 1997, 25: 305–327.
16. Chen, H, Geng, Z, Jia, J. Criteria for surrogate end points. *J. Royal Statist. Soc. Ser. B*, 2007, 69: 919–932.
17. Prentice, RL. Surrogate endpoints in clinical trials: Definition and operational criteria. *Stat. Medi.* 1989, 8: 431–440.
18. Geng, Z, Hu, YH. On statistical inference of interactions. *Chinese J. Epidemiol.*, 2002, 23: 221–224. (In Chinese)
19. Rothman, KJ, Greenland, S, Lash, TL. *Modern Epidemiology* (3rd edn.). New York: Lippincott Williams & Wilkins, 2008.
20. Pearl, J. (2001) Direct and indirect effects. 17th Conf. Uncertainty AI, 411–420.
21. Ding, P, Geng, Z. Identifiability of subgroup causal effects in randomized experiments with nonignorable missing covariates. *Statist. Med.*, 2014, 33: 1121–1133.
22. Zhang, JL, Rubin, DB. Estimation of causal effects via principal stratification when some outcomes are truncated by 'death'. *J. Edu. Behav. Statist.*, 2003, 28: 353–368.
23. Spirtes, P, Glymour, C, Scheines, R. *Causation, Prediction, and Search* (2nd edn.). The MIT Press, 2000.
24. Pearl, J. Causal diagrams for empirical research (with discussion). *Biometrika*, 1995, 83: 669–710.
25. Wang, X, Geng, Z, Chen, H, Xie, X. Detecting multiple confounders. *J. Stat. Plan. & Inf.* 2009, 139: 1073–1081.
26. Verma, T, Pearl, J. Equivalence and synthesis of causal models. *Uncertain. Artif. Intell.*, 1990, 6: 255–268.
27. Xie, X, Geng, Z, Zhao, Q. Decomposition of structural learning about directed acyclic graphs. AI, 2006, 170: 422–439.
28. Wang, CZ, Zhou, Y, Zhao, Q, Geng, Z. Discovering and orienting the edges connected to a target variable in a DAG via a sequential local learning approach. *Comput. Statist. & Data Analy.*, 2014, 77: 252–266.
29. He, Y, Geng, Z. Active learning of causal networks with intervention experiments and optimal designs. *JMLR*, 2008, 9: 2523–2547.

30. Guyon, I, Aliferis, C, Cooper, G, Elisseeff, A, Pellet, J, Spirtes, P, Statnikov, A. Design and analysis of the causation and prediction challenge. Challenges in causality (Vol. 1) WCCI Causation and Prediction challenge, 1–33, 2011.
31. Tsamardinos, I, Brown, L, Aliferis, C. The max-min hill-climbing Bayesian network structure learning algorithm. *Mach. Learn.*, 2006, 65: 31–78.
32. Burzykowski, T., Molenberghs, G. and Buyse, M. *The Evaluation of Surrogate Endpoints.* Springer, 2005.
33. Fisher, R. *Design and Experiments.* Oliver and Boyd, Edinburgh, 1935.
34. Heckman, J. Instrumental variables: a study of implicit behavioral assumptions used in making program evaluations. *Journal of Human Resources*, 1997, 32: 441–462.
35. Heckman, J. Econometric causality. *International Statistical Review*, 2008, 76: 1–27.
36. Lauritzen, S. L. Discussion on causality. *Scand. J. Statist.*, 2004, 31: 189–192.
37. Neyman, J. On the application of probability theory to agricultural experiments: Essay on principles, Section 9. *Ann. Agric. Sci. Translated in Statist. Sci.*, 1923, 1990, 5: 465–480.
38. Reintjes, R., de Boer, A., van Pelt, W., Mintjes-de Groot, J. Simpson's paradox: an example from hospital epidemiology. *Epidemiology*, 2000, 11: 81–83.
39. Robins, J. M., Mark, S. D. and Newey, W. K. Estimating exposure effects by modeling the expectation of exposure conditional on confounders. *Biometrics*, 1992, 48: 479–495.
40. Rubin, D. B. Estimating causal effects of treatments in randomized and nonrandomized studies. *J. Educ. Psychology.*, 1974, 66: 688–701.
41. Simpson, E. H. The interpretation of interaction in contingency tables. *J. Royal Statist. Soc. B*, 1951, 13: 238–241.
42. Spirtes, P. and Glymour, C. An algorithm for fast recovery of sparse causal graphs. *Social Science Computer Review*, 1991, 9: 62–72.
43. VanderWeele, T. J. Surrogate measures and consistent surrogates (with discussion). *Biometrics*, 2013, 69: 561–581.
44. Wu Z. G., He, P. and Geng, Z. Sufficient conditions for concluding surrogacy based on observed data. *Statistics in Medicine*, 2011, 30: 2422–2434.
45. Xie, X. and Geng, Z. A recursive method for structural learning of directed acyclic graphs. *J. Mach. Learn. Res.*, 2008, 9: 459–483.
46. Yule, G. U. Notes on the theory of association of attributes in statistics. *Biometrika*, 1903, 2: 121–134.

---

*For the introduction of the corresponding author, see the front matter.

CHAPTER 13

COMPUTATIONAL STATISTICS

Jinzhu Jia*

13.1. Random Number Generator[1]

Simulations or simulated experiments need a few random numbers from some specified distribution. Assume that the distribution function of a random variable X is $F(x)$, denoted by $X \sim F(x)$, we say that the numbers randomly drawn from distribution $F(x)$ are the random numbers from $F(x)$.

Statistical software or packages such as R and MATLAB could be used to produce a lot of random numbers from a few distributions, such as normal distribution, uniform distribution, binomial distribution and Poisson distribution. In fact, random numbers from any other distirbutions could be realized by transformations of random numbers from uniform distribution. A more general result is: special transformations of random numbers from one distribution give random numbers from another distribution.

Theorem 1. *Suppose that $F(x)$ is the distribution function of random variable X. Suppose further that its inverse function exists, denoted by $F^{-1}(x)$, then $F(X) \sim U[0,1]$.*

Theorem 2. *Suppose that random variable $X \sim U[0,1]F(x)$ is one distribution function, then the distribution of $F^{-1}(X)$ is $F(x)$.*

From Theorems 13.1.1 and 13.1.2, we could transform random numbers from one distribution to another distribution as follows. Suppose that $X \sim G(x)$, we get random numbers from $F(x)$ by the following two steps. (1) From 13.1.1 $G(X) \sim U$, (2) from 13.1.2, $F^{-1}(G(X)) \sim F(x)$. *Note*: We

*Corresponding author: jzjia@math.pku.edu.cn

need function $G(x)$ to be a continuous and strictly monotone function. Distribution function for a discrete random variable is not a good one.

We now introduce how to produce random numbers from uniform distributions. One could draw random numbers by throwing dices or from physical process. But these two ways cannot be used to generate many random numbers and these random numbers cannot be duplicated many times unless they are stored in a hard disk. Another generating way is via mathematical formula, which generates a series of numbers via recursive mathematical formula. When the generated series is long enough, it has the properties of random numbers and thus could be viewed as a set of random numbers. This method is very fast and takes only very small amount of storage and could be repeated many times. Almost all statistical packages are using this mathematical way to produce random numbers. Of course, it has its own flaws. The numbers generated are not real random numbers, and people call them pseudo-random numbers. Good pseudo random number cannot be distinguished from real random numbers and so we also call them random numbers.

The way random numbers are generated is called a random number generator. A good random number generator should have the following properties:

(1) The series of numbers should have the statistical property of the popularity, such as the randomness and the independence between numbers.
(2) The series should have a very long period.
(3) It should be very fast and it takes very few memories to generate the random numbers.

There are a few common random number generators, including (1) linear congruential generator (2) linear feedback shift register, and (3) combination generator. These are classical pseudo-random number generators and we omit the mathematical principles here.

13.2. Tests for Random Numbers[2]

The random numbers generated from mathematical formulas are not real random numbers and they are pseudo-random numbers. Good pseudo-random numbers should have the statistical properties of real random numbers, which could be tested through statistical hypothesis testing. To test random numbers from uniform distribution, there are a few common tests, including Kolmogorov–Smirnov (K–S) test, test for parameters, test for uniformity, test of independence and test for regular patterns in combinations of numbers.

(1) K–S test. K–S test is used to test if there are statistical differences between empirical distribution function and the population distribution function. The statistics in K–S test is defined as $\max_{i=1,\dots,n} |F_n(x_i) - F(x_i)|$, where $F_n(x)$ is empirical distribution and $F(x)$ is the population distribution function. When we test if random numbers are from $U[0,1]$, $F(x) = x, 0 \leq x \leq 1$.

(2) Test for parameters. It is known that the expectation of random variable from $U[0,1]$ is 1/2, and the variance is 1/12. So a good uniform random number should have mean value close to 1/2 and variance close to 1/12. We could construct test statistics via central limit theorem. Denote random numbers as $r_1, r_2, \dots, r_n$ Under null hypothesis that $r_1, r_2, \dots, r_n$ independent and identically distributed (i.i.d.) from $U[0,1]$, both

$$\frac{\bar{r} - \frac{1}{2}}{\sqrt{\text{var}(\bar{r})}} = \sqrt{12n}\left(\bar{r} - \frac{1}{2}\right)$$

and

$$\frac{s^2 - \frac{1}{12}}{\sqrt{\text{var}(s^2)}} = \sqrt{180n}\left(s^2 - \frac{1}{12}\right)$$

follow the standard normal distribution, where $\bar{r} = \frac{1}{n}\sum_{i=1}^{n} r_i$ and $s^2 = \frac{\sum_{i=1}^{n}(r_i - \bar{r})}{n-1}$.

(3) Test for uniformity. We first divide the interval $[0,1]$ into m smaller intervals with the same length. If random numbers from $U[0,1]$, then the probability of one random number from one of the m smaller intervals is $1/m$. We could apply χ^2 goodness-of-fit tests. Specifically, suppose that we have generated n random numbers and we denote by n_i the number of random numbers that is fall into the i-th small interval, then statistics

$$\sum_{i=1}^{m} \frac{(n_i - \mu_i)^2}{\mu_i} = \frac{m}{n}\sum_{i=1}^{m}\left(n_i - \frac{n}{m}\right)^2$$

follows $\chi^2(m-1)$ asymptotically, where $\mu_i = E(n_i) = \frac{n}{m}$.

(4) Test of independence. When random numbers are mutually independent, the theoretical autocorrelation is 0. Thus, we could use the sample autocorrelation to test if random numbers are mutually independent. Define

$$\rho(j) = \frac{\frac{1}{n-j}\sum_{i=1}^{n-j}(r_i - \bar{r})(r_{i+j} - \bar{r})}{\frac{1}{n}\sum_{i=1}^{n}(r_i - \bar{r})^2}, \quad j = 1, \dots, n.$$

When $n-j$ is large enough, $\rho(j)\sqrt{n-j}$ follows standard normal distribution asymptotically under the null hypothesis that random numbers are i.i.d. from $U[0,1]$.

We could also test the uniformity and independence of random numbers via dividing $[0,1] \times [0,1]$ into smaller blocks. Specifically, we pair the generated random numbers $r_1, r_2, \ldots, r_{2n}$, and form two-dimensional random vectors:

$$v_1 = (r_1, r_2), \ldots, v_n = (r_{2n-1} r_{2n}).$$

We divide $[0,1] \times [0,1]$ evenly into k^2 smaller square blocks. Denote by n_{ij} the number of random vectors that fall into the ij-th block. Then the following statistics follows $\chi^2(k^2-1)$ asymptotically:

$$V = \frac{k^2}{n} \sum_{i=1}^{k} \sum_{j=1}^{k} \left(n_{ij} - \frac{n}{k^2}\right)^2.$$

(5) Test for regular patterns in combinations of numbers. This is for testing if the numbers generated are random or not. In other words, random numbers should not have obvious regular patterns. For example, one could use the number of random numbers needed such that all of the 10 digits after the decimal point are just collected to test if the random numbers are random enough.

13.3. Calculation of Distribution Function[3,4]

For a continuous random variable, its distribution function is

$$F(x) = \int_{-\infty}^{x} f(t)dt.$$

For a discrete random variable, its distribution function is

$$F(x) = \sum_{x_i \leq x} p(x_i),$$

where $p(x_i) = P(X = x_i)$ So the calculation of distributions essentially is the calculation of integral or sum of series. There are a few commonly used numerical integration methods such as Integration via interpolation and Gaussian quadrature. We could also calculate some special distribution function via the relationship between different distributions. We focus on integration via interpolation and Gaussian quadrature here.

(1) Integration via interpolation

Consider the calculation of $\int_a^b f(x)dx$. We divide the interval $[ab]$ evenly into n smaller intervals. Denote the $n+1$ knot as $x_0 = a, \ldots, x_n = b$. Because of the equal length of each small interval, $x_k = a + k \cdot \frac{b-a}{n}$. We could use a polynomial with order n to approximate $f(x)$. The polynomial is defined as follows:

$$L_n(x) = \sum_{j=0}^{n} \frac{\prod_{k\neq j}(x - x_k)}{\prod_{k\neq j}(x_j - x_k)} f(x_j).$$

In practice, $[a,b]$ is divided into many smaller intervals. For example, $[a,b] = \bigcup_{i=1}^{m} I_i$, with m smaller intervals $I_i i = 1, 2, \ldots, m$ does not intersect with each other. Then, $\int_a^b f(x)dx = \sum_{i=1}^{m} \int_{I_i} f(x)dx$. On each small interval I_i, we could use a polynomial with very small order n, such as $n = 0, 1$ or 2.

Obviously, integration via interpolation could be represented as follows: $\int_a^b f(x)dx \approx \int_a^b L_n(x)dx = \sum_{j=0}^{n} A_j f(x_j)$, where $A_j = \int_a^b \frac{w(x)}{(x-x_j)w'(x)}dx$, $w(x) = \prod_{j=0}^{n}(x - x_j)$. When $f(x)$ is a polynomial with order not greater than n, $\int_a^b f(x)dx = \sum_{j=0}^{n} A_j f(x_j)$.

When the number of knots n is fixed, we could adjust the position of the n knots, and choose appropriate A_j's, such that $\int_a^b f(x)dx = \sum_{j=0}^{n} A_j f(x_j)$ holds for any polynomial with order not greater than $2n-1$. Gaussian quadrature chooses the positions of knots and A_j's.

(2) Gaussian quadrature

Gaussian quadrature uses orthogonal polynomials. Common used Gaussian quadratures are Gauss–Legender integral formula, Gauss–Lauguerer integral formula, Gauss-Hermite integral formula, etc. One could choose different formula according to different integral area. Gauss–Legender integral formula is

$$\int_{-1}^{1} f(x)dx \approx \sum_{k=1}^{n} A_k f(x_k),$$

where the n knots $x_1, \ldots, x_n$ are the roots of Legender polynomial L_n:

$$L_n(x) = \frac{1}{2^n n!} \frac{d^n[(x^2-1)^n]}{dx^n},$$

$$A_k = \frac{2}{(1-x_k^2)[L_n'(x_k)]^2}.$$

Gauss–Lauguerer integral formula is

$$\int_0^{\infty} e^{-x} f(x)dx \approx \sum_{k=1}^{n} A_k f(x_k),$$

where the n knots $x_1, \ldots, x_n$ are the roots of Lauguerer polynomial L_n:

$$L_n(x) = e^x \frac{d^n[e^{-x}x^n]}{dx^n},$$

$$A_k = \frac{(n!)^2}{x_k[L_n'(x_k)]^2}.$$

13.4. Stochastic Simulation[5,6]

Stochastic simulation is one method to solve problems by estimating parameters related to random variables. These parameters could be estimated by generating a few random numbers. Stochastic simulation is also called Monte Carlo method. The key of stochastic simulation is to generate random numbers from specified distribution and to estimate parameters using these generated random numbers.

We have already mentioned how to generate uniform random numbers and in fact there are mature software or packages to generate uniform random variables. If the specified distribution function is easy to calculate, then we could obtain the target random numbers by mathematical transformations. Here, we introduce more general methods, including acceptance–rejection method, transformation method, importance resampling method and importance sampling method.

(1) Acceptance–rejection method: We first introduce a simple acceptance–rejection method. Suppose the density function $f(x)$ is defined on interval $[a, b]$ and it is bounded from above $f(x) \leq M$. We could generate the random number with the density $f(x)$ through the following steps. (a) We generate one random number X from $U[a, b]$, (b) We generate one random number R from $U[0, 1]$; (3) If $R \leq \frac{f(x)}{M}$, we accept X, else we do not accept X and repeat the previous steps. In general, we do not need $f(x)$ to be bounded. Instead, we only need $f(x) \leq M(x)$ with $cM(x)$ a density function for some constant $c > 0$. We omit the details here.

(2) Transformation sampling: We introduce the transformation sampling via a few samples. (a) To generate a random number from $\chi^2(n)$, we could generate n i.i.d. random numbers from standard normal distributions and then produce a random number by taking the sum of squares of n i.i.d. random numbers. (b) By transforming two independent uniform random numbers X and Y from $U[0, 1]$, we could get two random numbers U and V

from independent standard normal distribution.

$$\begin{cases} U = \sqrt{-2\ln X}\cos 2\pi Y \\ V = \sqrt{-2\ln X}\sin 2\pi Y \end{cases}.$$

(3) Importance resampling: Consider sampling from the distribution with density function $f(x)$. If it is very hard to sample random variables directly from $f(x)$, we could sample random variables from other distributions first. For example, we sample random numbers from distribution with density function $g(x)$ and denote these random numbers as $y_1, \ldots, y_n$. Then, we resample random numbers from $y_1, \ldots, y_n$ and y_i is sampled with probability $\frac{w_i}{\sum_i w_i}$, where $w_i = \frac{f(x_i)}{g(x_i)}$. These resampled numbers have density $f(x)$ when n is large enough.

(4) Importance sampling: Importance sampling is a very powerful tool to estimate expectations. Consider the estimation of $E[g(X)]$. Suppose that the density of X is $\mu(x)$. If we could get the random numbers from distribution with density $\mu(x)$, we could estimate $E[g(X)]$ with $\frac{\sum_{i=1}^n g(x_i)}{n}$. When it is not easy to get the random numbers from distribution with density (x), we could estimate $E[g(X)]$ by the following importance sampling procedure. (a) We generate random numbers $y_1, y_2, \ldots, y_n$ with density $f(y)$, (b) We assign weights for each random number, $w_i = \frac{\mu(y_i)}{f(y_i)}$, (c) We calculate weighted average: $\frac{\sum_{i=1}^n g(y_i)w_i}{n}$ or $\frac{\sum_{i=1}^n g(y_i)w_i}{\sum_{i=1}^n w_i}$. Either of the two weighted averages is a good estimate of $E[g(X)]$.

(5) Practical examples: Stochastic simulation method could solve stochastic problems. It could also solve deterministic problems. Stochastic problems include the validation of statistical theories through simulations. A well-known deterministic problem is the stochastic approximation of integrals $\int_a^b g(x)dx$. Notice that $\int_a^b g(x)dx = \int_a^b \frac{g(x)}{f(x)} f(x)dx$. If we choose $f(x)$ to be a density function then $\int_a^b g(x)dx$ is the expectation of some random variables: $E(\frac{g(X)}{f(X)})$. We could use importance sampling to estimate the expectation.

13.5. Sequential Monte Carlo[6]

Sequential Monte Carlo is usually used to sample random numbers from a dynamic system.

We first introduce sequential importance sampling, which is usually used to sample high-dimensional random vectors. Consider drawing samples from density $\pi(x)$. We apply importance sampling method. We first draw samples from density

$$g(x) = g_1(x_1)g_2(x_2|x_1)\cdots g_d(x_d|x_1,\ldots,x_d).$$

The above decomposition makes sample generating much easier, since we could draw samples from lower-dimensional distribution. Note that x_j could be a multidimensional vector. If the target density $\pi(x)$ could also be decomposed in the way $g(x)$ was decomposed,

$$\pi(x) = \pi(x_1)\pi(x_2|x_1)\cdots\pi(x_d|x_1,\ldots,x_d),$$

then the weight in importance sampling could be defined as

$$w(x) = \frac{\pi(x_1)\pi(x_2|x_1)\cdots\pi(x_d|x_1,\ldots,x_d)}{g_1(x_1)g_2(x_2|x_1)\cdots g_d(x_d|x_1,\ldots,x_d)}.$$

The above weight could be calculated in a recursive way. Let $X_t = (x_1, \ldots, x_t)$, $w_1 = \frac{\pi(x_1)}{g_1(x_1)}$, $w(x)$ could be calculated as follows:

$$w_t(x_t) = w_{t-1}(x_{t-1})\frac{\pi(x_t|X_{t-1})}{g_t(x_t|X_{t-1})}.$$

Finally $w_d(x_d)$ is exactly $w(x)$.

In general, $\pi(x_t|X_{t-1})$ is hard to calculate. To solve this problem, we introduce an auxiliary distribution $\pi_t(X_t)$ which makes $\pi_d(X_d) = \pi(x)$ hold. With the help of this auxiliary distribution, we could have the following importance sampling procedure: (a) sample x_t from $g_t(x_t|X_{t-1})$; (b) calculate $u_t = \frac{\pi_t(X_t)}{\pi_{t-1}(X_{t-1})g_t(x_t|X_{t-1})}$ and let $w_t = w_{t-1}u_t$. It is easy to see that w_d is exactly $w(x)$.

We use state-space model (particle filter) to illustrate sequential Monte Carlo. A state-space model could be described using the following two formulas.

(1) Observation formula: $y_t \sim f_t(\cdot|x_t,\phi)$ and (2) State formula: $x_t \sim q_t(\cdot|x_{t-1},\theta)$. Since x_t could not be observed, this state-space model is also called as Hidden Markov Model. This model could be represented using the following figure:

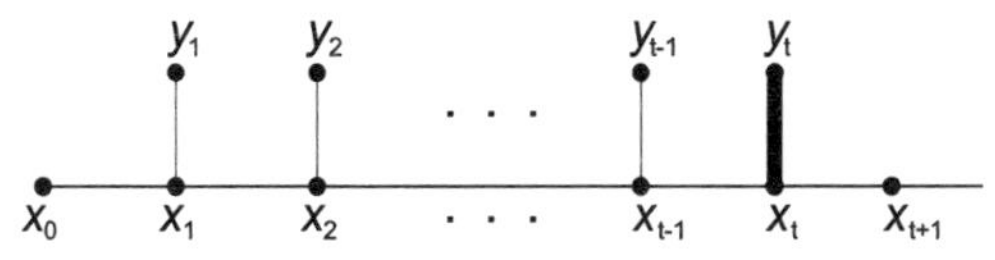

One difficulty in state-space model is how to get the estimation of the current state x_t when we observe $(y_1, y_2, \ldots, y_t)$. We assume all parameters ϕ, θ are known. The best estimator for x_t is

$$E(x_t|y_1, \ldots, y_t) = \frac{\int x_t \prod_{s=1}^{t} [f_s(y_s|x_s)q_s(x_s|x_{s-1})]dx_1 \cdots dx_t}{\int \prod_{s=1}^{t} [f_s(y_s|x_s)q_s(x_s|x_{s-1})]dx_1 \cdots dx_t}.$$

At time t, the posterior of x_t is

$$\pi_t(x_t) = P(x_t|y_1, y_2, \ldots, y_t) \propto \int q_t(x_t|x_{t-1})f_t(y_t|x_t)\pi_{t-1}(x_{t-1})dx_{t-1}.$$

To draw samples from $\pi_t(x_t)$, we could apply sequential Monte Carlo method.

Suppose at time t, we have m samples denoted as $x_t^{(1)}, \ldots, x_t^{(m)}$ from $\pi_t(x_t)$ Now we observe y_{t+1}. The following three steps give samples from $\pi_{t+1}(x_{t+1})$:

1. Draw samples $(x_{t+1}^{(*j)})$ from $q_t(x_{t+1}|x_t^{(j)})$.
2. Assign weights for the generated sample: $w^{(j)} \propto f_t(y_{t+1}|x_{t+1}^{(*j)})$.
3. Draw samples from $\{x_{t+1}^{(1)}, \ldots, x_{t+1}^{(m)}\}$ with probabilities $\{\frac{w^{(1)}}{s}, \ldots, \frac{w^{(m)}}{s}\}$ where $s = \sum_j w^{(j)}$. Denote these samples as $\{x_{t+1}^{(*1)}, \ldots, x_{t+1}^{(*m)}\}$.

If $x_t^{(1)}, \ldots, x_t^{(m)}$ are i.i.d. from $\pi_t(x_t)$, and m is large enough, then $x_{t+1}^{(1)}, \ldots, x_{t+1}^{(m)}$ are approximately from $\pi_{t+1}(x_{t+1})$.

13.6. Optimization for Continuous Function[7,8]

Optimization problem is one important problem in computational statistics. Many parameter estimation problems are optimization problems. For example, maximum likelihood estimation (MLE) is an optimization problem. Commonly used optimization methods include Newton method, Newton-like method, coordinate descent method and conjugate gradient method, etc.

(1) Newton method: Optimization is closely related to finding the solution of an equation. Let us first consider one-dimensional optimization problems. If $f(x)$ has a maximum (or minimum) point at $x = x^*$ and it is smooth enough (for example one order derivative function is continuous and second-order derivatives exists), then $f'(x^*) = 0$. Take the Taylor expansion at $x = x_0$,

we have

$$0 = f^{'}(x) \approx f^{'}(x_0) + f^{''}(x_0)(x - x_0),$$

from which, we have the Newton iteration:

$$x^{(t+1)} = x^{(t)} - \frac{f^{'}(x^{(t)})}{f^{''}(x^{(t)})}.$$

For multidimension problem, consider the maximization problem: $\max_\theta l(\theta)$, the Newton iteration is similar to one-dimensional problem:

$$\theta^{(t+1)} = \theta^{(t)}[1^{''}(\theta^t)]^{-1}l^{'}(\theta^t).$$

(2) Newton-like method: For many multidimensional problems, the Hessian matrix ($1^{''}(\theta^t)$) is hard to calculate and we could use an approximated Hessian ($[M^{(t)}]$) instead:

$$\theta^{(t+1)} = \theta^{(t)}[M^{(t)}]^{-1}l^{'}(\theta^t).$$

There are many reasons why Newton-like method is used instead of Newton method in some situation. First, Hessian matrix might be very hard to calculate. Especially, in high-dimensional problems, it takes too much space. Second, Hessian matrix does not guarantee the increase of objective function during the iteration, while some well-designed $M^{(t)}$ could.

Commonly used $M^{(t)}$ include identity matrix I, and scaled-identity matrix αI, where$\alpha \in (0, 1)$ is a constant.

(3) Coordinate descent: For high-dimensional optimization problems, coordinate descent is a good option. Consider the following problem:

$$\min_{\theta=(\theta_0,\theta_2,\ldots,\theta_p)} l(\theta_1, \theta_2, \ldots, \theta_p).$$

The principle of coordinate descent algorithm is that for each iteration, we only update one coordinate and keep all other coordinates fixed. This procedure could be described using the following pseudo-code:

```
Initialization: θ = (θ_2, ..., θ_p)
for j = 1, 2, ..., p
  update θ_j (keep al other θ_k fixed)
```

(4) Conjugate Gradient: Let us first consider a quadratic optimization problem:

$$\min_{X \in R^k} \frac{1}{2}x^{'}Gx + x^{'}b + c,$$

where G is a $k \times k$ positive definite matrix. If k vectors $q_1, q_2, \ldots, q_k$ satisfy $\langle q_i, Gq_j \rangle = 0, \forall_i \neq j$, we say that these vectors are conjugate respective to G. It could be proved that we could get the minimal point if we alternatively search on any k directions that are conjugate. There are many conjugate directions. If the first direction is negative gradient, and the other directions are linear combinations of already calculated directions, we have conjugate gradient method. Generalizing the above idea to a general function other than quadratic function, we have general conjugate gradient method.

13.7. Optimization for Discrete Functions[9–11]

Optimization for discrete functions is quite different from optimization for continuous functions. Consider the following problem:

$$\max_{\theta} f(\theta),$$

where θ could take N different values. N could be a bounded integer and it could also be infinity. A well-known discrete optimization problem is "Traveling Salesman" problem. This is a typical non-deterministic polynomial time problem (NP for short). Many discrete optimization problems are NP problems.

We use a classical problem in statistics to illustrate how to deal with discrete optimization problems in computations statistics. Consider a simple linear regression problem:

$$y_i = \sum_{j=1}^{p} x_{ij}\beta_j + \epsilon_i, \quad i = 1, 2, \ldots, n,$$

where for p coefficients β_j, only s non-zeros and the rest $p - s$ coefficients are zeros. In other words, among the p predictors, only s of them contribute to y. Now the problem is to detect which s predictors contribute to y. We could use AIC, and solve the following discrete optimization problem:

$$\min_{m} n \log \left[\frac{\text{RSS}(\beta, m)}{n} \right] + 2s,$$

where $\text{RSS}(\beta, m)$ is the residual sum of squares and m denotes a model, that is, which predictors contribute to y. There are 2^p possible models. When p is big, it is impossible to search over all of the possible models. We need a few strategies. One strategy is to use greedy method — we try to make the objective function decrease at each iteration by iteration method. To avoid local minimum, multiple initial values could be used. For the above-statistical problem, we could randomly select a few variables as the initial model and then for each iteration we add or delete one variable to make the objective function decrease. Forward searching and backward searching are usually used to select a good model. They are also called as stepwise regression.

Simulation annealing is another way to solve discrete optimization problems. Evolutionary algorithm is also very popular for discrete optimization problem. These two kinds of optimization methods try to find the global solution of the optimization problem. But they have the disadvantage that these algorithms are too complicated and they converge very slowly.

Recently, there is a new way to deal with discrete optimization problem, which tries to relax the original discrete problem to a continuous convex problem. We still take the variable selection problem as an example. If we replace s in the objective function as $\sum_{j=1}^{p} |\beta_j|$, we have a convex optimization problem and the complexity of solving this new convex problem is much lower than the original discrete problem. It also has its own disadvantage: not all discrete problems could be transfered to a convex problem and it is not guaranteed that the new problem and the old problem have the same solution.

13.8. Matrix Computation[12,13]

Statistical analysis cannot leave away from matrix computation. This is because data are usually stored in a matrix and a lot of statistical methods needs the operations on matrix. For example, the estimation in linear regression needs the inversion of a matrix and principal component analysis (PCA) needs singlular value decomposition (SVD) of a matrix.

We introduce a few commonly used matrix operation, including (1) triangular factorization, (2) orthogonal-triangular factorization and (3) singular value decomposition.

(1) Triangular factorization: In general, a matrix can be decomposed into product of a unit lower-triangular matrix (L) and an upper-triangular matrix. This kind of decomposition is called LR factorization. It is very useful in solving linear equations. When matrix X is symmetric and positive definite, it has special decomposition, that is $X = TT'$ where T' is the transpose of matrix T and T is a lower-triangular matrix and so T' is an upper-triangular matrix. This kind of decomposition for positive definite matrix is called as Cholesky decomposition. It can be proved that Cholesky decomposition for a symmetric and positive definite matrix always exists. If we further ensure that the diagonal matrix in triangular matrix (T) is

positive, then Cholesky decomposition is unique. Triangular factorization could be seen in solving linear equations and calculate the determinant of a matrix.

(2) Orthogonal-triangular factorization: The decomposition of a matrix to a product of an orthogonal matrix and a triangular matrix is called as orthogonal-triangular factorization or QR factorization. For a matrix with real values, if it is full column rank, the QR factorization must exist. If we further ensure the diagonal elements in the triangular matrix is positive, then the factorization is unique. Householder transformation and Given transformation could be used to get QR decomposition.

(3) Singular value decomposition: SVD for short of a matrix plays a very important role in computational statistics. The calculation of principal components in PCA needs SVD. SVD is closely related to eigenvalue decomposition. Suppose that A is a symmetric real matrix, then A has the following eigenvalue decomposition (or spectral decomposition):

$$A = UDU',$$

where U is an orthogonal matrix $UU^{'} = I$, D is a diagonal matrix. Denote $U = [u_1, \ldots, u_n]$ and $D = \text{diag}(\lambda_1, \ldots, \lambda_n)$, A could be written as

$$A = \sum_{i=1}^{n} \lambda_i u_i u_i^{'}.$$

The diagonal elements of D are called as the eigenvalues of A and u_i is called as the eigenvector of A in respect to the eigenvalue λ_i. In PCA, A is taken as sample covariance matrix $A = \frac{X^{'}X}{n}$ (*note*: X is the centralized matrix. The eigen vector of A in respect to the largest eigenvalue is the loading of the first principal component.

For a general matrix $X \in \mathbb{R}^{n \times m}$, it has a singular value decomposition that is similar as eigenvalue decomposition. SVD is defined as follows:

$$X = UDV',$$

where $U \in \mathbb{R}^{n \times r}, D \in \mathbb{R}^{r \times r}, V \in \mathbb{R}^{m \times r}$. r is the rank of X. $U^{'}U = V^{'}V = I$. D is a diagonal matrix and all of its diagonal elements are positive. By the following equations, we could see the relationship between SVD and eigenvalue decomposition:

$$X^{'}X = V^{'}DU^{'}UDV = V^{'}D^2V$$

$$XX^{'} = UDV^{'}VDU^{'} = UD^2U'.$$

That is, V is the eigenvector of $X^{'}X$ and U is the eigenvector of XX'. Iterative QR decomposition could be used to calculate the eigenvalues and eigenvectors of a symmetric matrix.

13.9. Missing Data[14]

Missing data is very common in real data analysis. We briefly introduce how to deal with missing data problems. We denote by Y the observed data, and by Z the missing data. The goal is to calculate the observational posterior $p(\theta|Y)$. Because of missing data, it is very hard to calculate this posterior. We could calculate it by iteratively applying the following two formulas:

$$p(\theta|Y) = \int p(\theta|Y, Z)p(Z|Y)dz$$

$$p(Z|Y) = \int p(Z|\theta, Y)p(\theta|Y)d\theta.$$

The iterative steps are described as follows:

a. Imputation:
   Draw samples $z_1, z_2, \ldots, z_m$ from $p(Z|Y)$.
b. Posterior update:

$$[p(\theta|Y)]^{(t+1)} = \frac{1}{m}\sum_{j=1}^{m} p(\theta|Y, z_j).$$

The sampling in Step (a) is usually hard. We could use an approximation instead:

(a1) Draw θ^* from $[p(\theta|Y)]^{(t)}$,
(a2) Draw Z from $p(Z|\theta^*, Y)$.

Repeating (a1) and (a2) many times, we obtain $z_1, z_2, \ldots, z_m$, which can be treated as samples from $p(Z|Y)$.

In the above iterations, it is hard to draw samples from $p(Z|Y)$ and it takes a lot of resources. To overcome this difficulty, more economic way is proposed and it is named as "Poor man's data augmentation (PMDA)". The simplest PMDA is to estimate θ first and denote by $\hat{\theta}$ the estimation. Then $p(Z|Y, \hat{\theta})$ is used to approximate $p(Z|Y)$. Another option is to have a more accurate estimation, for example second-order approximation. If $p(Z|Y)$ is easy to calculate, we could also use importance sampling to get exact posterior distribution. Note that

$$p(\theta|Y) = \int p(\theta|Y, Z)\frac{p(Z|Y)}{p(Z|Y, \hat{\theta})}p(Z|Y, \hat{\theta})dz.$$

By the following steps, we could get the exact posterior:

a. Imputation:

(a1) Draw samples $z_1, z_2, \ldots, z_m$ from $p(Z|Y, \hat{\theta})$.
(a2) Calculate the weights

$$w_j = \frac{p(z_j|Y)}{p(z_j|Y, \hat{\theta})},$$

b. Posterior update:

$$p(\theta|Y) = \frac{1}{\sum_j w_j} \sum_{j=1}^{m} w_j p(\theta|Y, z_j).$$

The above data augmentation method is based on Bayes analysis. Now, we introduce more general data augmentation methods in practice.

Consider the following data:

$$\begin{pmatrix} Y_1 \\ X_1 \end{pmatrix}, \ldots, \begin{pmatrix} Y_{n_1} \\ X_{n_1} \end{pmatrix}, \begin{pmatrix} ? \\ X_{(1)} \end{pmatrix}, \ldots, \begin{pmatrix} ? \\ X_{(n_0)} \end{pmatrix},$$

where "?" denotes missing data. We could use the following two imputation methods:

(1) Hot deck imputation: This method is model free and it is mainly for when X is discrete. We first divide data into K categories according to the values of X. For the missing data in each category, we randomly impute these missing Ys from the observed ones. When all missing values are imputed, complete data could be used to estimate parameters. After a few repetitions, the average of these estimates is the final point estimator of the unknown parameter(s).

(2) Imputation via simple residuals: For simple linear model, we could use the observed data only to estimate parameters and then get the residuals. Then randomly selected residuals are used to impute the missing data. When all missing values are imputed, complete data could be used to estimate parameters. After a few repetitions, the average of these estimates is the final point estimator of the unknown parameter(s).

13.10. Expectation–maximum (EM) Algorithm[15]

When there are missing data or even where there is no missing data, but when hidden variable is introduced, the likelihood function becomes quite simpler, EM algorithm might make the procedure to get the MLE much easier.

Denote by Y the observation data and Z the missing data θ is the target parameter. The goal is to get the MLE of θ:

$$\max_{\theta} P(Y|\theta).$$

EM algorithm is an iterative method. The calculation from θ_n to θ_{n+1} can be decomposed into E step and M step as follows:

1. E step. We calculate the conditional expectation $E_n(\theta)E_{Z|Y,\theta_n} \log P(Y,Z|\theta)$.
2. M step. We maximize the above conditional expectation

$$\theta_{n+1} = \arg\max_{\theta} E_n(\theta).$$

EM algorithm has the property that the observation likelihood $P(Y|\theta)$ increases from $\theta = \theta_n$ to $\theta = \theta_{n+1}$. EM algorithm usually converges to the local maximum of the observation likelihood function. If the likelihood function has multiple maximums, EM algorithm might not get the global maximum. This could be resolved by using many initial points.

For exponential family, EM algorithm could be treated as updating sufficient statistics. We briefly explain this phenomenon. Exponential family has the following type of density:

$$p(Y,Z|\theta) = \phi(Y,Z)\psi(\xi(\theta))\exp\{\xi(\theta)^T t(Y,Z)\},$$

where Y denotes the observed data, Z denotes the missing data and θ is the parameter. $t(Y,Z)$ is sufficient statistics. In EM algorithm, E step is:

$$\begin{aligned} E_n(\theta) &\triangleq E_{Z|Y,\theta_n} \log P(Y,Z|\theta) \\ &= E_{Z|Y,\theta_n}\phi(Y,Z) + \psi(\xi(\theta)) + \xi(\theta)^T E_{Z|Y,\theta_n}(t(Y,Z)). \end{aligned}$$

M step is to maximize $E_n(\theta)$, which is equivalent to maximize the following function:

$$\psi(\xi(\theta)) + \xi(\theta)^T E_{Z|Y,\theta_n}(t(Y,Z)).$$

Comparing the above function with the likelihood function using both Y and Z, we see that in EM algorithm, we only have to calculate the conditional expectation of sufficient statistics $E_{Z|Y,\theta_n}(t(Y,Z))$.

We take two–dimensional normal data with missing values as an example. $(X_1, X_2) \sim N(\mu_1, \mu_2, \sigma_1^2, \sigma_2^2, \rho)$. Sufficient statistics is the vector of $(\sum_i x_{i1}, \sum_i x_{i2}, \sum_i x_{i1}x_{i2}, \sum_i x_{i1}^2, \sum_i x_{i2}^2)$. The estimate of the five parameters in the two–dimensional normal distribution is the function of the sufficient statistics. For example, $\hat{\mu}_1 = \frac{1}{n}\sum_i x_{i1}$. When some value is missing, for example x_{i1} is missing, we need to replace the items that contains x_{i1} with the conditional expectation. Specifically, we need $E(x_{i1}|x_{i2}, \theta^{(t)}), E(x_{i1}x_{i2}|x_{i2}, \theta^{(t)})$ and $E(x_{i1}^2|x_{i2}\theta^{(t)})$ to replace $x_{i1}, x_{i1}x_{i2}$, and x_{i1}^2, respectively, in the sufficient statistics. $\theta^{(t)}$ is the current estimation of the five parameters. The whole procedure could be described as follows:

1. Initialize $\theta = \theta^{(0)}$.
2. Calculate the conditional expectation of missing items in the sufficient statistics.
3. Update the parameters using the completed sufficient statistics. For $j = 1, 2$,

$$\hat{\mu_j} = \frac{1}{n}\sum_i x_{ij}, \hat{\sigma}_j^2 = \frac{1}{n}\sum_i (x_{ij} - \hat{\mu}_j)^2,$$

$$\hat{\rho} = \frac{\frac{1}{n}\sum_i (x_{i1} - \hat{\mu}_1)(x_{i2} - \hat{\mu}_2)}{\hat{\sigma_1}\hat{\sigma_2}}.$$

4. Repeat 2 and 3 until convergence.

13.11. Markov Chain Monte Carlo (MCMC)[16,17]

MCMC is often used to deal with very complicated models. There are two commonly used MCMC algorithms, Gibbs sampling and Metropolis method.

(1) Gibbs sampling: It is usually not easy to draw samples from multi-dimensional distributions. Gibbs sampling tries to solve this difficulty by drawing samples from one-dimensional problems iteratively. It constructs a Markov chain with the target distribution as the stable distribution of the constructed Markov chain. The detailed procedure of Gibbs sampling is as follows. Consider drawing samples from $p(\theta_1, \theta_2, \ldots, \theta_d)$. We first give initial values of $\theta^{(0)} = (\theta_1^{(0)}, \theta_2^{(0)}, \ldots, \theta_d^{(0)})$,

1. draw $\theta_1^{(i+1)}$ from $p(\theta_1|\theta_2^{(i)}, \ldots, \theta_d^{(i)})$,
2. draw $\theta_2^{(i+1)}$ from $p(\theta_2|\theta_1^{(i+1)}, \theta_3^{(i)}, \ldots, \theta_d^{(i)})$,

   ...

d. draw $\theta_d^{(i+1)}$ from $p(\theta_d|\theta_1^{(i+1)}, \theta_2^{(i+1)}, \ldots, \theta_{d-1}^{(i+1)})$.

This procedure makes $(\theta^{(0)}, \theta^{(1)}, \ldots, \theta^{(t)}, \ldots)$ a Markov chain, and its stable distribution is the target distribution $p(\theta_1, \theta_2, \ldots, \theta_d)$.

(2) Metropolis method: Different from Gibbs sampling, Metropolis method provides a simpler state transferring strategy. It first moves the current state

of random vector and then accepts the new state with well-designed probability. Metropolis method also construct a Markov chain and the stable distribution is also the target distribution. The detailed procedure of Metropolis method is as follows. Consider drawing samples from $\pi(x)$. We first design a symmetric transfer probability function $f(x, y) = f(y, x)$. For example, $f(y, x) \propto \exp(-\frac{1}{2}(y - x)^T \Sigma^{-1}(y - x))$ the probability density function of a normal distribution with mean x and covariance matrix Σ.

1. Suppose that the current state is $X_n = x$. We randomly draw a candidate state (y^*) from $f(x, y)$;
2. We accept this new state with probability $\alpha(x, y^*) = \min\{\frac{\pi(y^*)}{\pi(x)}, 1\}$. If the new state is accepted, let $X_{n+1} = y^*$, else, let $X_{n+1} = x$.

The series of $(X_1, X_2, \ldots, X_n, \ldots)$ is a Markov chain, and its stable distribution is $\pi(x)$.

Hastings (1970)[32] extended Metropolis method. They pointed out the transfer probability function does not have to be symmetric. Suppose the transfer probability function is $q(x, y)$, then the acceptance probability is defined as

$$\alpha(x, y) = \begin{cases} \min\left\{\frac{\pi(y)q(y,x)}{\pi(x)q(x,y)}, 1\right\}, & if\ \pi(x)q(x, y) > 0 \\ 1, & if\ \pi(x)q(x, y) = 0. \end{cases}$$

It is easy to see that if $q(x, y) = q(y, x)$, the above acceptance probability is the same as the one in the Metropolis method. The extended method is called as Metropolis–Hastings method.

Gibbs sampling could be seen as a special Metropolis–Hastings method. In Metropolis–Hastings method, if the transfer probability function is chosen as the fully conditional density, it is easy to prove that $\alpha(x, y) = 1$, that is, the new state is always accepted.

Note that MCMC does not provide independent samples. But because it produces Markov chains, we have the following conclusion:

Suppose that $\theta^{(0)}, \theta^{(1)}, \ldots, \theta^{(t)}, \ldots$ are random numbers (or vectors) drawn from MCMC, then for a general continuous function $f(\cdot)$,

$$\lim_{t \to \infty} \frac{1}{t} \sum_{i=1}^{t} f(\theta^{(t)}) = E(f(\theta)),$$

where θ follows the stable distribution of the MCMC. So we could use the samples from MCMC to estimate every kind of expectations. If independent samples are really needed, independent multiple Markov chains could be used.

13.12. Bootstrap[18,19]

Bootstrap, also known as resampling technique, is a very important method in data analysis. It could be used to construct confidence intervals of very complicated statistics and it could also be used to get the approximate distribution of a complicated statistics. It is also a well-known tool to check the robustness of a statistical method.

The goal of Bootstrap is to estimate the distribution of a specified random variable ($R(x, F)$) that depends on the samples ($x = (x_1, x_2, \ldots, x_n)$) and its unknown distributions (F). We first describe the general Bootstrap procedure.

1. Construct the empirical distribution $\hat{F}: P(X = x_i) = 1/n$.
2. Draw n independent samples from empirical distribution $\hat{F}$. Denote these samples as $x_i^*, i = 1, 2, \ldots, n$. In fact, these samples are randomly drawn from $\{x_1, x_2, \ldots, x_n\}$ with replacement.
3. Calculate $R^* = R(x^*, \hat{F})$.

Repeat the above procedures many times and we get many R^*. Thus, we could get the empirical distribution of R^*, and this empirical distribution is used to approximate the distribution of $R(x, F)$. This is Boostrap. Because in bootstrap procedure, we need to draw samples from the observation, this method is also called as re-sampling method.

The above procedure is the classic non-parametric bootstrap and it is often used to estimate the variance of an estimator. There are parametric versions of Bootstrap. We take regression as an example to illustrate the parametric bootstrap. Consider the regression model

$$Y_i = g_i(X, \beta) + \epsilon_i, \quad i = 1, 2, \ldots, n,$$

where $g(\cdot)$ is a known function and β is unknown; $\epsilon_i \sim F$ i.i.d. with $E_F(\epsilon_i) = 0$ and F is unknown.

We treat X deterministic. The randomness of data comes from the error term ϵ_i. β could be estimated from least squares,

$$\hat{\beta} = \arg\min_{\beta} \sum_{i=1}^{n} (Y_i - g(x_i, \beta))^2.$$

If we want to get the variance of $\hat{\beta}$, parametric Bootstrap could be used.

1. Construct the empirical distribution of residuals $\hat{F}: P(\epsilon_i = \hat{\epsilon}_i) = \frac{1}{n}$, where $\hat{\epsilon}_i = Y_i - g(x_i, \hat{\beta})$.
2. Resampling. Draw n i.i.d. samples from empirical distribution $\hat{F}$ and denote these samples as $\epsilon_i^*, i = 1, 2, \ldots, n$.

3. Calculate the "resampled" value of Y:

$$Y_i^* = g(x_i, \beta) + \epsilon_i^*.$$

4. Re-estimate parameter β using $(x_i, y_i^*), i = 1, 2, \ldots, n$.
5. Repeat the above steps and get multiple estimate of β. These estimations could be used to construct the confidence interval of β, as well as the variance of $\hat{\beta}$.

Bootstrap can also be used to reduce bias of statistics. We first estimate the bias $(\hat{\theta}(x) - \theta(F))$ using bootstrap, where $\hat{\theta}(x)$ is the estimate of $\theta(F)$ using observed samples and $\theta(F)$ is the unknown parameter. Once the bias is obtained, deducting the (estimated) bias from $\hat{\theta}(x)$, we have a less-biased estimator. The detailed procedure is as follows:

1. Construct the empirical distribution $\hat{F}$: $P(X = x_i) = 1/n$.
2. Randomly draw samples from $\{x_1, x_2, \ldots, x_n\}$ with replacement and denote these samples as $x^* = (x_1^*, x_2^*, \ldots, x_n^*)$.
3. Calculate $R^* = \hat{\theta}(x^*) - \theta(\hat{F})$.

Repeat the above three steps and we get the estimate of bias, that is, the average of multiple R^*'s denoted as $\bar{R}^*$. The less-biased estimate of $\theta(F)$ is then $\hat{\theta}(x) - \bar{R}^*$.

In addition to Bootstrap, cross-validation, Jackknife method and permutation test all used the idea of resampling.

13.13. Cross-validation[19,20]

Cross-validation is a very important technique in data analysis. It is often used to evaluate different models. For example, to classify objects, one could use linear discriminant analysis (LDA) or quadratic discriminant analysis (QDA). The question now is: which model or method is better? If we have enough data, we could split the data into two parts: one is used to train models and the other to evaluate the model.

But what if we do not have enough data? If we still split the data into train data and test data, the problem is obvious. (1) There are not enough train data and so the estimation of the model has big random errors; (2) There are not enough test data and so the prediction has big random errors. To reduce the random errors in the prediction, we could consider using the sample many times: for example, we split the data many times and take the average of prediction errors. K-fold cross-validation is described as follows:

Suppose each element in the set of $\{\lambda_1, \lambda_2, \ldots, \lambda_M\}$ corresponds to one model and our goal is to select the best model. For each possible values,

1. Randomly split the data into K parts; every part has the same size.
2. For each part, we leave the data for prediction and use the remainder $K-1$ parts of data to estimate a model.
3. Use the estimated model to predict ions on the reserved data and calculate the prediction errors (sum of residual squares).
4. Finally, we choose the λ that makes the sum of errors the smallest.

In the K-fold cross-validation, if K is chosen as the number of sample size n, the cross-validation is called as Leave one out cross-validation (LOO). When sample size is very small, LOO is usually used to evaluate models.

Another method very closely related to LOO is Jackknife. Jackknife also removes one sample every time (could also remove multiple samples). But the goal of Jackknife is different from LOO. Jackknife is more similar to Bootstrap and it is to get the property of an estimator (for example, to get the bias or variance of an estimator), while LOO is to evaluate models. We briefly describe Jackknife.

Suppose $Y_1, \ldots, Y_n$ are n i.i.d. samples. We denote by $\hat{\theta}$ the estimate of parameter θ. First, we divide data into g groups, and we assume that each group has h observations, $n = gh$. For one special case, $g = n, h = 1$. Let $\hat{\theta}_{-i}$ denote the estimate of θ after the ith group of data deleted. Now, we find a few values:

$$\tilde{\theta}_i = g\hat{\theta} - (g-1)\hat{\theta}_{-i}, \quad i = 1, \ldots, g.$$

Jackknife estimator is

$$\hat{\theta}_J = \frac{1}{g}\sum_{i=1}^{g}\tilde{\theta}_i = g\hat{\theta} - \frac{g-1}{g}\sum_{i=1}^{g}\hat{\theta}_{-i}$$

and the estimated variance is

$$\frac{1}{g(g-1)}\sum_{i=1}^{g}(\tilde{\theta}_i - \hat{\theta}_J)^2 = \frac{g-1}{g}\sum_{i=1}^{g}(\hat{\theta}_{-i} - \hat{\theta}_{(\cdot)})^2,$$

where $\hat{\theta}_{(\cdot)} = \sum_{i=1}^{g}\hat{\theta}_{-i}$.

It can be seen that Jackknife estimator has the following good properties: (1) the calculation procedure is simple; (2) it gives the estimated variance of the estimator. It has another property — reduce bias.

13.14. Permutation Test[21]

Permutation test is a robust non-parametric test. Compared with parametric test, it does not need the assumption on distribution of data. It constructs statistics using resampled data based on the fact that under the null hypothesis, two groups of data have the same distribution.

By a simple example, we introduce the basic idea and steps of using permutation test. Consider the following two-sample test: the first sample has five observations denoted as $\{X_1, X_2, X_3, X_4, X_5\}$. They are i.i.d. samples and have distribution function $F(x)$; the second sample has four observations denoted as $\{Y_1, Y_2, Y_3, Y_4\}$. They are i.i.d. samples and have distribution function $G(x)$. The null hypothesis is $H_0\colon F(x) = G(x)$, and the alternative is $H_1\colon F(x) \neq G(x)$.

Before considering permutation test, let us consider parameter test first. Take T-test for example. T-test has a very strong assumption that $F(x) = G(x)$ and both of them are distribution function of one normal random variable. This assumption cannot even be tested when sample size is very small. Test statistics for T-test is defined as follows:

$$T = \frac{\bar{X} - \bar{Y}}{S\sqrt{\frac{1}{5} + \frac{1}{4}}}.$$

where $\bar{X} = \frac{1}{5}\sum_{i=1}^{5} X_i$, $\bar{Y} = \frac{1}{4}\sum_{i=1}^{4} Y_i$, $S^2 = \frac{\sum_{i=1}^{5}(X_i-\bar{X})^2+\sum_{j=1}^{4}(Y_i-\bar{Y})^2}{5+4-2}$. When $|T| > c$, we reject the null hypothesis and treat the two data from two different distributions. c is decided by the level of test. We usually choose the level to be $\alpha = 0.05$. In T-test, $c = |T_7(0.025)| = T_7(1 - 0.025)$, where $T_7(0.025) < 0$ denotes the 0.025 quantile of t distribution with degree of freedom 7, that is $P(T \leq T_7(p) = p)$.

We have to point out one more time that the chosen c in T-test depends on a strong assumption that data are from normal distribution. When this assumption is very hard to verify, we could consider permutation test.

Permutation test only uses the assumption that data are from the same distribution. Since they have the same distribution, we could treat them as i.i.d. samples. So T defined above should have the same distribution of T' defined as follows:

(1) We randomly choose five elements from $\{X_1, X_2, X_3, X_4, X_5, Y_1, Y_2, Y_3, Y_4\}$ without replacement and let them be the first sample. Denote these five elements as $\{X_1', X_2', X_3', X_4', X_5'\}$ The remaining four elements denoted by $\{Y_1', Y_2', Y_3', Y_4'\}$ are treated as the second sample.
(2) We calculate T' using the same formula as T.

For this small data set, we could calculate the distribution of T. Under the null hypothesis, T uniformly takes values on $(9/5) = 126$ possible numbers. If we use the level of test $\alpha = 0.05$, we could construct the rejection area $\{T\colon |T| > |T|_{(120)}\}$, $|T|_{(120)}$ denotes the 120 largest values of 126 possible $|T|$s. It is easy to know that $P_{H_0}(|T| > |T|_{(120)}) = \frac{6}{126} = 0.0476$.

In general, if the first sample has m observations, and the second sample has n observations when both m and n are very large, it is impossible to get the exact distribution of T and at this situation, we use Monte Carlo method to get the approximate distribution of T and calculate its 95% quantile, that is, the critical value c.

13.15. Regularized Method[11,22,23]

Regularized method is very popular in parameter estimation. We first take the ridge regression as an example. Consider least squares,

$$\min_{\beta} ||Y - X\beta||_2^2.$$

When X^TX is invertible, the solution is $(X^TX)^{-1}X^TY$; when X^TX is not invertible, usually regularized method is used, for example,

$$\min_{\beta} ||Y - X\beta||_2^2 + \lambda||\beta||_2^2,$$

where $\lambda > 0$, and $||\beta||_2^2$ is called the regularized term. The above regularized optimization problem has a unique solution:

$$(X^TX + \lambda I)^{-1}X^TY.$$

Even if X^TX is invertible, regularized method always gives more robust estimator of β.

$||\beta||_2^2$ is not the only possible regularized term. We could also choose $||\beta||_1 \triangleq \sum_{j=1}^{p} |\beta_j|$ as the regularized term and it is called L1 regularization. L1 regularization is very popular in high-dimensional statistics and it makes the estimation of β sparse and so could be used for variable selection.

L1 regularized least square is also called as Lasso and it is defined as follows:

$$\min_{\beta} ||Y - X\beta||_2^2 + \lambda||\beta||_1.$$

When $\lambda = 0$, the solution is exactly the same as least squares. When λ is very big, $\beta = 0$. That is, none of these variables is selected. λ controls the size of selected variables and in practice, it is usually decided by cross-validations.

Regularized terms can also be used for other optimization problems than least squares. For example, L1 regularized Logistic regression could be used for variable selections in Logistic regression problems. In general, L1 regularized maximum likelihood could select variables for a general model.

There are many other regularized terms in modern high-dimensional statistics. For example, group regularization could be used for group selection.

Different from ridge regression, general regularized methods including the Lasso do not have closed-form solutions. They usually have to depend on numerical methods. Since a lot of regularized terms including L1 term are not differentiable at some points, traditional methods like Newton methods cannot be used. There are a few commonly used methods, including coordinate descent and Alternating Direction Method of Multipliers (ADMM).

The solution of general regularized method, especially for convex problem, can be described by KKT conditions. KKT is short for Karush–Kuhn–Tucker. Consider the following constrained optimization problem:

$$\begin{aligned} &\text{minimize } f_0(x), \\ &\text{subject to } f_i(x) \leq 0, \quad i = 1, 2, \ldots, n, \\ &h_j(x) = 0, \quad j = 1, 2, \ldots, m. \end{aligned}$$

Denote by x^* the solution of the above problem. x^* must satisfy the following KKT conditions:

1. $f_i(x^*) \leq 0$ and $h_j(x) = 0, i = 1, 2, \ldots, n; j = 1, 2, \ldots, m$.
2. $$\nabla f_0(x^*) + \sum_{i=1}^{n} \lambda_i \nabla f_i(x^*) + \sum_{j=1}^{m} \nu_j \nabla h_j(x^*) = 0.$$
3. $\lambda_i \geq 0, i = 1, 2, \ldots, n$ and $\lambda_i f_i(x^*) = 0$.

Under a few mild conditions, it can be proved that any x^* satisfying KKT conditions is the solution of the above problem.

13.16. Gaussian Graphical Model[24,25]

Graphical model is used to represent the relationships between variables. A graph is denoted by (V, E) where V is the set of vertices and $E \subset V \times V$ is the set of edges. When we use graphical model to represent the relationship between variables, V is usually chosen as the set of all variables. That is, each vertex in the graph denotes one variable. Two vertices (or variables) are not connected if and only if they are conditionally independent given all other variables. So, it is very easy to read conditional independences from the graph.

How to learn a graphical model from data is a very important problem in both statistics and machine learning. When data are from multivariate normal distribution, the learning becomes much easier. The following Theorem gives the direction on how to learn a Gaussian graphical model.

Theorem 3. *Suppose that* $X = (X_1, \ldots, X_p)$ *follows a joint normal distribution* $N(0, \Sigma)$*, where* Σ *is positive definite. The following three properties are equivalent:*

1. *In the graphical model, there is no edge between* X_i *and* X_j*.*
2. $\Sigma^{-1}(i, j) = 0$.
3. $E(X_j | X_{V \setminus X_j}) = \sum_{k \neq j} \beta_{jk} X_k, \beta_{ji} = 0$.

Theorem 3 tells us that, to learn a Gaussian graphical model, we only need to know if the element in the inverse covariance matrix is zero or not. We could also learn Gaussian graphical model via linear regression method. That is, run regression of one variable, (for example X_j), on all other variables, if the coefficient is zero (for example, the coefficient of X_i is 0), then there is no edge between X_i and X_j on the graphical model.

When there are only very few number of variables, hypothesis test could be used to tell which coefficient is zero. When there are many variables, we could consider L1 regularized method. The following two L1 regularized methods could be used to learn a Gaussian graphical model.

(1) Inverse covariance matrix selection: Since we know that the existence of one edge between two vertices is equivalent if the corresponding element in inverse covariance matrix is 0 or not. We could learn sparse Gaussian graphical model by learning a sparse inverse covariance matrix. Note that the log likelihood function is

$$\ell\left(\sum\right) = \log\left(|\Sigma^{-1}|\right) - tr\left(\Sigma^{-1} S\right),$$

where S is the sample covariance matrix. To get a sparse Σ^{-1}, we could solve the following L1 regularized log likelihood optimization problem:

$$\min_{\theta} - \log(|\Theta|) + tr(\Theta S) + \lambda \sum_{i \neq j} |\Theta_{ij}|,$$

The solution of Θ is the estimate of Σ^{-1}. Because of L1 regularized term, many elements in the estimate of Θ are 0, which corresponds to non-existence of edges on the graphical model.

(2) Neighborhood selection: L1 regularized linear regression could be used to learn the neighborhood of a variable. The neighborhood of a variable (say X_j) is defined as the variables that are connected to the variable (X_j) on the graphical model. The following Lasso problem could tell which variables are the neighborhood of X_j.

$$\theta^{j,\lambda} = \arg\min_{\theta} \|X_j - X_{V\backslash X_j}\theta\|_2^2 + \lambda\|\theta\|_1.$$

The neighborhood of X_j is the set of variables that has non-zero coefficient in the estimate of $\theta^{j,\lambda}$. That is,

$$ne(j,\lambda) = \{k: \theta^{j,\lambda}[k] \neq 0\}.$$

It is possible that X_i is chosen in the neighborhood of X_j, while X_j is not chosen in the neighborhood of X_i. For this situation, we could assign an edge between X_i and X_j on the graphical model.

In the above two regularized methods, λ is a tuning parameter and it could be decided by cross-validation.

13.17. Decision Tree[26,27]

Decision tree divides the space of predictors into a few rectangular areas, and on each rectangular area, a simple model (for example a constant) is decided. Decision tree is a very useful nonlinear statistical model. Here, we first introduce regression tree, then introduce classification tree, and finally, we introduce random forest.

(1) Regression tree: Suppose now we have N observations $(x_i, y_i), i = 1, 2, \ldots, N$, where x_i is a p-dimensional vector, y_i is a scalar response. Regression tree is to decide how to divide the data and to decide the values of response on each part. Suppose that we have already divided the data into M parts, denoted by $R_1, R_2, \ldots, R_M$. We take simple function on each part, that is, a constant on each part. This simple function could be written as $f(x) = \sum_{m=1}^{M} c_m I(x \in R_m)$. Least squares could be used to decide the constants:

$$\hat{c}_m = \text{avg}(y_i | x_i \in R_m).$$

In practice, every part in not known and we have learnt the partition from observed data. To remove complexity, greedy learning could be used.

Specifically, we consider splitting some area by one predictor only iteratively. For example, by considering the value of predictor X_j, we could divide the data into two parts:

$$R_1(j,s) = \{X|X_j \leq s\} \quad \text{and} \quad R_2(j,s) = \{X|X_j > s\}.$$

We could find the best j and s by searching over all possible values:

$$\min_{j,s}\left[\min_{c_1}\left[\sum_{x_i \in R_1(j,s)} (y_i - c_1)^2\right] + \min_{c_2}\left[\sum_{x_i \in R_2(j,s)} (y_i - c_2)^2\right]\right].$$

Once we have a few partitions, in each part, we take the same procedure as above and divide the parts into two parts iteratively. This way, we get a few rectangular areas and in each area, a constant function is used to fit the model. To decide when we shall stop partitioning the data, cross-validation could be used.

(2) Classification tree: For classification problems, response is not continuous but takes K different discrete values. We could use the similar procedures of regression tree to partition the observed data. But the difference is that we could not use least squares as the objective function. Instead, we could use misclassification rate, Gini index or negative log likelihood as the loss function and try to minimize the loss for different partitions and for different values on each partition of the data. Let us take misclassification as an example to see how to learn a classification tree. For the first step to divide the data into two parts, we are minimizing the following loss:

$$\min_{j,s}\left[\min_{c_1}\left[\sum_{x_i \in R_1(j,s)} I(y_i \neq c_1)\right] + \min_{c_2}\left[\sum_{x_i \in R_2(j,s)} I(y_i \neq c_2)\right]\right].$$

The procedures of classification tree and regression tree are quite similar.

(3) Random forest: Random forest first constructs a few decision trees by a few Bootstrap samples and then it combines the results of all of these trees. Below is the procedure of random forest.

1. For $b = 1$ to B:
   (a) draw Bootstrap samples,
   (b) construct a random tree as follows: randomly select m predictors, and construct a decision tree using these m predictors.

2. We obtain B decision trees $T_b(x), b = 1, 2, \ldots, B$. We combine the results of these B trees:
   (a) for regression, $\hat{f}(x) = \frac{1}{B}\sum_{b=1}^{B} T_b(x)$,
   (b) for classification: do prediction using each of these B trees and then vote

$$\hat{Y}(x) = \arg\max_k \#\{b: T_b(x) = k\}.$$

13.18. Boosting[28,29]

Boosting was invented to solve classification problems. It iteratively combines a few weak classifiers and forms a strong classifier.

Consider a two-class problem. We use $Y \in \{-1, 1\}$ to denote the class label. Given predictor values for X, one classifier $G(X)$ takes values -1 or 1. On the training data, the misclassification rate is defined as

$$\text{err} = \frac{1}{N}\sum_{i=1}^{N} I(y_i \neq G(x_i)).$$

A weak classifier means that the misclassification is a little bit better than random guess, that is *err* <0.5. Boosting repeatedly applies a weak classifier on weighted training data and produces a series of weak classifiers. It finally combines these weak classifiers and gives a good classifier. Below is a detailed description.

1. Assign equal weights for all train data points $w_i = \frac{1}{N}, i = 1, \ldots, N$.
2. Repeat the following steps for M times:
   (a) Train a weak classifier ($G_m(x)$) using the weighted data
   (b) Calculate the weighted classification error

$$\text{err}_m = \frac{\sum_{i=1}^{N} w_i I(y_i \neq G_m(x_i))}{\sum_{i=1}^{N} w_i}.$$

   (c) Calculate the coefficient

$$\alpha_m = \log\frac{1 - \text{err}_m}{\text{err}_m}.$$

   (d) Update

$$w_i = w_i \exp[\alpha_m \cdot I(y_i \neq G_m(x_i))].$$

3. Combine the M weak classifiers and give a final classifier: $G(x) = \text{sign}\left[\sum_{m=1}^{M} \alpha_m G_m(x)\right]$.

The above classifier could solve two-class classification problems very well and the procedure is called as Adaboost. But it does not provide the probability of $P(Y_i = 1|x_i)$. For the purpose of getting the probability, we could consider Logitboost. Logitboosting is an extension of Adaboos. In fact, both Adaboost and Logitboost could be seen as additive logistic regression. The difference is that they have different objective functions. Adaboost minimizes $E(e^{-yF(x)})$ and Logitboost minimizes $E(\log(1+e^{-2yF(x)}))$. Logitboost is described as follows:

1. Assign equal weights for all train data points $w_i = \frac{1}{N}, i = 1, \ldots, NF(x) = 0$. $p(x_i) = 1/2$.
2. Repeat the following steps for M times:
   (a) calculate new responses and their weights
   $$z_i = \frac{y_i - p(x_i)}{p(x_i)(1 - p(x_i))},$$
   $$w_i = p(x_i)(1 - p(x_i)).$$
   (b) get $f_m(x)$ by weighted least squares
   $$f_m(x) = \arg\min_f \sum_{i=1}^{N} w_i(z_i - f(x_i))^2$$
   and update $F(x)$ and $p(x)$: $F(x) = F(x) + \frac{1}{2}f_m(x), p(x) = \frac{e^{F(x)}}{e^{F(x)}+e^{-F(x)}}$.
3. Finally, output the final classifier and the probability
   $$G(x) = sign[F(x)],$$
   $$p(x) = \frac{e^{F(x)}}{e^{F(x)} + e^{-F(x)}}.$$

Logitboost has a very natural objective and it is very easy to extend Logitboost to other problems. For example, for multi-class classification problems, we could replace the objective function in Logitboost with the log likelihood function.

13.19. R Software[30]

Computational statistics and statistical simulation cannot leave computation tools. C and Fortran languages are quite useful languages. These languages have the property of being very fast. But they also have the disadvantage that they are too complex and cannot combine with stochastic simulations very well.

Recently there are well-designed software or packages for statistical computing and stochastic simulations. They could generate random numbers very fast. SAS, MATLAB, python and R belong to this category.

We briefly introduce R here. It has the following advantages: (1) R is for free. (2) It is very easy to install and use R. (3) There are many R users all over the world and a lot of classic or newly developed statistical method has R packages.

Of course, R has its own limitations. For example, R is not that fast as C. A better way is to combine R and C — leave complicated computing to C and call C from R.

We now introduce R in the following aspects: (1) data types that R deals with, (2) the way R generates random numbers, (3) the function for matrix operations, (4) classical statistical analysis in R, (5) how to use packages and (6) statistical plot.

1. Data types that R deals with: The basic types in R include numeric, character and time. R could deal with many scientific computing problems and it could also deal with text data. Data in R usually are stored in vector, list, data frame or matrix.
2. The way R generates random number: R could generate many random numbers very fast. In R, one could generate random numbers from a distribution using the following command: r+distribution name+parameters. For example, rnorm() produces normal random numbers; runif() gives random numbers from uniform distribution: "d+distribution name+parameters" gives the value of density function for some distribution; "p+distribution name+parameters" gives the value of distribution function for some distribution; "q+distribution name+parameters" gives quantiles. For detailed description of each command, one could type "? + command" in R window. For example "?rnorm" tells us how to use rnorm() in R to generate random numbers from normal distribution.
3. The function for matrix operations: R could deal with many scientific computing problems. For example, QR factorization(qr(X)), inversion of a matrix(solve(X)), calculate the determinant of a matrix(det(X)), eigenvalue decomposition(eigen(X)) and SVD decompostion(svd(X)).
4. Classical statistical analysis in R: Almost all classical statistical analysis could be realized in R. For example, linear regression (lm), generalized

linear models (glm), anova (anova), t-test(t.test) and principal component analysis (princomp).

5. R packages: R has a lot of functions for data analysis. It also has a lot of packages. For example, LARS package could be used to solve L1 regularized least squares problem. To use R packages, we have to install them first. For this purpose, type "install.packages (pkgname)" is enough, where pkgname is the name of package that we want to install. To use a package in R, type "library(pkgname)" in R, then we could use all of the functions defined in this package.
6. Statistical plot: R software has a very rich plotting tools. In general, two-dimensional plot could use the command "plot". Special statistical plot such as histogram (R command: hist), boxplot (R command: boxplot) can be produced very conveniently in R.

13.20. Statistics Toolbox in MATLAB[31]

MATLAB is a very powerful commercial software for scientific computing. It has many special toolboxes, including numerical analysis, signal computing, digit image process, digital signal process and scientific and engineer plot, etc. It also has a powerful statistical toolbox. We introduce statistical toolbox in MATLAB in the following aspects. (1) data types that MATLAB deals with, (2) the way MATLAB generates random numbers, (3) matrix computation in MATLAB (4) classical statistics in MATLAB, (5) statistical plot, and (6) extension of MATLAB toolbox.

1. Data types that MATLAB deals with: Matlab mainly deals with vector and matrix, where vector is treated as a one-dimensional matrix. For statistical analysis, MATLAB has a special data structure called as dataset or Dataset Arrays. This data structure is similar to data frame in R Each row in a dataset denotes one observation and each column denotes one variable. One column in a dataset must have the same basic data type, but different columns do not require the same basic data type (for example, numeric or character).
2. The way MATLAB generates random numbers: MATLAB could produce many random numbers very fast. A general command for random number generating in MATLAB is "distribution name + rnd + parameters". For example, normrnd() produces random numbers from normal distribution and poissrnd() gives random numbers from Poisson distribution. "distribution name + pdf + parrameters" gives the value of a density function. "distribution name +cdf+parameters" gives the value of a cumulative

distribution function. "distribution name +inv+parameters" gives quantiles. For detailed description of each method (function or command) in MATLAB, one could type "help+command" in MATLAB window. For example, "help normrnd" tells us how to use normrnd() in MATLAB to generate random numbers from normal distribution; it also gives a few related commands, such as normcdf, normfit, norminv, normlike, normpdf, normstat, random, randn.

3. Matrix computing: MATLAB is very fast in the computation of matrix. Many matrix computations have very simple command in MATLAB. For example, QR factorization(qr(X)), inversion of a matrix(inv(X)), computation of the determinant(det(X)), eigenvalue decomposition (eig(X)) and SVD decomposition (svd(X))
4. Classical statistics in MATLAB: Many classical statistical methods are realized and have simple command in MATLAB. For example, linear regression (regres LinearModel.fit), generalized linear models (glmfit), classification (classification tree), anova (anova, anova1, anova2, anovan), variable selection (stepwisefit, Lasso), ridge regression (ridge), hypothesis test (ztest, ttest, kstest, chi2gof), principal component analysis (pca), clustering (kmeans), factor analysis (factoran), non-negative matrix factorization (nnmf) etc.
5. Statistical plot: Statistical plot tools in MATLAB are also very rich. For example, scatter plot (gscatter), box-plot (boxplot) and qqplot, etc. For two-dimensional plot, the general command is "plot", and for three-dimensional surf plot, the command is "surf".
6. Extension of matlab toolbox: MATLAB constantly updates every year, and many newly developed statistical methods are gradually included in the statistics toolbox. One could also use the MATLAB to develop his own method very conveniently. A simple approach is to write his own functions through the m file. If it is a large project, you can use the mex file, which combines C language. When necessary, you could use the MATLAB parallel computing toolkit for multi-core parallel computing.

References

1. Gentle, JE. *Random Number Generation and Monte Carlo Methods.* New York: Springer, 1998.
2. Kendall, MG, Smith, BB. Randomness and random sampling numbers. *J. R. Stat. Soc.*, 1983, 101:1 147–166.
3. Lange, K. *Numerical Analysis for Statisticians.* New York: Springer, 1999.

4. Pozrikidis, G. *Numerical Computation in Science and Engineering.* New York: Oxford University Press, 1998.
5. Chen, MH, Shao, QM, Ibrahim, JG. *Monte Carlo Methods in Bayesian Computation.* New York: Springer, 2000.
6. Liu, JS. *Monte Carlo Strategies in Scientific Computing.* New York: Springer, 2001.
7. Atkinson, KA. *An Introduction to Numerical Analysis* (2nd edn.). Hoboken: John Wiley and Sons, 1988.
8. Snyman, JA. *Practical Mathematical Optimization: An Introduction to Basic Optimization Theory and Classical and New Gradient-Based Algorithms.* Berlin: Springer Publishing, 2005.
9. Dowsland, KA. Simulated annealing. In CR Reeves (ed.), *Modern Heuristic Techniques for Combinatorial Problems.* New York: Wiley, 1993.
10. Back, T. *Evolutionary Algorithms in Theory and Practice.* New York: Oxford University Press, New York, 1996.
11. Tibshirani, R. Regression shrinkage and selection via the lasso. *J. R. Stat. Soc. B*, 1996, 58(1): 267–288.
12. Golub, GH, Van Loan, CF. *Matrix Computations.* Baltimore: JHU Press, 2012.
13. Horn, RA, Johnson CR. *Matrix Analysis.* Cambridge: Cambridge University Press, 2012.
14. Tanner, MA. *Tools for Statistical Inference: Methods for Exploration of Posterior Distribution and Likelihood Functions.* (3rd edn.). Berlin: Springer, 1996.
15. Dempster, AP, Laird, NM, Rubin, DB. Maximum likelihood from incomplete data via the EM algorithm. *J. R. stat. Soc. B*, 1977: 1–38.
16. Casella, G, George, EI. Explaining the Gibbs sampler. *Amer. Statist.*, 1992, 46(3): 167–174.
17. Chib, S, Greenberg, E. Understanding the metropolis–hastings algorithm. *Amer. Statist.*, 1995, 49(4): 327–335.
18. Efron, B. Bootstrap methods: Another look at the jackknife. *Ann. Stat.*, 1979, 7(1): 337–374.
19. Efron, B. *The Jackknife, the Bootstrap and Other Resampling Plans.* Philadelphia: Society for Industrial and Applied Mathematics, 1982.
20. Efron, B, Gong, G. A leisurely look at the bootstrap, the Jackknife, and Cross-Validation. *Am. Stat.*, 1983, 37: 36–48.
21. Higgins, J. *Introduction to Modern Nonparametric Statistics.* Pecific Grove: Duxbury Press. 2003.
22. Boyd, S, Vandenberghe, L. *Convex Optimization.* Cambridge: Cambridge University Press, 2004.
23. Yuan, M, Lin, Y. Model selection and estimation in regression with grouped variables. *J. R. Stat. Soc. B*, 2006, 49–67.
24. Meinshausen, N, Bühlmann, P. High-dimensional graphs and variable selection with the Lasso. *Ann. Stat.*, 2006, 34: 1436–1462.
25. Yuan, M, Lin, Y. Model selection and estimation in the Gaussian graphical model. *Biometrika*, 2007, 94(1): 19–35.
26. Breiman, L. Random forests. *Mach. Learn.*, 2001, 45(1): 5–32.
27. Hastie, T, Tibshirani, R, Friedman, J. *The Elements of Statistical Learning* (2nd edn.). Berlin: Springer-Verlag, 2009.
28. Freund, Y. Boosting a weak learning algorithm by majority. *Inform. Comput.*, 1995, 121(2): 256–285.
29. Friedman, J, Hastie, T, Tibshirani, R. Additive logistic regression: A statistical view of boosting (with discussion). *Ann. Stat.*, 2000, 28: 337–374.

30. Crawley, MJ. *Statistics: An Introduction Using R.* Hoboken: John Wiley & Sons, 2014.
31. http://www.mathworks.com/help/stats/index.html.
32. Hastings, W.K. Monte Carlo sampling methods using Markov chains and their applications. *Biometrika.* 1970, **57**(1): 97–109.

About the Author

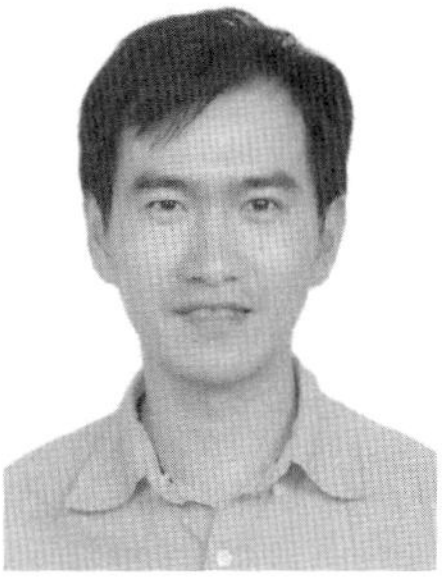

Jinzhu Jia is an Assistant Professor at the School of Mathematical Sciences and Center for Statistical Science. He got his Bachelor's degree in June 2004 from Wuhan University and Ph.D on January 2009 from Peking University. He did his post-doctoral research from January 2009 to December 2010 in UC Berkeley. He joined the faculty group in Peking University in January 2011. His research interests include high-dimensional statistics, statistical machine learning and causal inference. He has published many papers in the fields of variable selection, applications of high-dimensional statistics and causal inference. He is the PI of two funds from National Scientific Funding of China.

CHAPTER 14

DATA AND DATA MANAGEMENT

Yongyong Xu*, Haiyue Zhang, Yi Wan, Yang Zhang, Xia Wang,
Chuanhua Yu, Zhe Yang, Feng Pan and Ying Liang

14.1. Data Dictionary[1,2]

Data dictionary is a metadata repository to describe the meaning and content of data. Data dictionary is an essential integral part in the process of building a database, which is to ensure the sharing, security, integrity, consistency, validity, recoverability and scalability of the database.

Data dictionary is an important part of the database, which aims to make detailed instructions on each of the elements in data flow diagram. In design phase of database, data dictionary is used to describe the design of the base table in the database, mainly including content of description on table properties, such as field name, data type, primary key, foreign key, etc. In the data analysis phase, data dictionary is used to query the definition and explanation of all the elements in data flow diagram, which can be used for the second development of data, such as data extraction, data collection, data interface design, etc.

Data dictionary normally contains five parts, including data item, data structure, data flow, data storage and processing procedure. Its core content is the definition and description of data item, such as the identifier, name, code, alias, abbreviation of data item, the length of data item, scope and classification code of data item, etc.

Some commercial statistical analysis softwares use variable labels and value labels to define and describe data item. For example, if there are no instructions on data items for the five variables (X1 $\sim$ X5) in Table 14.1.1,

*Corresponding author: xuyongy@fmmu.edu.cn

Table 14.1.1 Fifty-eight live birth records data matrix.

X1	X2	X3	X4	X5
XT0368	1	34.1	3.27	48.6
XT1132	2	34.8	4.31	50.7
:	:	:	:	:
XT2005	1	34.5	3.86	50.3

Table 14.1.2 SPSS variable review.

The name of the metadata	Note
Name	
Type	Numerical values, comma segmentation, segmentation, index, date, dollar, other currencies, string
Width	
Decimal	
Label	
Value	{Code value, meaning of the value}
Missing	
Column	
Align	Left-aligned, right-aligned
Measure	Quantitative classification, grade, name

Table 14.1.3 SPSS Table 14.1.1 data display (for instance).

Metadata name	Note			
Variable name	X1	X2	...	X6
Data type	String	Numerical values	...	Numerical values
Data length	4	1	...	3
Decimal digits	0	0	...	1
Variable labels	Serial number	Gender	...	Body length (cm)
Value label		{1, male} {2, female}	...	
Missing data show			...	
Data matrix columns	4	1	...	4
Data alignment	Align at left	Align at left	...	Align at left
Measurement type	Nominal group	Nominal group	...	Quantitative measurement

except the researcher himself, no one knows the meaning of each data in the Table, and the data cannot be used for analysis.

Table 14.1.2 is the content for definition and description of the data items in the SPSS Variable Review window, which has a total of 10 description items.

Table 14.1.3 shows the results of data items in Table 14.1.1 which are described by the metadata in Table 14.1.2.

14.2. Data Coding[3,4]

Data coding refers to the transformation of verbal data, such as gender, occupation, name of disease and questionnaire answers, into category and code which is easy to be identified and computer processed. The classification name, code value and value meaning of data coding are the metadata needed to be importantly described by data dictionary.

Coding principle: (1) uniqueness; (2) scalability; (3) briefness; (4) consistent format; (5) adaptability; (6) interpretiveness ; (7) stability; (8) identifiability; (9) operability.

Coding method: Coding is a classifying process for a particular object or thing, or it is a classification set with multiaxis classification for things. In most categories, code is used for expression. Code can be letters, numbers, or mixed code with both (such as ICD-10). Commonly used classification methods include: (1) qualitative classification, such as social gender classification and code: male = M, female = F; (2) rank classification, such as, the self-evaluation of health (in descending order) in SF-36 scale: perfect = 5, very good = 4, good = 3, normal = 2, poor = 1; (3) quantitative classification, such as, age group classification and code in Table 14.2.1.

Encoding type: Common types of codes are shown in Figure 14.2.1.

Unified code is the basic measure to share data, such as "GB/T2261.1-2003 personal general information classification and code" provides a person's gender, marital status, health status and working status codes. "The International Statistical Classification of Diseases and Related Health Problems 10th Revison" specifies the classification and code of disease diagnosis name and causes of death.

Table 14.2.1 Age group code table of the national health service (NHS) survey.

Code	Age range (years)
01	0–4
02	5–14
03	15–24
04	25–34
05	35–44
06	45–54
07	55–64
08	65–

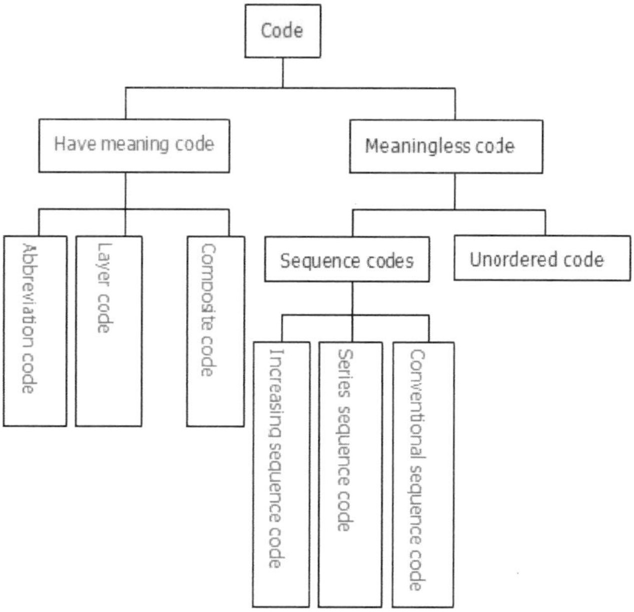

Fig. 14.2.1 Schematic diagram for common types of codes.

Object Identifier (OID): OID, its purpose is to find the object in information system. Unlike data coding, OID coding should absolutely have no meaning, to ensure the stability of the OID. OID can be used for all object identification methods including one-dimension code, two-dimension code, RFID, IC card, etc., which is the basis for achieving "one code for one thing" in the Internet era. The OID identification allocation scheme and registration management system have been established, and the OID registration parsing management system has developed.

14.3. Data Management[5,6]

Data management refers to the overall management of enterprises (institutions) data, including data availability, usability, integrity, and data security. A perfect data management system is constituted by data management institution (personnel), data management system and specific management process (Figure 14.3.1).

The purpose of data management: (1) supporting decision making, such as to determine clinical treatment effect; (2) reduction of conflicting operations; (3) protection of the interests of the data related parties; (4) standardization training of the data management owners, managers, and operators; (5) forming a standardized data processing flow; (6) reducing

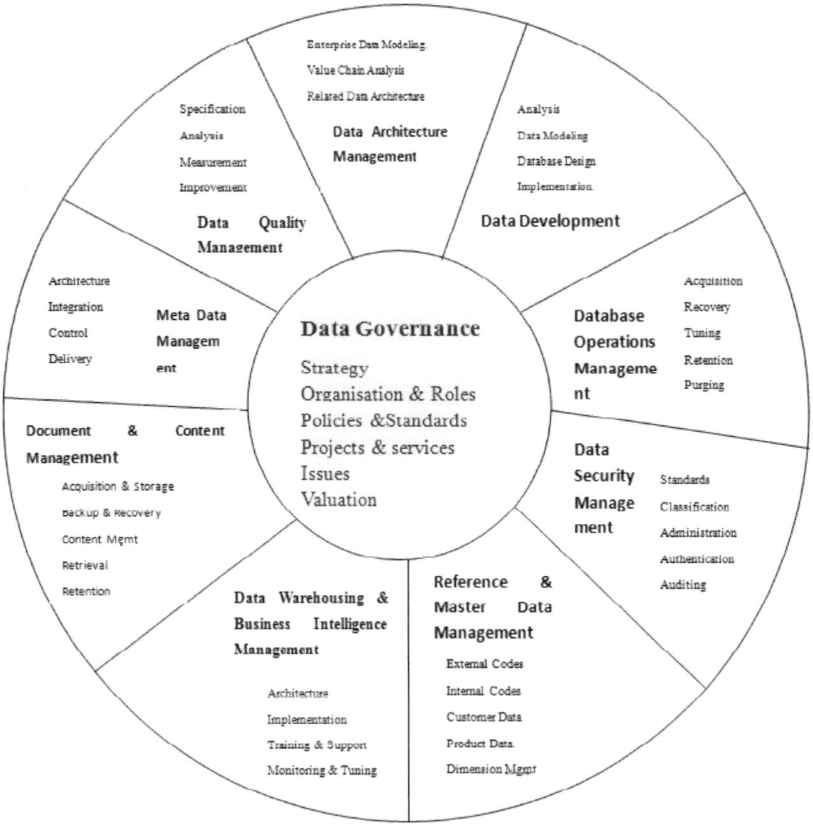

Fig. 14.3.1 Data management process.

cost and increasing efficiency by improving coordination among data related parties; (7) improving transparency of data management.

The basic requirement of data management:

(1) Policies, norms and strategies of data management, such as reliability of data management system, traceability of data, administrative authority and management by authority.
(2) Data quality management, including establishment of quality guarantee system, such as determination of data management organization and personnel responsibilities, the qualification requirements, responsibilities and rights of data management personnel, equipping with corresponding resources (personnel, equipment, facilities, fund, technology and methods), strict operation according to standard operation procedure (SOP), etc. The data quality of clinical trial is usually controlled from CRF quality, the inspection of quality control includes data entry

system verification, data valid range verification, logic verification, safety inspections, etc.

(3) Privacy protection and data security, such as privilege management, identity, level management on information system security, response and disposal plans on information security incident of information system, etc.
(4) Data architecture and information integration, such as master data management, metadata management, data dictionary management, code management, data document management, etc.
(5) Data warehouse and intelligent management, such as business intelligence (BI), data mining, knowledge management, etc.

Clinical Data Management: The "Good Clinical Data Management Practice, GCDMP" developed by the Society of Clinical Data Management (SCDM) provides relevant operation process for clinical trial data management, including data management participants and their responsibilities and qualifications, clinical trial data management information system development and usage, data standardization, basic management content (CRF design, data entry, data verification, data storage and privacy protection, etc.), and data quality assurance, etc.

14.4. Data Element[7,8]

Data elements are the fundamental units of data. Within a certain context, it is usually used to construct a specific information unit which is semantically correct, independent and without any ambiguous interpretations. It is a minimized unit of data whose values are assigned through a series of attributes/properties including definition, identification, representation, permissible values, etc., for which further subdivision is impossible.

A data element is generally composed of the three parts listed below:

(1) Object class: A set of ideas, concepts, or objects in the real world, which are assigned with explicit boundaries and meanings, and whose properties and behaviors follow the same rules.
(2) Property: An obvious characteristic possessed by all members of an object class, which is highly distinctive and noticeable.
(3) Representation: The way of description through which data is expressed.

Object classes are things whose relevant data are expected to be studied, collected and stored, such as person, household, medical institution, observation and intervention. Different classification and naming methods can be adopted based on various types of roles within different contexts, which form a variety of specified object classes, such as, "persons" can be divided into doctors, patients, nurses, inspectors, directors, investigators, etc., according to their roles in health service.

Property is a characteristic of an object class. For example, the object class *Person* can have many characteristics, such as color, name, sex, date of birth, height, occupation, and health condition, etc. Property may be described by a number of phrases depending on the chosen natural language. Based on their similarity with each other, properties are combined to form property groups, such as physical characteristics, educational characteristics and labor characteristics, etc.

Representation is closely related to the value domains of data elements. A value domain is the set of all permissible values of data elements. Representation is composed of value domain and data type. Units of measure and representation class will also be included, if necessary. It illustrates the data type of data element concept and the range of possible values. There are many methods to represent data element. Representation class is the classification scheme for representation, such as name, date, count, currency, picture, etc.

A data element concept is composed of an object class and a property. Therefore, a data element is composed of a data element concept and a representation. Figure 14.4.1 shows the structural model of data elements.

A data element is a combination of data element concept and representation. According to the figure, there is a many-to-one relationship between the data element and the data element concept, that is, a data element must have a data element concept, while many data elements may

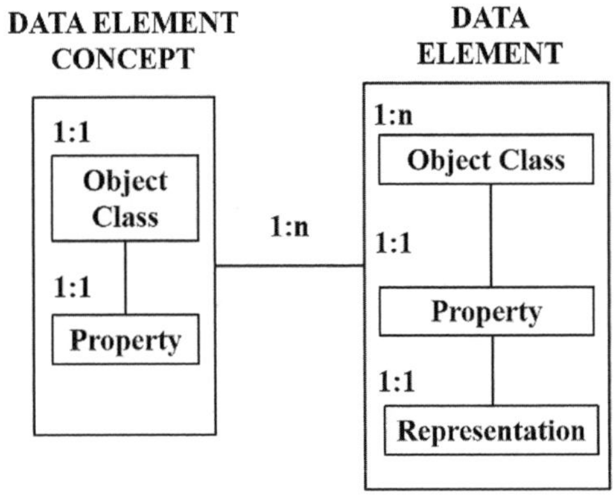

Fig. 14.4.1 Structural model of data elements.

share the same data element concept. Taking *person-weight* as a data element concepts (object class + property), based on different representation methods, it corresponds to more than one data element, such as *person-weight* (lb), *person-weight* (g), *person-weight* (kg), *person-weight* (jin), etc.

14.5. Data Set[9,10]

Data set is a set of data collected for a specific purpose, and it is a group of data elements. The common types of data sets include:

(1) Data Set Specification (DSS) refers to the data collection and standardized output identified by stakeholder. The most important feature of DSS is implementing and collecting standards. It aims to provide a unified definition of data items related to data collection to ensure the standardization of data collection.
(2) Minimum Data Set (MDS) is a set of selective core data, which is collected for a specific purpose, minimum, and recognized by users and interest-related persons. MDS do not rule out the collection of additional data to meet the needs of individual health agencies or local areas.
(3) National Minimum Data Sets (NMDS) refer to the national data that must be collected throughout the country. It relies on national agreements to collect and provide the core data.

At present, the standardization research institutes of many countries focus on a particular field of data sets (minimum data sets) research. A good representative is the Australian National Diabetes data set, which includes 37 data items and is divided into four sections: patient's basic information, diagnostic information, clinical information and personal medical history. For the national health survey data set, representatives are the British health survey data sets, United States health survey data sets and Australian health survey data sets, etc.

The researches on the data set of the Chinese health field are mainly released by the National Health and Family Planning Commission of the People's Republic of China. The purpose is to solve the problems of health information standardization in different health institutions and different professional fields, and to promote the development of health information. There are "Standard for basic data set of person information for health records", "Standard for basic data set of birth certificate", "Standard for basic data set of children's physical examination", "Standard for basic data set of immunization", "Standard for basic data set of infectious disease report", "Standard for basic data set of outpatient service", "Standard for basic data set of inpatient service", "Standard for basic data set of medical certificate of death", etc.

Each data set has common attributes and specific attributes. Common attributes are also called "basic attributes", which include data set subject, identity, entity, and data item. Subject is the core attribute of the data set, which is the conclusion, abstraction and generalization of the essential content of the data set. Identity is the data set's Chinese name, English name, identifier, etc. Entity is the collection of similar information of a data set. Data item is the collection of elements within a data set. The specific attributes include the data set's subject, area, institution where it was submitted, time when it was established, diseases involved and so on. The specific attributes are the personalized identification of the same data set in common attributes.

Data set has two main functions. The first is to express things which need to be expressed by a number of data elements. Such as the full list of a person's name, including his/her current name, nickname, alias, pen name, Chinese name, English name, former name, use time of the former name and abandoned time, etc. The second is to standardize the national minimum data set for regional health care, disease surveillance, statistical investigation and reporting, etc., such as inpatient survey data sets, death report minimal data sets and tumor registry data sets.

14.6. Data Type[11–13]

In ISO/IEC 11404, a data type is defined as a set of distinct values characterized by properties of those values, and by operations on those values.

Data type is the smallest unit to construct message and semantic document, which is key to the practical value of any general model, and is the basis of document exchange, data collection, storage, transmission and information technology personnel programming. For example, the address description, in addition to describing the location of the address, its usage and duration of validity also need to be illustrated. An example of data type is shown in Table 14.6.1.

Defining and using data type is an indispensable link in the development of information standard. Data dictionary, data set, bibliographic data element directory, data element code, formulation of the standards of shared files-all are related to data type. Currently, the international standards for the data type include ISO11404, HL7 V3 Data Types, ISO 21090, open EHR Data Types Information Model, ISO/IEC 11179, etc.

Table 14.6.1 Examples for data type (address).

Description item	Description content
Valid time range	Begin time, end time
Use	Home address, work place, school address, emergency contact address, temporary address
Address name	Province, city, district (county), street (town) residents' committee (village), house number

ISO 11404 is the data type for information expression of all disciplines. Other existing international standards focusing on the field of health information are using ISO 11404 definitions of data types. Different standards draw lessons from each other and maintain a high degree of coordination.

Definition of the data type proposed by HL7 V3 is completely independent from the applied technology, whose purpose is to express health information with qualified accuracy and scope by using a minimized amount of data types. The data type defines a wide variety of various countries around the world about Person Name (PN), Entity Name Part (ENXP), Instance Identifier (II), Monetary Amount (MO), etc. ISO 21090 is the standard that is comprehensively used to coordinate the specification of various data types. It extends the semantics of the ISO 11404 data type and maintains its continuity. By using the terms, concepts and types defined in V2.0 UML, UML class definition for the same data type is provided and the data type definition is also made to be more explicit and structured.

Open EHR data type keeps consistency with the HL7 V3 data type. However, the design method is obviously different, which is expressed in terms of naming, identification, processing of the nested types, and the use of vacant identifications.

Data type specification is one of the basic problems of data standardization. For both the international and domestic data type standards, the ultimate goal is to better understand and express electronic data and information of the medical field, facilitating the sharing of information and promoting the exchange of information.

14.7. Meta Data[7]

Data element is the fundamental unit of data. In order to have a proper understanding and application of data element, comprehensive description and interpretation for each data element is necessary. Metadata is the data defining and interpreting other data, which is the explanation of the data, and providing information needed for accurately understanding and interpretation of the data.

Therefore, metadata could be interpreted as defining data element from different perspectives or based on different properties. These different perspectives or properties constitute different forms of metadata. For example, the basic components of a data element are object class, property and representation. By providing definitions of the object class, property and representation which correspond to the data element, data elements could be precisely described. Metadata related to data elements and their relationships are shown in Figure 14.7.1.

Metadata has five basic properties, which are identifying and definition, collection and usage guide, source and reference, relation, and administration, respectively. The registration meta model and basic attribute metadata description formulated by ISO/IEC 11179-3 are divided into 10 categories and 45 basic attributes to standardize the various types of data, that is, the formulation of data standards (Table 14.7.1).

A standardized description of a series of data elements, namely, the collection of metadata, is called a data dictionary. The national health data

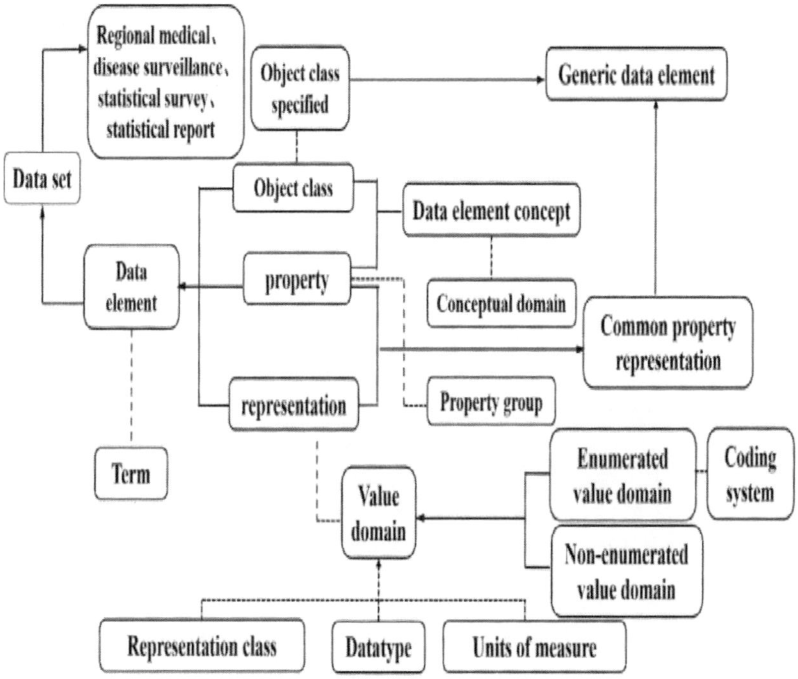

Fig. 14.7.1 Structure chart of metadata.

Table 14.7.1 Basic attributes of metadata.

Metadata category (number)	Basic attributes
Identifying (8)	Name, Context name, Context identifier, Context description, Item identifier, Item identifier-data identifier, Item identifier-item registration authority identifier, Version
Definitional (3)	Definition, Definition language identifier, Definition source reference
Administrative (4)	Comments, Registration status, Responsible organization name, Submitting organization name
Relational (7)	Classification scheme name, Classification scheme identifier, Classification scheme type name, Classification scheme item type name, Classification scheme item value, Related metadata reference, Type of relationship
Data element concepts (4)	Object class name, Object class identifier, Property name, Property identifier
Data elements (8)	Value domain name, Value domain identifier, Data type name, Data type scheme reference, Layout of representation, Representation class, Maximum size, Minimum size
Conceptual domains (1)	Dimensionality
Value domains (3)	Data type name, Datat ype scheme reference, Unit of measure name
Permissible values (3)	Value, Permissible value begin date, Permissible value end date
Value meanings (4)	Value meaning description, Value meaning identifier, Value meaning begin date, Value meaning end date

dictionary is a metadata repository containing definitions and representations of data elements with the goal of allowing users to have easy access to data elements and metadata which describes the former.

14.8. Data Warehouse[14,15]

Data warehouse is a data set which could be data subject oriented, integrated, non-volatile, and reflection of time variant, with the purpose of data mining and decision making support.

The characteristics of the data in the data warehouse are:

(1) Subject oriented: In the operational system, data collection is deposited specially with a separate application center, data is application transaction oriented, such as, Hospital Information System (HIS) only supplies diagnosis and treatment information of patients, Laboratory Information System (LIS) only provides test result of patients. And the data are deposited in the data warehouse according to the business subjects, such as, infectious disease monitoring, clinical pathway, single-disease clinical pathway, treatment effect comparison of single diseases, etc. Different medical institutions have different business subjects in different periods.
(2) Integration: Data is derived from different operating systems, of which file layout, encoding, naming habits, and metrics may be different. In a number of enterprises, in addition to access to internal data from the operating system, external system data are also very important. Therefore, before storing the data from different sources into a data warehouse, these different data elements must be standardized, and data should be cleaned, transformed and integrated.
(3) Time character: Data stored in the operating system generally contains the current value, reflects the current information. However, data warehouse is used for analysis and decision making. Decision makers must make decisions based on the trend of the data, which requires not only the current data but also historical data. Therefore, the purpose of the data warehouse requires that it contains current data, also including historical data.
(4) Stability: The data in operational system is updated in real time. However, the data in warehouse is almost no longer updated after loading, and it is used only for query analysis.

Clinical Data Warehouse (CDW) is to form relationships or hierarchical Clinical Data Repository (CDR) according to demographic characteristics, clinical laboratory results, imaging reports and images, progress notes, admission information, ICD-9 diagnosis codes, prescription, medication, discharges and referral information, discharge summary and other topics, which come from different sources, such as HIS, LIS, Radiology Information System (RIS), Clinical Information System (CIS), Population Information System (PIS) and other information system. Then CDW does statistical analysis and data mining through analysis platform (Figure 14.8.1).

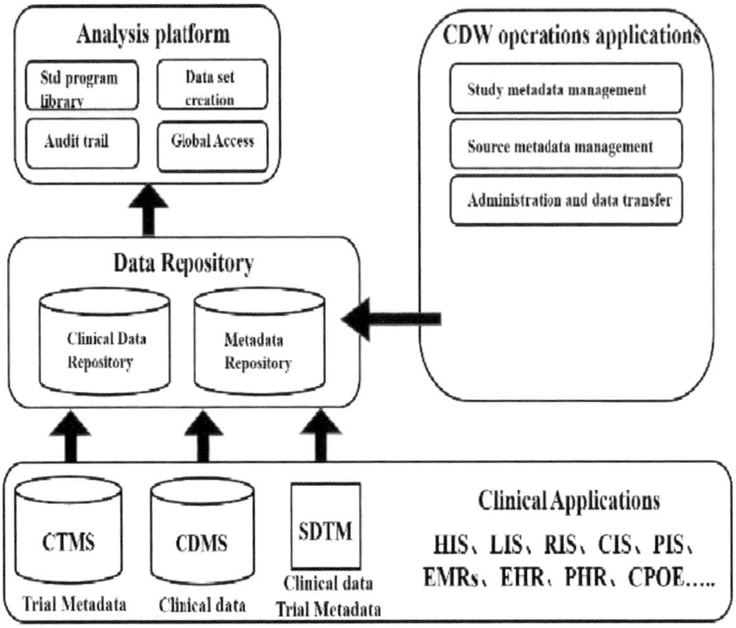

Fig. 14.8.1 Elements of the in-process CDW.

14.9. Extensible Markup Languages (XML)[16,17]

XML is the abbreviation for extensible markup language, which is a new language to describe structured data. It is a common language specification which was developed by W3C in 1998. It is similar to HTML, however, XML does not concern about how the data is arranged and displayed in a browser, but concerns about how to describe the organization and structure of data content for the exchange and processing on the network. XML is used to meet the growing demand for network applications, to ensure good interoperability when data interaction and cooperation take place through the network. XML can define file types, so it is conducive to the expression and structuring of information in a consistent manner, which can format and transmit data for different platforms and systems data exchange.

XML has the following four main features:

(1) Simplicity: XML provides a friendly environment for the programmer and author of document. Strict definitions and rules of XML enable the human and machine to easily read the document. XML document syntax contains a very small set of rules so that developers can start work immediately. The XML document based on a core set of basic nested structure. When a layer of detail is increased and the structure becomes

more complex, the authors or the developers only need to use internal structures to represent complex information set without changing its structure.

(2) Extendibility: XML allows developers to create their own Document Type Definition (DTD), effectively create “extensible” symbol set that can be used for a variety of applications. Furthermore, using several additional criteria can expand the XML.

(3) Interoperability: XML can be used on multiple platforms, and can be explained by a variety of tools. XML can be used in many different computing environments in the world because it supports many primary standards with the use in character encoding. XML is a very good supplement to Java, many of the early XML developments were carried out using Java.

(4) Openness: The XML standard itself is completely open in Web, and it can be obtained free of charge. Anyone can parse an XML document with good structure. If it has a DTD, anyone can also check this document. For instance, the following is the XML document for describing the clinical diagnosis of right knee osteoarthritis by using SNOMED:

```
<code code=‘396275006’ codeSystem=‘2.16.840.1.113883.19.6.96’
codeSystemName=‘SNOMED CT’ displayName=‘Osteoarthritis’>
<originalText> osteoarthritis of the right knee</originalText>
<qualifier>
<name code=‘363698007’ codeSystem=‘2.16.840.1.113883.19.6.96’
codeSystemName=‘SNOMED CT’ displayName=‘finding site’/>
<value code=‘6757004’ codeSystem=‘2.16.840.1.113883.19.6.96’
codeSystemName=‘SNOMED CT’ displayName=‘right knee’/>
</qualifier>
</code>
```

14.10. HL7 Standards[11,18,19]

Health level seven (HL7) is the famous medical information standard development organization (SDO) in the United States. It has developed for more than 20 years. The purpose of the organization is to solve how to realize the information exchange and data sharing within information systems developed by different manufacturers. As the information exchange standard, HL7

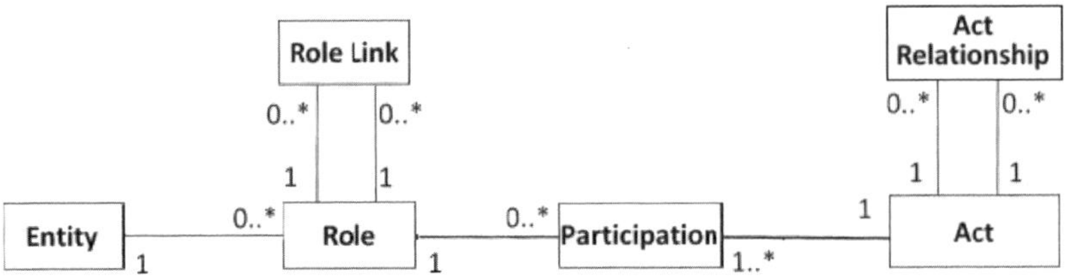

Fig. 14.10.1 HL7 RIM six core classes and relationship.

released version 1.0 in 1987, followed by v2.0, v2.1, V2.2, v2.3 and V2.3.1. In 2000, HL7 released the latest version 3.0. The core part is Reference Information Model (RIM). HL7 RIM is a static information model about health and healthcare. The purpose is to realize the semantic connection and coordinating constraint information provider and receiver through information model to ensure correct information and unambiguous exchanging. The current health information standards and health information systems construction in many organizations are following HL7 and HL7 RIM.

HL7 RIM abstracts the health information into six core classes, respectively for act, entity, role, participation, act relationship, and role link. The relationship description among core classes uses Unified Modeling Language (UML) to express, as shown in Figure 14.10.1.

HL7 CDA is the document markup standard for clinical information exchanging between different information systems developed by HL7. It includes clinical document architecture and semantic standards based on CDA. And the latest version is the CDA release 2. CDA content comes from HL7 RIM, using the HL7 data type representing data element value format and content. Furthermore, CDA uses Logical Observation Identifiers Names and Codes (LOINC) and Systematized Nomenclature of Medicine-Clinical Terms (SNOMED CT) as its coding system for domain value. At present, CDA has been applied to many research fields and used to construct information exchange specifications or standards.

HL7 V3 datatype: HL7 RIM uses 29 data types from HL7 V3 datatype. For example, four data types about coding value are coded simple (CS), coded value (CV), coded with equivalents (CE), and concept descriptor (CD).

14.11. International Classification of Diseases[20]

International Statistical Classification of Diseases and Related Health Problems (ICD) adopts line classification method to use combination of letter and number for classification of diseases on the basis of diseases property. ICD's history can be dated back to 1853, Jacques Bertillon, the France medical statistician, put forward the Bertillon statistical classification of diseases on causes of death, which was used for classification of registration and statistics of causes of death. In 1893, Bertillon, who was the president of the International Statistical Association, developed "the international list of causes of death", which was the first edition of ICD. Since then, ICD was named as the "international list of causes of death" for the second to the fifth edition by the International Statistical Conference in Paris in 1900, 1920, 1929, and 1938. In 1948, the World Health Organization (WHO) was responsible for the professional maintenance of international classification of causes of death, and changed its name to the "international statistical classification of diseases, trauma, and causes of death" for the sixth edition. Under the

Table 14.11.1 Blocks codes of ICD-10.

Chapter	Blocks codes	Blocks contents
I	A00-B99	Certain infectious and parasitic diseases
II	C00-D48	Neoplasms
III	D50-D89	Diseases of the blood and blood-forming organs and certain disorders involving the immune mechanism
IV	E00-E90	Endocrine, nutritional and metabolic diseases
V	F00-F99	Mental and behavioral disorders
VI	G00-G99	Diseases of the nervous system
VII	H00-H59	Diseases of the eye and adnexa
VIII	H60-H95	Diseases of the ear and mastoid process
IX	I00-I99	Diseases of the circulatory system
X	J00-J99	Diseases of the respiratory system
XI	K00-K93	Diseases of the digestive system
XII	L00-L99	Diseases of the skin and subcutaneous tissue
XIII	M00-M99	Diseases of the musculoskeletal system and connective tissue
XIV	N00-N99	Diseases of the genitourinary system
XV	O00-O99	Pregnancy, childbirth and the puerperium
XVI	P00-P96	Certain conditions originating in the perinatal period
XVII	Q00-Q99	Congenital malformations, deformations and chromosomal abnormalities
XVIII	R00-R99	Symptoms, signs and abnormal clinical and laboratory findings, not elsewhere classified
XIX	S00-T98	Injury, poisoning and certain other consequences of external causes
XX	V01-Y98	External causes of morbidity and mortality
XXI	Z00-Z99	Factors influencing health status and contact with health services
XXII	U00-U99	Codes for special purposes

organization and leadership of WHO, the ICD-10 took effect on January 1, 1993, and more than 38 countries had used or planned to use it. According to the WHO's advice, the use of ICD-10 would no longer take 10 years as revision period, and it may last for 20 years or longer. The latest version is ICD-10 which has 22 chapters, and the contents of chapters are shown in Table 14.11.1.

ICD is used to transform the diseases and related health problems terms description into alphanumeric character encoding, which is easy for data storage, retrieval and analysis. The four digits codes of ICD-10 can cover 14,400 diseases coding, and it can accommodate 16,000 diseases coding through expanding four digits coding for five or six digits. However, the latter belongs to local standards.

The operations of ICD-10 can find a coding for a name of disease in the indexes of the Chinese version of ICD-10, or look up in the contents catalogues in Table 14.11.1 according to the disease name, such as, chronic type B viral hepatitis is an infectious disease, its coding range in contents catalogues is A00-B99, and its corresponding code for B18.1 can be reconfirmed.

14.12. LOINC[21]

Logical Observation Identifiers Names and Codes, LOINC provides a set of universal Identifier codes for identifying laboratory and clinical test results. LOINC facilitates the exchange and sharing of results, such as blood hemoglobin, serum potassium, or vital signs, for clinical care, outcomes management, and research between different electronic medical record systems. LOINC developed by the Indiana Regenstrief Institute in 1994 was funded by the U.S. Centers for Disease Control and Prevention (CDC), American Health Policy Research Office and the National Library of Medicine, and has been cooperating with international LOINC Committee, assistant mapping program maintenance and update within LOINC database, support documents and regenstrief LOINC mapping assistant (RELMA). In recent years, LOINC has carried out collaboration and cooperation with other international well-known medical terminology standards, such as SNOMED. Naming and encoding of medical observation generally adopt LOINC standard system, such as the observation index report message standard of ASTM, E1238 HL7, CENTC251 and DICOM in international representation and exchange of clinical medical information. LOINC was adopted successfully in America, also in France, Canada, Germany, Switzerland, South Korea, Brazil, Argentina, Mexico, Spain, etc. Hong Kong and Taiwan of China had adopted and used LOINC in the actual work.

The core content of LOINC concept is mainly composed of one code, six concept definition axes (or a full name composed of six database field values, that is, definition of LOINC concept), and abbreviation. Each LOINC concept is made up of some basic concepts and conceptual combination (LOINC Parts). The basic concept has a corresponding concept hierarchy and the preferred term, synonyms and related name. Each LOINC record corresponds to only one test results or group results (panel, combination). The following are the six concept definition axes of LOINC:

(1) Component, e.g. potassium, hemoglobin, hepatitis C antigen.
(2) Property Measured, e.g. a mass concentration, enzyme activity.
(3) Timing, that is, whether the measurement is an observation at a moment of time, or an observation integrated over an extended duration of time, e.g. 24-hour urine sample.
(4) Type of sample, e.g. urine, venous blood.
(5) Type of scale, that is, whether the measurement is quantitative (a true measurement) ordinal (a ranked set of options), nominal (e.g. *E. coli*; *Staphylococcus aureus*), or narrative (e.g. dictation results from X-rays).
(6) Method: Where relevant, the method is used to produce the result or other observation results.

LOINC International: LOINC has also developed multiple languages database and related supporting documents in non-English speaking countries, including Simplified Chinese (China), German (Germany, Switzerland), Estonian, French (France, Switzerland), Korean (South Korea), Portuguese (Brazil), Spanish (Argentina, Mexico, Spain). The languages using the RELMA to search and map include Chinese (China), Korean (Korea) and Spanish (Argentina, Spain).

14.13. SNOMED[22]

SNOMED was initially proposed by College of American Pathologists (CAP). In 1999, CAP and NHS combined SNOMED Reference Terms in American and Clinical Terms Version 3 (CTV3, or Read Codes) in England as Systematized Nomenclature of Medicine — Clinical Terms (SNOMED CT).

The main objective of SNOMED CT is to be used as clinical terminology systems standard when exchanging documents between different CISs. SNOMED CT is the basic of electronic information exchange among computers, covering most aspects of clinical information, such as diseases, clinical finding, operation, microorganisms, drugs, environment, physical activity,

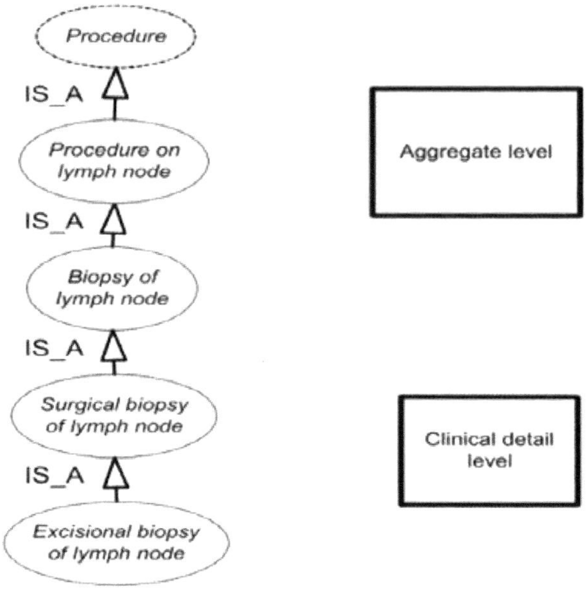

Fig. 14.13.1 Concept granularity.

etc., can be implemented in a coordinated manner between different disciplines, professions and locations for clinical care data indexing, storage, retrieval and aggregation, to facilitate computer processing.

SNOMED CT builds terms description by concept coding, description and relationship.

(1) Concept identifier: The identifier uses 8–18 digits as unique identifier of a clinical concept, and 8 or 9 digits are the most common. For example, 22298006 is the concept identifier for "myocardial infarction", and 399211009 is the concept identifier for "history of myocardial infarction".
(2) Description: Human readable natural language description (Fully Specified Name, FSN). Each concept identifier has one unique FSN, such as "history of myocardial infarction".
(3) Relationship: Each concept in SNOMED CT is logically defined through its relationship to other concepts. The Concept Granularity is showed as in Figure 14.13.1.

SNOMED CT is a comprehensive clinical terminology, providing clinical content and presentation for clinical documentation and reporting, where each concept has a unique identifier and a variety of descriptions; all descriptions of the same concept have correlation. It is connected by hierarchy relationship between one concept and another concept, and the same concept can exist in multiple hierarchies. SNOMED CT includes existing approximately 280,000 concept codes, 730,000 existing terms (description) and 920,000 existing definition type relationships. These concepts, terminologies and relationships can: (1) grab more detailed medical information (diagnostic information as different from ICD), (2) share medical information across agencies and regions, (3) reduce information system (electronic medical record) error, (4) improve the standardization degree of information system, (5) improve the retention and retrieval efficiency of clinical data.

Currently, SNOMED CT has no official Chinese version.

14.14. Clinical Data Interchange Standards Consortium Foundational Standards, CDISC[23,24]

The CDISC is a global, open, multidisciplinary, non-profit organization to develop standards which was founded in 1997. The CDISC standards are serial standards on acquisition, exchange, submission and archive of clinical research data and metadata. The basic standards include the following three categories:

(1) Standard data tabulation model for clinical trial data (SDTM) aims at original clinical trial data collection.
(2) Analysis data model (ADaM) aims at analysis of data set.
(3) Other standards, such as, clinical data acquisition standards harmonization for CRF standards (CDASH) aims at the standard CRF table in clinical trial.

SDTM: A data list with subjects as observational objects, including three categories: interventions, events, and findings. Interventions are interventions based on study protocol (such as, treatment drug), concomitant medication, and other substances with self-exposure of subjects (such as, alcohol, tobacco, coffee, etc.), which include three lists of exposure prescription (EX), concomitant medications (CM), and substance use (SU). Events refer to presuppose iconic event and independent events or status of evaluation occurring during test in research program (such as, adverse events), the events or status before the test (such as, history of diseases), including three lists of adverse events (AE), disposition (DS), and medical history (MH). Findings are observational data for treatment effect evaluation in the study protocol, which include seven lists of ECG test, inclusion/exclusion criteria (IE), Laboratory tests (LB), questionnaires (QS), physical examination (PE), subject characteristics (SC), vital signs (VS).

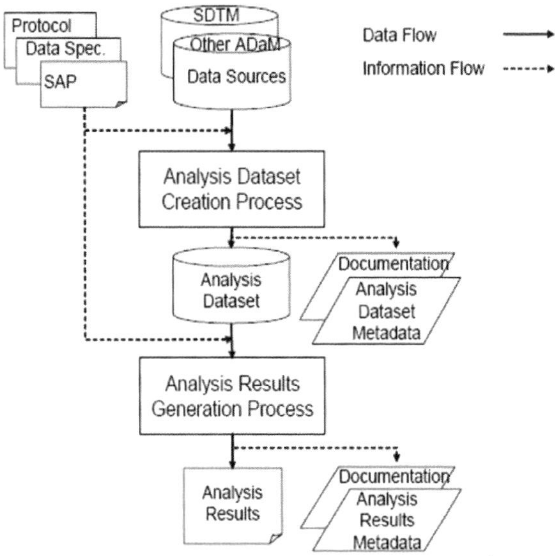

Fig. 14.14.1 ADaM statistical analysis of data flow and information flow.

ADaM standardizes the data flow and information flow in statistical analysis of clinical trial (Figure 14.14.1). The information flow includes study protocol, data standards, statistical analysis plan (SAP), metadata document of analysis data sets, and metadata document of analysis results.

ADaM metadata: ADaM regulates four kinds of metadata, including metadata of analysis data set, metadata of analysis variables, metadata of analysis parameters, and metadata of analysis results, respectively.

There is no formal Chinese version of CDISC currently.

14.15. Digital Imaging and Communications in Medicine, (DICOM)[25]

DICOM is an international standard (ISO 12052) on medical imaging and related information, which defines the format of medical imaging with quality meeting clinical needs and data exchange.

With the development of CT technology in the 1970s and the introduction of other digital diagnostic imaging modes, as well as the clinical growing application of computer use, the America Radiological Society (ACR) and the National Electronic Manufacturers Association (NEMA) realized that it was necessary to establish a standardization method for transmission of imagines and related information among devices manufactured by different manufacturers which had different digital image format.

Since DICOM 1.0 was published in 1985, the production and use of medical imaging equipment with substitution of X-ray film by full digital image has a general standard to follow, and the standard is more and more widely applied in the field of radiology, such as cardiovascular imaging equipment, radiation medical diagnostic imaging equipment (X-ray, CT, MRI, ultrasound, etc.), eye imaging and dental imaging equipment, etc. More than 10,000 medical imaging equipment adopt DICOM standard around the world. In 1993, DICOM 3.0 issued by the ACR–NEMA joint committee consisted of 20 parts:

Part 1: Introduction and Overview
Part 2: Conformance
Part 3: Information Object Definitions
Part 4: Service Class Specifications
Part 5: Data Structures and Encoding
Part 6: Data Dictionary
Part 7: Message Exchange
Part 8: Network Communication Support for Message Exchange
Part 9: Retired (formerly Point-to-Point Communication Support for Message Exchange)
Part 10: Media Storage and File Format for Media Interchange
Part 11: Media Storage Application Profiles
Part 12: Media Formats and Physical Media for Media Interchange
Part 13: Retired (formerly Print Management Point-to-Point Communication Support)
Part 14: Grayscale Standard Display Function
Part 15: Security and System Management Profiles
Part 16: Content Mapping Resource
Part 17: Explanatory Information
Part 18: Web Services
Part 19: Application Hosting
Part 20: Imaging Reports using HL7 Clinical Document Architecture

DICOM standard does not do provision on the following aspects:

(1) The detailed realization functions of equipment with the DICOM standard in declaration of conformity;
(2) The overall features of the system of equipment with the DICOM standard in declaration of conformity;
(3) Test and evaluation of the DICOM standard;
(4) DICOM standard gives a specification on the information exchange between medical imaging equipment and other systems. Due to the interaction between these equipment and other medical equipments, the DICOM standard will overlap with the scope of other medical

information fields. DICOM standard does not norm equipment in other medical information fields.

14.16. Anatomical Therapeutic Chemical Classification System (ATC)[26]

ATC drug classification system is a drug classification system used for basis of drug treatment, efficacy, and chemical properties in the organs and systems of main ingredient. The WHO Collaborating Centre for Drug Statistics Methodology formulated the ATC system, and released the first edition in 1976. In 1996, the ATC system became an international standard. Now the ATC system has released the 2013 edition.

The ATC system, namely the anatomy therapeutics and Chemical classification system, is the WHO official classification system about drug. ATC includes the following meaning of abbreviation, A (anatomical) means anatomy, which shows the drug for the body organ systems; T (therapeutic) means therapeutics, which shows drug treatment purposes; C (chemical) means chemical, which shows the classification of drugs.

ATC code has a total of seven digitals including first, fourth, fifth digitals for letters and second, third, sixth, seventh digitals for numbers.

The drug code of ATC system is divided into five levels:

The first directory is one letter code based on anatomic classification, including a total of 14 categories (Table 14.16.1), such as, C for cardiovascular system. The second directory is two numerical code based on classification of therapeutics, such as, C03 for diuretics. The third directory is one letter code according to pharmacology classification on the basis of therapeutics classification, such as, C03C for potent diuretics. The fourth directory is one letter code, which is classified by chemical composition, such as, C03CA for sulfonamides. The fifth directory is two numerical code according to the compound classification, such as, C03CA 01 furosemide.

ATC/DDD Index: The WHO Collaborating Center for Drug Statistics methodology provides online retrieval tool for ATC code and Defined Daily Dose (DDD) of official drug statistics (http://www.whocc.no/atc_ddd_index/), such as, search result for ATC code C03CA 01:

C CARDIOVASCULAR SYSTEM
C03 DIURETICS
C03C HIGH-CEILING DIURETICS
C03CA Sulfonamides, plain

ATC code	Name	DDD	U	Adm.R
C03CA01	furosemide	40	mg	O
		40	mg	P

Table 14.16.1 The first directory of drug code in ATC system.

A	Alimentary tract and metabolism
B	Blood and blood forming organs
C	Cardiovascular system
D	Dermatologicals
G	Genito-urinary system and sex hormones
H	Systemic hormonal preparations, excluding sex hormones and insulins
J	Anti-infectives for systemic use
L	Antineoplastic and immunomodulating agents
M	Musculo-skeletal system
N	Nervous system
P	Anti-parasitic products, insecticides and repellents
R	Respiratory system
S	Sensory organs
V	Various

In 2010, the Beijing Municipal Health Bureau had completed the Chinese version of ATC/DDD classification catalogues, and listed the generic names, name of commodity, specifications, dosage forms, the DDD value, administration route and the manufacturer information of drugs used in the city with ATC code on the base of ATC coding order.

14.17. International Classification of Functioning, Disability and Health (ICF)[27]

The International Classification of Functioning, Disability and Health, known more commonly as ICF, is a classification of health and health-related domains. As the functioning and disability of an individual occurs in a context, ICF also includes a list of environmental factors. ICF is the WHO framework for measuring health and disability at both individual and population levels. ICF was officially endorsed by all 191 WHO member states in the fifty-fourth World Health Assembly on May 22, 2001 (resolution WHA 54.21) as the international standard to describe and measure health and disability.

The following Figure 14.17.1 is one representation of the model of disability that is the basis for ICF.

The classification is organized in two parts, each comprising two components. Part 1 — Functioning and Disability — includes Body Functions and Structures and Activities and Participation; Part 2 — Contextual Factors —

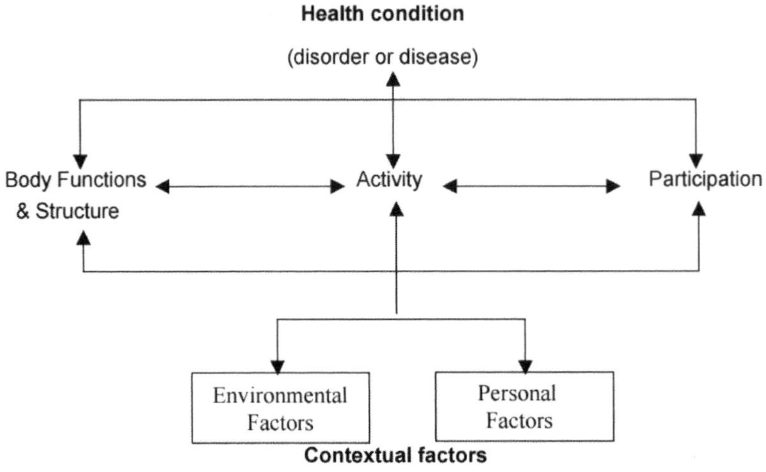

Fig. 14.17.1 ICF concept model.

incorporates Environmental Factors and Personal Factors, though Personal Factors are not yet classified in the ICF. Each component is subdivided into domains and categories at varying levels of granularity (up to four levels), each represented by a numeric code.

The prefix to an ICF code is a single letter (b, s, d, or e) representing the component in ICF where the code appears. The prefix "b" represents the Body Function component, "s" represents the Body Structure, "d" represents the Activities and Participation, and "e" represents the Environmental Factors, although the user may choose to use the more granular, optional a (for Activities), or p (Participation), depending on their specific user needs. The following are prefixes for the sub-groups of the Body Function component: "b1" Ch.1 Mental Function,"b2" Ch.2 Sensory Function and Pain, "b3" Ch.3 Voice and Speech Function, "b4" Ch.4 Functions of the Cardiovascular, haematological, Immunological and Respiratory System, "b5" Ch.5 Functions of Digestive, Metabolic and Endocrine Systems, "b6" Ch.6 Genitourinary and Reproductive Functions , "b7" Ch.7 Neuromusculoskeletal and Movement-related Functions, "b8" Ch.8 Functions of Skin and Related Structures. The third, fourth and fifth levels of directory are coded by integers, such as, b210 represents visual function, b2102 represents visual quality, b21022 represents visual contrast sensitivity.

The rating level uses one integer place as the code. 0 represents no problem, 1 represents mild problem, 2 represents moderate problem, 3 represents severe problem, 4 represents the most serious problem, 8 represents no assessment, and 9 represents inapplicability. Integrity of the ICF code is constituted by the rating item code and rating level coding. For example, as for visual function, b210.0, b210.1, b210.2, b210.3, b210.4 and b210.8, respectively represent no problem (no, not appearing, can be ignored, or loss of 0–4%), mild problem (mild, low level, loss of 5–24%), moderate problem (medium, general, loss of 25–49%), severe problem (high, very high, loss of 50–95%) and no assessment (current information cannot determine the severity of vision loss).

Combining disease classification framework (e.g. ICD-10), ICF provides an evaluation framework for the measurement result of individual and community health under the WHO "biology–psychology–social" medical mode, which has changed the content of data acquisition, statistical description, analysis model and health assessment method of "biological" medical mode with diseases as symbol over the past century. ICF is widely used in clinical medicine, preventive medicine, community health services, and other fields. Different researchers can create practical ICF Core Sets according to their needs, such as physical function evaluation data set for annual physical examination subjects, etc.

14.18. Data Security and Privacy Protection[29,30]

Whether paper or electronic data, government data, business data or personal data, data security and privacy protection is the most important. Security of data and information includes three aspects, the first is confidentiality, which ensures that unauthorized information will not be acquired by others for illegal use, such as, personal information of patients, diagnostic information, behavioral information, physical defects, etc.; the second is integrity, which protects the information from tampering by unauthorized institutions and individuals in the process of recording, transmission, storage, analysis and use, while preventing inappropriate modification, faulty operation and data loss by data administrators and authorized users; the third is availability, which ensures the access and use of information when it is needed by authorized users.

The direct target of information security and protection is the specific information, information system and information network. The security measures include:

(1) Authentication, such as, setting up accounts, passwords, phone confirmation and other measures;
(2) Authority, setting access permission according to user's role;

(3) Accountability, keeping save, modify, and access trail records to ensure accountability;
(4) Non-repudiation, carrying the unique identifier or information of the operator during operating which cannot be copied by others.

Data security and privacy protection includes three aspects: organizational management personnel management and technical measures. Organizational management includes regulatory agencies, such as security management agencies, post setting, staff responsibilities. Personnel management includes laws, regulations, personnel training, etc. Technical measures include environmental security, network security, hardware security, software security, data encryption, disaster recovery, etc.

Classified criteria for security protection of computer information system: The protection objects include:

(1) Legitimate rights and interests of citizens, legal persons and other organizations;
(2) Social order and public interests;
(3) National security.

The security protection of information system has five levels according to the damage size after being destroyed.

The first level, damage on the legitimate rights and interests of the citizens, legal persons and other organizations, with no harm on national security.

The second level, serious damage on the legitimate rights and interests of the citizens, legal persons and other organizations, or damage on social order and public interests, with no harm on national security.

The third level, serious damage on social order and public interests, or damage on national security.

The fourth level, particularly serious damage on social order and public interests, or serious damage on national security.

The fifth level, particularly serious damage on national security.

Privacy protection is one of the legitimate rights and interests of patients. De-identification should be applied during analysis and secondary use of data, that is, information relating to personal status, address, contact, etc. should be withheld to avoid adverse consequences for subject's money, employment, credit, insurance, reputation and other aspects.

References

1. Chan, HC, Wei, KK. A system for query comprehension. *Inf. Soft. Technol.*, 1997, 3: 141–148.
2. Guo, SH, Sun, YF. The information system design based on the dictionary database. *JOC*, 2000, 4: 26–29.
3. About Universal Decimal Classification (UDC) [EB/OL]. http://www.udcc.org/about.htm. Accessed on September 24, 2015.
4. Lewis-Beck, MS. *The Sage Encyclopedia of Social Science Research Methods.* London: Sage, 2004.
5. Thomas, G. The DGI Data Governance Framework [EB/OL]. http://www.datagovernance.com/wp-content/uploads/2014/11/dgi_framework.pdf. Accessed on September, 28, 2015.
6. Wang, J, Wang, YZ, Huang, Q. Interpretation of "Technical Guidance for Clinical Trial Data Management". *Chinese J. Clin. Pharmacol.*, 2013, 11: 874–876.
7. GB/T 18391.1-2009/ISO/IEC 11179-1: Information technology — metadata registry (MDR) Part 1: framework. Standardization Administration of China, 2009.
8. WS/T 303-2009. *Health Information Data Elements Standardization Rules.* Beijing: China Standard Press, 2009.
9. Data set specifications [EB/OL]. http://www.aihw.gov.au/data-set-specifications. Accessed on September 29, 2015.
10. National Minimum Data Sets [EB/OL]. http://www.aihw.gov.au/national-minimum-datasets. Accessed on September 29, 2015.
11. Dolin, RH, Alschuler, L, Boyer, S, *et al.* HL7 Clinical document architecture, release 2.0. *J. Amer. Med. Inf. Assoc.*, 2006, 13(1): 30–39.
12. ISO/TC 215, ISO/DIS 210909. Health Informatics — Harmonized data types for information interchange. ISO, 2011.
13. Open EHR Data Types Information Model [EB/OL]. http://www.openEHR.org. Accessed on September 23, 2015.
14. Arfaoui, N, Akaichi, J. Datawarehouse: Conceptual and logical schema. Int. J. Enterprise Computing and Business Systems 2, 2012: 1–31.
15. Li, CB, Li, SJ, Li, XC. *Data Warehouse and Data Mining Practice.* Beijing: Electronic Industry Press, 2014.
16. A Technical Introduction to XML [EB/OL]. http://www.xml.com/pub/a/98/10/guide0.html. Accessed on September 20, 2015.
17. Zhang, Y. XML and its application in library and information retrieval. *New Technology of Library and Information Service*, 2001, 2: 30–35.
18. Health Level seven [EB/OL]. http://www.hl7.org/. Accessed on September 20, 2015.
19. HL7 Reference Information Model. Health Level seven [EB/OL]. http://www.hl7.org/implement/standards/rim.cfm. Accessed on September 20, 2015.
20. Dong, JW, *et al. The Tenth Revision of ICD-10 — Instruction Manual.* Beijing: People's Medical Publishing House, 2008.
21. Logical Observation Identifiers Names and Codes (LOINC®) Users' Guide [EB/OL]. http://loinc.org/downloads/files/LOINCManual.pdf. Accessed on September 29, 2015.
22. SNOMED CT Starter Guide [EB/OL]. http://www.ihtsdo.org/fileadmin/user_upload/doc/download/doc_StarterGuide_Current-en-US_INT_20141202.pdf. Accessed on September 29, 2015.
23. CDISC Analysis Data Model Team. Analysis Data Model (ADaM) http://www.cdisc.org/adam-v2.1-%26-adamig-v1.0. Accessed on October 29, 2015.

24. CDISC Vision and Mission [EB/OL]. http://www.cdisc.org/CDISC-Vision-and-Mission. Accessed on September 29, 2015.
25. ISO 12052. Health informatics — Digital imaging and communication in medicine (DICOM) including workflow and data management. ISO, 2011.
26. International language for drug utilization research [EB/OL]. http://www.whocc.no/.
27. How to use the ICF: A practical manual for using the International Classification of Functioning, Disability and Health (ICF) [EB/OL]. http://www.who.int/ classifications/drafticfpracticalmanual2.pdf.
28. WHO ICF Browser [EB/OL]. http://apps.who.int/classifications/icfbrowser/Default.aspx.
29. GB/T 22240-2008. Information security technology — Classification guide for classified guide for classified protection of information system. Standardization Administration of China, 2008.
30. ISO/IEC 27001. Information technology — Security techniques — Information security management systems. ISO, 2013.

---

*For the introduction of the corresponding author, see the front matter.

CHAPTER 15

DATA MINING

Yunquan Zhang and Chuanhua Yu*

15.1. Big Data[1-3]

Data mining is always inseparable from large amounts of data, known as big data. Big data is a term for data sets that are so large or complex that traditional data processing applications or tools are inadequate and unable to achieve the goals of data capture, data storage, data management, and data analysis in a limited time. Big data, in healthcare, for instance, are usually characterized by large-scale, complicated, and linked data information. In addition to genomic information, big data can also include medical, environmental, financial, geographic, and social media information, etc. Big data in healthcare are measurable data information which is associated with health maintenance, sub-health status, or diseases. These data include lifestyle and behavior pattern, genetic factors, healthcare system, and social environmental factors, etc.

The characteristics of big data can be summarized as 4 "V": volume (huge volumes), variety (wide diversity of database types), velocity (dynamic and fast updated), and value (low value density).

(1) Volume: Available data volume is increasing so rapidly with an exponential growth that data volume has been currently accumulated to the scale of TB to PB. Global data size will reach 35.2 ZB by 2020 as expected. (1 Byte can store one letter, e.g., 'A' or 'x'. $1\,B=2^{0}B$, $1\,kB=2^{10}B$, $1\,MB=2^{20}B$, $1\,GB=2^{30}B$, $1\,TB=2^{40}B$, $1\,PB=2^{50}B$, $1\,EB=2^{60}B$, $1\,ZB=2^{70}B$, $1\,YB=2^{80}B$, $1\,BB=2^{90}B$, $1\,NB=2^{100}B$, $1\,DB=2^{110}B$.)

*Corresponding author: yuchua@163.com

(2) Variety: Database types are diverse and miscellaneous, which include not only structured data such as relational data, unstructured data such as text, e-mail, and multimedia data, but also semi-structured data. Moreover, unstructured data are growing far more rapidly than structured data.
(3) Velocity: Multiple sources of data are updated so fast that we must have access to data capture, and interactive and *quasi*-real-time data analysis. Thus, decisions based on data can be made in a fraction of a second.
(4) Value: Big data are of great value but low value density (sometimes referred to as "Veracity"). To discover the value, the core purpose of data mining, is the process of discovering interesting patterns and knowledge from a tremendous amount of data, which is similar to panning gravel for gold and dredging for a needle in the sea.

Analyses for big data mainly include association rule mining, classification and regression tree (CART), web mining, social network analysis, machine learning, pattern recognition, support vector machine (SVM), artificial neural networks (ANNs), evolutionary computation, deep learning, and data visualization.

There are three major shifts in the concepts of data mining in the age of big data: (1) from part (sample) to whole (population): all data can be included into our analyses rather than only the data obtained from random sampling, (2) more efficient rather than absolutely accurate: it will lead to greater insight and benefits when appropriately ignoring microcosmic accuracy of data analysis, (3) more focus on correlation rather than causality.

Internet data are the original sources of big data, which are most widely accessed and accepted. In addition to internet data, different departments in all fields may generate a number of big data sources, for example, the sources of death data can be from the National Electronic Disease Surveillance System (NEDSS), Cause-of-death Information from Civil Registration, the Maternal and Child Health Information System (MCHIS), the Death Case Reporting System in county and above levels' medical institutions, etc.

15.2. Data Preprocessing[4,5]

Data preprocessing is the data processing before data mining, the purpose of which is to help improve the quality of the data and the efficiency and ease of the mining process.

Accuracy, completeness, and consistency define the three elements of data quality. In the real world, large databases and data warehouses are commonly inaccurate (containing errors or values that deviate from the expected), incomplete (lacking attribute values or certain attributes of interest), and inconsistent (e.g., containing discrepancies in the department codes used to categorize items). In addition, timeliness, believability, and interpretability are also the factors affecting data quality. Thus, it is of significance and necessity to conduct data preprocessing to improve data quality.

There are four major steps involved in data preprocessing, namely, data cleaning, data integration, data reduction, and data transformation.

(1) Data cleaning routines work to "clean" the data by filling in missing values, smoothing noisy data, identifying or removing outliers, and resolving inconsistencies, and so on.
(2) Data integration merges and integrates data from multiple data sources and data formats using unified storage in order to build a data warehouse.
(3) Data reduction obtains a reduced representation of the data set that keeps the original completeness but is much smaller in data volume, yet produces the same (or almost the same) analytical results, thus helps in improving the efficiency of data mining process.

Data reduction strategies include dimensionality reduction, numerosity reduction, and data compression. (a) Dimensionality reduction excludes or removes irrelevant, weakly relevant, and redundant attributes or dimensions, applying dimensionality reduction methods of wavelet transforms and principal components analysis. (b) Numerosity reduction replaces the original data volume by alternative, smaller forms of data representation by parametric or non-parametric techniques. For parametric methods, a model, such as linear regression and log-linear models, is used to estimate the data, so that typically only the data parameters need to be stored, instead of the actual data. Non-parametric methods for storing reduced representations of the data include histograms, sampling, and clustering. (c) Data compression obtains a reduced or "compressed" representation of the original data using data encoding scheme, in the process of which the original data are reconstructed from the compressed data without any information loss.

(4) Data transformation transforms or consolidates the data into forms appropriate for data mining. Strategies for data transformation include:

    (a) Smoothing, which works to remove noise from the data. Techniques include binning, regression, and clustering.

(b) Aggregation, where summary or aggregation operations are applied to the data. For example, the data of daily outpatient hospital admissions may be aggregated so as to compute monthly and annual total amounts.
(c) Attribute construction, where new attributes are constructed and added from the given set of attributes to help the mining process.
(d) Normalization, where the attribute data are scaled so as to fall within a smaller range, such as -1 to 1, or 0 to 1, in order to eliminate influence of dimension.
(e) Discretization, where the raw values of a numeric attribute (e.g., age) are replaced by interval labels (e.g., 0–14, 15–59, etc.) or conceptual labels (e.g., youth, adult, senior). One numeric attribute can be redefined as several conceptual groups according to actual need.
(f) Concept hierarchy generation, where attributes of nominal data such as street can be generalized to higher-level concepts, like city or country.

15.3. Anomaly Detection[6–8]

Anomaly detection, also known as outlier detection, is the process of finding data objects that are very different from most other data points, namely to detect outliers or anomalies.

In a given statistical process used to generate a set of data objects, an outlier is a data object that deviates significantly from the rest of the objects, as if it was generated by a different mechanism. In general, outliers can be classified into three categories, namely global outliers, contextual (or conditional) outliers, and collective outliers. Outliers usually result from data sources from different clusters, natural variability, and errors of data measurement and collection, etc.

Two orthogonal ways are presented below to categorize outlier detection methods.

(1) According to whether domain expert-labeled examples of normal and/or outlier objects can be clearly obtained when building an outlier detection model, the outlier detection methods can be divided into supervised methods, semi-supervised methods, and unsupervised methods. The tasks to examine and label a sample of the underlying data (normal or outlier) are done by domain experts, we then classify the unlabeled data objects into normal objects or outliers based on expert-labeled examples.

(2) According to statistical methods used, the outlier detection methods can be categorized into three types: model-based methods, proximity-based methods, and clustering-based methods.

(a) Model-based methods for outlier detection assume that normal objects in a data set are generated by a stochastic process (a generative probability distribution model), and then identify those objects in low-probability regions of the model as outliers. Model-based methods can be divided into parametric methods and non-parametric methods, according to how the models are specified and learned.
A parametric method assumes that normal data objects are generated by a parametric distribution with parameter Θ. Probability density function of the parametric distribution $f(x, \Theta)$ gives the probability that object x is generated by the distribution. The smaller this value is, the more likely x is an outlier. The simplest example is to detect outliers based on univariate or multivariate normal distribution. A non-parametric method tries to determine the model based on input data flexibly (completely parameter-free) instead of assuming a priori statistical model. Examples of non-parametric methods include histogram and kernel density estimation.

(b) Proximity-based methods assume that the proximity of an outlier object to its nearest neighbors significantly deviates from the proximity of the object to most of the other objects in the data set. There are two types of proximity-based outlier detection methods: distance-based and density-based methods. A distance-based outlier detection method consults the neighborhood of an object, which is defined by a given radius. An object is then considered as outlier if its neighborhood does not have enough other points. A density-based outlier detection method investigates the density of an object and that of its neighbors, and an object is identified as an outlier if its density is much lower relative to that of its neighbors.

(c) Clustering-based methods detect outliers by examining the relationship between objects and clusters. Intuitively, an outlier is an object that belongs to a small and remote cluster, or does not belong to any cluster. Moreover, if the object belongs to a small cluster or sparse cluster, all the objects in the cluster are outliers (namely, collective outliers).

15.4. Association Rule Mining[9–11]

Association rule mining is used to detect interesting associations between variables (itemsets) in the databases and data warehouses. A typical example of association rule mining is the correlation analysis between beers and diapers in Wal-Mart Supermarket of the United States.

For all transactions (or observations), the set of all items (or variables) is called itemset. Association rule mining should follow two major steps as below:

(1) Identify all large frequent itemsets from the transaction database (Table 15.4.1). The occurrence frequency of an itemset I is the number of transactions that contain the itemset I, which is also known as the support of itemset I. Let $\{A, B\}$ be an itemset (a 2-itemset), we have Support $(A \Rightarrow B) = P(A \cup B)$, which implies that support of the rule $A \Rightarrow B$ is the percentage of all transactions that contain $A \cup B$ (this is taken to be the probability). If the support of item $\{A, B\}$ satisfies a prespecified minimum support threshold, then $\{A, B\}$ is a frequent itemset.
(2) Generate strong association rules from the frequent itemsets. Confidence of the rule $A \Rightarrow B$ is the percentage of transactions containing A that also contain B (this is taken to be the conditional probability), namely Confidence $(A \Rightarrow B) = P(B|A)$. If the confidence of $A \Rightarrow B$ satisfies a prespecified minimum confidence threshold, then A, B are associated items. Rules that satisfy both a minimum support threshold and a minimum confidence threshold are called strong association rules. Minimum support and confidence thresholds are usually specified according to the need of data mining.

Table 15.4.1. A hypothetical example of association rule.

Case number	Diabetes (A)	Arteriosclerosis (B)	Obesity	Hypertension
1	0	1	1	1
2	1	1	0	0
3	1	0	1	0
4	1	0	0	0
5	1	1	0	0
6	1	1	1	0

Based on Table 15.4.1, we have

$$\text{Support}(A \Rightarrow B) = P(A \cup B) = 3/6 = 0.5$$

$$\text{Confidence}(A \Rightarrow B) = P(B|A) = 3/5 = 0.6.$$

The association rule can be expressed as

$$\text{diabetes} \Rightarrow \text{arteriosclerosis[support=50\%; confidence=60\%]}.$$

Frequent itemset mining methods:

(1) Apriori algorithm is based on an important property that all non-empty subsets of a frequent itemset must also be frequent. That is also to say, if a k-itemset is not frequent (does not satisfy the minimum support threshold), then the resulting $k+1$-itemset is not frequent either. To find L_k, a set of candidate k-itemsets is generated by joining L_{k-1} with itself. This set of candidates is denoted as C_k. C_k is a superset of L_k, that is, its members may or may not be frequent, but all of the frequent k-itemsets are included in C_k. A database scan to determine the count of each candidate in C_k would result in the determination of L_k.

(2) FP-growth algorithm is short for frequent pattern growth and compresses the database representing frequent items into a frequent pattern tree (FP-tree). FP-growth algorithm scans the database twice. The first scan derives the set of frequent items (1-itemsets) and their support counts (frequencies). The set of frequent items is sorted in the order of descending support count. In the second scan of the database, the items in each transaction are processed in the order of descending support count, and a branch is created for each transaction. In this way, the problem of mining frequent patterns in databases is transformed into that of mining the FP-tree.

15.5. Data Classification[12,13]

Data classification is widely applied in data mining. It is a technique that constructs a classifier based on previous data, and uses this classifier to predict new data that class labels are unknown.

Data classification is a two-step process, consisting of a learning step (where a classification model is constructed) and a classification step (where the model is used to predict class labels for given data).

If the class label of each training tuple is known, this learning step is also known as supervised learning (e.g., decision tree). It contrasts with unsupervised learning (e.g., clustering), in which the class label of each training

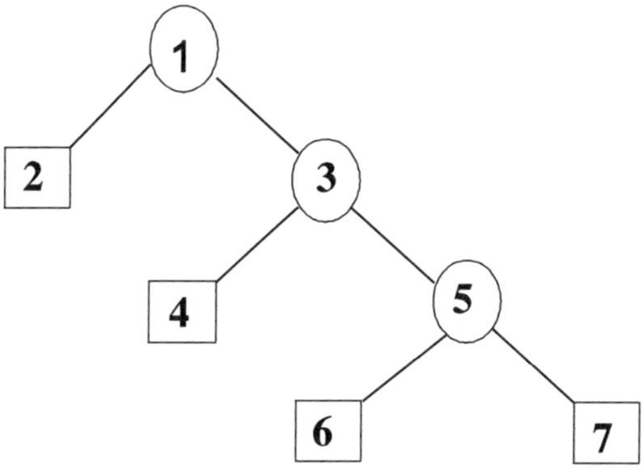

Fig. 15.5.1. Schematic diagram of tree structure.

tuple is not provided, and the number or set of classes to be learned may not be known in advance. In the classification step, the predictive accuracy of the classifier is estimated. If we were to use the training set to measure the classifier's accuracy, the classifier tends to overfit the data. Therefore, a test set is used, which is independent of the training set. In practice, cross-validation and bootstrap sampling method are often used to evaluate the accuracy of the classification model. When two or more classification models are generated, it is necessary to use statistical hypothesis test and ROC curve to select the best classification model.

Several commonly used classification algorithms are listed as below:

(1) A decision tree is a flowchart-like upside-down tree structure. The decision tree presented in Figure 15.5.1 has four knot layers (including the root knot ①). The squares represent the leaf node, and each leaf node holds only one class label value. Each root node (presented as circles) can be divided into two or more branches, each of which denotes an outcome of the test. The methods for node splitting in decision tree include Entropy method, Pearson Chi-square test, and Gini index method.

Classification and regression trees (CART) and C4.5 algorithm are two of the most commonly used decision tree algorithms. CART is the basis of many integrated classification algorithms and can not only construct a classification tree but also a regression tree. Iterative Dichotomiser 3 (ID3) algorithm and C4.5 algorithm are both based on Entropy theory and information gain theory, while C4.5 is an improved algorithm of ID3. Although the current C5.0 algorithm further improves the operation efficiency, it is often for commercial use. Thus, C4.5 algorithm is still a popular decision tree algorithm.

Random forest is a common combination of classification method, in which each classification is a decision tree, and the set of classifications generate a "forest".

(2) Bayes classification methods (Bayes classifiers) predict the posterior probability that a given tuple belongs to a particular class based on the prior probability and Bayesian formula, and then classify the object into the category that is of a maximum *posteriori* probability. Bayesian classifiers have the minimum error rate in comparison to all other classifiers. Bayes classification methods include naive Bayesian classification, Bayesian belief network, and the expectation maximization (EM) algorithm.

Additionally, k-nearest neighbor (KNN), artifical neural network (ANN), and SVM are also commonly used classification techniques in data mining.

15.6. Web Mining[14–16]

Web mining aims to discover useful information or knowledge from the web hyperlink structure, page content, and usage data. Although web mining uses many data-mining techniques, it is not purely an application of traditional data-mining techniques due to the heterogeneity and semi-structured or unstructured nature of web data.

Three major steps involved in web mining include data collection and preprocessing, pattern discovery, and pattern analysis. Based on the primary kinds of data used in the mining process, web mining tasks can be categorized into three major types: web-structure mining, web-content mining, and web-usage mining.

(1) Web-structure mining

Web-structure mining discovers useful knowledge from hyperlinks, which represent the structure of the web. Web-structure mining includes hyperlink analysis and web crawling. PageRank and HITS, both of which were originated from social network analysis, are the two most influential hyperlink based search algorithms. They both exploit the hyperlink structure of the web to rank pages according to their levels of "prestige" or "authority". Apart from search ranking, hyperlinks are also useful for finding web communities, namely, community discovery. A web crawler is a program that automatically accesses the web's hyperlink structure, collects and saves the information of each linked page for the analysis and mining procedures. Crawling is often the first step of web mining. There are two main types of crawlers: universal crawlers (download all pages irrespective of their contents) and topic crawlers (download only pages of certain topics).

2. Web-content mining

Web-content mining extracts or mines useful information or knowledge from web page contents. It includes two steps: data extraction from web and information integration. Data extraction step achieves structured data extraction by supervised and unsupervised learning methods, or extracts useful information from unstructured text, for instance, mining of the user's point of view or attitude from product comments, forum discussion, and blog and micro-blog communication. Information integration step needs to semantically integrate the data/information extracted from multiple sites in order to produce a consistent and coherent database. Intuitively, integration means: (1) to match columns in different data tables that contain the same type of information and (2) to match data values that are semantically the same but expressed differently at diversified sites.

3. Web-usage mining

Web-usage mining mainly refers to the automatic analysis of web usage logs, including search time, search words, retrieval paths, as well as which retrieval results were viewed by users. By mining these usage logs, we can discover a lot of potential and common search behavioral patterns of users. Studying on these patterns can be useful to solve customer feedback on search results, and to further improve the search engine.

Large scale web mining has been unable to rely on individual computing nodes, while using dedicated parallel computer hardware is of high cost. With the emergence of new technologies, such as big data, cloud computing, and internet of things, distributed file systems can take the advantages of distributed processing parallel architecture, and can also avoid the problem of reliability. This makes it possible for ordinary users to conduct web mining in big data era.

15.7. Text Mining[17–19]

Text mining, also known as knowledge discovery from text database, extracts potential and understandable patterns and knowledge that are unknown in advance from the collection of massive text or corpus.

Text mining tasks include text retrieval, text feature selection, text categorization, text clustering, topic detection and tracking, and text filtering.

(1) Text retrieval: Text retrieval, also called full-text retrieval, aims to locate the document sets according to the user's information needs.
(2) Text feature selection: Text feature selection calculates the score of each text feature based on a certain evaluation function of text feature, then sorts the features in the order of descending scores, and the feature words with the highest scores are selected.
(3) Text categorization: Under a given classification system, text categorization automatically categorizes text associations based on the contents and maps of the text unlabeled by categories to those labeled by categories. This mapping relationship can be one to one and one to many, because a text document can be associated with multiple categories. Text categorization is a typical process of supervised machine learning, which generally includes two steps: training and classification. Algorithms of text categorization include decision trees, Bayesian networks, neural networks, and SVM, etc.
(4) Text clustering: Text clustering is an unsupervised machine learning method. The main methods of text clustering include hierarchical clustering algorithms represented by BIRCH algorithm and partitional clustering algorithms represented by k-means algorithm.
(5) Topic detection and tracking (TDT): TDT is an information processing technology, and aims to automatically identify new topics and keep track of known topics from the media information flow. According to different application requirements, TDT can be divided into five kinds, namely, segmentation report, topic tracking, topic detection, first reported detection, and association detection.
(6) Text filtering: Text filtering is a method or process that extracts information the user needs or filters useless information from the dynamic text information flow based on a certain standard. Spam filtering is a typical application of text filtering. The commonly used methods of spam filtering include the Bogofilter method based on the Bayes principle and the DMC/PPM method using statistical data compression technique.

The general flow of text mining is shown in Figure 15.7.1.

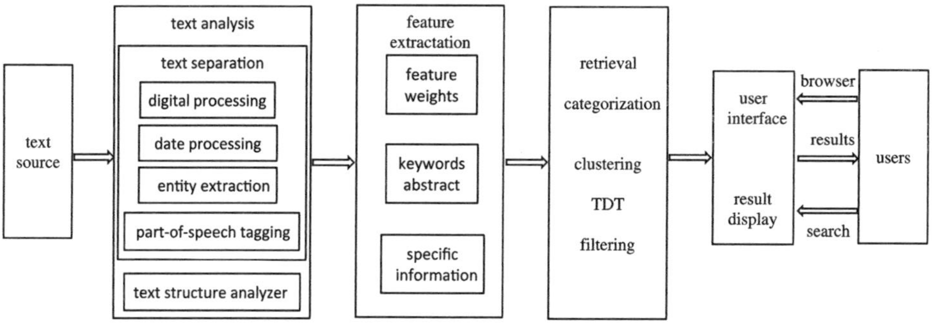

Fig. 15.7.1. The general flow of text mining.

15.8. Social Network Analysis[20–22]

Social network refers to the assemblages of social actors themselves (individuals, groups, and organizations) and relationships between social actors. Examples of social network include interpersonal relationship network, the internetwork, ecological network, neural network, science citation network, author collaboration network, and so on. Social network analysis is a research method to study the relationships between groups of social actors. Social network analysis focuses on relationship patterns of the actors, which can be individuals, communities, groups, organizations, and countries, etc. From the point of view of social network, the interaction between individuals in social environment can be expressed as a pattern or rule based on the relationship. Regular patterns of these relationships are helpful to understand the social structure, quantitative analyses of which is the basic point of social network analysis.

A social network is mainly demonstrated in the form of sociograms and sociomatrixes.

(1) Sociogram: A sociogram generally consists of points (social actors) and lines (the relationship between social actors). Sociograms can be divided into: categories of directed graphs (or digraphs) and undirected graphs based on the direction of relationship lines; categories of binary graphs, signed graphs and valued graphs based on close degree of the relationships; categories of complete graphs and non-complete graphs based on completeness of the relationships, etc.

(2) Sociomatrix: Rows and columns in the matrix represent social actors, and elements of the corresponding rows and columns represent the relationships between social actors. Thus, the relationships between social actors can be

studied using matrix manipulation, and correlation and regression relationships between different sociomatrixes can be used to discover associations between different social networks.

Connections and distances between social actors are two basic concepts of social networks. Connection related concepts include the sub-graphs, connected graphs, components, dyads and triads, etc. Dyads and triads are the basis of a variety of network models. Distance related concepts include nodal degree, walks, trails, paths, cycles, and density, etc. These concepts comprehensively describe the roles of social actors in the network and the structure of the whole network.

Methods of social network analysis mainly include centrality analysis and cohesive subgroups analysis.

(1) Centrality analysis: Centrality analysis is the key point of social network analysis. What roles ("prestige" or "authority") social actors play in a social network, has great impact on communication patterns and effects of information in the whole network. Centrality has two important indicators: point centrality and graph centrality. Point centrality measures the authority or prestige degree of a node in the network, while graph centrality describes the close degree or coherence of the whole sociography.

(2) Cohesive subgroups analysis: Cohesive subgroups are subsets of actors among whom there are relatively strong, direct, intense, frequent, or positive ties. Cohesive subgroups analysis can reveal internal sub-structures within a social network and quantify these structures. When conducting cohesive subgroups analysis, we should first analyze well-defined subgroups (such as cliques), and then loosely defined subgroups (such as n-cliques).

15.9. Machine Learning[23,24]

Machine learning is a multi/interdisciplinary science of artificial intelligence, which involves many disciplines, such as probability theory, statistics, approximation theory, convex analysis, and computational complexity theory, etc. Machine learning is widely defined as below: a computer program is said to learn from experience E with respect to some class of tasks T and performance measure P, if its performance at tasks in T, as measured by P, improves with experience E.

Generally speaking, machine learning is devoted to studying how computers can simulate or realize learning behaviors of human, so as to acquire new knowledge or skills, reorganize the existing knowledge structure and gradually improve its performance. Process of human learning is time consuming, easily forgotten, and cannot be copied (learning ability is highly dependent on the individual). Contrarily, the process of machine learning is efficient, easily copied, and the knowledge learned can be permanently retained.

Methods of machine learning can be divided into three categories: supervised learning, unsupervised learning, and reinforcement learning.

The general theorems and rules applied to machine learning include the Principle of Majority Decision, Occam Razor, and No Free Lunch Theorem. Algorithms of machine learning can be evaluated by methods of Minimum Description Length, analysis of predictive accuracy, and cross-validation.

Classical algorithms of machine learning include C4.5 algorithm in decision tree algorithms, k-means algorithm in clustering algorithms, SVM, Apriori algorithm in association rule mining used to identify frequent itemsets, EM algorithm, PageRank algorithm, AdaBoost iterative algorithm, k-nearest neighbor algorithm, naive Bayes algorithm, and classification and regression tree (CART).

The basic structure of a learning system mainly includes four parts: the environment, learning process, knowledge database, and execution and evaluation (shown in Figure 15.9.1). As for a whole learning system, the environment provides some information, which is learned and used by learning process to modify the knowledge database. These modifications can drive the execution step more efficiently. The execution step then feeds something back to the learning process when the task is completed.

The most important factor that affects the design of a learning system is the information that the environment provides to the system, more specifically, is the quality of the information, which directly determines design difficulty of the learning process. Knowledge in knowledge database has a variety of expression ways, such as feature vector, first-order logic statements, production rule, and semantic network, etc. In the choices of expression ways, we should ensure: (1) strong expression ability; (2) easy ratiocination; (3) knowledge database is easy to modify; (4) knowledge is easy to expand.

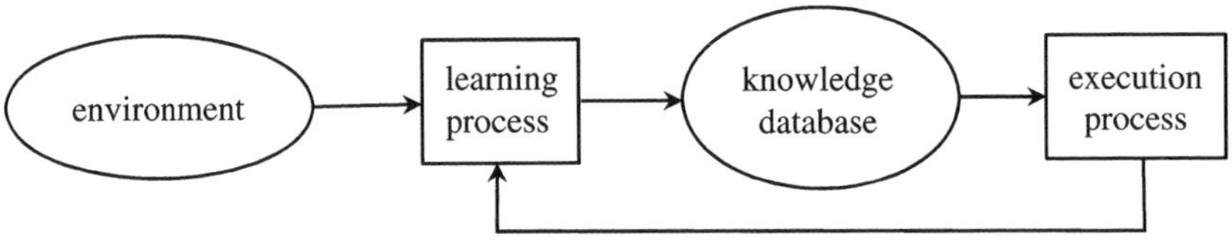

Fig. 15.9.1. The basic structure of a learning system.

Machine learning has a wide range of applications in many fields, including data mining, computer vision, natural language processing, biological feature recognition, search engines, medical diagnosis, credit card fraud detection, securities market analysis, DNA sequencing, speech and handwriting recognition, strategy games and robot application, etc.

15.10. Pattern Recognition[25–27]

Pattern is the regular relationship between components or influencing factors of an object. Pattern recognition, also known as pattern classification, is the process that divides a sample into a certain category by characteristic learning of the sample.

Pattern recognition is an important part of information science and artificial intelligence. It is widely used in many fields, such as text recognition, speech recognition, fingerprint recognition, remote sensing image recognition, and medical diagnosis, etc.

According to whether the training data have been hand-labeled or not in learning procedure, pattern recognition is generally categorized as supervised pattern recognition and unsupervised pattern recognition. A system of pattern recognition usually includes four major parts: raw data acquisition and preprocessing, feature extraction and selection, classification or clustering, and postprocessing (shown in Figure 15.10.1).

Methods of pattern recognition mainly include syntactic pattern recognition and statistical pattern recognition.

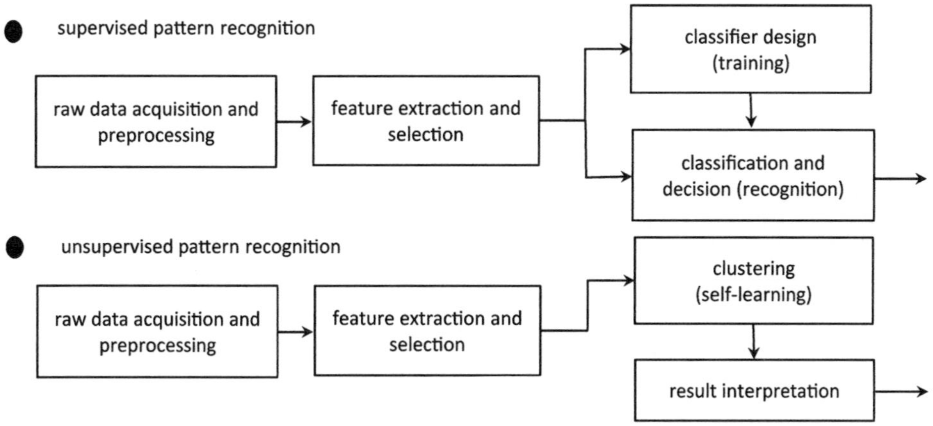

Fig. 15.10.1. Typical process of pattern recognition.

(1) Syntactic pattern recognition

Syntactic pattern recognition decomposes objects into a series of basic units expressed as certain symbols, then describes relationships between basic units of objects as syntactic relationships between respective symbols, and classifies the objects into certain patterns using the principles of formal language and syntactic analysis.

(2) Statistical pattern recognition

Statistical pattern recognition establishes mathematical models based on statistical theories and applies these models to predict the classifications of sample objects. Generally, so-called pattern recognition is namely statistical pattern recognition.

(a) Statistical decision

Statistical decision, also known as Bayesian decision, is an important theory and method of pattern recognition. On condition that conditional probability and priori probability of certain categories are known or could be estimated, statistical decision compares posterior probabilities of a sample object belonging to each category using the Bayesian formula, and then classifies the sample object into a category with the highest probability.

(b) Linear discriminant analysis

Linear discriminant analysis makes decisions by constructing a linear discriminant function, that is to say, it divides a feature space into several decision regions by a hyperplane. The commonly used linear discriminant methods include the classical Fisher linear discriminant, the perceptron criterion function, the least square error criterion and linear SVM, etc.

(c) Nonlinear discriminate analysis

Nonlinear discriminate analysis is developed on the basis of linear discriminant method. It has a variety of more applicable methods, which include the classical piecewise linear discriminant function, quadratic discriminant function, nonlinear SVM, Kernel machine, and multilayer perceptron neural network method, etc.

Other pattern recognition methods also include nearest neighbor method, decision tree and random forest, and logistic regression, etc.

15.11. SVM[28–30]

SVM, proposed and published by Vapnik *et al.* in 1995, is one of the research hotspots in the field of machine learning. SVM is a machine learning method

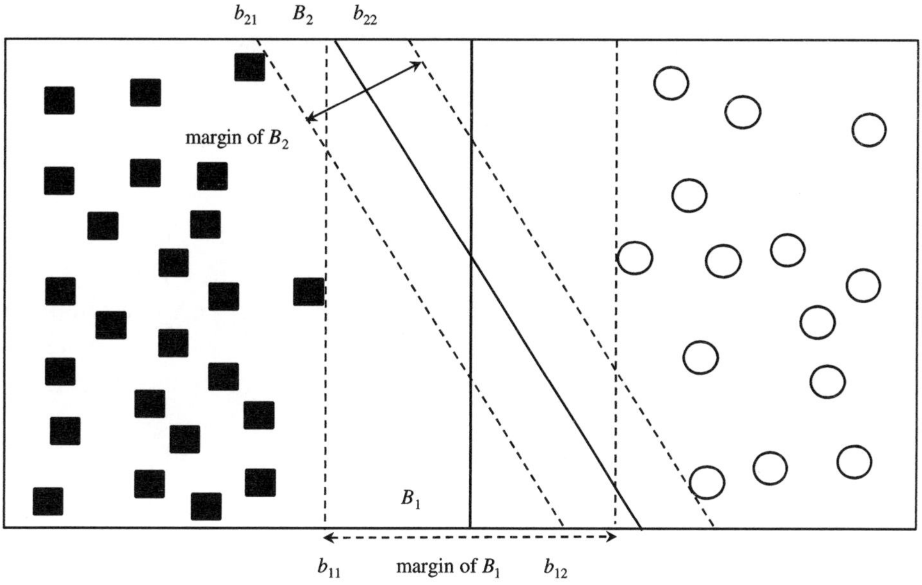

Fig. 15.11.1. Margins of decision boundaries.

which is based on structure risk minimum criterion and can be used for classification of linear and nonlinear data. According to whether the data can be linearly separable or not, SVM can be divided into linear SVM and nonlinear SVM.

Linear SVM searches for optimal separating hyperplane in the original space (shown in Figure 15.11.1). Circles and squares in the figure represent two samples from different categories, all of which can be completely separated by an infinite number of hyperplanes. Although there are no training errors using these hyperplanes, we cannot ensure that they perform equally well in classification predicting of unknown samples.

As shown in Figure 15.11.1, two decision boundaries B_1 and B_2 can both accurately divide the training samples into their respective categories. Each decision boundary B_i corresponds to a pair of hyperplanes b_{i1} and b_{i2}. By parallel shifting a hyperplane which is parallel to a decision boundary (B_1 or B_2) until reaching the nearest square, thus we can obtain b_{i1}. Similarly, b_{i2} can be also obtained by parallel shifting a hyperplane which is parallel to a decision boundary (B_1 or B_2) until reaching the nearest circle. Distance between the two hyperplanes (b_{i1} and b_{i2}) is called margin. As we can see, the margin of B_1 is larger than that of B_2. In this case, B_1 is just the maximal margin hyperplane, which is the optimal separating hyperplane that SVM searches for.

If the margin is small, any slight disturbance of the decision boundary may have a great impact on classification. Therefore, decision boundaries with small margins are prone to overfitting the classification model, resulting in very poor generalization ability in unknown samples; while large margins will improve classification accuracy of the corresponding hyperplanes.

In order to adapt to nonlinear data, linear SVM method can be further extended to nonlinear SVM. This process includes two steps: (1) transforming the original training set into a higher dimensional space using nonlinear mappings; (2) searching the new space for the nonlinear separating hypersurface, which corresponds to the maximal margin hyperplane in original space.

The disadvantages of SVM include large training sets and slow training process. However, SVM is more applicable to complex modeling of nonlinear decision boundaries and less prone to overfitting the model compared with other methods. SVM is mainly used for prediction and classification, which has been successfully applied in many fields, such as handwritten numeral recognition, object recognition, speaker recognition, and benchmark time series prediction, etc.

15.12. ANN[31–33]

ANN is a family of models inspired by neural networks of human brain and is artificially constructed to achieve certain functions based on the view of information processing.

ANN is composed of a large number of connected input nodes and output nodes, each of which represents a specific activation function. Connections between every two nodes represent weighted values (namely, weights) of the connected signals, which are memory connections of ANN. Outputs of ANN vary greatly by connection modes, weights, and activation functions. The learning process of most neural network models is to minimize errors between model outputs and the actual outputs based on training samples by constant adjustment of weight parameters.

ANN can be generally divided into two categories: feedforward neural network and feedback neural network.

Neural network inputs a number of nonlinear models, as well as weighted interconnections between different models, and ultimately gets an output model. Specifically, input layers are a number of independent variables, which are combined into the middle hidden layers. Hidden layers mainly consist of

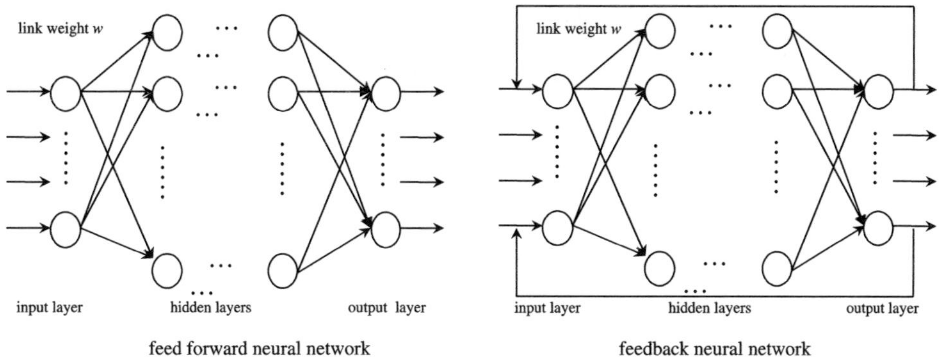

Fig. 15.12.1. Two typical structures of neural network.

many nonlinear functions, also known as transition functions or squeezing functions. Hidden layers are the so-called black boxes and almost no one can find out how these independent variables are combined together by nonlinear functions of hidden layers in all cases. This is a typical case that computers think instead of humans (see Figure 15.12.1).

There are five factors affecting the results when constructing neural network models:

(1) The number of hidden layers: For certain input layers and output layers, we should try a variety of parameter settings for the number of hidden layers to find out a satisfactory model structure.
(2) The number of input variables in each layer: Overabundant independent variables may cause model overfitting, so inputting variables should be selected before modeling process.
(3) Network connection types: Inputting variables of neural network models can be connected by different types (e.g., forward, backward, and parallel), which may result in different model results.
(4) Connection degree: Elements of a certain layer can be completely or partially linked to elements of other layers. Incomplete connection can reduce the risk of overfitting, while it can weaken the predictive ability of neural network models.
(5) Transition functions: Transition functions can squeeze all the inputting variables that range from negative infinity to positive infinity into a small range. Thus, model stability and reliability can be improved using transition functions, which generally include threshold logic function, hyperbolic tangent function, S-curve function, etc.

15.13. Evolutionary Computation[34–36]

Evolutionary computation is a subdomain of intelligent computing which involves combinatorial optimization. Evolutionary computation algorithms are based on natural selection mechanism of "survival of the fittest" and transmission of genetic information in the process of biological evolution. The algorithms regard problems to be solved as the natural environment, and search for the optimal solution among populations composed of possible solutions through the process of iterative simulation, which is similar to natural evolution.

Essentially, evolutionary algorithms are methods searching for the optimal solution. The search strategy is not blind search or exhaustive search, but objective function oriented search methods. Using a natural parallel structure, evolutionary algorithms constantly generate new individuals through the process of crossover and mutation. By constantly expanding the search scope, evolutionary algorithms are not easy to run into locally optimal solution, and can find out globally optimal solution with a high probability.

In the searching process, evolutionary algorithms make use of structured and random information, and makes it possible to obtain the maximum survival probability for the most satisfying decision. Thus, evolutionary algorithm is a probabilistic algorithm. In general, evolutionary computation involves the following steps: (1) give a set of initial solutions, (2) evaluate the performance of given solutions, (3) select a certain number of solutions from current solutions as initial iterative solutions, (4) repeat the above operation and obtain next iterative solutions based on the previous iterative solutions, (5) if these solutions satisfy the convergence criterion, then terminate the iteration process; otherwise repeat the above steps.

Evolutionary computation includes four main branches, namely, genetic algorithm, evolutionary strategy, evolutionary programming, and genetic programming. Genetic algorithm is the first evolutionary computation algorithm, and was proposed in 1975 by Professor JH Holland from the United States. Genetic algorithms apply encoding technologies to strings of binary numbers (also called chromosome), and simulate the biological evolution process of populations composed of these number strings, then evaluate the fitness of each chromosome and conduct genetic operations (e.g., selection, crossover, and mutation operations) so as to find out the optimal solution with the maximum fitness (shown in Table 15.13.1 and Figure 15.13.1).

Evolutionary computation has a very wide range of applications, and has been successfully applied into many fields, such as pattern recognition,

Table 15.13.1. Corresponding relationships between basic concepts of biogenetics and genetic algorithm.

Biogenetics	Genetic algorithm
Individual and group	Solution and solution space
Chromosomes and genes	Coding of solutions and elements in coded strings
Survival of the fittest	A solution with the maximum fitness will be of highest probability to survive
Population	A set of solutions selected based on fitness function
Mating and mutation	A genetic operator and methods generating new solutions

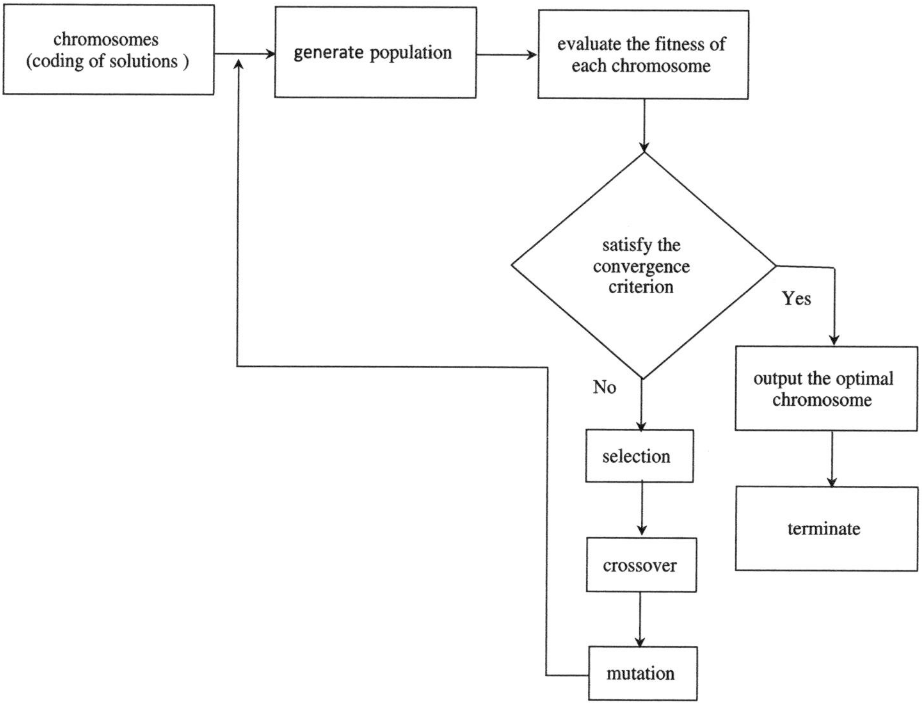

Fig. 15.13.1. Basic operation process of genetic algorithm.

image processing, artificial intelligence, economic management, mechanical engineering, electrical engineering, communication engineering, biology, etc.

15.14. Deep Learning[37–39]

The applications of deep learning have made a breakthrough since deep learning proposed by Hinton *et al.* in 2006. Up to now, in addition to

Stanford University, four business giants including Baidu, IBM, Google, and Microsoft, have set up a research institute for deep learning.

Deep learning, developed from artificial neural network, is a kind of learning method based on unsupervised feature learning and feature hierarchy.

Deep learning has a similar hierarchical structure to neural network: The system is a multilayer network that consists of an input layer, hidden layers (single layer or multilayer), and only the nodes in adjacent layers are connected with each other, while interlayer and trans-layer nodes are not. The development lies in: neural network adjusts the parameters using back propagation (BP) algorithm (iterative algorithm is used to train the whole network), while deep learning is based on layer by layer training mechanism, which can avoid occurrence of diffusion gradient using BP algorithm when dealing with deep networks.

Specifically, training process of deep learning includes the following two steps:

(1) Top-down unsupervised learning: Single layer neurons are constructed layer by layer; through layer-wise fine-tuning using wake–sleep algorithm (tuning one layer at a time), training results are used as input of the higher layer. This step is essentially an initialization process of network parameters. Different from random initialization of traditional neural networks, initial parameters of deep learning models are obtained through the unsupervised learning process after inputting the data structure. Thus, these initial values are more close to the global optimum and deep learning models can thus achieve better results.
(2) Bottom-up supervised learning: Based on parameters of each layer obtained from unsupervised learning, this process adds a classifier to the top of the coding layer (e.g., logistic regression, SVM). Through supervised learning with labeled data, parameters of the whole network are fine-tuned using gradient descent methods.

Concerned with deep learning, shallow learning models include traditional neural network models (number of layers is usually less than three), SVM containing only one hidden layer, Boosting, and maximum entropy method without hidden layer nodes (e.g., logistic regression), etc. The biggest limitation of shallow learning models is relying on artificial extraction of sample features, while deep learning models can deal with feature learning process automatically.

Compared with traditional shallow learning, deep learning has several characteristics: (1) depth enhancement of the model structure (usually with

5–10 hidden layers); (2) clear highlight of the importance of feature learning. Through layer-wise feature transformation, sample features in the original space are transformed to a new feature space, thus making it easier to classify or predict.

Models or methods commonly used in deep learning include automatic encoding, sparse encoding, restricted Boltzmann machine, deep belief network, and convolutional neural network, etc.

Deep learning has been successfully applied in a number of fields, such as computer vision, speech recognition, and natural language processing (e.g., machine translation, semantic mining, etc.).

15.15. Other Data Mining Methods[13,40]

In addition to methods previously described in this chapter, commonly used methods of data mining include data clustering, Bayesian methods, time-series data mining, etc.

(1) Data clustering

Clustering methods can be classified into the following five categories: (a) Partitioning methods: Given a set of n objects, a partitioning method constructs k-partitions of the data, then uses an iterative relocation technique that attempts to improve the partitioning by moving objects from one group to another. Commonly used algorithms include k-means, k-medoids and CLARANS, etc. (b) Hierarchical methods: A hierarchical method creates a hierarchical decomposition of the given set of data objects, and can be divided into the top-down approach (the divisive approach) and the bottom-up approach (the agglomerative approach). Algorithms of hierarchical methods include BIRCH algorithm, CURE algorithm, and CHAMELEON algorithm, etc. (c) Density-based methods: Density-based clustering algorithms can overcome the shortcoming that distance-based algorithms can only find out spherical-shaped clusters. Representative algorithms include Density-Based Spatial Clustering of Application with Noise (DBSCAN), OPTICS, DENCLUE, etc. DBSCAN defines a cluster as a set of density connected points, and divides regions of sufficiently high density into clusters. Such a method can discover clusters of arbitrary shape from spatial database containing noise. (d) Grid-based methods: Grid-based methods quantize the object space into a finite number of cells that form a grid structure and perform all the clustering operations on each cell of the grid structure. Representative algorithms include STING, CLIQUE, WAVE-CLUSTER, etc. (e) Model-based methods: Model-based methods specify the model of each cluster and discover the data objects appropriate for certain models. Model-based methods can be usually conducted using statistical models (e.g., COBWEB) and neural network models.

(2) Bayesian methods

Bayesian methods are probability-based learning algorithms, which are based on Bayes theorem and mainly used for classification and regression. (a) Bayes optimal classification method: Bayes optimal classification method obtains the most probable classification of new samples using weighted-average posterior probability of each hypothesis. The method is theoretically optimal, while it is of high computation cost. (b) Gibbs algorithm: Gibbs algorithm is an alternative non-optimal approach for Bayes optimal classification method. Gibbs algorithm randomly selects a certain hypothesis from all the hypotheses based on current distribution of posterior probabilities, then classifies new samples using the selected hypothesis. Other Bayes methods also include naive Bayes, Bayes belief network, and EM algorithm.

(3) Time-series data mining

Time-series data mining includes two major fields, namely, dimensionality reduction and pattern detection. (a) Dimensionality reduction: The main purpose of dimensionality reduction is to express the information of time series in a brief way, which is used for further analysis. Descriptive statistics are commonly used for dimensionality reduction, but may filter out a lot of information. Other methods of dimensionality reduction include discrete Fourier transform, discrete wavelet transform, singular value decomposition, etc. (b) Pattern detection: Pattern detection can discover the internal pattern of a certain time series or patterns across multiple time series. Similarity analysis can be used to measure the similarity of multiple time series, and can also be used for clustering and classification analysis of time series with different lengths. Pattern detection has been successfully applied in the fields of fraud detection, prediction of new product, etc.

15.16. Data Visualization[41–43]

Data visualization refers to a variety of methods that enhance the intuitive perception of data using interactive and visual representations of data. Data visualization maps data that are invisible or difficult to display directly into perceptible graphics, symbols, colors, and textures, which improve the efficiency of data identification and transmission of effective information.

According to the way of information transmission, traditional visualization methods can be divided into two categories, namely, exploratory visualization and interpretative visualization. In data analysis stage, information contained in the data is not clear and we hope to quickly discover the characteristics, trends, and anomalies through data visualization. And exploratory visualization is just the process that transfers data information to the designers and analysts of visualization. Interpretative visualization refers to the process in visual presentation stage that transfers the information or knowledge obtained from data analysis to the public in a visible way.

From the application point of view, data visualization has multiple objectives: effective presentation of important features, revelation of objective laws, quality control for simulation and measurement, to help understanding false concepts and processes, to improve the efficiency of scientific research and development, to promote communication and cooperation, etc.

According to data objects involved in visualization, data visualization includes two branches: scientific visualization and information visualization. Scientific visualization deals with data in the fields of science and engineering (e.g., three-dimensional measurement data containing information of spatial coordinates and sets, computational simulation data, and medical imaging data, etc.) and focuses on how to use geometry, topology, and shape features to present the law contained in the data. While information visualization deals with abstract data that are unstructured and non-geometric (e.g., financial data, social network data, and text data, etc.), and the core challenge of visual information is to reduce the interference of visual confusion on useful information extracted from high dimensional, complex, and massive data. Visual analytics is the science of analytical reasoning that integrates graphics induced by visualization and data analysis, data mining, and human-computer interaction techniques.

Data visualization is a combination of many disciplines including statistics, data mining, graphic design, and information visualization. The process of data visualization can be generalized as the following seven stages: acquire (obtain the data, whether from a file on a disk or a source over a network), parse (provide some structure for the data's meaning, and order it into categories), filter (remove all but the data of interest), mine (apply methods from statistics or data mining as a way to discern patterns or place the data in mathematical context), represent (choose a basic visual model, such as a bar graph, list, or tree), refine (improve the basic representation to make it clearer and more visually engaging), and interact (add methods for manipulating the data or controlling what features are visible). Each step of the process is inextricably linked because of the potential interactions between steps (see Figure 15.16.1).

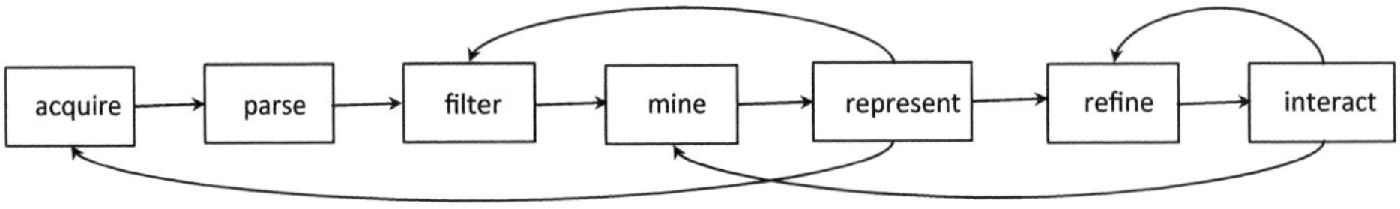

Fig. 15.16.1. Interactions between the seven stages of data visualization.

High-dimensional data need to be dealt with data transformation or statistical dimension reduction techniques (see item 4.19) before being processed by visualization conducted in low dimensional space using information display modes (e.g., color, brightness). See item 7.15 for spatial and temporal data visualization.

There are various types of tools for data visualization. Microsoft Excel is the most commonly used entry-level tool for data visualization analysis. Online data visualization tools (e.g., Google Charts, Data-Driven Documents, and Gephi, etc.) are popular with ordinary users due to the simple and convenient operation. Additionally, interactive graphical user interface (GUI) tools (e.g., JavaScript library Crossfilter and Tangle, etc.), map tools and visual programming environments (e.g., Processing, NodeBox, and R) can also be used for data visualization.

15.17. Tools and Software of Data Mining[44]

According to the application scope, data mining tools can be divided into two categories, namely, specialized mining tools and generalized mining tools: (1) Specialized mining tools provide solutions to problems in a particular field, and optimize the algorithms based on full consideration on particularity of data and customer demand. (2) Generalized mining tools do not distinguish the meanings of specific data and deal with common data types using generalized mining algorithms. Users can conduct data mining of multiple patterns using generalized mining tools and decide themselves what to mine and how to mine the data according to their applications.

There are a wide variety of data mining tools in the market. In practical application, we usually choose an appropriate data mining tool based on comprehensive consideration of the following aspects: (1) pattern types (e.g., classification, clustering, association, etc.) that data mining tools can conduct; (2) ability to solve complex problems; (3) operating performance; (4) data access capability; and (5) interfaces with other data products.

In addition to R software (see item 15.18), other common data mining tools including QUEST system developed by Almaden research center of IBM company, MineSet system co-developed by SGI company and Stanford University, DBMiner system developed by Simon Fraser University in Canada, Intelligent Miner developed by IBM, SAS Enterprise Miner developed by North Carolina State University, SPSS Clementine developed by Stanford University, Weka which is open-source, and various integrated mining tools by database vendors. Here, we only give a brief introduction of several data mining tools, including MineSet, SAS Enterprise Miner, SPSS Clementine, and Weka.

(1) MineSet system is well known for its advanced display and visualization methods. It supports a variety of relational databases and can read data directly from the Oracle, Informix, and Sybase. It can execute query using SQL command and carry out data transformation into multiple types. It is easy to operate, supports international characters, and can be released directly to web.
(2) SAS Enterprise Miner is a specialized module of statistical analysis system (SAS). It is a generalized mining tool and conducts data mining process in accordance with the method of "sampling, exploration, transformation, modeling, and evaluation". SAS Enterprise Miner can be integrated with SAS data warehouse and online analytical processing (OLAP) and conduct data mining towards the end-to-end knowledge discovery process, which includes the process from data entry and data capture to solution obtaining.
(3) Clementine SPSS is an open data mining tool. It not only supports the entire data mining process (from data acquisition, transformation, modeling, assessment to the final deployment), but also supports industry standards for data mining, that is CRISP-DM. Visual data mining of Clementine SPSS makes the "thinking" analysis possible, which focuses on the problem to be solved, rather than some technical work (e.g., writing codes).
(4) Weka (Environment for Knowledge Analysis Waikato) is a free software for machine learning and data mining, which is non-commercial, Java-based, and open-source. As an open data mining platform, Weka integrates a large number of machine learning algorithms to undertake the tasks of data mining, which include data preprocessing, classification, regression, clustering, association rules, and visualization on the new interactive interface, etc. Moreover, users can also develop more data mining algorithms based on Java language and Weka architecture.

15.18. R and Data Mining[45,46]

As a free, open-source software for statistical analysis, R is not only of small size, but can also support cross-platform operations, and has a strong advantage in terms of data mining: (1) R has a strong function of mathematical and statistical analysis, and new algorithms and techniques can be updated and implemented very fast in R. (2) R has more than 5,000 high-quality packages, which involve various fields, including statistical computing, machine learning, financial analysis, biological information, social network analysis, natural language processing, etc. (3) R has powerful capabilities for data visualization, and provides a fully programmable graphics language. (4) R has strong expansibility, which can not only easily read data outputted by SAS, SPSS, and other software, but also provide interactive interfaces for data mining software (e.g., MySQL and Weka).

R provides a wealth of packages for data mining. In this item, we give a brief introduction of some packages and functions in R, which can be used to implement several data mining methods that are commonly used.

(1) Association rules and frequent item sets

"arules" and "arulesViz" are two packages that are dedicated to association analysis. "arules" is used for the digital generation of association rules, and provides two functions (Apriori and Eclat) which can be used for algorithm implementation of fast mining of frequent itemsets and association rules. "arulesViz" is an expansion package of "arules", and provides several practical and novel visualization technologies for association rules, which makes association analysis an integration from algorithm running to result presentation.

2. Clustering analysis

There are a wide variety of clustering algorithms, the vast majority of which can be implemented in R. Packages used for clustering in R mainly include "stats", "cluster", "fpc", and "mclust", etc. "stats" mainly contains some basic statistical functions used for statistical calculation and generation of random numbers. "cluster" is dedicated to cluster analysis, and contains a number of cluster-related functions and data sets. "fpc" contains the algorithm functions used for fixed point clustering and linear regression clustering. "mclust" is mainly used for clustering, classification, and density estimation, which can be complemented based on Gaussian mixture model and the EM algorithm.

3. Discriminant analysis

Fisher discriminant, Bayes discriminant, and distance discriminant are the three main types of mainstream algorithms for discriminant analysis. R Packages and respective functions used for discriminant analysis mainly include: (a) "MASS" package (functions of lda and qda used for linear discriminant analysis and quadratic discriminant analysis, respectively); (b) "klaR" package (NaiveBayes function for naive Bayes classification); (c) "class" package (knn function for k-nearest neighbor classification) and (d) "kknn" package (knn function for weighted k-nearest neighbor classification).

4. Decision tree

CART algorithm of decision tree can be implemented using packages of "rpart" (functions of rpart, prune.part, and post), "rpart.plot" (rpart.plot function) and "maptree" (draw.tree function), and C4.5 algorithm can be implemented using function J48 in "RWeka" package. Specifically, "rpart" is mainly used to establish the classification tree and related recursive partitioning algorithm; "rpart.plot" is used to draw a decision tree for rpart model; "maptree" is used to prune and draw a tree structure; "RWeka" provides the interface between R and Weka.

In addition, packages of "e1071" (core function is svm) and "nnet" (core function is nnet) in R can be used for model analysis of SVM and BP neural network, respectively.

15.19. Hadoop and Data Mining[47–49]

Hadoop is an open source distributed computing platform affiliated with the Apache software foundation. It is based on Hadoop distributed file system (HDFS) and MapReduce (open source implementation of Google MapReduce), and provides users with a transparent and detailed distributed infrastructure in bottom system.

Given a large-scale file of distributed storage in a number of computers with Hadoop installed, we do not need to consider how to store data and which computers the data should be stored in, and HDFS will automatically deal with these. Advantages of HDFS (e.g., high fault tolerance, high scalability, etc.) make it possible for users to deploy Hadoop in low-price hardware and to construct distributed systems. And distributed programming models of MapReduce allow users to develop parallel applications without understanding the underlying details of the distributed system. Thus, users can use Hadoop to easily organize computer resources so as to build their own

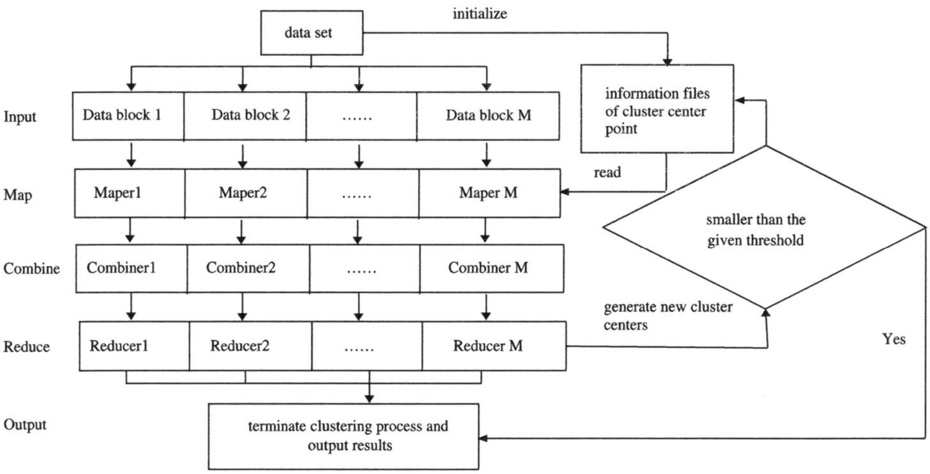

Fig. 15.19.1. Parallel processing flow chart of k-means clustering algorithm.

distributed computing platforms, and can make full use of the capacity of computing and storage to conduct the massive data processing and mining.

The applications of Hadoop in data mining are briefly introduced as below based on the example of k-means algorithm used for clustering analysis.

MapReduce-based parallel algorithm of k-means clustering mainly includes the following two parts: (1) Initialize information files of cluster center point and divide the data set into M blocks of equal size for parallel processing. (2) Start tasks of Map and Reduce to conduct parallel computing of the algorithm and obtain the clustering results (algorithm flowchart shown in Figure 15.19.1).

Each iteration of the MapReduce needs to restart the computing process, each of which in return consists of multiple tasks of Map and Reduce. Each Map task needs to read the data block information and the current information file of clustering center point. Map task is mainly to calculate the distance between each data object and the cluster center point, and then to distribute data objects to the nearest cluster. Reduce task aggregates data objects in each cluster to find out the new cluster center points, and determines whether to terminate the clustering process. Adding Combine task is to calculate the average value of each cluster in distributed blocks and transmit local results to the Reduce task, which can thus reduce communication load between nodes.

Hadoop distributed computing platform has prominent advantages when dealing with massive data, which thus makes Hadoop widely applicable in the internet field. For instance, Yahoo supports their research on advertising system and web search through cluster operation of Hadoop; Facebook uses cluster operation of Hadoop to conduct data analysis and machine learning; Baidu uses Hadoop for web log analysis and web mining; Hadoop system of Taobao net affiliated to Alibaba is used for data storage and processing of electronic commerce transaction; BigCloud system of China Mobile Research Institute is based on Hadoop and provides international services of data analysis. It is believed that in the future, Hadoop will be widely applied in more fields of big data, such as biopharmaceutics, telecommunications, banking, e-commerce, etc.

References

1. Huang, H, Hao, Y, Wang, Y, *et al.* *Taming the Big Data.* Beijing: People's Posts and Telecommunications Press, 2013. (in Chinese)
2. Meng, RT, Luo, Y, Yu, CH, *et al.* Application and challenges of healthy big data in the field of public health. *Chinese Gen. Pract.* 2015, 18(35): 4388–4392. (in Chinese)
3. Schonberger, VM, Cukier, K. *Big Data: A Revolution That Will Transform How We Live, Work and Think.* London: John Murray, 2013.
4. García, S, Luengo, J, Herrera, F. *Data Preprocessing in Data Mining.* New York: Springer, 2014.
5. Han, J, Kamber, M, Pei, J. *Data Mining: Concepts and Techniques.* (3rd edn.). Burlington: Morgan Kaufmann Publishers, 2012.
6. Bhattacharyya, DK, Kalita, JK. *Network Anomaly Detection: A Machine Learning Perspective.* Boca Raton: Chapman and Hall/CRC, 2013.
7. Dunning, T, Friedman, E. *Practical Machine Learning: A New Look at Anomaly Detection.* Sebastopol: O'Reilly Media, 2006.
8. Gianvecchio, S. *Application of Information Theory and Statistical Learning to Anomaly Detection.* Ann Arbor: Proquest, Umi Dissertation Publishing, 2011.
9. Rao, CR, Wegman, EJ, Solka, JL. *Handbook of Statistics: Data Mining and Data Visualization.* Amsterdam: Elsevier/North Holland, 2005.
10. Tao, ZP. *Constraint-based Association Rule Mining.* Hangzhou: Zhejiang Gongshang University Press, 2012. (in Chinese)
11. Zhang, C, Zhang, S. *Association Rule Mining: Models and Algorithms.* (1st edn.). New York: Springer, 2002.
12. Fan, M, Fan, HJ. *Introduction to Data Mining.* Beijing: People's Posts and Telecommunications Press, 2011. (in Chinese)
13. Tan, P, Steinbach, M, Kumar, V. *Introduction to Data Mining.* London: Pearson, 2005.
14. Linoff, GS, Berry, MJA. *Mining the Web: Transforming Customer Data into Customer Value.* Hoboken: Wiley, 2002.
15. Liu, B. *Web Data Mining: Exploring Hyperlinks, Contents, and Usage Data.* (2nd edn.). New York: Springer, 2011.
16. Yu, Y, Xue, GR, Han, DZ. *Web Data Mining.* Beijing: Tsinghua University Press, 2009. (in Chinese)
17. Cheng, XY, Zhu, Q. *Principles of Text Mining.* Beijing: Science Press, 2010. (in Chinese)

18. Feldman, R, Sanger, J. *The Text Mining Handbook: Advanced Approaches in Analyzing Unstructured Data.* Cambridge: Cambridge University Press, 2006.
19. Munzert, S, Rubba, C, Meiner, P, Nyhuis, D. *Automated Data Collection with R: A Practical Guide to Web Scraping and Text Mining.* Hoboken: Wiley, 2010.
20. Liu, J. *Introduction to Social Network Analysis.* Beijing: Social Sciences Literature Press, 2004. (in Chinese)
21. Ting, I, Hong, T, Wang, SL. *Social Network Mining, Analysis and Research Trends: Techniques and Applications.* Hershey: Information Science Reference, 2012.
22. Wu, YL, Li, P, Wang, YM, *et al.* The application of social network analysis in veterinary epidemiology. *Chinese J. Animal Health Inspection*, 2013, 30(8): 43–49. (in Chinese)
23. Cleophas, TJ, Zwinderman, AH. *Machine Learning in Medicine — Cookbook.* New York: Springer, 2014.
24. Harrington, P. *Machine Learning in Action.* New York: Manning Pubns, Co, 2012.
25. Bishop, CM. *Pattern Recognition and Machine Learning.* New York: Springer, 2010.
26. Yang, SY, Zhang, H. *Pattern Recognition and Intelligent Computation: Applications of MATLAB.* (3rd edn.). Beijing: Electronic Industry Press, 2015. (in Chinese)
27. Zhang, XG. *Pattern Recognition.* (3rd edn.). Beijing: Tsinghua University Press, 2010. (in Chinese)
28. Deng, N, Tian, Y, Zhang, C. *Support Vector Machines: Optimization Based Theory, Algorithms, and Extensions.* Boca Raton: Chapman and Hall/CRC, 2012.
29. Steinwart, I, Christmann, A. *Support Vector Machines.* New York: Springer, 2008.
30. Wang, JG, Zhang, WX. *Modeling and Intelligent Optimization of Support Vector Machines.* Beijing: Tsinghua University Press, 2015. (in Chinese)
31. Dybowski, R, Gant, V. *Clinical Applications of Artificial Neural Networks.* Cambridge: Cambridge University Press, 2007.
32. Ma, R. *Principles of Artificial Neural Network.* Beijing: China Machine Press, 2014. (in Chinese)
33. Taylor, BJ. *Methods and Procedures for the Verification and Validation of Artificial Neural Networks.* New York: Springer, 2006.
34. Ashlock, D. *Evolutionary Computation for Modeling and Optimization.* New York: Springer, 2006.
35. Fogel, DB. *Evolutionary Computation: Toward a New Philosophy of Machine Intelligence.* Hoboken: Wiley-IEEE Press, 2005.
36. Wang, YP. *Theory and Method of Evolutionary Computation.* Beijing: Science Press, 2011. (in Chinese)
37. Hall, ML. Deep Learning: A Case Study Exploration. Saarbrücken: VDM Verlag, 2011.
38. Ohlsson, S. *Deep Learning: How the Mind Overrides Experience.* Cambridge: Cambridge University Press, 2011.
39. Wen, N. *7 Powerful Strategies in Deep Learning.* Shanghai: East China Normal University Press, 2010. (in Chinese)
40. Dean, J. *Big Data, Data Mining, and Machine Learning: Value Creation for Business Leaders and Practitioners.* Hoboken: Wiley, 2014.
41. Chen, C, Härdle, WK, Unwin, A. *Handbook of Data Visualization.* New York: Springer, 2008.
42. Chen, W, Shen, ZQ, Tao, YB. *Data Visualization.* Beijing: Publishing House of Electronics Industry, 2013. (in Chinese)
43. Fry, B. *Visualizing Data: Exploring and Explaining Data with the Processing.* Sebastopol: O'Reilly Media, Inc., 2008.
44. Witten, IH, Frank, E, Hall, MA. *Data Mining: Practical Machine Learning Tools and Techniques.* (3rd edn.). Burlington: Morgan Kaufmann, 2011.

45. Huang, W, Wang, ZL. *Data Mining: R in Action.* Beijing: Publishing House of Electronics Industry, 2014. (in Chinese)
46. Zhao, Y, Cen, Y. *Data Mining Applications with R.* Cambridge: Academic Press, 2013.
47. Lam, C. *Hadoop in Action.* Greenwich: Manning Publications, 2010.
48. Prajapati, V. *Big Data Analytics with R and Hadoop.* Birmingham: Packt Publishing, 2013.
49. Zhang, LJ, Fan, Z, Zhao, YL, *et al.* Hadoop Practice of Big Data Analysis and Mining. Beijing: China Machine Press, 2015. (in Chinese)

About the Author

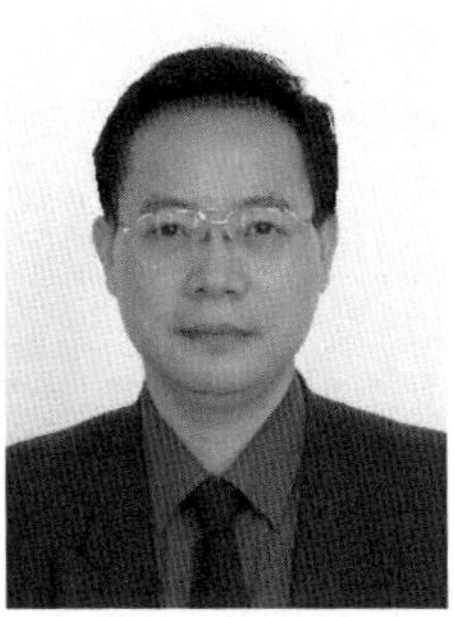

Chuanhua Yu, Ph.D. supervisor, is a Professor of the Department of Epidemiology and Biostatistics in School of Public Health, Wuhan University; the Global Health Institute, Wuhan University. He was a visiting scholar at Department of Biostatistics of the University of Washington (Seattle) in the year 2007 to 2008. He holds a Bachelor's and Master degree from Tongji Medical College at Huazhong University of Science and Technology. He is a member of the Steering Committee on Higher School of Medical Humanities Education Department, a member of the Second National Committee of experts on Animal Epidemic Prevention in the Agriculture Ministry, a Standing Committee Member in the International Biometric Society of China Branch Committee, and vice president of the Health Statistics and Information Society of Hubei Province. He also sits on the editorial board of the journals "Chinese Journal of Health Statistics" and "Journal of Public Health and Preventive Medicine".

He has published more than 140 scientific papers, among which are more than 30 SCI papers. In nearly two years, he published more than 10 ESI high cited papers in the Lancet and other top magazines. He was the person in charge of the National Natural Science Foundation of China, China Postdoctoral Fund and other research projects. There are nearly 50 books published, including as main editor "the Excel and Data Analysis (3rd Edition)", "the SPSS and Statistical Analysis (2nd Edition)", and translation book "Statistical Methods in Diagnosis Medicine" and so on. Main research interest are quantitative methods and applications of the global burden of disease, diagnostic test evaluation and related statistical methods, statistical evaluation of health services, data mining technology and software development and so on.

CHAPTER 16

MEDICAL RESEARCH DESIGN

Yuhai Zhang* and Wenqian Zhang

16.1. Experimental Design[1]

The design of experiments is defined as the design of any task that aims to describe or explain the variation of information under conditions that are hypothesized to reflect the variation. The British statistician R.A. Fisher described the basic theories and methods of experimental design in his monograph "The Design of Experiments" in 1935.

The basic content of experimental design includes: (1) Establish a research hypothesis and identify the main and minor issues in the research. (2) Determine the scope and number of subjects (sample size estimation). (3) Determine the treatment and non-treatment factors. (4) Determine the design scheme and method of randomization. (5) Select observed indicators and statistical analysis methods.

The key components of experimental design include: (1) An experimental unit: the object to which a treatment or condition is independently applied, such as a biological specimen, animal, organ or patient. It is necessary to establish inclusion and exclusion criteria when the experimental unit is a patient. (2) Treatment factor: the experimental conditions (single or multiple factors) set by researchers. For example, experimental subjects are divided into two groups. One group is the experimental group (intervention group) and the other group is the control group. (3) Non-treatment factors, also known as block factors: the experimental control conditions set by researchers, such as the weight, strains of animals, or the age, sex, and conditions of patients. (4) The treatment effect: the main observed indicator

*Corresponding author: zhyh@fmmu.edu.cn

of the experimental results, including qualitative observations (e.g. the death of animals) and quantitative observations (e.g. the survival time of animals).

The principles of experimental design, also known as Fisher's principles, are:

(1) Control: A group of experimental units set by researchers as the reference for comparison between groups. There is no intervention in the control group.
(2) Randomization: Each experimental unit has the same probability of being assigned to the experimental group and the control group.
(3) Replication: Both the experimental and control group must have enough experimental units for repeating observations.

The frequently used forms of control include:

(1) Blank control, which refers to the control group without any intervention.
(2) Experimental control, which refers to the control group without the studied intervention, but some experimental activities related to the treatment are conducted in the control group, such as perfusion or surgery.
(3) Standard control, which refers to the control group with a standard or conventional intervention, such as standard therapy for patients.
(4) Mutual control, which refers to the experimental groups compared with each other without a special control group.
(5) Self control, which refers to when the experimental and control treatments are conducted on the same subject, such as a comparison before and after therapy.

Researchers should select an appropriate experimental design model according to the treatment and control factors. For example, a completely randomized design is selected when there is only a treatment factor and there are no block factors.

16.2. Types of Research[2]

Medical research is the process of obtaining data, information, and facts for extending human knowledge in the biomedical field. The purpose of medical research is to explore the laws of disease occurrence, development, and prognosis, and provide scientific evidence for the treatment and prevention of diseases.

In 2001, the nine most common types of medical research were listed in the Evidence Pyramid (Figure 16.2.1) developed by the Medical Research Library of Brooklyn, State University of New York Downstate Medical

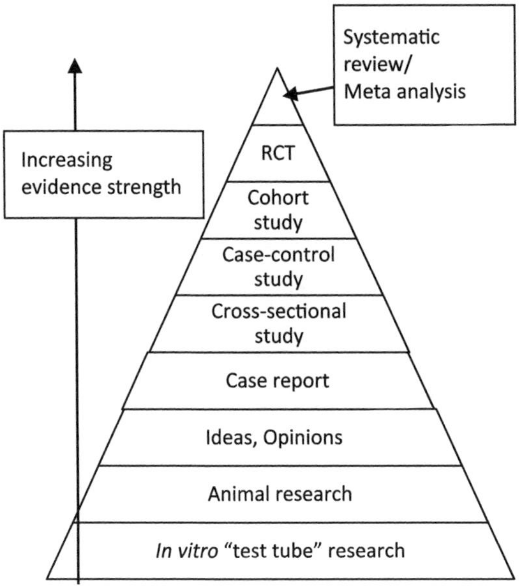

Fig. 16.2.1. The evidence pyramid.

Center. The closer to the bottom of the evidence pyramid the more studies there are, but there is a weaker level of evidence for clinical applications. Conversely, closer to the top of the evidence pyramid there are fewer studies but there is a stronger evidence level for clinical applications. The bottom of the evidence pyramid is preclinical research, including basic medical research, *in vitro* "test tube" research (e.g. physiology, pathology, biochemistry, microbiology, and genomics), and animal research. Clinical research with people (patients) as study subjects is located in the middle part of the pyramid of evidence, including expert ideas, opinions, case reports, cross-sectional studies, case-control studies, cohort studies, and randomized control trials (RCT). The top of the evidence pyramid is the systematic review/meta-analysis, which is based on multiple RCT studies.

There are many different types of medical research. The research can be divided by its purpose into exploratory research and confirmatory research. It can be divided by its field into basic research, clinical research, and field studies. It can be divided by its research subjects into clinical research, animal research or laboratory research. It can be divided into experimental or observational according to whether there are active interventions and random grouping. It can be divided into longitudinal studies or cross-sectional studies according to its timeline. Longitudinal studies can also be divided into prospective and retrospective studies.

16.3. Sample Size[3]

Sample size is the number of observations or replicates in a study. The research indicators are not stable and the test efficiency is low if the sample size is too small; if the sample size is too large, it will waste human power and material resources and increase the difficulty of controlling the study conditions. Therefore, it is essential to estimate the necessary minimum number of observations in the design phase of the study, with the premise of ensuring the research conclusion with certain accuracy and test efficiency. This process is called the sample size estimation.

Because the purposes of experimental and observational studies are different, the sample size estimation is also different. The purpose of an experimental study is to compare the effects among different treatments, so it is necessary to estimate the sample size according to the requirements of the hypothesis test. The purpose of an observational study is generally to estimate the population parameters (rate or mean), so it is also necessary to estimate a sample size that allows these parameters to be estimated.

An appropriate sample size generally depends on six study-design parameters:

(1) Minimum expected difference (also known as the effect size, δ): This parameter is the smallest measured difference between groups that the investigator would like the study to detect. As the minimum expected difference is made smaller, the sample size needed to detect statistical significance increases. The selection of this parameter is subjective and is based on judgment and experience with the problem being investigated. In general, for the same treatment effect, the size of quantitative indicators is smaller than that of qualitative indicators.
(2) Estimated measurement variability: This parameter is represented by the expected σ in the measurements made within each comparison group. As statistical variability increases, the sample size needed to detect the minimum difference increases. Ideally, the estimated measurement variability should be determined on the basis of preliminary data collected from a similar study population.
(3) Types of experimental design: The more rigorous the experimental design, the smaller the sample size required. For example, the sample size requirement of a complete randomized design is larger than a paired design or a randomized block design. When three factors are considered, a Latin square design can require a smaller sample size than a three independent groups design.

(4) Type of statistical analysis: One-tailed statistical analysis requires a smaller sample size for detection of the minimum difference than does a two-tailed analysis.
(5) Significance criterion (α): This parameter is the maximum P value for which a difference is to be considered statistically significant. As the significance criterion is decreased (made more strict), the sample size needed to detect the minimum difference increases. The significance criterion is customarily set to 0.05.
(6) Statistical power ($1-\beta$): This parameter is the power that is desired from the study. As power is increased, sample size increases. In randomized controlled experiments, the statistical power is customarily set to a number greater than or equal to 0.80, with many experts now advocating a power of 0.90.

When parameters of a population are estimated, the sample size depends on the following three parameters:

(1) Confidence level ($1-\alpha$): As the confidence level is increased, the sample size increases. Confidence level is usually set to 0.95.
(2) Standard deviation of the population (σ): As the standard deviation increases, the sample size increases. The standard deviation is usually obtained from previous studies or pre-investigation experiments.
(3) Tolerance error (δ): The estimated maximum difference between the sample statistics and population parameters. As the value gets larger, the sample size becomes smaller.

When the sample size obtained through the above three parameters is n, the possibility that the difference between the sample statistic and the population parameter is not more than δ is $1-\alpha$.

16.4. Completely Randomized Design[4]

A completely randomized design (CRD) is one where the treatments are assigned completely at random so that each experimental unit has the same chance of receiving any one treatment. For the CRD, any difference among experimental units receiving the same treatment is considered to be caused by experimental error.

A CRD is probably the simplest experimental design. It involves only one treatment factor (but there can be multiple levels), so it is also called a single factor design.

A CRD relies on randomization to control for the effects of extraneous variables. The experimenter assumes that, on average, extraneous factors will affect treatment conditions equally, so any significant differences between conditions can fairly be attributed to the independent variable. In addition, randomization provides a basis for making a valid estimate of random fluctuations, which is essential in testing of the significance of real differences.

CRDs do not restrict the number of groups. The experimental units in each treatment group can be equal (called a balanced design) or not equal (called an unbalanced design), but the test efficiency is higher when the design is balanced.

The concrete steps of a CRD are:

(1) Numbering: assign a number to each experimental unit in any convenient manner; for example, consecutively from 1 to n.
(2) Assigning a random number: assign a number randomly to each experimental unit using a table of random numbers or a random number generator. Random numbers obtained for each experimental unit can have 1, 2 or 3 digits.
(3) Ranking: rank the n random numbers obtained in ascending or descending order.
(4) Grouping: divide the derived n ranks into t groups, each consisting of r numbers, according to the sequence in which the random numbers appeared. For example, the first n_1 ranks were assigned to group 1. The $n_1 + 1$ to $n_1 + n_2$ ranks were assigned to group 2 and so on.

For CRD data, the statistical analysis methods most commonly used include:

(1) For two groups with a small sample size, a t test or non-parametric test (Wilcoxon rank sum test) can be used to compare the difference of effects between the groups.
(2) For two groups with a large sample size, a u test can be used.
(3) For multiple groups, a one-way analysis of variance (ANOVA) or a non-parametric test (Kruskal–Wallis test) can be used.

A major advantage of the CRD is the simplicity of design and statistical analysis, especially when the number of replications is not uniform for all treatments. The disadvantage of the CRD is that the efficiency is lower than for more complicated designs. Moreover, the homogeneity of the experimental units must be better in a CRD. Hence, a CRD is appropriate only for experiments with homogeneous experimental units, such as laboratory experiments, where environmental effects are relatively easy to control. For other experiments, where there is generally larger variation among experimental units, the CRD is rarely used.

16.5. Paired Design[4]

A paired design is a special case of a randomized block design. It can be used when the experiment has only two treatment conditions and subjects can be grouped into pairs, based on some pairing variables. Then, within each pair, subjects are randomly assigned to different treatments.

Pairing variables are the main non-treatment factors that are under control. In animal experiments, factors such as sex, and weight can be used as pairing variables, and then within each pair, animals are randomly assigned to the experimental or control group. In clinical trials, factors such as sex, age, severity of disease, and occupation of patient can be used as pairing variables. Although the pairs are independent, within each pair there is dependency. In fact, the more dependency within a pair, the greater the reduction in experimental error.

There are two main forms of paired design:

1. Heterogeneous paired design: Two same or similar subjects are matched into a pair, and then each receives a different treatment. For example, to study the effect of vitamin E deficiency on the content of vitamin A in the liver, rats of the same species were matched into pairs by same sex, age, and similar weight, and then the rats in each pair were randomly fed either a normal diet or a vitamin E deficient diet.

2. Self-controlled design: In a self-controlled design, as the name implies, each subject serves as his or her own control. For example, from one blood sample, the hemoglobin value is measured using two different kinds of instruments; or pre and post-treatment observations are collected for each subject.

The steps of a paired design: Randomly select n-paired experimental units from the reference population. Within a pair, randomly assign one of the pair to treatment 1 and the other to treatment 2. The experiment (study) is run for a pre-assigned time and during this time all other variables are kept under control. At the end of the assigned time, we measure the responses for the n-paired experimental units. Letting X and Y denote the responses for treatments 1 and 2, respectively, the data are in the paired form: $(X_1, Y_1), \ldots, (X_n, Y_n)$.

Statistical analysis methods for paired design data:

(1) Quantitative data: If the difference between the pairs is normally distributed, then a paired t-test can be used. Otherwise, variable

transformation should be considered or a non-parametric test (Wilcoxon signed rank sum test) should be used to compare the differences between the treatment groups.

(2) Qualitative data: Depending on the analysis purposes, a paired t-test, Bowker test or Kappa consistency test can be used.
(3) Ranked data: A correlation analysis can be performed by using the Wilcoxon signed rank sum test or Kendall coefficients.

The advantage of the paired design is that it can enhance the balance between treatment groups. In particular, in a case when it is not easy to make some non-treatment factors balance between two groups by a CRD, a paired design can improve the balance of these factors between groups. The disadvantage of a paired design is that the matching variables are not easy to strictly control and it reduces the efficiency when matching is poor or has failed.

The advantage of the paired design in clinical trials is that the two patients in each pair are more similar and individual variation of patients has less effect on the experimental effect, which can improve the efficiency of the test. However, in clinical trials, it is often difficult to match patients when the source of the cases is insufficient.

16.6. Randomized Block Design[5]

Because the paired design is only applied in research with two groups, to solve the problem of studies with multiple groups, R.A. Fisher proposed the randomized block design in 1926. It can be seen as an expansion of the paired design.

With a randomized block design, the experimenter divides subjects into subgroups called blocks, such that the variability within blocks is less than the variability between blocks. Typically, a blocking factor is a source of variability that is not of primary interest to the experimenter. An example of a blocking factor might be the weight of animals. Then, subjects within each block are randomly assigned to treatment conditions (Figure 16.6.1). Compared with a CRD, this design reduces variability within treatment conditions and potential confounding factors, producing a better estimate of treatment effects.

Statistical analysis methods for randomized block design data:

(1) Quantitative data: If the data are normally distributed and variance homogeneity is assured, two-way ANOVA can be used; if the data do not meet the above requirements, it is necessary to conduct variable

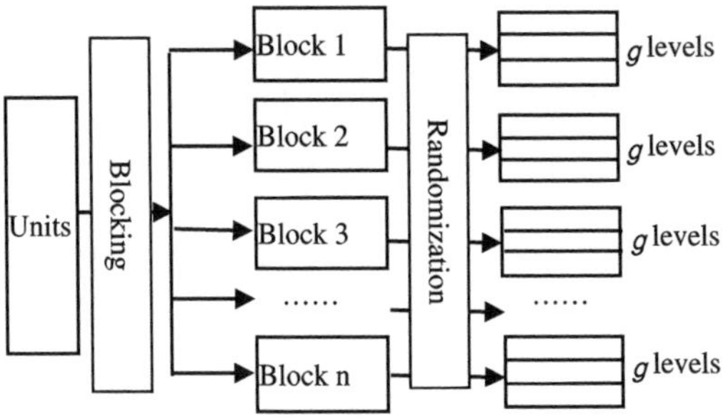

Fig. 16.6.1. Randomized block design.

transformations (such as logarithmic transformations) or use a non-parametric test (e.g. the Friedman M test).

(2) Qualitative data: Logistic regression analysis or a logarithm linear model can be used.

(3) Ranked data: The Friedman M test can be used.

The randomized block design is characterized by the times of random distribution repeated several times. The subjects are randomly assigned within the same block and the number of subjects in each treatment group is the same.

The advantage of the randomized block design is simple: the units within blocks are as uniform as possible, so that the balance among treatment groups is better. Particularly in the case when it is not easy to make the non-treatment factors balance among groups in a CRD, a randomized block design can achieve the goal of reducing the random error and improving the experiment efficiency. The disadvantages of the randomized block design include: the design does not allow for many treatment groups; when the block size increases, the error also increases, and then the efficiency is reduced; the number of subjects in each block must be the same; if missing data exist, the statistical analysis becomes more difficult.

It should also be noted that if a blocking factor is of interest to the experimenter, it is necessary that there be no interaction between the two factors. Otherwise, experiments must be done under the combination of each level of the two-factors, that is, a two-factor factorial design.

16.7. Latin Square Design[6]

The Latin square design allows for two blocking factors. In other words, this design is used to simultaneously control (or eliminate) two sources of nuisance variability. This method was developed by R.A. Fisher in 1926.

		columns		
		one	two	three
row	one	A	B	C
	two	B	C	A
	three	C	A	B

Fig. 16.7.1. 3×3 Latin square diagram.

A Latin square is a square matrix with r rows, r columns, and r letters, and each letter appears only once in each row and each column. The treatment factor levels are the Latin letters in the Latin square design. Such a square matrix is called an r order Latin square or an $r \times r$ Latin square. A three-order Latin square or a 3×3 Latin square is shown in Figure 16.7.1.

In a Latin square design, the experimental units are blocked according to two factors (non-treatment factors). Each row is the level of the row factor, and each column is the level of the column factor; that is, each experimental unit not only belongs to a row block, but also belongs to a column block. Therefore, the basic unit of a Latin square design is a "square." There are $r \times r$ experimental units in r rows and r columns, and r treatments are arranged in each block.

Basic requirements for a Latin square design: (1) Three factors with the same levels. (2) No interaction between columns, rows or treatments. (3) Homogeneity of variances in rows, columns and treatments.

Steps of a Latin square design:

(1) Select a basic Latin square according to the number of treatments.
(2) Perform the basic Latin square randomization. Permute the rows and the columns.
(3) Specify the letters to represent treatment factors.
(4) Arrange experiments and statistical analysis according to the last Latin square.

Statistical analysis methods used for Latin square design data:

(1) Quantitative data: A three-way ANOVA can be used. The total variation is divided into treatment group variation, row block variation, column block variation, and error.
(2) Qualitative data: Logistic regression analysis for two classification and multiclassification responses can be used.
(3) Ranked data: Ordinal logistic regression analysis can be used.

The Latin square design is an extension of the randomized block design. The advantages of the Latin square design are that the number of experiments is greatly reduced, the method is particularly suitable for animal experiments and laboratory studies, and two non-treatment factors are under-controlled, so the error is smaller and the efficiency is higher. The disadvantages are that the number of treatments must equal the number of replicates; the experimental error is likely to increase with the size of the square; small squares have very few degrees of freedom for experimental error; interactions between treatments, rows, and columns cannot be evaluated; and missing data will increase the difficulty of statistical analysis.

16.8. Factorial Design[7]

A factorial experiment is an experiment that includes two or more factors, each with discrete possible values or "levels", and the experimental units can take on all possible combinations of these levels across all such factors. Factorial design is often used to study the effect of each factor on the response variable, as well as the effects of interactions between factors on the response variable in medical research.

Factorial design was first proposed by John Bennet Lawes and Joseph Henry Gilbert in the 19th century. R.A. Fisher and Frank Yates also made important contributions to the development of this design. In particular, Yates played an important role in the statistical analysis of this design.

Factorial design requires two or more treatment factors, each with at least two levels, and each treatment is a combination of the levels of factors. The total treatments are all possible combinations of the levels of factors.

The factorial design requires the number of subjects in each treatment group to be equal and there must be at least two subjects in each group, otherwise the interactions between the factors cannot be analyzed.

There are two arrangement methods for subjects in a factorial design: a CRD or a randomized block design. The most simple factorial design is the 2×2 factorial design where four treatment groups are formed from comprehensive combinations of two levels of two factors; see Table 16.8.1.

Data from a factorial experiment can be analyzed using ANOVA or regression analysis.

(1) Quantitative data: In general, multifactor analysis of variance can be used. The ANOVA model includes the main effects of each factor and the interaction effects between factors.

Table 16.8.1. 2 × 2 factorial design.

Factor A	Factor B	
	b_1	b_2
a_1	a_1b_1	a_1b_2
a_2	a_2b_1	a_2b_2

(2) Qualitative data: For analysis purposes, logistic regression analysis of two or more classifications can be used, and the main effect of each factor and the corresponding interaction effects enter the model at the appropriate scale.
(3) Ranked data: Non-parametric tests or ordinal logistic regression analysis can be used, and the main effect of each factor and the corresponding interaction effects enter the model at the appropriate scale.

The advantages of factorial designs are: a greater precision can be obtained in estimating the overall main factor effects; interactions between different factors can be explored; additional factors can help to extend the validity of conclusions derived.

Some disadvantages of factorial experiments include: the total possible number of treatment level combinations increases rapidly as the number of factors increases and higher order interactions (three-way and four-way) are very difficult to interpret. A large number of factors greatly complicates the interpretation of results. Therefore, an experiment with more factors and levels generally uses a non-comprehensive combination of factorial design, such as an orthogonal design, which can greatly reduce the number of experiments.

16.9. Cross-over Design[8]

A cross-over design is a repeated measurements design such that each experimental unit (patient) receives different treatments during the different time periods, i.e. the patients cross over from one treatment to another during the course of the trial. This is in contrast to a parallel design, in which patients are randomized to a treatment and remain on that treatment throughout the duration of the trial. The cross-over design is commonly used in bioequivalence or clinical equivalence tests.

There are several specific concepts in the cross-over design:

(1) Run in: Over a period of time without any treatment it is confirmed that the subjects are in a natural state and can be tested.

Table 16.9.1. 2 × 2 Cross-over design.

subjects	Phase I		wash out		Phase II
1	treatment A	→	no treatment	→	treatment B
2	...		...		...
⋮	⋮		⋮		⋮
n_1	treatment A	→	no treatment	→	treatment B
1	treatment B	→	no treatment	→	treatment A
2	...		...		...
⋮	⋮		⋮		⋮
n_2	treatment B	→	no treatment	→	treatment A

(2) Wash out: The time between treatment periods. It is intended to prevent continuation of the effects of the trial treatment from one period to another.
(3) Carry-over effect: Also known as a delayed effect, a carry-over effect is defined as an effect of the treatment from the previous time period on the response during the current time period; that is, the previous period effect cannot be fully eliminated by a washout period.

The simplest form of cross-over design is the completely randomized cross-over design with a two treatment, two period, 2 × 2 cross-over design; see Table 16.9.1.

The advantages of a cross-over design: (1) One advantage of using a cross-over design is that sample sizes are smaller than for a parallel group trial design. Therefore, it is suitable in a situation where subjects are difficult to recruit, such as patients with rare diseases. (2) A cross-over design reduces the between-patient variability, because the comparison of treatment A versus B is made on the same patient; thus, the trial efficiency is high. (3) Every subject receives two treatments in one clinical trial, so the possible benefits for every patient are equal.

The disadvantages of a cross-over design: (1) Each treatment period cannot be very long or the subjects may drop out of the trial. (2) When the state of the subjects radically changes, such as death or a cure, the latter stage of treatment will not be able to be conducted. For example, if treatment A cures the patient during the first period, then treatment B will not have the opportunity to demonstrate its effectiveness. (3) How to confirm whether the subjects returned to the initial state is difficult. (4) If someone dropped out of the trial in a certain stage, missing data will increase the difficulty

		subjects		
		one	two	three
order	one	A	B	C
	two	B	C	A
	three	C	A	B

Fig. 16.9.1. 3 × 3 Latin square.

of statistical analysis. (5) This design is not suitable for a trial in which the disease has a self-healing tendency or has a short course.

The multiple treatments and multiple stages cross-over design is an extension of the simple cross-over design. It can be applied in a trial with three or more treatment factors, such as a 3×3 cross-over design. In a 3×3 crossover design, there are more than two ways to represent the order. The basic building block for the crossover design is the 3×3 Latin square; see Figure 16.9.1.

To achieve replicates, this design could be replicated several times. In this Latin square, we have each treatment occurring in each period. Even though the Latin square guarantees that treatment A occurs once in the first, second, and third period, we do not have all sequences represented. It is important to have all sequences represented when doing clinical trials with drugs.

A replicated cross-over design is a design where there are more treatment periods than there are treatments and at least one treatment is repeated for each individual trial subject. For example, if there are two treatments (A and B), the test sequence may be a balanced design ABAB, BABA, or an unbalanced design such as ABA, BAB. The replicated cross-over design can analyze the carrying effect and provide greater power for an average biological equivalence assessment.

16.10. Split-block Design[9,10]

Split-block design is a design method invented by Fisher in 1925 for use in agricultural experiments. In simple terms, a split-plot experiment is a blocked experiment where the blocks themselves serve as experimental units for a subset of the factors. Thus, there are two levels of experimental units. The blocks are referred to as whole plots, while the experimental units within blocks are called split plots. Corresponding to the two levels of experimental units are two levels of randomization.

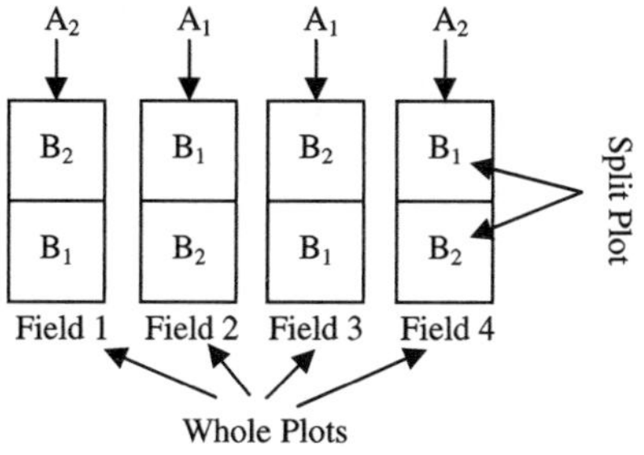

Fig. 16.10.1. Split-plot agricultural layout (Factor A is the whole-plot factor and factor B is the split-plot factor).

As a simple illustration, consider a study of the effects of two irrigation methods (factor A) and two fertilizers (factor B) on the yield of a crop, using four available fields as experimental units. In this experiment, it is not possible to apply different irrigation methods (factor A) in areas smaller than a field, although different fertilizer types (factor B) could be applied in relatively small areas. For example, if we subdivide each whole plot (field) into two split plots, each of the two fertilizer types can be applied once within each whole plot, as shown in Figure 16.10.1. In this split-plot design, a first randomization assigns the two irrigation types to the four fields (whole plots); then within each field, a separate randomization is conducted to assign the two fertilizer types to the two split plots within each field.

Depending on whether the first level experimental unit can be formed as a block, a split-plot design can be divided into a completely randomized split-plot or a randomized complete block split-plot design.

1. Completely randomized split-plot design

(1) The first level units are randomly divided into I groups, and the number of cases in each group is $n(n \geq 2)$, respectively receiving $a_1, a_2, \cdots, a_I$ levels of treatment.

(2) The second-level units within the first-level units are randomly assigned to receive J treatments $b_1, b_2, \cdots, b_J$.

For example, when $I = 3$ and $J = 2$, the experimental design of a completely randomized split-plot is shown in Table 16.10.1.

2. Randomized complete block split-plot design

If the first-level units can form blocks, then a randomized complete block split-plot design can be used following these steps:

(1) The first level experimental units are matched to$r$ whole plots, each whole plot having$I$ split plots. (2) I split plots within the blocks (first level

Table 16.10.1. Completely randomized split-plot design.

Factor A	Split plot (randomization)	Factor B (randomization)	
a_1	1	a_1b_1	a_1b_2
	3	a_1b_2	a_1b_1
a_2	6	a_2b_2	a_2b_1
	5	a_2b_1	a_2b_2
a_3	2	a_3b_1	a_3b_2
	4	a_3b_2	a_3b_1

Table 16.10.2. Randomized complete block split-plot design.

Whole plots	First level experimental unit	Spit plots
I	$(a_3b_2\ \ a_3b_1)$	$(a_1b_2\ \ a_1b_1)$
	$(a_2b_1\ \ a_2b_2)$	$(a_4b_1\ \ a_4b_2)$
II	$(a_2b_1\ \ a_2b_2)$	$(a_3b_2\ \ a_3b_1)$
	$(a_1b_2\ \ a_1b_1)$	$(a_4b_1\ \ a_4b_2)$
III	$(a_1b_2\ \ a_1b_1)$	$(a_2b_2\ \ a_2b_1)$
	$(a_4b_1\ \ a_4b_2)$	$(a_3b_1\ \ a_3b_2)$

experimental unit) are randomly assigned to I treatments with A factors. (3) rI split plots are randomly assigned to J treatment with B factors.

For example, when $I = 4$ and $J = 2$, the experimental design of a randomized complete block split-plot is shown in Table 16.10.2.

The restriction on the randomization mentioned in the split-plot designs can be extended to more than one factor. For the case where the restriction is on two factors the resulting design is called a split-split-plot design. These designs usually have three different levels of experimental units.

The analysis of a split-plot experiment is more complex than that for a completely randomized experiment due to the presence of both split-plot and whole-plot random errors. When the split-plot experiment is balanced and the ANOVA sums of squares are orthogonal, a standard, mixed-model, ANOVA-based approach to the analysis is possible.

16.11. Nested Design[11]

A nested design (sometimes referred to as a hierarchical design) is used for experiments in which there is an interest in a set of treatments and

Table 16.11.1. Nested design.

A	Sugar-coated tablets		Capsule	
B	0.5 b_{11}	1.0 b_{12}	0.8 b_{21}	1.5 b_{22}

the experimental units are sub-sampled. A nested design is generally not a comprehensive combination of the levels of each factor, but of various factors grouped according to their affiliation system, and each level of experimental factors is not crossed.

For example, consider a drug toxicity study where set A is the dosage regimen and there are two levels, a_1 represents sugar-coated tablets and a_2 represents a capsule; set B is the dose and its level depends on A's level. When A $= a_1$, B has two dose levels, 0.5 mg and 1.0 mg; when A $= a_2$, B has two dose levels, 0.8 mg and 1.5 mg. Thus, there are a total of four treatment groups; see Table 16.11.1.

The application conditions of the nested design are: (1) the subject itself has affiliations. There are various factors that can be subdivided. As previously mentioned, it is not a comprehensive combination of the levels of the dosage regimen (A factor) or dose (B factor). Here, two levels of factor B are nested in two levels of factor A. (2) The subject itself is not an affiliation, but the importance of these factors is different in the experiment. For example, consider an effect of antibacterial drugs on mice. There are three factors to consider. Factor A is the drug, factor B is the mouse strain, and factor C is the sex of the mice. According to expert knowledge, the important order for the three factors is A $\rightarrow$ B $\rightarrow$ C. Therefore, in the design of the experiments, factor B can be nested under factor A, and factor C can be nested under factor B, thereby forming a nested design.

The difference between a nested design and a factorial design is whether the status of the factors is equal. Equal is the factorial design; inequality is the nested design. In the application of the nested design, the important sequence of experimental factors should be based on previous knowledge and expertise and should not be set arbitrarily.

In the nested design with two factors, according to the importance sequence of factors, the two factors A and B serve as the primary and secondary treatment factors, respectively. In a nested design with three factors A, B, and C, the three factors serve as primary, secondary, and third treatment factors, respectively. The minimum treatment groups are the aggregate of the minimum level of factors. For example, in the nested design with two factors, factor A has I levels, and under the ith level, factor B has J_i levels $(i = 1, 2, \ldots, I)$; then, the total treatment groups are $g = \sum_{i=1}^{I} J_i$.

ANOVA can be used in the analysis of a nested-design experiment and the total variation and degree of freedom should be decomposed into the first-level experimental unit factors and second-level experimental unit. Note that in the nested design, factors cannot freely cross into comprehensive combinations; therefore, the interaction effect between the factors cannot be examined. If the interaction effect is important, a nested design is not appropriate.

16.12. Repeated Measures Design[12]

The repeated measures design takes measurements on the same subject over time ($m \geq 3$) or under different conditions. The key point of the repeated measures design is that the same subject is measured multiple times under different conditions. In general, any experiment can be designed as a repeated measure study.

Data obtained by the repeated measures design are called repeated measurement data and are used to analyze the changes of one outcome at different points of time. Repeated measurement data tracking the same sample at different points in time is also called longitudinal data or sometimes referred to as panel data.

The repeated measures design can be seen as an extension of the parallel design. It has the following characteristics: the measurement values have change trends over time; the measurement values from the same subject at different times are related; generally, the closer the observation point intervals the greater the correlation between the measured values; multiple measurements of different subjects are independent; and time is not randomly assigned to the subjects.

The advantages of repeated measures designs include: each subject can be act as its own control and fewer subjects are required. The design takes out error variance that is caused by individual differences, resulting in more sensitivity/power for the treatment's main effect.

The disadvantages of repeated measures designs include: it may not be feasible; it may not give realistic assessments of treatment effects; the analyzes are more difficult and usually there is a need to take into account associations between observations taken from the same individual. If there is any potential carry-over effect, latent effect, or learning effect, the repeated measures design should be used with caution.

Response variables of a repeated measurements design may be continuous, discrete, or dichotomous, among which the continuous variables are the most common. Traditional analysis methods should be used with caution because the multiple measurements of subjects at different time points are dependent. For univariate repeated measurements data, ANOVA is appropriate. Measurements data from one subject at different time points can be seen as a block when the sphericity assumption is met. Sphericity is an important assumption of repeated measures ANOVA. It refers to the condition where the variances of the differences between all possible pairs of groups (i.e. levels of the independent variable) are equal.

For multiple variables repeated measurements data, it should be analyzed by complicated statistical models, such as a mixed linear model or generalized estimating equations. If the response variable is discrete or dichotomous, generalized linear mixed models are appropriate. A mixed model is a statistical model containing both fixed effects and random effects. It provides a general, flexible approach for repeated measurements on each subject over time or by condition, because it allows for a wide variety of correlation patterns (or variance–covariance structures) to be explicitly modeled.

16.13. Balanced Incomplete Block Design[13]

Block designs usually have each treatment occurring at least once per block. However, in some cases, the blocks are not large enough to contain all treatments because of the limitations of the experimental conditions. Balanced incomplete block designs can solve this problem. When the block size is smaller than the number of treatments, this design may still be able to make comparisons between treatments as a randomized block design.

Assume that there are b blocks of k plots each, and t treatments each replicated r times. Thus,

$$N = bk = tr.$$

Also assume that blocks are incomplete in the sense that (i) $k < t$ and (ii) no treatment occurs more than once in any block.

For distinct treatments i and j, the concurrence λ_{ij} of i and j is the number of blocks which contain both i and j.

An incomplete block design is balanced if there is an integer λ such that $\lambda_{ij} = \lambda$ for all distinct treatments i and j. The name "balanced incomplete

Table 16.13.1. Balanced incomplete block design.

Block	Treatment A	B	C	D
1	Δ	Δ		
2			Δ	Δ
3	Δ		Δ	
4		Δ		Δ
5	Δ			Δ
6		Δ	Δ	

"Δ" denotes acceptance of treatment

block design" is often abbreviated to BIBD. In a balanced incomplete-block design, $\lambda = r(k-1)/(t-1)$.

For example, consider a study of the effects of four eye drops. Since the effects may be different in different subjects, two eyes of each subject are matched as a block. The size of each block is 2 and therefore cannot be assigned to all of the four treatments. The six blocks of this design with $t = 4$, $r = 3$, $b = 6$, and $k = 2$ are as follows: $\lambda = r(k-1)/(t-1) = 3(2-1)/(4-1) = 1$

In this Table 16.13.1, we can find the characteristics of BIBD: (1) each treatment appears at most once in each block; (2) each treatment appears in the same number of blocks as any of other treatments; and (3) each pair of treatments appears in the same number of blocks as any other pairs of treatments.

The advantages of BIBD include: small blocks are more homogeneous than large blocks, so experimental error is lower; it can be used to reduce block size in single factor experiments when the number of treatments is large; it can be used when there is variability within larger blocks; and it can be used to increase precision.

Disadvantages of BIBD include: designs can require a fixed number of treatments, a fixed number of subjects, or both; more subjects are needed; and the complexity of the analysis is increased and there is unequal precision for certain comparisons of treatment means.

Fisher and Yates developed design tables for BIBD in 1953. Researchers can select an appropriate design table according to the number of treatments and block size in order to design their experiment.

If the experimental data meet the normality assumption, ANOVA can be used to analyze BIBD. Because the treatments are implemented in different blocks for which experimental conditions may be different, the results of the experiment cannot be used to directly add or calculate the mean to describe treatment effects. They should be adjusted according to different experimental conditions of blocks before performing ANOVA.

If the experimental data obtained from BIBD do not meet the normality assumption, a non-parametric method should be used to analyze them, such as the Durbin test, which was developed by Durbin in 1951.

16.14. Orthogonal Design[6]

The orthogonal design is a type of general fractional-factorial design used to test the comparative effectiveness of multiple intervention components. It is not a comprehensive combination of all intervention components, but a specific set of combinations of them according to the orthogonality principal. The critical advantage of the orthogonal design is that it allows the researcher to test the effectiveness of many interventions simultaneously in a single experiment (and possibly identify some of their interactions) with far fewer experimental units than it would take to exhaust all possible intervention combinations. This feature makes it particularly valuable for testing the best way to implement complex interventions with many facets. For example, it can be applied in testing ways to implement the numerous components or activities involved in complex formula of medicine, multiple parameters of medical instruments, and culture conditions of biosomes. Variations across units in how interventions are implemented will occur regardless of whether the variants are tested; explicit testing as part of the experimental design allows the program operator to learn which variant is best for each intervention.

The combinations of intervention components must comply with the orthogonal design matrix. Each orthogonal design matrix has a symbol $L_N(m^k)$, where N is the number of experiments, k is the number of interventions, and m is the number of levels of interventions. For example, $L_8(2^7)$ consists of two tables; one is the orthogonal matrix (see Table 16.14.1). In this table, each column can arrange one intervention with two levels and it can arrange at most seven interventions and requires at least eight experimental units.

Another table is the top-design table, which is used to determine how to arrange interventions (see Table 16.14.2).

Suppose there are four factors A, B, C and D. If the researcher does not care about interactions between factors, there are many schemes to arrange the four factors according to Table 16.14.2. If first-order interactions must be

Table 16.14.1. $L_8(2^7)$ orthogonal design matrix.

Experimental unit	Intervention 1	2	3	4	5	6	7
1	1	1	1	1	1	1	1
2	1	1	1	2	2	2	2
3	1	2	2	1	1	2	2
4	1	2	2	2	2	1	1
5	2	1	2	1	2	1	2
6	2	1	2	2	1	2	1
7	2	2	1	1	2	2	1
8	2	2	1	2	1	1	2

Table 16.14.2. $L_8(2^7)$ top design table of orthogonal design.

Number of interventions	Row 1	2	3	4	5	6	7
3	A	B	AB	C	AC	BC	ABC
4	A	B	AB=C D	C	AC=B D	BC=A D	D

considered, columns 3, 5 and 6 in the table cannot arrange factors. Column 7 is used to analyze second-order interactions of ABC, and only under the assumption of not considering the second-order interactions can column 7 be used to arrange the D factor. In this case, A, B, C, and D factors must be arranged in columns 1, 2, 4, and 7. Once an experimental factors arrangement scheme is determined, it cannot be changed. The subsequent analysis is based on this arrangement scheme.

An orthogonal design is a fractional-factorial design at the expense of the analysis of any interactions between factors. Therefore, an orthogonal design is only used when the main effect and important first-order interactions are based on expert considerations.

Experimental analysis of an orthogonal design is usually straightforward because you can estimate each main effect and interaction independently. The effect of an individual intervention is calculated by comparing the mean outcome over all subjects for experimental units that provide one variant to the mean for subjects among those who provide the other. ANOVA can be used if the researcher considers interaction effects between factors.

16.15. Uniform Design[14]

Uniform design is an experimental design method proposed by Chinese mathematicians Fang Kaitai and Wang Yuan in 1978. Uniform design is also a kind of non-comprehensive experimental design. It overcomes the shortcomings of orthogonal design, which is not applicable to experiments with too many factor levels. The advantages of the uniform design include: fewer experiments, the factors can be adjusted, and it can prevent experimental accidents or too slow reaction speeds. Uniform design has been widely used in various fields, such as the pharmaceutical, biological, chemical, aerospace, electronics, and military engineering fields.

Orthogonal design has two characteristics: "uniform and dispersive, regular and comparable." In order to ensure the characteristic "regular and comparable", the orthogonal design requires that the experiments be repeated at least q^2 times (assuming each factor has a q level). When the q value is larger, more experiments are required. If we want to further reduce the number of experiments, the requirement "regular and comparable" must be removed. Uniform design is a method that only considers the requirement "uniform and dispersive". Uniform design has a significant characteristic that each level of each factor is used in only one experiment.

Similar to orthogonal design, uniform design arranges experiments through the use of a carefully designed table. Each design table has a symbol, $U_n(q^S)$ or $U_n^*(q^s)$, where * means better uniform property with a priority to choose, U means "uniform", n means n experiments, q means q levels of each factor, and s means s columns of the table. Each uniform design table has an instruction table that indicates how to choose the applicable columns from the design table and provides an indicator of uniform degree for each experimental plan. Below is an example that explains how to use the $U_6^*(6^4)$ design table (Table 16.15.1).

Table 16.15.1. $U_6^*(6^4)$ design table.

	1	2	3	4
1	1	2	3	6
2	2	4	6	5
3	3	6	2	4
4	4	1	5	3
5	5	3	1	2
6	6	5	4	1

Table 16.15.2. $U_6^*(6^4)$ instruction table.

S	Row				D
2	1	3			0.1875
3	1	2	3		0.2656
4	1	2	3	4	0.2990

Table 16.15.1 means that there are six experiments that should be done and each factor has six levels. Four columns of the table mean that at most four factors can be arranged. The instruction table is shown in Table 16.15.2.

If there are two factors, then columns 1 and 3 of Table 16.15.1 can be used to arrange the experiment. If there are three factors then columns 1, 2, and 3 of Table 16.15.1 should be used. The rest can be done in the same manner. The last column of Table 16.15.2 shows the deviation of uniform degree. Less deviation means a better uniform degree, which can be used as an indicator for choosing a design table.

Usually, there are two methods to analyze the data obtained from a uniform design: (1) Intuitive analysis: Because uniform design allows more degrees of each factor, the interval between degrees is small, the experimental points are distributed uniformly across the whole experimental range, and the results of the experiment have better representation. The best experimental point is closer to the optimal condition of a comprehensive experiment. (2) Regression analysis: Linear models, quadratic polynomial models, and nonlinear models can be used to screen variables by stepwise regression.

16.16. Sequential Experiment Design[15]

Sequential experiment design is also called a non-fixed sample experiment. One stage will be completed, followed by another, then another, and so on, with the aim that each stage will build upon the previous one until enough data are gathered over an interval of time to test your hypothesis. The sample size is not predetermined. The corresponding statistical analysis is called a sequential analysis.

The initial work on sequential designs was done by Wald in the 1940s. The closed modifications came from work by Bross and Armitage. In 1975, British statistician Peter Armitage systematically described the different types of sequential design in clinical trials. According to whether the maximum sample size was predetermined, it can be divided into open and closed sequential designs. According to whether one-sided or two-sided tests are used, it can be divided into one-way and two-way sequential designs. According to the data type, it can be divided into quantitative and qualitative response sequential designs.

The advantages of the sequential design include: (1) In clinical trials and epidemiological research, because sample size depends on the number of cases and the enrollment rate of subjects, regarding sample size as a variable will be more reasonable than viewing it as a constant in the design phase. (2) When a difference really exists between treatment groups, sequential analysis can reach conclusions earlier than a fixed sample size experiment; accordingly, this design can reduce sample size and can shorten the experimental period. In some situations, such as expensive animal experiments, sequential design is very applicable. (3) In clinical trials, when significant results are observed, the experiment is stopped. Sequential design conforms more to the requirements of ethics than a fixed sample size trial because it avoids ineffective or even harmful therapy for patients. The disadvantages of a classical sequential design are that it is only applicable for acute experiments for which results can be acquired quickly. The interval between two subjects entering the experiment should not be too long. Moreover, the sequential design is not applicable for experiments with multiple response variables.

In recent years, increasing attention has been paid to the group sequential method, which can be used for medium and long-term clinical trials. This method was proposed by SJ Pocock in 1977.

In clinical trials, the group sequential method requires that the whole trial be divided into k continuous periods. Each period is called a group and $2n$ subjects enter the trial in each group. When the ith ($i = 1, 2, \ldots, k$) period is completed, an interim analysis is performed. If the p value is smaller than the significance level, which is specified in advance, the trial is stopped; otherwise, the trial continues until the next planned interim analysis. When the outcome is still not significant after the last period, the trial is stopped and considered to support the null hypothesis.

In this process, multiple tests are performed. Each test will add to the probability of a type I error, and then the total significance level α will increase. Skovlund's study showed that if the significance level was used for each test, the total significance level will increase to 0.19 after 10 tests.

To maintain the total significance level as a constant α, common strategies for interim analyzes are different adjustments of the nominal significance level. The nominal level is chosen such that the desired overall significance level (e.g. 0.05) is maintained.

A group sequential method is appropriate for a long-term trial or the situation in which the whole trial process can be divided into several continuous periods. It retains the advantages of the traditional sequential method, avoids its limitations, and matches the interim analysis just in time. For a double blind trial, a group sequential method cannot be used because of the need to perform unblinding processes. However, computer-assisted unblinding may be used for statistical analysis, which can overcome this difficulty.

16.17. Response Surface Methodology[16]

Response surface methodology (RSM) is a method for optimizing factors of the chemical industrial process that was introduced by G.E.P. Box and K.B. Wilson in 1951. The main idea of RSM is to use a sequence of designed experiments to obtain an optimal response. In general, RSM assumes that the problem to be solved is an optimization problem with conditional limitations and the form of the objective function is unknown:

$$Y = f(X_1, X_2, \ldots, X_k) + \varepsilon.$$

X indicates the experimental factors (independence variables), Y is the response (dependence variables), ε is the error. RSM can resolve the optimization problem under this assumption and the conditional limitations of the application system. In RSM, response is represented as a surface in three-dimensional space, called the response surface.

The advantages of RSM include fewer experiments, a shorter experimental period, and high precision. RSM has been widely used in the chemical, food, medicine, and biology domains.

RSM can be divided into two stages: response surface design and response surface optimization.

There are three common design methods of RSM:

(1) Plackett–Burman design: Plackett–Burman designs are experimental designs presented in 1946 by Robin L. Plackett and J.P. Burman. Their goal was to find experimental designs for investigating the dependence of some measured quantity on a number of independent variables (factors), each taking L levels (which generally refers to two levels) in such a way as to minimize the variance of the estimates of these dependencies using a limited number of experiments. Interactions between the factors were considered negligible. The solution to this problem is to find an experimental design where each combination of levels for any pair of factors appears the same number of times, throughout all of the experimental runs. A complete factorial design would satisfy this criterion, but the idea was to find smaller designs.

For the case of more than two levels, Plackett and Burman rediscovered designs that had previously been developed by Raj Chandra Bose and K. Kishen. Plackett and Burman gave specifics for designs having a number of experiments equal to the number of levels L to some integer power, for L = 3, 4, 5, or 7.

When interactions between factors are not negligible, they are often confounded with the main effects in Plackett–Burman designs, meaning that the designs do not permit one to distinguish between certain main effects and certain interactions.

Plackett–Burman designs are often used in primary experiments to screen for the important factors.

(2) Central composite design: A central composite design is the most commonly used response surface designed experiment. Central composite designs are a factorial or fractional-factorial design with center points, augmented with a group of axial points (also called star points) that can be used to estimate curvature.

Central composite designs are especially useful in sequential experiments because you can often build on previous factorial experiments by adding axial and center points.

When possible, central composite design has the desired properties of orthogonal blocks and rotatability.

After the designed experiment is performed, a multivariate quadratic equation is used, sometimes iteratively, to obtain results.

$$y = \beta_0 + \sum_{i=1}^{k} \beta_i x_i + \sum_{i=1}^{k} \beta_{ii} x_i^2 + \sum_{i<j}\sum \beta_{ij} x_i x_j + \varepsilon.$$

According to the results of regression and ANOVA, we can evaluate the effects of each factor and their interactions to the response, describe the response surface with a contour map, and then find the influencing factors under the optimal response condition.

(3) Box–Behnken Design: A Box–Behnken design is a type of response surface design that does not contain an embedded factorial or fractional-factorial design. These designs are rotatable (or near rotatable) and require three levels of each factor. The designs have limited capability for orthogonal blocking compared to the central composite designs. Box–Behnken designs have treatment combinations that are at the midpoints of the edges of the experimental space and require at least three continuous factors.

These designs allow efficient estimation of the first and second order coefficients. Because Box–Behnken designs often have fewer design points, they can be less expensive to perform than central composite designs with the same number of factors. However, because they do not have an embedded factorial design, they are not suited for sequential experiments.

Box–Behnken designs can also prove useful if you know the safe operating zone for your process. Box–Behnken designs also ensure that all factors are not set at their high levels at the same time.

The design and data analysis of RSM can be conducted by using the software Design Expert and Minitab.

References

1. Krauth, J. *Experimental Design: A Handbook and Dictionary for Medical and Behavioral Research.* Amsterdam: Elsevier Science & Technology Books, 2000.
2. Machin, D, Campbell, MJ. The design of studies for medical research. John Wiley & Sons, 2005.
3. Lohr, S. *Sampling: Design and Analysis.* Cengage Learning, 2009.
4. Armitage, P, Berry, G, Matthews, JN. *Statistical Methods in Medical Research.* Hoboken: John Wiley & Sons, 2008.
5. Caliński, T, Kageyama, S. *Block Designs: A Randomization Approach.* New York: Springer, 2000.
6. Fisher, RA. *The Design of Experiments.* London: Oliver & Boyd, 1935.
7. Douglas, MC. *Design and Analysis of Experiments.* Hoboken: John Wiley & Sons, 2005.
8. David, A, Ratkowsky, M, Evans, A. *Cross-over Experiment: Design, Analysis, and Application.* New York: Marcel Dekker, 1993.
9. Federer, WT, King, F. *Variations on Split Plot and Split Block Experiment Designs.* Hoboken: John Wiley & Sons, 2007.
10. Fisher, RA. *Statistical Methods for Research Workers.* Edinburgh: Oliver and Boyd, 1925.
11. Gerry, PQ, Keough, MJ. *Experimental Design and Data Analysis for Biologists.* Cambridge: Cambridge University Press, 2002.
12. Vonesh, EF, Chinchilli, VG. *Linear and Nonlinear Models for the Analysis of Repeated Measurements.* London: Chapman and Hall, 2007.
13. Campbell, BF, Sengupta, S, Santos, C, Lorig, KR. Balanced incomplete block design: Description, case study, and implications for practice. *Health Educ. Q.* 1995, 22(2): 201–210.
14. Kaitai Fang. *Uniform Design and Uniform Design Table.* Beijing: Science Press, 1994.
15. Stuart, JP. Group sequential methods in the design and analysis of clinical trials. *Biometrika*, 1977, 64(2): 191–199.
16. Box, GE, Wilson, KB. On the experimental attainment of optimum conditions. *J. R. Stat. Soc. B.* 1951, 13(1): 1–45.

About the Author

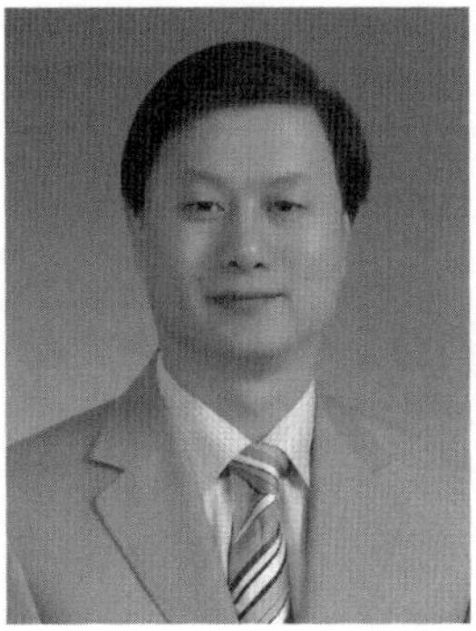

Yuhai Zhang is an Associate Professor at the Department of Health Statistics, Fourth Military Medical University, Xi'an, Shaanxi Province, China. Research interests include data mining, neural network and longitudinal data analysis.

CHAPTER 17

CLINICAL RESEARCH

Luyan Dai* and Feng Chen

17.1. Clinical Trial[1–3]

17.1.1. *Phases of clinical trial*

Clinical trial is the prospective research of drug, medical device or other interventions on human body (patient or the healthy volunteer) to demonstrate the effectiveness, adverse reaction of drugs and/or the regularity of administration, distribution, metabolism and elimination of a drug in human. It is to investigate or confirm the efficacy and safety of the treatment intervention. There are four phases of clinical trials for the new drug development.

Phase I Clinical Trials: The primary objective is to screen and assess the clinical pharmacology and safety. A series of trials are conducted to observe the tolerability and pharmacokinetics of the new drug and to provide the evidence for the design of dosing regimens.

Phase II Clinical Trials: One of the main objectives is to establish the efficacy of the investigational drug. By conducting a series of trials, phase II is aimed to explore the efficacy of a drug, to further evaluate the safety in patients from the target indication population, to explore the dose regiments and to provide the evidence for phase III trial designs. The designs may vary, including randomized controlled trial (RCT).

Phase III Clinical Trials: The objective is to confirm the efficacy and safety for the benefit risk assessment of a drug. Multiple trials may be conducted in the target population to provide sufficient evidence for the new

*Corresponding author: luyan.dai@boehringer-ingelheim.com

drug application (NDA) submission and approval for the drug registration. The RCT with adequate sample size is generally required in this phase.

Phase IV Clinical Trials: The phase is referred to the studies conducted by sponsors for research in the post-marketing setting. The objective is to delineate additional information for the treatment efficacy and safety after the drug is widely used, to assess the relationship of benefits and risks for the common or the special patient populations, and to optimize the dose administration in the clinical setting.

17.1.2. *Clinical trial principles*

The RCT shall strictly follow the principles of randomization for treatment allocation, comparison with control and reproducibility of the results (refer to Secs. 17.2, 17.4 and 16.4). The efficacy evaluation (including the method of blinding, refer to Sec. 17.3) shall be implemented following the study design and conducted to control the potential confounding and bias to guarantee the trustworthy and reliable results. Nowadays, RCT has been an important research method to demonstrate and confirm the safety and efficacy of the drug, medical device or clinical interventions.

The first published RCT in history appeared in 1984, for which Geoffrey Marshall, etc., issued the paper *Streptomycin Treatment for Pulmonary Tuberculosis* on the *Journal of the Medical Research Council* (*British Medical Journal, BMJ*). The efficacy of streptomycin in treating pulmonary tuberculosis was demonstrated in the study. The contribution made by the statistician AB Hill has been the scientific breakthrough in driving the clinical trial development and improving the quality of the clinical trials substantially. The confounding factors were firstly controlled by randomization, and the bias was reduced by using blinding, which made the significant impact on the clinical research and created a new era of RCT.

Study ethics must be complied in clinical trials. A good clinical trial must have a rigorously sound study design, strictly implemented SOPs, and seriously conducted operation to guarantee scientificity and reliability of the trials.

17.2. Randomization[4,5]

17.2.1. *Randomization*

In order to minimize the allocation bias and balance the distribution of known or unknown prognostic factors among treatment groups, randomized allocation is the important method used in statistics, also called as randomization, in which the subjects will be allocated into treatment group with certain probabilities. Randomization is one of the primary principles of the clinical trial design.

RA Fisher was the first person who introduced the concept of randomization in his book "*The Design of Experiments*" in 1935[4], in which he pointed out that randomization should be a prerequisite of the application of hypothesis testing. Since then, it has been widely used in crop breeding in agriculture research. The first published clinical trial in medicine using randomization was to study streptomycin treatment of pulmonary tuberculosis by AB Hill in 1948 (refer to Sec. 17.1 RCT).

Proper randomization can balance the subject characteristics (known or unknown, observed or unobserved) among treatment groups. Although randomization cannot guarantee that all the subject characteristics will be distributed exactly the same, with the increase of sample size, the distribution will tend to be balanced. The larger the sample size, the more balanced is the distribution. It therefore generates the comparable treatment groups.

17.2.2. *Randomization operation*

There are many methods to operate randomization. The lot-drawing and coin-tossing are the intuitive and simple methods. Nowadays, the randomization is implemented by the random number generator via computer.

(1) Fixed randomization, in which the subjects will be allocated to treatment groups at a fixed probability throughout the study. It includes (a) Complete randomization, in which the subjects will be allocated according to the pre-specified probability without any constraints. (b) Blocked randomization (also called permuted block randomization) in which sequential blocks will be used according to the time when subjects join the study. Each block will be completely randomized. (c) Stratified randomization, in which some important prognostic factors are pre-specified as stratification factors and well balanced among treatment groups. Within each stratum, the complete randomization will be implemented. If blocked randomization is implemented within each stratum, it is called as stratified block randomization. It is generally not recommended to include too many stratification factors and 1–3 factors are commonly considered. The stratified block randomization is implemented using the central randomization system.

(2) Adaptive randomization, in which the subjects will be allocated at an unfixable probability. It includes (a) Baseline adaptive randomization, in which the probability will be adjusted according to the baseline characteristics of the subject. (b) Response adaptive randomization, in which

the probability will be adjusted according to the test result of the previous subject.

In the clinical trials, the treatment allocation of subject will be implemented by randomizing the test drugs or treatments. In order to ensure the proper and effective randomization, the allocation process must comply with the SOPs strictly.

17.3. Blinding[4,5]

To avoid the influence on the results from the testers' preferences or expectations, blinding is usually used in clinical trials. Blinding methods include double-blind and single-blind methods while the unblinded one is called as open label.

In clinical trials, the investigators and researchers performing the treatment evaluation, and personals involved in the data management, and statistical analysis are considered as observers. The subjects or relatives or guardians of subjects can be considered as participants. The double-blind means both observers and participants are blinded, not knowing the treatment during trial conduct. The single-blind means the participant is blinded, while the open label means both researcher and participant know about the treatment carried out in the study.

17.3.1. *Double-blind trial*

Double-blind should be used whenever possible in the clinical trial, especially when the measurements are the variables which could be greatly impacted by the subjective assessment, e.g. questionnaires used in psychiatry areas (MMSE scale, NFDS, quality of life, etc.). When the double-blind is not feasible, the single-blind should be considered as appropriate.

In the double-blinded clinical trials, the blinding shall be kept to the researchers and participants throughout the trial conduct including the procedure of generating the random number, setting the random number seed, blinding the codes, content of the emergency unblinding, dispensing the trial medications, administrating the drugs, recording the measurements, performing statistical analysis to evaluate the efficacy and safety, and monitoring, cleaning and querying the data entries. The data can be unblinded only after the database is locked, and before performing the statistical analysis. The release of the unblinding codes without the pre-specified conditions is called as "breaking of blindness".

The double-blinding trial must comply with the SOPs, to avoid the unnecessary disclosure of the blinding codes. If all or majority of the cases are broken during the conduct, the trial should be considered as failure and a new trial should be conducted.

17.3.2. *Unblinded trial*

For trials that can not implement the blinding, they can only be carried out in an unblinded fashion. If it is an unblinded one, due to the subjective perception of researchers or participants to the treatment, the expectation or pre-judgment may influence the recording of measurements, especially for those subjectively assessed. If the researcher knows the drug that the participant is taking, his/her attention or care about the participant may increase. For example, the frequency of examinations could increase. The nurse could pay more attention to the participant. Such behaviors might impact the attitude of participants, and then influence the objectiveness of treatment outcomes. On the other hand, when the participant knows about what he/she is taking, e.g. drug or placebo, there could be a psychological effect to disturb or interfere with the cooperation with researchers during the trial conduct, leading to bias. Therefore, even for the unblinded experiment, the researchers and the researchers performing the assessment should not be the same person ideally. If the researcher performing the assessment is kept blinded during the trial conduct, the bias can be controlled to the minimum.

17.4. Selection of Control[1,6]

Difference is verified via comparison. A control should be designed in the clinical trial. The balance between the treatment and control groups should be maintained, which is one of the main methods to exclude the confounding factors and differentiate the treatment efficacy in the trial.

17.4.1. *Controlled design*

A controlled design can be parallel, or crossover. There can be one or more different control groups in the same clinical trial. Below summarizes five basic types of controlled designs.

(1) Placebo control: The placebo is a dummy medication of the test drug without active substance. The dosage, size, color, weight, odor and flavor should be identical to the test drug if possible. The purpose of designing the placebo control is to reduce the bias caused by the psychological effects from the researcher and participants when evaluating the efficacy and safety to minimize the expectant effect and control the placebo effect. The design

of placebo control can also eliminate the influence of the natural disease progression, and highlight the real effectiveness and adverse reaction of test drug. By doing that, the difference between test drug and placebo can be read directly under the trial condition.

(2) No-treatment control: The design does not have any drug or treatment as control. Therefore, it is unblinded, which may impact the objective assessment of the test result. It is applicable to the cases as follows: (a) due to the very special treatment, placebo control cannot be implemented or very difficult to carry out; (b) the adverse reaction of test drug is very unique preventing the researcher or participant from staying in the blind status. In such cases, the placebo control may add little values.

(3) Active control or positive control which uses the marketed drug that is efficacious as control. The positive control should be effective, accepted by medical society and recorded in the pharmacopoeia.

(4) Dose-response control which includes multiple doses of the test drug. The subjects are randomly allocated to the dose groups. The placebo control group (zero-dose group) can be either included or not included in the trial.

(5) External control (i.e. historical control). The test drug will be compared to the results from subjects in other studies. The external control can be a group of patients treated at an earlier time (i.e. historical control) or a group treated during the same time period but in another setting. Due to the limitation of comparability across studies, the method has the limitation in its application. It is generally not recommended except for certain circumstances as needed.

Furthermore, the selection of control types as described above can be used in combination. It may include: (1) three arms study, in which the trial uses placebo and positive control at the same time, usually for the non-inferiority trial. (2) add-on treatment, in which the standard treatment is added to each subject for ethical considerations in the placebo-controlled studies. The subjects in the test group are administered with the investigational drug while those in the control group are administered with the placebo afterwards.

17.5. Endpoint[1,5]

17.5.1. *Primary endpoint*

Endpoints are from clinical outcomes. Primary outcome is sometimes called as primary endpoint. It is a variable which has direct and essential relationship with the study objective, and can properly reflect the efficacy or safety of drugs. The primary outcome should have the features of easy quantification, objectivity, low variation, higher reproducibility according to the study objective and shall have the accepted criterion in the corresponding research flied. The primary outcome must be well defined in the clinical trial protocol and be used for the evaluation of sample size. Generally, there is only one primary outcome in a clinical trial. If several primary outcomes shall be evaluated at the same time, the method of controlling type-I errors shall be considered in the study design (refer to Sec. 17.7 multiplicity).

17.5.2. *Secondary endpoint*

Secondary outcomes are the supportive measures related to the study objective. There are commonly multiple secondary outcomes in a clinical trial and the number should be still controlled. Same as the primary endpoints, the secondary outcomes shall be well defined in the protocol. Its impact to the interpretation of the study results and relative importance should be described and reported.

In a confirmatory clinical trial, especially in the phase III, only after the statistical significance has been established for primary outcome(s), the statistical testing of secondary outcome(s) can be carried out in the confirmatory fashion. In an exploratory trial, results of both primary and secondary outcomes are used as hypothesis generating for future studies.

17.5.3. *Composite endpoint*

Composite endpoint can be derived using the predefined algorithm with the integration or combination of multiple outcomes to form a complex one. It is used if it's difficult to select the primary outcome from the multiple related to the primary objectives of the study.

17.5.4. *Global assessment endpoint*

Global assessment endpoint is one used to assess the overall safety, efficacy and/or feasibility of a treatment. It could be a combination of the objective outcomes and the subjective assessment from the researchers.

17.5.5. *Surrogate Endpoint*

Surrogate endpoints are those outcomes representing the clinical efficacy indirectly; it will be used when it is difficult or impossible to get the ultimate clinical outcomes during the trial. To be a surrogate, it depends on: (1) whether the parameter is related to the study objectives biologically, (2) whether the surrogate in disease epidemiology has the predictive effect to the clinical outcomes, (3) the magnitude of drug efficacy based on the surrogate endpoints should be consistent with that based on clinical outcomes. In some oncology clinical trials, tumor shrinkage and prolongation of PFS are not consistent with the prolongation of overall survival. It is followed that the selection of surrogate endpoint shall be comprehensively evaluated based on biology, epidemiology and clinical results. Therefore, the surrogate endpoint should be cautiously selected and communicated under supervision in the timely manner.

17.5.6. *Dichotomization of variable*

The continuous variable and ordinal variable can be dichotomized into a binary variable, which is quite useful in the clinical practice. Nevertheless, the judgment whether the treatment is efficacious or futile is usually made from a continuous parameter. The criterion used for dichotomization should be well defined in the protocol because it may commonly lead to information loss, and therefore reduce the study power and have impact on the sample size evaluation.

17.6. Analysis Set[1,5]

In the clinical trials, different endpoints represent different aspects. Some endpoints describe the treatment compliance. Some are used to describe efficacy and some measures the safety of the test drug. It is difficult to find one endpoint to comprehensively measure the overall effect of the drug effect in the clinical trials. Therefore, the analysis set may vary among the different types of endpoints. Nevertheless, two principles shall be followed to select the analysis sets, i.e.

(1) minimization of bias;
(2) control of type-I error.

17.6.1. *Intention to treat (ITT)*

Randomization is a method to minimize the bias. In order to control the bias, the subjects should be randomly allocated to the treatment for comparison. ITT, as one of the most important analysis set, is therefore followed by the randomization. ITT is an analysis dataset and statistical analysis policy that the subject is analyzed according to the planned protocol based on randomization, regardless of the treatment that the subject is actually treated and the compliance the subject is followed. Sometimes, it is also called as randomized set.

ITT is just a principle. In clinical trials, the subject after randomization may withdraw the informed consent before they receive the treatment or have no baseline records. It may not add much information to include these patients into the analysis set. In such cases, the analysis set may be modified according to the actual scenarios following the ITT principle. Such analysis set is named as modified ITT (mITT).

Given that there's neither unified definition of mITT, nor a guiding principle with consensus, the bias may be introduced due to the modification. Therefore, it is important to describe the definition when developing the statistical analysis plan. The definition should not be easily changed during the trial conduct. The result of mITT should be cautiously explained, and the potential bias of the results should be evaluated.

17.6.2. *Classification of analysis set*

Full analysis set (FAS) is the ideal analysis set closest to the ITT principle. It is a set that reasonably exclude subjects from the randomized set at a minimum. It is one type of mITT sets.

Per-protocol set (PPS) sometimes refers to the analysis set including "adequate cases" or "assessable cases". It is a subset of FAS including those subjects without important protocol violations which may potentially have significant impact on study conclusions. The subjects who are not compliant with the protocol, take the forbidden medication, or have the incomplete data collection on case report form (CRF) per protocol instruction may be excluded from PPS.

Safe set (SS) refers to the set including patients who receive at least one administration of the treatment as documented.

There is no consensus reached on the analysis set to be used for the primary efficacy endpoint(s). In principle, ITT is considered to be conservative for primary efficacy endpoints for the type-I error protection in superiority trials. In practice, FAS and PPS can be used to analyze the primary endpoints respectively. If the consistent conclusions are made based from the two sets, the reliability of the results and conclusions can be verified and enhanced. If the two lead to different results, reasons should be investigated. The analysis set definition used for the primary analysis should be clearly pre-specified in the protocol.

17.7. Multiplicity[7–9]

Multiplicity in clinical trials refers to the multiple testing, which means multiple hypotheses are formulated in one trial. The results of m hypotheses in the trial can be illustrated as shown in Table 17.7.1, in which m is known, R is observed, S, T, U, V are unobserved, and m_0 is a fixed but unknown.

False discovery rate (FDR) was proposed by Benjamini and Hochberg (1995) and is used to describe the expected rate of rejecting H_0 when H_0 is true, i.e.

$$FDR = \begin{cases} E(V/R) & R \neq 0 \\ 0 & R = 0 \end{cases}.$$

Family-wise error rate (FWER) is the probability of making one or more type-I errors among the m hypothesis tests, i.e.

$$FWER = P(V > 0).$$

The FWER is controlled in the strong sense if the FWER control at level α is guaranteed only when all null hypotheses are true in the multiple hypothesis tests.

The weak control of FEWR refers to the rate is controlled at level α for any configuration of true and non-true null hypotheses (including the global null hypothesis).

FWER control exerts a more stringent control over false discovery compared to FDR. If all the hypotheses are true, that is $m_0 = m$, FDR is equal to FWER, if $m_0 < m$, FDR < FWER. Meanwhile, the FWER control guarantees the control of FDR while FDR control procedure may not be able to necessarily control FWER.

In principle, FDR can be commonly controlled in the exploratory trials while FWER should be controlled for confirmatory trials.

Multiplicity should be considered for the trials with design features like multiple primary endpoints, interim analysis, multiple treatment comparison and subgroup analysis. The type-I error rate should be controlled properly.

Table 17.7.1. Results of multiple hypothesis tests.

Null hypothesis	Fail to reject H_0	Reject H_0	Total
True	U	V	m_0
False	T	S	$m - m_0$
Total	W	R	m

A variety of methods can be used for multiplicity adjustment. Depending on the specification of testing order, the methods can be divided into two main categories including single step procedure (e.g. Bonferroni and Dunnett) and stepwise procedure (e.g. Hochberg and Holm). Based on the distribution assumptions, the adjustment methods can be classified into three main types including (a) methods based on P values or non-parametric methods (e.g. Bonferroni and Holm method); (b) parametric methods (e.g. Dunnett method when a multivariate normal distribution or multivariate t-distribution holds); (c) methods based on re-sampling (e.g. Bootstrap or permutation test).

17.8. Group Sequential Design and Interim Analysis[5,10]

17.8.1. *Interim analysis*

Interim analysis refers to the analysis conducted prior to the trial completion. The interim analysis requires to be pre-specified in the protocol.

There are three types of interim analysis: (a) one to timely monitor for the protection of patient safety. If there is any safety concerns of a serious type that interfere with patient wellness, the trial should be terminated earlier due to safety; (b) one to stop the trial early due to efficacy. If the interim results suggest the trial meet the pre-specified criteria of stopping earlier, the trial may be terminated earlier either for the promising or futile efficacy. In the trial for dose selection, the inefficacious treatment group may be dropped at the interim; (c) one to re-estimate sample size. The interim analysis is usually conducted by a third party independent of trial team and study investigators.

In order to control the inflation of type-I errors introduced by the interim analysis, multiplicity should be adjusted per the objectives of interim analysis. Several statistical methods are commonly used including Pocock method, Peto method and O'Brien–Fleming method. Lan and Demets proposed a more flexible framework, i.e. $\alpha(t)$ spending function, (refer to Table 17.8.1). t refers information time, which is the percentage of the information collected at the interim to the total information. α is the overall type-I error rate. It is straightforward that $\alpha(0) = 0, \alpha(1) = \alpha$.

17.8.2. *Group sequential design*

The conception of group sequential design was proposed by Armitage and Bross as early as 1950s. In 1977, Pocock, etc. further studied its theory, and proposed the guiding principle for the implementation of group sequential

Table 17.8.1. Several α spending functions.

Spending methods	Form of function
Pocock	$\alpha(t) = \alpha[\log(1 + (e - 1)t)]$
O'Brien–Fleming	$\alpha(t) = 2 - 2\Phi(\frac{Z_{\alpha/2}}{\sqrt{t}})$
Exponential family	$\alpha(t) = \alpha t^{\rho}(\rho > 0)$
Gamma family	$\alpha(t) = \begin{cases} \frac{\alpha(1-e^{\gamma t})}{1-e^{-\gamma}}(\gamma \neq 0) \\ \alpha t(\gamma = 0) \end{cases}$

design. There are two types of group sequential design including parallel group design with control and single arm design without control.

The idea of group sequential design is to divide the trial into several phases. The interim analysis may be conducted at the end of each phase to decide whether the trial should be continued or stopped early.

The stopping rules for either efficacy or futility should be pre-specified. When the superiority can be confirmed and claimed based on the interim data with sufficient sample size and fulfill the criteria for early stop of efficacy, the trial can be stopped early. Meanwhile, the trial may also be stopped due to the futile interim results.

17.8.3. *Conditional power* (*CP*)

CP refers to the conditional probability that the final result will be statistically significant, given the data observed thus far at the interim and a specific assumption about the pattern of the data to be observed in the remainder of the study, such as assuming the original design effect, or the effect estimated from the current data, or under the null hypothesis.

17.8.4. *Predictive probability*

Predictive probability refers to the probability of achieving trial success at the end of the trial upon the data accumulated at the interim time point t.

17.9. Equivalence Design[1,11]

The equivalence design includes two types, i.e. bioequivalence and clinical equivalence.

Bioequivalence refers to the comparable or similar efficacy and safety for the same drug in different formulations or different drugs with similar efficacy as the reference. In that case, bioavailability (absorptivity and absorbance) of the drugs should be the same *in vivo*, and has the similar pharmacokinetic parameters of AUC, $C_{\max}$ and $T_{\max}$. The equivalence design is commonly used for the comparison between the generic and reference drug.

Clinical equivalence refers to the different formulations of the same drug or different drugs with the similar clinical efficacy and safety. For some drugs, the concentration or the metabolites cannot be clearly measured and or the drug is administrated locally which may not be able to enter into blood circulation completely. In these cases, it is not straightforward to measure the *in vivo* metabolism. Sometimes, the new drug may have the different administration route or mechanism of action. In these scenarios, the bioequivalence may not be able to conclude the equivalence of these drugs, in which the clinical trials are needed to demonstrate the clinical equivalence.

Compared to the clinical equivalence trials, bioequivalence trial may differ in four main aspects: (a) requirement on test drugs; (b) measurement criteria; (c) study design; (d) equivalence margin.

17.9.1. *Analysis for equivalence*

The analysis methods for equivalence can be categorized into two types: (1) those based on confidence interval and (2) those based on hypothesis test.

(1) Confidence interval: The 95% confidence interval can be used to assess the difference or ratio of the endpoints between two groups. If both upper and lower bounds of the confidence interval are within the equivalence zone, the conclusion can be made that the two treatment groups are equivalent. By doing that, the type-I error rate α can be controlled within 5%. The confidence interval can be generated by the estimation functions or models by adjusting the covariates. As illustrated in Figure 17.9.1, scenarios B and C can be concluded as being equivalent while other scenarios fail.

(2) Two one-side test: For treatment difference, the hypotheses may look like:

$$H_{0L}\colon \pi_T - \pi_S \le -\Delta \quad \text{versus } H_{1L}\colon \pi_T - \pi_S > -\Delta,$$

$$H_{0U}\colon \pi_T - \pi_S \ge \Delta \quad \text{versus } H_{1U}\colon \pi_T - \pi_S < \Delta.$$

Where $(-\Delta, \Delta)$ is the equivalence interval ($\Delta > 0$).

For the comparison using ratio, the hypotheses may look like:

$$H_{0L}\colon \pi_T/\pi_S \le \Delta \quad \text{versus } H_{1L}\colon \pi_T/\pi_S > \Delta,$$
$$H_{0U}\colon \pi_T/\pi_S \ge 1/\Delta \quad \text{versus } H_{1U}\colon \pi_T/\pi_S < 1/\Delta.$$

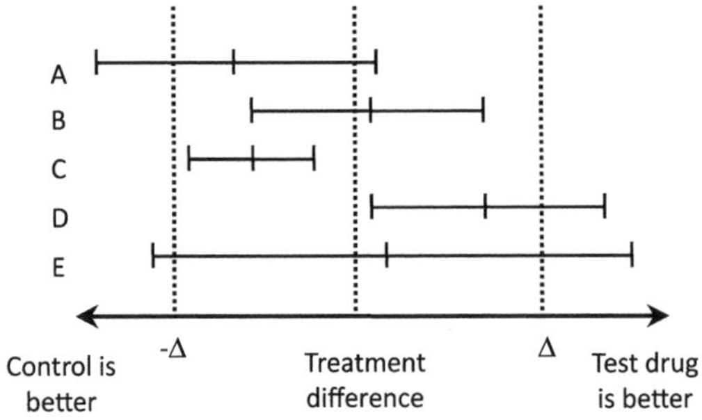

Fig. 17.9.1. An illustration-equivalence based on confidence interval.

Where $(\Delta, 1/\Delta)$ is the equivalence interval $(\Delta > 0)$. If both null hypotheses are rejected at the same significance level α, it can be concluded that the two drugs are equivalent.

17.9.2. *Equivalence margin*

The determination of equivalence margin Δ should be carefully evaluated and jointly made by the clinical expert, regulator expert and statistician according to trial design characteristics (including disease progression, efficacy of the reference drug, target measurements, etc.). For bioequivalence, $\Delta = 0.8$ is commonly used, that is, 80–125% as the equivalent interval.

17.10. Non-inferiority Design[1,12,13]

The objective of non-inferiority trial is to show that the difference between the new and active control treatment is small, small enough to allow the known effectiveness of the active control to support the conclusion that the new test drug is also effective. In some clinical trials, the use of placebo control may not be ethical when efficacious drug or treatment exists for the disease indications and the delay of the treatment may result in death, disease progression, disability or irreversible medical harms.

17.10.1. *Non-inferiority margin*

The non-inferiority margin Δ is a value with clinical meanings which indicate that difference may be ignorable in the clinical practice if difference is smaller than the margin. In other words, if the treatment difference is less than Δ, it is considered that the test drug is non-inferior to the active control. Similar as the determination of equivalence margin, the non-inferiority margin should be discussed and decided jointly by peer experts and communicated with the regulatory agency in advance and clearly specified in the study protocol.

The selection of non-inferiority margin may be based on the effect size of the active control. Assume P is the effect of placebo and C is the effect of active control. Without loss of generality, assume that a higher value describes a better effect and the limit of 97.5% one-sided confidence interval of $(C - P)$ is $M(M > 0)$. If the treatment effect of an active control is $M_1(M_1 \leq M)$, the non-inferiority margin $\Delta = (1 - f)M_1, 0 < f < 1$. f is usually selected among 0.5–0.8. For example, for drugs treating cardiovascular diseases $f = 0.5$, is sometimes taken for the non-inferiority margin.

The non-inferiority margin can also be determined based on the clinical experiences. For example, in clinical trials for antibacterial drugs, because the effect of active control drug is deemed to be high, when the rate is the endpoint type, the non-inferiority margin Δ can be set as 10%. For drugs treating antihypertension, the non-inferiority margin Δ of mean blood pressure decline is 0.67 kPa (3 mmHg).

17.10.2. *Statistical inference*

The statistical inference for non-inferiority design may be performed using confidence intervals. Followed by the scenario above, the inference is therefore to compare the upper bound of 95% confidence interval (or the upper bound of 97.5% one-sided confidence interval) of C-T to the non-inferiority margin.

In Figure 17.10.2.1, because the upper bound of confidence interval in trial A is lower than the non-inferiority margin M_2, the test drug is non-inferior to the active control. In other cases (B, C and D), the non-inferiority claim cannot be established.

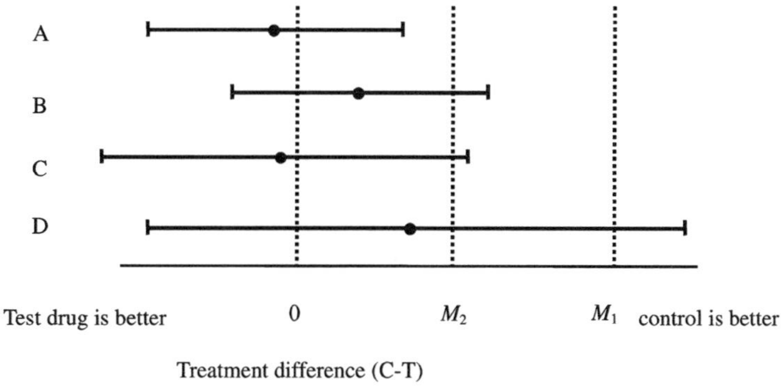

Fig. 17.10.2.1. Confidence intervals and non-inferiority margin.

The inference of non-inferiority design can also be performed using hypothesis tests. Based on different types of efficacy endpoints, the testing statistics may be selected and calculated for the hypothesis testing. Take the treatment difference as the effect measure:

$$H_0\colon C - T \geq \Delta, \quad H_1\colon C - T < \Delta,$$

where $\alpha = 0.025$ in the trial that a higher endpoint value measures a better effect.

17.11. Center Effect[1,5]

17.11.1. *Multiple center clinical trial*

Multicenter clinical trial refers to the trials conducted in multiple centers concurrently under one protocol with oversight from one coordinating investigator in collaboration with multiple investigators. Multicenter clinical trials are commonly adopted in phase II and III so that the required number of patients can be recruited within a short period. Because of the broader coverage of the patients than the single center trial, the patients entered may be more representative for generalizability of trial conclusions.

The section focuses on the multicenter clinical trials conducted in one country. The trials conducted in multiple countries or regions can be referred to in Sec. 17.15.

17.11.2. *Center effect*

In multicenter trials, the baseline characteristics of subjects may vary among centers and clinical practice may not be identical. It may introduce the potential heterogeneity or variation to the observed treatment effect among centers, which is called as center effect. Therefore, the considerations on center effect may need to be taken into account. If a big magnitude of center effect is seen, pooling data from all centers by ignoring the heterogeneity may have impact on the conclusion.

If every center have sufficient number of subjects and center effect is statistical significant, it is suggested to conduct the treatment-by-center interaction test and perform the consistency evaluation of effect estimation among centers in order to generalize the results from the multicenter trials. If such interaction exists, careful evaluation and explanation should be cautiously conducted. The factors introducing the heterogeneity like trial operation practices cross-centers, baseline characteristics of subjects, clinical practices, etc. should be thoroughly investigated.

17.11.3. *Treatment-by-center interaction*

There are two types of interactions, i.e. quantitative and qualitative interactions. The first one describes the situation where the magnitude of the treatment effect varies among centers but the direction of the effect remains the same. A qualitative interaction refers to the situation when both the magnitude and direction of the treatment effect differ among centers. If a quantitative interaction exists, an appropriate statistical method may be used to estimate the treatment effect for the robustness. If a qualitative interaction is observed, additional clinical trials may be considered for the reliability of the evaluation.

The statistical analysis by including treatment-by-center interactions is usually used for the evaluation of heterogeneity among centers. However, it is generally not suggested to include interaction in the primary analysis model because the power may be reduced for the main effect by including the term. Meanwhile, it is important to acknowledge that clinical trials are designed to verify and evaluate the main treatment effect.

When many centers are included, each center may only enroll a few subjects. The center effect is generally not considered in the analyses for primary and secondary endpoints.

The handling of center effect in the analysis should be pre-specified in the protocol or statistical analysis plan.

17.12. Adjustment for Baseline and Covariates[14,15]

17.12.1. *Baseline*

The baseline and covariates are the issues that should be considered in study design and analysis.

Baseline refers to the measurements observed prior to the start of the treatment. A broad definition of baseline may include all measurements recorded before the start of the treatment, including demographic characteristics, observations from physical examinations, baseline diseases and the severity and complication, etc. These measurements may reflect the overall status of the subject when entering into the trial. A specific definition of baseline sometimes refers to the measurements or values of the endpoints specified in the protocol before the start of the treatment. Such baseline values will be used directly for the evaluation of primary endpoint.

To balance the baseline distribution between treatment groups is critical for clinical trials to perform a valid comparison and draw conclusions. In randomized clinical trials because the treatment groups include subjects from the same study population, distribution of baseline is balanced in theory if randomization is performed appropriately. If an individual baseline value differs significantly among treatment groups, it might possibly happen by chance. Therefore, in general, there is no necessity to perform statistical testing for baseline values. It is not required by ICH E9 either.

However, in non-randomized clinical trials, the subjects in treatment and control groups may not come from the same population. Even if the collected baseline values appear to be balanced, it is unknown whether the other subject characteristics that are not collected or measured in the trial are balanced between treatment groups. In this case, the treatment comparison may be biased and the limitation of conclusions should be recognized.

To evaluate the primary endpoint, the baseline may be usually be adjusted for the prognosis of post-baseline outcomes. The commonly used method is to calculate the change from baseline, which is the difference between on-treatment and baseline values, either absolute or relative differences.

17.12.2. *Covariate*

Covariate refers to the variables related to the treatment outcomes besides treatment. In epidemiological research, it is sometimes called as confounding factor. The imbalance of covariate between treatment groups may result in bias in analysis results. Methods to achieve the balance of covariates include (1) simple or block randomization; (2) randomization stratified by the covariate; (3) control the values of covariates to ensure all subjects to carry the same value. Because the third method restricts the inclusion of subjects and limits the result extrapolation, applications are limited.

However, even if the covariate is balanced between treatment groups, trial results may still be impacted by the individual values when the variation is big. Therefore, covariates may be controlled and adjusted for the analysis. The common statistical methods may include analysis of covariance, multivariate regression, stratified analysis, etc.

17.13. Subgroup Analysis[16,17]

Subgroup analysis refers to the statistical analysis of subgroups defined based on the certain baseline characteristics, e.g. age, disease history, with/without some complication, indication subtype, genotype, etc. Subgroup analysis can be categorized into two types depending on timing of the analysis, i.e. pre-specified and post-hoc analyses.

The objective of pre-specified subgroup analysis is to perform the statistical inference for treatment effect in the subgroup from the whole population. The analysis results may be the supportive evidence for the drug approval. Therefore, these subgroup analyses should be specified and well defined in the protocol in advance.

The post-hoc analysis refers to the analysis without pre-specification. It is usually performed after knowing the trial results and exploratory in nature. The objectives of such subgroup analyses include but are not limited to: (a) sensitivity analysis to evaluate robustness of the overall conclusions; (b) internal consistency within the trial; (c) exploration of the prognostic or predictive factors for treatment effect. The post-hoc analysis is data-dependent and may not completely avoid data fishing. It can serve for the purpose of hypothesis generating. Confirmation of the findings requires additional trials for the further extrapolation and acceptance by regulatory agency.

In principle, the assessment of efficacy and safety is for the overall trial population. Nevertheless, the treatment effect may differ among subpopulations and result in heterogeneity. The subgroup analysis is important to understand the variation and investigate the heterogeneity. The subgroup should be defined based on the baseline measures, rather than the on-treatment outcomes.

Several common aspects should be considered statistically for subgroup analysis:

(1) whether the subgroup analysis is exploratory or confirmatory;
(2) whether the randomization is maintained within the subgroup;
(3) whether the sample size or power of subgroup analysis is adequate if hypothesis testing is performed;
(4) whether multiplicity adjustment is considered if multiple subgroups are involved;
(5) whether the difference in baseline characteristics has an impact to the treatment effect and the difference between subgroup and overall populations;
(6) analysis methods of subgroup;
(7) heterogeneity assessment across subgroups and treatment-by-subgroup interaction; and
(8) result presentation and interpretation of subgroup analysis.

17.14. Adaptive Design[18–21]

An adaptive design is defined as a study including prospectively planned opportunity for modification of one or more specified aspects of the study design and hypotheses based on analysis of data from subjects in the study while keeping trial integrity and validity. The modification may be based on the interim results from the trial or external information for the investigation and update of the trial assumptions. An adaptive design also allows the flexibility to monitor the trial for patient safety and treatment efficacy, reduce trial cost and shorten the development cycle at a timely manner.

The concept of adaptive design was proposed as early as 1930s. The comprehensive concept used in clinical trial was later proposed and promoted by PHRMA working group on adaptive design.

CHMP and FDA have issued the guidance on adaptive design for drugs and biologics. The guidance covers topics including (a) points to consider from the perspectives of clinical practices, statistical aspects, regulatory requirement; (b) communication with health authorities (e.g. FDA) when designing and conducting adaptive designs; and (c) the contents to be covered for FDA inspection. In addition, clarification is provided to several critical aspects in the guidance, such as type-I error control, the minimization of bias for efficacy assessment, inflation of type-II errors, simulation study, statistical analysis plan, etc.

The adaptive designs commonly adopted in clinical trials may include: group sequential design, sample size re-estimation, phase I/II trials, phase II/III seamless design, dropping arms, adaptive randomization, adaptive dose escalation, biomarker-adaptive; adaptive treatment-switching, adaptive-hypothesis design, etc.

In addition, trials may also include adaptive features including the revision of inclusion and exclusion criterion, amendment of treatment administration, adjustment for hypothesis test, revision of endpoints, adjustment of equivalence/non-inferiority margin, amendment of trial timelines, increasing or reducing the number of interim analyses, etc.

An adaptive design may not be limited to the ones mentioned above. In practice, multiple features may be included in one trial at the same time. It is generally suggested not to include too many which will significantly increase the trial complexity and difficulty in result interpretation.

It should be also emphasized that adjustment or amendment for adaptive designs must be pre-specified in the protocol and thoroughly planned. Any post-hoc adjustment should be avoided.

17.15. International Multi-center Clinical Trial[5]

An international multicenter random clinical trial (MRCT) refers to the trial conducted in multicenters and multiple countries or regions under the same protocol concurrently. MRCTs can greatly facilitate NDAs in several countries or regions simultaneously.

17.15.1. *Bridging study*

If a new drug has been approved in the original region, an additional trial may be needed for the extrapolation of treatment efficacy and safety to the new region for drug registration. Such an additional trial is called as bridging study.

17.15.1.1. *Bridging method*

Several methods or strategies accepted by health authorities may include:

PMDA Method 1: The probability of preserving a percentage of treatment effect in region J to overall treatment effect greater than some fixed value (π) should be no less than $1-\beta$. It can be written as

$$P(D_J|D_{\text{all}} > \pi) \geq 1 - \beta,$$

where D_J describes the observed effect in region J and D_{all} represents the overall effect. Here, $\pi > 50\%$, $\beta < 20\%$.

PMDA Method 2: The probability of having effect observed in every region is greater than 0 should be no less than $1-\beta$, that is

$$P(D_i > 0,\ for\ all\ i) \geq 1 - \beta.$$

SGDDP approach: Huang, *et al.* (2012) proposed a framework of global drug development program (SGDDP), in which trial has two phases: an MRCT and a local clinical trial (LCT). The MRCT is conventional confirmatory phase III trials conducted in multiple regions or countries, while LCT is a bridging study separate from the MRCT. In this program, two types of populations may be included: target ethnic group (TE) and non-target ethnic group (NTE). The test statistic Z of the TE can therefore be constructed as

$$Z = \sqrt{1-w}Z_1 + \sqrt{w}Z_2,$$

where Z_1 is the test statistic of TE and Z_2 is the test statistic of NTE assuming Z_1 and Z_2 are independent. If both Z_1 and Z_2 follow the normal distribution, Z is a weighted average and follows the normal distribution as well.

Bayesian methods can be used for bridging trials including Bayesian predictive methods, empirical Bayes methods and Bayesian mixed models, etc.

17.15.2. *Evaluation of consistency*

The commonly used consistency criteria include (1) reproducibility probability (PR), a probability of reproducing the same result conclusion by repeating the same trial among the same trial population. The three calculation methods may include the estimated power approach, the confidence interval approach and Bayesian approach; (2) generalizability probability (PG), a probability of observing the positive treatment effect in the new region given that treatment effect may vary among regions.

17.16. Clustered Randomized Controlled Trial (cRCT)[22]

A cRCT is one to randomize subjects as a cluster (or group). A cluster, sometimes called as a unit, can be a community, class, family and manufactory site. If a cluster is allocated into one treatment, all subjects in the cluster will receive the same treatment or intervention. The cRCT is sometimes used for the large scale of vaccine trials or community intervention trials.

Because the subjects in one cluster may share some similar characteristics, they are not independent of each other. For example, the students in one class receive the same course education and tend to have the similar level of knowledge; family members may tend to share similar preference or habit of food intake; the workers in the same manufactory site may share the similar working environment. Therefore, the outcome measures may share similar patterns correspondingly. In conventional setting, independence is an assumption required for many statistical analysis methods. Since the assumption may not hold for cRCTs, these statistical analysis methods may not be applicable.

According to the design features of cRCTs, the aspects below are important to be considered for design, conduct, analysis and report.

(1) Quality control: Because the randomization is based on clusters, the blinding of a cRCT should be kept during the conduct. In addition, the potential bias introduced by subject inclusion and exclusion, loss to follow-up, etc., should be minimized.
(2) Sample size: In cRCTs, sample size calculations shall be performed by considering the correlation coefficient in clusters. For example, the number of clusters from the treatment and control groups may be calculated by

$$m = \frac{[1 + (k-1)\rho]}{k} \frac{2 \times (z_{1-\alpha/2} + z_{1-\beta})^2 \sigma^2}{\delta^2},$$

where ρ is the intra-class correlation coefficient, m is the number of clusters, k is average number of subjects in the cluster. The total sample size in treatment group is therefore $n = m \times k$.

Denote N as the sample size required for a conventional randomized trial sharing the same trial assumptions. There is a formula describing the relationship with the required sample size for cRCTs, i.e.

$$mk = [1 + (k - 1)\rho]N.$$

As seen from the formula, only if the correlation coefficient in the cluster is larger than 0, the total sample size of a cRCT is generally bigger than a conventional RCT.

(3) Analysis method: For cRCTs, analysis methods of generalized estimation equation (GEE) and multilevel model are often used to handle the correlation within the clusters (Refer to Secs. 3.18 and 4.19).
(4) Result and report: The suggestions and recommendations in CONSORT should be taken.

17.17. Pragmatic Research[23,24]

Pragmatic research is the trial to determine the effectiveness of treatment in the real world and make clinical decisions. The design of pragmatic trial should ensure that the participants and patients in the real world are as similar as possible, in order to verify the external validity. Such studies will also try to ensure that treatment in the trial can be carried out in the real clinical trials, in order to obtain clinical outcomes and effectiveness assessments that are accepted by clinicians, patients, regulators and government agencies.

The conventional clinical trials are aimed to explore and confirm the treatment effect (i.e. efficacy and safety) in the controlled settings. The bias and confounding factors should be carefully controlled for an efficient trial. The trials are commonly conducted with the control group (placebo or active control).

CONSORT makes several suggestions to report the trial results from a pragmatic trial in addition to those recommended for a conventional trial.

Limitations of a pragmatic trial may include: (1) the cost of a pragmatic trial may be higher than a conventional clinical trial with the complexity of design, analysis and result interpretation introduced by the flexible treatment; (2) no clear cut or definition to differentiate whether a trial is completely pragmatic or controlled. In most cases, trials may combine certain characteristics from a pragmatic and controlled trial; and (3) pragmatic trial

Table 17.17.1. Comparison between pragmatic trials and conventional clinical trials.

	Pragmatic research	Clinical trials
Population	Patients in the real world; diversity and heterogeneity for the external validity	Relatively homogeneous subjects under trial protocol to maximize the internal validity
Treatment	Flexible treatment	Clearly defined treatment in protocols
Control	Active control	Determined by trial objectives and endpoints
Follow-up	Relatively long-term follow up	Relatively short-term follow up
Blinding	May not be able to use blinding in general	Use blinding as much as possible
Endpoint	Broader, patients-centered outcomes	Measurable symptoms or clinical outcomes
Randomization	Can be randomized, but the design can also consider the patient preference	Feasibility evaluation; Randomization is the gold standard
Phase	Mostly phase IV	Phase I, II or III
Sample size	Relatively big	Relatively small

Table 17.17.2. Two points to consider for the report of pragmatic trial results.

	Points to consider
Population	To include a good spectrum of patients in the various clinical settings and reflect in the trial inclusion/exclusion criteria for the population representativeness.
Treatment	To describe the additional resources on top of regular clinical practices.
Outcome	To describe the rationale of selecting the clinical endpoints, relevance and the required follow-up period, etc.
Sample size	To describe the minimally clinically important difference if the sample size calculation is based on that assumption.
Blinding	To describe the reasons and rationales why blinding cannot be adopted and implemented.
Generalizability	To describe the design considerations in determining the measure outcomes and discuss the potential variation introduced by the different clinical settings.

is not recommended for early clinical studies to explore biological effects of a new treatment.

Pragmatic trial maintains a good external validity on the basis of certain level of internal validity, provides a reasonable compromise between observational trials and controlled clinical trials. Pragmatic trials are increasingly valued by the scientific community, clinicians and regulators, however, they cannot replace conventional clinical trials. Both concepts play important roles in generating and providing evidence in medical research.

17.18. Comparative Effectiveness Research (CER)[5,24]

CER is sometimes called as outcome research. It is to evaluate medical interventions in the real world. In CER, "medical intervention" refers to the treatment or interventions that patients actually receive; "final outcome" may include the measurements with patient centricity including the outcomes that patients feel and care (e.g. recovery, quality of life, death, etc.) and the cost of the intervention (e.g. time, budget and cost and etc.); "real medical environment" emphasizes the real world setting which may differ from the "controlled setting" in RCTs for the evaluation of new drugs, medical devices or medical techniques.

The notion of "outcome" was firstly introduced by a few researchers in evaluating healthcare quality in 1966. Carolyn Clancy and John Eisenberg published a paper in "Science" in 1998[23] and addressed the importance of outcome research. The conception of CER was later proposed in 2009 which provides more detailed elaboration than outcome research. It takes patients as care center to systematically research the effect of different interventions and treatment strategies including diagnosis and monitoring the treatment and the patient health in the real world. It evaluates the health outcomes of various patient clusters by developing, expanding and using all sources of data for the basis of decision making by patient, medical personnel, government and insurance agencies. The concept has been successfully implemented in health economics and policy research. The analysis methods are similar to those used in big data analytics, which are exploratory in nature and data driven.

The comparative strategies or measures may include comparison between different types of drugs or interventions, administration, disease and genotype, surgery, hospitalization and outpatient treatment. It may also include comparison among interventional devices and medicine treatment and different nursing model (e.g. patient management, technical training).

The types of analysis methods may include but are not limited to the systematic review or meta-analysis, decision analysis, retrospective analysis and prospective analysis covering registry studies in which patients may not enter into clinical controlled trials or pragmatic trials.

The key principles of selected methods are to explore the data for accumulative knowledge, including data mining and machine learning methods while controlling and adjusting the confounding and bias (e.g. propensity score matching).

CERs are aimed to evaluate the effectiveness of the intervention in the real world. However, the real environment could be very complex. Several critical questions remain including the selection of the outcome measures, the control and adjustment of confounders and bias, the standardization of various databases and the collaborative platforms for data integrity and quality, the generalizability and representativeness of the study results, etc.

In medical research, RCT and CER are complementary to each other. RCT are primarily in pre-marketing settings prior to drug approval, and CERs are having the increasing importance in the post-marketing settings.

17.19. Diagnostic Test[1,5]

A diagnostic test is a kind of medical test to aid in the diagnosis or detection of a disease. The basic statistical methods may include the comparison to a gold standard test to assess the quality.

17.19.1. *A gold standard test*

A gold standard test is the diagnosis method widely accepted and acknowledged as being reliable and authoritative in the medical society. It may rely on the conclusion of histopathology inspection, imaging inspection, culture and identification of the isolated pathogen, long-term follow-up, and other common confirmation approach used in clinical practice.

The possible result from a diagnosis test may be summarized in Table 17.19.1.

Common statistical measures used in diagnosis tests may include (refer to Table 17.19.1):

(1) Sensitivity and specificity:

$$Se = P(T_+|D_+) = a/(a+c),$$

$$Sp = P(T-|D-) = d/(b+d).$$

Table 17.19.1. The fourfold table of diagnosis test.

Result of center diagnosis test	Gold standard		In total
	Diseased D_+	Not diseased D_-	
Positive T_+	a(true positive)	b(false positive)	$a+b$
Negative T_-	c(false negative)	d(true negative)	$c+d$
In total	$a+c$	$b+d$	$N=a+b+c+d$

(2) Mistake diagnostic rate and omission diagnostic rate:

$$\text{Mistake diagnostic rate } \alpha = b/(b+d),$$

$$\text{Omission diagnostic rate } \beta = c/(a+c).$$

(3) Positive predictive value (PV_+) and negative predictive value (PV_-):

$$PV_+ = \frac{a}{a+b}, \quad PV_- = \frac{d}{c+d}.$$

And the relationship is

$$PV_+ = \frac{prevalence \times Se}{prevalence \times Se + (1 - Sp) \times (1 - prevalence)},$$

$$PV_- = \frac{Sp \times (1 - prevalence)}{Sp \times (1 - prevalence) + prevalence \times (1 - Se).}$$

(4) Accuracy (π),

$$\pi = (a+d)/N.$$

Another expression of Accuracy is

$$\pi = \frac{a+c}{N} Se + \frac{b+d}{N} Sp.$$

(5) Youden index (YI):

$$YI = Se + Sp - 1.$$

(6) Odd product (OP):

$$OP = \frac{Se}{1-Se} \frac{Sp}{1-Sp} = \frac{ad}{bc}.$$

(7) Positive likelihood ratio (LR_+) and negative likelihood ratio (LR_-):

$$LR_+ = \frac{P(T_+|D_+)}{P(T_+|D_-)} = \left(\frac{a}{a+c}\right) \Big/ \left(\frac{b}{b+d}\right) = Se/(1 - Sp),$$

$$LR_- = \frac{P(T_-|D_+)}{P(T_-|D_-)} = \left(\frac{c}{a+c}\right) \Big/ \left(\frac{d}{b+d}\right) = (1 - Se)/Sp.$$

LR_+ and LR_- are the two important measures to evaluate reliability of a diagnosis test which incorporates sensitivity (*Se*) and specificity (*Sp*) and will not be impacted by prevalence. They are more stable than *Se* and *Sp*.

In the comparison of two diagnosis tests, receiver operating characteristic curve (ROC) and area under the ROC curve (AUC) also commonly used.

17.20. Statistical Analysis Plan and Report[1,5]

17.20.1. *Statistical analysis plan*

A statistical session is an important component in a protocol. It describes overview of the statistical considerations and methods to analyze the trial data. A statistical analysis plan can be an independent document including more detailed, technical and operational contents of statistical specifications than that in a protocol. The statistical analysis plan may include:

(1) Study overview: The session includes study objectives and design, selection of control, randomization scheme and implementation, blinding method and implementation, definition of primary and secondary endpoints, type of comparison and hypothesis test, the sample size calculation, definition of analysis data sets, etc.
(2) Statistical analysis method: It may describe descriptive statistics, analysis models for parameter estimation, confidence level, hypothesis test, covariates in the analysis models, handling of center effect, the handling of missing data and outlier, interim analysis, subgroup analysis, multiplicity adjustment, safety analysis, etc.
(3) Display template of analysis results: The analysis results need to be displayed in the form of statistical tables, figures and listings. The table content, format and layout need to be designed in the plan for clarity of result presentation.

17.20.2. *Statistical analysis report*

A statistical analysis report is a report of summarizing the complete analysis results according to a statistical analysis plan. It is an important document to interpret analysis results and serves as an important basis for writing the study report. The general contents may include:

(1) study overview (refers to that in the statistical analysis plan),
(2) statistical analysis method (refers to that in the statistical analysis plan),
(3) Result and conclusion of statistical analysis including:
    - Subject disposition (including number of recruited subjects, screening failures, concomitant medication use, compliance summary, summary of analysis sets, etc.), (Refer to Figure. 17.20.1).

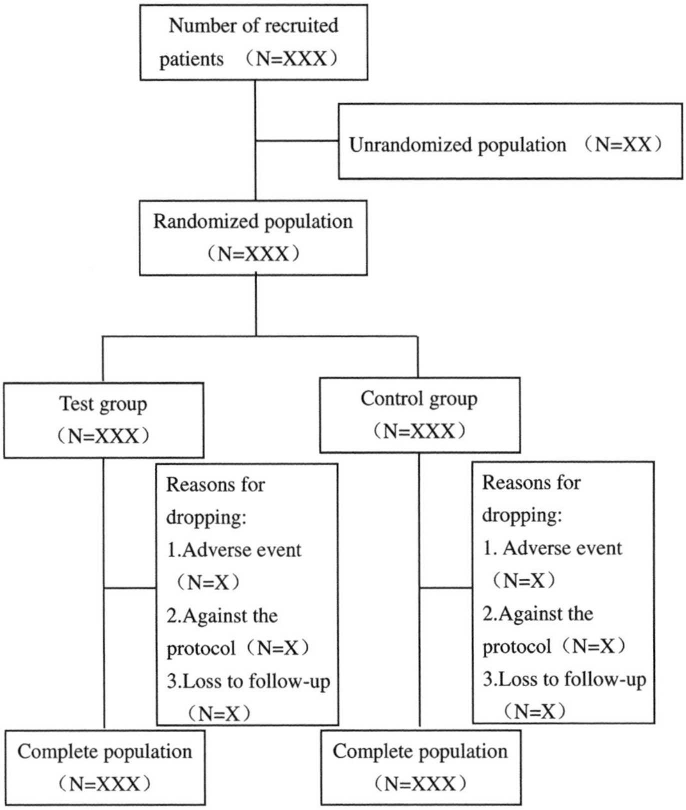

Fig. 17.20.1. Flowchart of a clinical trial.

— Comparison of baseline characteristics (including demographic distribution, medical history, drug, baseline medication, etc.)
— Analysis of primary and secondary endpoints (including descriptive and inferential analysis, e.g. point estimate and confidence interval, *p*-values of hypothesis test, etc.)
— Safety summary (including adverse events, serious adverse events, AEs leading to treatment discontinuation, abnormal laboratory findings, worsening of disease conditions during the treatment, the safety outcomes in relationship to the treatment administration, etc.)

17.21. Introduction to CONSORT[25,26]

Given the importance of RCTs as the important research methods to draw conclusions in medical research, several worldly reputed editors of medical journals formulated a team including clinical epidemiologists, clinical specialists and statisticians to reach a consensus for the standardization of reporting RCT results in mid-1990s.

A consolidated standard of reporting trials (CONSORT statement) was issued after 2 years of comprehensive research on RCTs. The statement was published in 1996 and was applied by the *Journal of Clinical Pharmacology.* Later, the standard was revised in 2001 and 2010, respectively, and now is widely used by many highly reputed journals worldwide.

According to a paper structure, CONSORT statement is consists of six parts: title and abstract, introduction, methods, result, discussion and other information. It includes 25 terms, 37 provisions. (refer to Table 17.21.1).

Nowadays, CONSORT statement has been widely used in different types of research, including the cRCTs (refer to Sec. 17.16), etc.

Table 17.21.1. CONSORT statement (Version in 2010).

Section/topic	Item no.	Checklist item
Title and abstract	1a	Identification as a randomized trial in the title
	1b	Structured summary of trail design, methods, results and conclusions
Introduction		
Background and objectives	2a	Scientific background and explanation of rationale
	2b	Specific objectives or hypotheses
Methods		
Trial design	3a	Description of trial design (such as parallel, factorial), including allocation ratio
	3b	Important changes to methods after trial commencement (such as eligibility criteria) with reasons
Participants	4a	Eligibility criteria for participants
	4b	Settings and locations where the data were collected
Interventions	5	The interventions for each group with sufficient details to allow replication, including how and when they were actually administered
Outcomes	6a	Completely defined prespecified primary and secondary outcomes measures including how and when they were assessed
	6b	Any changes to trial outcomes after the trial commenced with reasons
Sample size	7a	How sample size was determined
	7b	When applicable, explanation of any interim analyses and stopping guidelines

(*Continued*)

Table 17.21.1. (*Continued*)

Section/topic	Item no.	Checklist item
Randomization	8a	Method used to generate the random allocation sequence
Sequence generation	8b	Type of randomization, details of any restriction (such as blocking and block size)
Allocation concealment mechanism	9	Mechanism used to implement the random allocation sequence (such as sequentially numbered containers), describing any steps taken to conceal the sequence until interventions were assigned
Implement	10	Who generated the random allocation sequence, who enrolled participants, and who assigned participants to interventions
Blinding	11a	If done, who was blinded after assignment to interventions (for example, participants, care providers, those assessing outcomes) and how
	11b	If relevant, description of the similarity of interventions
Statistical methods	12a	Statistical methods used to compare groups for primary and secondary outcomes
	12b	Methods for additional analyses, such as subgroup analyses and adjusted analyses
Results		
Participant flow (a diagram is strongly recommended)	13a	For each group, the numbers of participants who were randomly assigned, received intend treatment, and were analyzed for the primary outcome
	13b	For each group, losses and exclusions after randomization, together with reasons
Recruitment	14a	Dates defining the periods of recruitment and follow-up
	14b	Why the trial ended or was stopped
Baseline data	15	A table showing baseline demographic and clinical characteristics for each group
Numbers analyzed	16	For each group, number of participants (denominator) included in each analysis and Whether the analysis was by original assigned groups
Outcomes and estimation	17a	Assessment effect of each primary and secondary outcomes for each group and its precision (such as 95% confidence interval).
	17b	For binary outcomes, presentation of both absolute and relative effect sizes is recommended
Ancillary analyses	18	Results of any other analyses performed, including subgroup analyses and Adjusted analyses, distinguishing prespecified from exploratory
Adverse evens	19	All adverse events or unintended effects in each group (for specific guidance, See CONSORT[26])

(*Continued*)

Table 17.21.1. (*Continued*)

Section/topic	Item no.	Checklist item
Discussion		
Limitations	20	Trial limitations, addressing sources of potential bias, imprecision; and, if relevant, Multiplicity of analyses
Generalizability	21	Generalizability (external validity, applicability) of the trial findings
Interpretation	22	Interpretation consistent with results, balancing benefits and harms, and considering other relevant evidence
Other information		
Registration	23	Registration number and name of trial registry
Protocol	24	Where the full trial protocol can be accessed, if available
Funding	25	Sources of funding and other support (such as supply of drugs), role of funders

References

1. China Food and Drug Administration. *Statistical Principles for Clinical Trials of Chemical and Biological Products*, 2005.
2. Friedman, LM, Furberg, CD, DeMets, DL. *Fundamentals of Clinical Trials.* (4th edn.). Berlin: Springer, 2010.
3. ICH E5. Ethnic Factors in the Acceptability of Foreign Clinical Data, 1998.
4. Fisher, RA. The Design of Experiments. New York: Hafner, 1935.
5. ICH. E9. Statistical Principles for Clinical Trials, 1998.
6. ICH E10. Choice of Control Group and Related Issues in Clinical Trials, 2000.
7. CPMP. Points to Consider on Multiplicity issues in clinical trials, 2009.
8. Dmitrienko, A, Tamhane, AC, Bretz, F. *Multiple Testing Problems in Pharmaceutical Statistics.* Boca Raton: Chapman & Hall, CRC Press, 2010.
9. Tong Wang, Dong Yi on behalf of CCTS. Statistical considerations for multiplicity in clinical trial. *J. China Health Stat.* 2012, 29: 445–450.
10. Jennison, C, Turnbull, BW. *Group Sequential Methods with Applications to Clinical Trials.* Boca Raton: Chapman & Hall, 2000.
11. Chow, SC, Liu, JP. *Design and Analysis of Bioavailability and Bioequivalence Studies,* New York: Marcel Dekker, 2000.
12. FDA. Guidance for Industry: Non-Inferiority Clinical Trials, 2010.
13. Jielai Xia *et al.* Statistical considerations on non-inferiority design. *China Health Stat.* 2012, 270–274.
14. Altman, DG, Dor'e, CJ. Randomisation and baseline comparisons in clinical trials. *Lancet,* 1990, 335: 149–153.
15. EMA. Guideline on Adjustment for Baseline Covariates in Clinical Trials, 2015.
16. Cook, DI, Gebski, VJ, Keech, AC. Subgroup analysis in clinical trials. *Med J.* 2004, 180(6): 289–291.
17. Wang, R, Lagakos, SW, Ware, JH, *et al.* Reporting of subgroup analyses in clinical trials. *N. Engl. J. Med.,* 2007, 357: 2189–2194.
18. Chow, SC, Chow, M. *Adaptive Design Methods in Clinical Trials.* Boca Raton: Chapman & Hall, 2008.

19. FDA. Guidance for Industry: Adaptive Design Clinical Trials for Drugs and Biologics, 2010.
20. Tunis, SR, Stryer, DB, Clancy, CM. Practical clinical trials: Increasing the value of clinical research for decision making in clinical and health policy. *JAMA*, 2003, 291(4): 425–426.
21. Mark Chang. *Adaptive Design Theory and Implementation Using SAS and R*. Boca Raton: Chapman & Hall, 2008.
22. Donner, A, Klar, N. *Design and Analysis of Cluster Randomization Trials in Health Research*. London: Arnold, 2000.
23. Clancy, C, Eisenberg, JM. Outcome research: Measuring the end results of health care. *Science*, 1988, 282(5387): 245–246.
24. Cook, TD, Campbell, DT. *Quasi-Experimentation: Design and Analysis Issues for Field Settings*. Boston: Houghton-Mifflin, 1979.
25. Campbell, MK, Elbourne, DR, Adman, DG. CONSORT statement: Extension to cluster randomized trials. *BMJ*, 2004, 328: 702–708.
26. Moher, D, Schuh, KF, Altman, DG *et al.* The CONSORT statement: Revised recommendations for improving the quality of reports of parallel-group randomized trials. *Lancet*, 2001, 357: 1191–1194.

About the Author

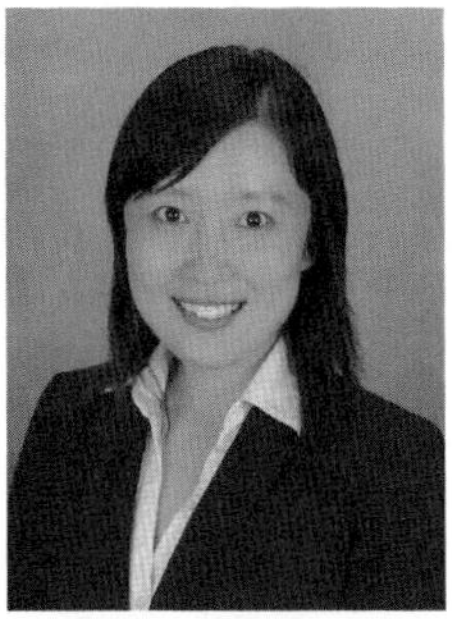

Dr. Luyan Dai is currently heading the statistics group based in Asia as a regional function contributing to the global development at BI. She was relocated to Asia in 2012 to build up the statistics team in Shanghai for Boehringer Ingelheim. Prior to this, she worked at Boehringer Ingelheim in the U.S.A. since 2009. She was the statistics leader for several phase II/III programs for hepatitis C and immunology. She was also the leading statistician for a respiratory product in COPD achieving the full approval by FDA.

In the past years, she has accumulated solid experience with various regulatory authorities including FDA, China FDA, Korea FDA, in Asian countries. She has gained profound statistical insights across disease areas and development phases. Her main scientific interests are in the fields of Bayesian statistics, quantitative methods for decision making and Multi-Regional Clinical Trials.

Dr. Luyan Dai received her PhD in statistics at the University of Missouri-Columbia, the U.S.A. She started her career at Pfizer U.S. as clinical statistician in the field of neuroscience after graduation.

CHAPTER 18

STATISTICAL METHODS IN EPIDEMIOLOGY

Songlin Yu* and Xiaomin Wang

18.1. Measures of Incidence Level[1,2]

Various measures are considered to quantify the seriousness of a disease spread in a population. In this term, we introduce some indices based on new cases. They are incidence, incidence rate and cumulative incidence.

1. Incidence: It is supposed that in a fixed population consisting of N individuals, the number of new cases D occurs during a specified period of time. The incidence F is calculated by using the equation $F = (D/N) \times 10^n$. The superscript n is a proportional constant used for readability. Incidence expresses a disease risk of an individual during the period. It is an estimate of incidence probability. This indicator is also known as incidence frequency. Because of population movement, it is not possible for all persons in the population to remain in the observation study throughout. Some people may withdraw from the observation study for some reasons. Let the number of withdrawn persons be C, then the adjusted equation becomes $F = [D/(N - C/2)] \times 10^n$. The adjusted formula supposes that the withdrawn people were all observed half of the period.

We can subgroup the start population and new cases by sex or/and age. Then the incidence by sex or/and age group can be obtained.

Incidence F belongs to a binomial distributed variable. Its variance $\mathrm{Var}(F)$ is estimated by using the equation: $\mathrm{Var}(F) = F(1 - F)/N$.

2. Incidence rate. As opposed to incidence, which is an estimate of probability of disease occurrence, the incidence rate is a measure of probabilistic

*Corresponding author: slyu6153@hotmail.com

density function of disease occurrence. Its numerator is the number of new cases D, its denominator is the observed/exposed amount of person-time T. The incidence rate is calculated by using the equation $R = (D/T) \times 10^n$, where the superscript n is a proportional constant chosen for readability. The observational unit of T can be day, week, month or year. If year is used as observational unit, the indicator is called incidence rate per person-year. The indicator is used usually to describe the incidence level of chronic disease. Person-time should be collected carefully. If you are lacking precise person-time data, the quantity (population at midterm)×(length of observed period) may be used as an approximation of the amount of person-time T.

When D is treated as a Poisson random variable with theoretical rate λ, then $D \sim Poisson(\lambda T)$, where λT is the expectation *of* D, and $\text{Var}(D) = \lambda T$. The variance of rate R *is* calculated by using the formula: $\text{Var}(R) = \text{Var}(D/T) = D/T^2$. Incidence rate is a type of incidence measures. It indicates the rate of disease occurrence in a population. This indicator has its lower bound of 0, but no upper bound.

3. Cumulative incidence. Let $F_i(i = 1, \ldots, c)$ be the incidence of a disease in a population with age group i, and the time span of the age group is l_i. The cumulative incidence p_i is calculated as $p_i = F_i \times l_i$ for a person who is experienced from the start to the end of the age group. For a person who is experienced from the age group 0 up to the age group c, the cumulative incidence P is calculated as $P = 1 - \prod_{i=0}^{c}(1 - p_i)$. It is the estimated value of disease probability a person experienced from birth to the end of c. If the incidence rate is r_i for age group i, its cumulative incidence is then estimated as $p_i = 1 - \exp(r_i \times l_i)$. This formula can be used to calculate the cumulative incidence P.

18.2. Prevalence Level[3–5]

It is also known as prevalence rate. The quantity reflects the load of existing cases (unhealed and newly occurred cases) on a population. If a researcher is interested in exploring the load of some attributes like smoking or drinking in a community, the prevalence level can also be used to describe the level of the event. There are three kinds of indices used to describe prevalence level as follows:

1. Point prevalence proportion: It is also known as point prevalence. This is a measure often used to describe the prevalence level. Simple point prevalence proportion (p_t) at time t is estimated as the proportion of the number of prevalent cases C_t over the study population of size N at time

t. The quantity is calculated by the following equation: $p_t = (C_t/N_t) \times k$, where k is a proportional constant, for example, taking the value of 100% or $100,000/10^5$.

Point prevalence proportion is usually used in cross-sectional study or disease screen research.

2. Period prevalence proportion: Its numerator is the diseased number at the beginning of the period plus the new disease cases occurring in the whole period. The denominator is the average number of population in the period. The quantity is calculated as

$$P_p = \frac{C_s + C_p}{\text{Average number of population in the period}} \times k,$$

where C_s is the number of cases at the beginning of the period, C_p is the number of new cases occurring in the period.

Expanding the period of the period prevalence proportion to the life span, the measure becomes life time prevalence. Life time prevalence is used to describe the disease load at a certain time point for remittent diseases which recur often.

The level of prevalence proportion depends on both the incidence, and the sustained time length of the disease. The longer the diseased period sustains, the higher the level of the prevalence proportion, and vice versa. When both prevalence proportion and the sustained time length of a disease are stable, the relationship between the prevalence proportion and the incidence can be expressed as

$$\text{Incidence} = \frac{\text{Point prevalence proportion}}{\text{Average sustained time period of the disease}},$$

where the average period of disease is the sustained length from diagnosis to the end (recovery or dead) of the disease. For example, the point prevalence proportion of a disease is 2.0%, and the average length of the disease is 3 years. The disease incidence is estimated as

$$\text{Incidence per year} = \frac{0.02}{(1 - 0.02) \times 3} = 0.0068(6.8‰).$$

If the prevalence proportion of a disease is low its incidence is estimated approximately by the following equation:

$$\text{Incidence} = \frac{\text{Point prevalenc proportion}}{\text{Average sustained time period lasted of the disease}}.$$

There are two methods to estimate 95% confidence intervals for prevalence proportion.

(1) Normal approximation methods. The formula is

$$95\%\mathrm{CI} = P \pm 1.96\sqrt{P(1-P)/(N+4)},$$

where P is the prevalence proportion and N the number of the population.

(2) Poisson distribution-based method: When the observed number of cases is small, its 95% CI is based on the Poisson distribution as

$$95\%\mathrm{CI} = P \pm 1.96\sqrt{D/N^2},$$

where D is the number of cases, N defined as before.

Because prevalent cases represent survivors, prevalence measures are not as well suited to identify risk factors as are the incidence measures.

18.3. Distribution of Disease[2,6,7]

The first step of epidemiological research is to explore the disease distribution in various groups defined by age, gender, area, socio-economic characteristics and time trend by using descriptive statistical methods. The purpose of this step is to identify the clustering property in different environments in order to provide basic information for further etiological research of the disease. The commonly used descriptive statistics are the number of cases of the disease and its derived measures like incidences, rates or prevalences.

1. Temporal distribution: According to the characteristics of a disease and the purpose of research the measurement unit of time can be expressed in day, month, season, or year. If the monitoring time is long enough for a disease, the so-called secular trend, periodic circulation, seasonal change, and short-term fluctuation can be identified. Diseases which produce long-term immunity often appear during peak year and non-epidemic year. Diseases related with meteorological condition often display seasonal characteristics. In order to test the clustering in time of a disease, it is necessary to collect accurate time information for each case. Let T be the length of the observational period and D the total number of cases occurred in the period $(0 \sim T)$ in an area. If T is divided into discontinuous m segments $(t_1, t_2, \ldots, t_m)$, and the number of cases in the i-th segment is $d_i (i = 1, 2, \ldots, m)$, and $D = d_1 + d_2 + \ldots + d_m$, we rescale the occurrence time as $z_i = t_i/T$ $i = 1, \ldots, m$. Then the test hypothesis can be established as H_0: the time of the disease occurrence is randomly distributed in the period $(0 \sim T)$; H_a : the time of the disease occurrence is not randomly distributed in the period of $(0 \sim T)$. The multinomial distribution law is used to test the probability of the event occurrence as

$$\Pr\{D_1 = d_1, \ldots, D_m = d_m | (p_1, \ldots, p_m)\} = \prod_{i=1}^{m} p_i^{d_i},$$

where $p_i = 1/m$ is a fraction of m segments in time length.

2. Geographic distribution: The term of geography here is a generic term indicating natural area, not restricting the defined administrative area only. Some chronic diseases like endemic goiter, osteoarthrosis deformans endemica are influenced severaly by local geometrical environment. The variety of disease distribution from place to place can be displayed with geographic maps, which can provide more information about geographic continuity than the statistical table. Usually, the homogeneous Poisson process can be used to characterize the geographic distribution. This process supposes that the frequency of an event occurring in area A follows the Poisson distribution with its expectation λ. The estimate of λ is

$$\hat{\lambda} = \frac{\text{Number of events occurred in area } A}{\text{Number of population in that area}}.$$

If, for example, area A is divided into m subareas, the number, R_i, of the population and the number, D_i, of the events in subarea $i (i = 1, 2, \ldots, m)$ are counted, the expectation of the events is calculated as $E_i = R_i \times \hat{\lambda}$ for subarea i. Then, a Chi-square test is used to identify if there exists some clustering. The formula of the Chi-square statistic is

$$\chi^2 = \sum_{i=1}^{m} (D_i - E_i)^2 / E_i, \quad \chi^2 \sim \chi^2_{(m-1)}.$$

3. Crowed distribution: Many infectious and non-infectious diseases have high-risk population.

The phenomenon of disease clustering provides important information for etiological research and preventive strategy. There are many statistical methods aimed at testing disease clustering.

18.4. Cross-sectional Study[8,9]

It is also called prevalence proportion study or simply prevalence survey. The method is applied to obtain data of disease prevalence level and suspected factors in a fixed population at a time point or a very short time interval. The main purpose of the study is aimed at assessing the health needs of local residents, exploring the association between disease and exposure. It is also used to establish database for cohort study. This research method is a static survey. But if multiple cross-sectional studies are conducted at different time points for a fixed population, these multiple data sets can be concatenated as a systematic data come from cohort study. Owning to its relatively easy and economic characteristic, cross-sectional study is a convenient tool used to explore the relationship between disease and exposure in a population which have some fixed characteristics. It is also used in etiological research for sudden break-out of a disease. In order to obtain observational data with high quality, clearly-defined research purpose, well-designed questionnaire, statistically-needed sample size, and a certain response proportion are needed.

Steps of cross-sectional study are:

1. **Determination of study purpose**: The purpose of an investigation should be declared clearly. The relationship between disease and susceptible risk factor(s) should be clarified. The specific target should be achieved, and the evidence of the association should be obtained.
2. **Determination of objects and quantity**: Research object is referred to the population under investigation. For example, in order to explore the extent of health damage caused by pollution, it is necessary to investigate two kinds of people, one who is exposed to the pollutant, and the other who is not exposed to the pollutant. It is also needed to consider the dose–response association between the degree of health damage and the dose exposed. The minimum necessary sample size is estimated based on the above consideration.
3. **Determination of observed indicators**: It is necessary to define the exposure, its dose, monitoring method, and its standard; to define the health damage, its detecting method and standard. It is also necessary to record every result accurately, and to maintain accuracy during the whole course of field performance.
4. **Statistical analysis**: The primary statistical index used in cross-sectional study is the disease prevalence measure in both exposed and unexposed populations, respectively. The ratio of the two prevalences, namely relative risk, is used to describe the association between disease and exposure. For example, Table 18.4.1 shows an artificial data organized in a 2×2 form resulted from a cross-sectional study.

From Table 18.4.1, the ratio of prevalence proportion of exposed group to that of unexposed group is $\mathrm{PR} = (0.2/0.02) = 10.0$. If there is no difference in

Table 18.4.1. An artificial 2 × 2 table resulted from cross-sectional study.

Risk factor	Health status		Total	Prevalence proportion
	Ill: Y	Healthy: $\bar{Y}$		
Exposed: X	50	200	250	0.20
Unexposed: $\bar{X}$	10	490	500	0.02

prevalence proportions between the two groups, the ratio would be 1.0 when ignoring measurement error. This ratio is an unbiased estimate of relative risk. But if the exposed level influences the disease duration, the ratio should be adjusted by the ratio of the two average durations (D_+/D_-) and the ratio of the two complementary prevalence proportions $(1 - P_+)/(1 - P_-)$. Prevalence proportion and relative risk have a relationship as follows:

$$\mathrm{PR} = \mathrm{RR} \times \frac{D_+}{D_-} \times \frac{(1 - P_+)}{(1 - P_-)},$$

where (D_+/D_-) is the ratio of the two average durations for the two groups with different exposure levels respectively, and P_+ and P_- are the prevalence proportions for the two groups, respectively too. When the prevalence proportions are small, the ratio of $(1 - P_+)/(1 - P_-)$ is close to 1.0.

Cross-sectional study reflects the status at the time point when observation takes place. Because this type of study cannot clarify the time-sequence for the disease and the exposure, it is not possible to create a causal relationship for the two phenomena.

18.5. Cohort Study[5,8]

It is also termed prospective, longitudinal or follow-up study. This type of study is designed to classify persons into groups according to their different exposure status at the beginning of the study; then follow-up the target subjects in each group to obtain their outcome of disease status; finally analyze the causal relation between disease and exposure. This is a confirmatory course from factor to outcome and is broadly used in the fields of preventive medicine, clinical trials, etiological research, etc. Its main weakness is that it requires more subjects under investigation and much longer time to follow up. As a consequence, it needs more input of time and money. That the subjects may easily be lost to follow-up is another shortage.

1. Study design: The causal and the outcome factors should be defined clearly in advance. The causal factor may exist naturally (such as smoking

Table 18.5.1. Data layout of cohort study.

Exposure	Observed subjects at the beginning (n_i)	Diseased number in the period (d_i)
Exposed: X	n_1	d_1
Unexposed: X	n_0	d_0

behavior, occupational exposure), or may be added from outside (such as treatment in clinical trial, intervention in preventive medicine). The outcome may be illness, death or recovery from disease. For convenience, in the following text, the term exposure is used as causal factor and disease as outcome.

The terms exposure and disease should be defined clearly with a list of objective criteria. At the beginning of a research, the baseline exposure and possible confounding factors should be recorded. One should also be careful to record the start time and the end time when disease or censoring occurs.

2. Calculation of incidence measures: If the observed time period is short, or the time effect on outcome can be ignored, the exposure situation can be divided into two groups: exposed and unexposed. The disease status can also be divided into two categories: diseased and not diseased, data are organized in a 2 by 2 table shown in Table 18.5.1.

The incidence of exposed group is $F_1 = d_1/n_1$, and the incidence of unexposed group is $F_0 = d_0/n_0$. The ratio of the two risks or relative risk is $RR = F_1/F_0$. If the data contain censored events, the adjusted incidence with censored number can be obtained. The whole follow-up period can be divided into several smaller segments. Then the segmental and cumulative incidences can be calculated.

If the observational unit is person-year, the total number of person-years can be obtained. Let the total numbers of person-years be T_1 and T_0 for the exposed and the unexposed group, respectively. The incidence rate of exposed group is calculated by $R_1 = d_1/T_1$, and that of unexposed group by $R_0 = d_0/T_0$. The denominators T_1 and T_0 represent the observed total numbers of person-years of exposed and non-exposed group, respectively. The relative risk is obtained by $RR = R_1/R_0$. If the total period is divided into several segments under the condition that the incidence rate in each segment remains unchanged and that the disease occurrence follows exponential distribution, the conditional incidence rate $R_{(k)}$ and the conditional incidence frequency $F_{(k)}$ have the relation by $F_{(k)} = 1-\exp(R_{(k)}\Delta_{(k)})$, where $\Delta_{(k)}$ is the time length of segment k.

If the follow-up time lasts even longer, the aging of subjects should be taken into account. Because age is an important confounding factor in some disease, the incidence level varies with age.

There is another research design called historical prospective study or retrospective cohort study. In this research, all subjects, including persons laid off from their posts, are investigated for their exposed time length and strength as well as their health conditions in the past. Their incidence rates are estimated under different exposed levels. This study type is commonly carried out in exploring occupational risk factors.

Unconditional logistic regression models and Cox's proportional hazard regression models are powerful multivariate statistical tools provided to analyze data from cohort study. The former model applies data with dichotomous outcome variable: the latter applies data with person-time. Additional related papers and monographs should be consulted in detail.

18.6. Case-control Study[2,8]

Case-control study is also termed retrospective study. It is used to retrospectively explore possible cause of a disease. The study needs two types of subjects: cases and non-cases who serve as controls. According to the difference between the exposed proportion of the case group and that of the proportion of the control group, a speculation is made about the association between disease and suspicious risk factor.

1. Types of designs: There are two main types of designs in case-control study. One type is designed for group comparison. In this design, case group and control group are created separately. The proportions of exposed history of the two groups are used for comparison. The other type is designed for comparison within matched sets. In each matched set, 1 case matches 1 to m controls who are similar to the corresponding case with respect to some confounding factors, where $m \leq 4$. Each matched set is treated as a subgroup. The exposure difference in each matched set is used for comparison. In classical case-control design, both cases and controls are from a general population. Their exposed histories are obtained via retrospective interview.

Nested case-control design is a newly developed design in case-control study realm. With this design, the cases and controls come from the same cohort, and their exposed histories can also be obtained from a complete database or a biological sample library.

2. Analytical indices: Data from case-control study cannot be made available to calculate any incidence indices, but are available to calculate odds

Table 18.6.1. Data layout of exposure from case–control study with group comparison design.

	Level of exposure			
Group	Yes	No	Total	Odds
Cases	a	b	n_1	a/b(odds1)
Controls	c	d	n_0	c/d(odds2)

Table 18.6.2. Data layout of exposure among N pairs from case-control study with 1:1 matching design.

Exposure of case	Exposure of control		
	+	−	Total
+	a	b	$a+b$
−	c	d	$c+d$
Total	$a+c$	$b+d$	N

ratio (OR). The index OR is used to reflect the difference of exposed proportions between cases and controls. Under the condition of low incidence for a disease, the OR is close to its relative risk. If the exposed level can be dichotomously divided into "Yes/No", the data designed with group comparison can be formed into a 2×2 table as shown in Table 18.6.1.

In view of probability, odds is defined as $p/(1-p)$, that is, the ratio of the positive proportion p to negative proportion $(1-p)$ for an event. With these symbols in Table 18.6.1, the odds of exposures for the case group is expressed as

$$\text{odds}_1 = (a/n_1)/(b/n_1) = a/b.$$

And the odds of exposures for the control group is expressed as

$$\text{odds}_0 = (c/n_0)/(d/n_0) = c/d.$$

The OR of the case group to the control group is defined as

$$\text{OR} = \frac{\text{odds}_1}{\text{odds}_0} = \frac{a/b}{c/d} = \frac{ad}{bc},$$

namely the ratio of the two odds.

For matching designed data the data layout varies with m, the control number in each matched set. Table 18.6.2 shows the data layout designed with 1:1 matching comparison. The N in the table represents the number of matched sets. The OR is calculated by b/c.

3. Multivariate models for case-control data analysis: The data layout is shown in Tables 18.6.1 and 18.6.2 are applied to analyze simple disease-exposure structure. When a research involves multiple variables, a multivariate logistic regression model is needed. There are two varieties of logistic regression models available for data analysis in case-control studies. The unconditional model is suitable for data with group comparison design and the conditional model is suitable for data with matching comparison design.

18.7. Case-crossover Design[9,10]

The case-crossover design is a self-matched case-control design proposed by Maclure.[10] The design was developed to assess the relationship between transient exposures and the acute adverse health event. The role of the case-crossover design is similar to the matched case-control study but the difficulties from selection for controls in matched case-control study have been avoided. In a general matched case-control study, the selection of controls is a difficult issue because the similarity between the case and the control in a matched set is demanded. Otherwise, it may introduce so-called "selection bias" into the study. In the case-crossover design, however, the past or future exposed situation of a subject serves as his/her own control. In this way, some "selection bias" like gender, life style, genetics, etc., can be avoided. At the same time, work load can be reduced. This kind of study is recently used in many research areas like causes of car accidents, drug epidemiology and relation between environmental pollution and health.

1. Selection of exposure period: In case-crossover design, the first step is to identify the exposure or risk period (exposure window), which is defined as the time interval from exposing to some risk substances until disease onset. For example, a person falls ill after 6 days since his exposure to some pollutant, the exposure period is 6 days. The health condition and the exposure situation 7 days before the person can be used as his/her own control. The control and the case automatically compose a matched set. Therefore, the key of the case-crossover design is that the exposure level of the control is used to compare with the exposure level of the case automatically.

2. Types of case-crossover designs: There are two types of case-crossover designs:

(1) **Unidirectional design**: Only the past exposed status of the case is used as control.

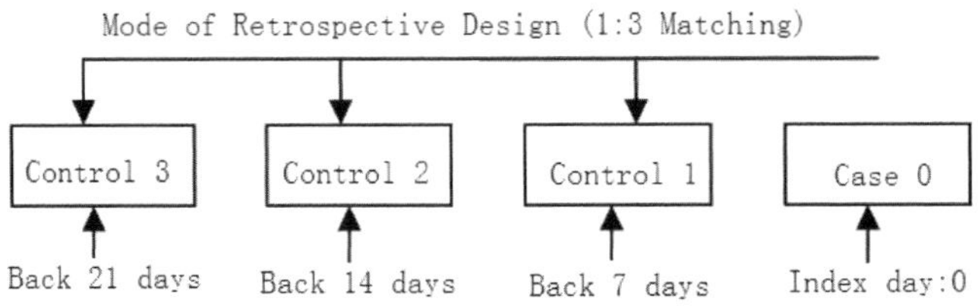

Fig. 18.7.1.

Table 18.7.1. Data layout of 1:1 matched case-crossover design.

	Control	
Case	Exposed	Unexposed
Exposed	a	b
Unexposed	c	d

(2) Bidirectional design: Both the past and the future exposed statuses of the case serve as controls. In this design, it is possible to evaluate the data both before and after the event occurs, and the possible bias which is generated by the time trend of the exposure could be eliminated.

In addition, based on how many time periods are to be selected, there exist 1:1 matched design and 1: $m(m > 1)$ matched design. Figure 18.7.1 shows a diagram of retrospective 1:3 matched case-crossover design.

3. Data compilation and analysis: The method of data compilation and analysis used for case-crossover design is the same as for general matched case-control study. For example, the data from 1:1 matched case-crossover design can form a fourfold table as shown in Table 18.7.1. The letters b and c in the table represent the observed inconsistent pairs. Like the general 1:1 matched case-control design, the OR is calculated with the usual formula by $\text{OR} = b/c$. Conditional logistic regression model can be applied for multivariate data coming from case-crossover design.

18.8. Interventional Study[5,11]

The interventional study is the research where an external factor is added to subjects in order to change the natural process of a disease or health status. Clinical trial for treatment effects is an example of intervention study that is based on hospital and patients are treated as subjects who receive the interventional treatment. Interventional study in epidemiology is a kind of study in which healthy people are treated as subjects who receive intervention, and the effects of the intervention factor on health are to be evaluated.

Interventional study has three types according to its different level of randomization in design.

1. Randomized controlled trial: This kind of trial is also called clinical trial owing to its frequent use in clinical medicine. The feature is that all eligible subjects are allocated into intervention group or control group based on complete randomization. Steps of the trial are:

Formulation of hypothesis → selection of suitable study population → determination of minimal necessary sample size → receiving subjects → baseline measurement of variables to be observed → completely randomized allocation of subjects into different groups → implementation of intervention → follow-up and monitoring the outcome → evaluation of interventional effects. But it is sometimes hard to perform complete randomization for intervention trial based on communities. In order to improve the power of the research, some special design may be used, such as stratified design, matching, etc.

2. Group randomized trial: This type of trial is also called randomized community trial in which the groups or clusters (communities, schools, classes, etc.), where subjects are included, are randomly allocated into experimental group or control group. For example, in a research on preventive effects of vaccination, students in some classes are allocated vaccine immunization group, while students in other classes are allocated control group. If the number of the communities is too small, the randomization has little meaning.

3. Quasi-experimental study: Quasi-experimental study is an experiment without random control group, even without independent control group. Pretest — post-test self-controlled trial and time series study belong to this kind of study. There is another trial called natural trial. It is used to observe the naturally progressive results between disease and exposure. There are many untypical trials like

(1) One-group pre-test–post-test self-controlled trial: The process of the trial is

Baseline measurements before intervention begins → intervention → follow-up and outcome measurements.

Because this kind of trial has no strict control with the observed difference in outcomes between pre-test and post-test, one cannot preclude the effects from confounding factors, including time trend.

(2) Two-group pre-test — post-test self-controlled trial: This trial is a modification of one-group pre-test–post-test self-controlled trial. Its trial processes are

Intervention group: Baseline measurements before intervention begins → intervention → follow-up and outcome measurements.

Control group: Baseline measurements before intervention begins → no intervention → follow-up and outcome measurements.

Because of no randomization, the control is not an equal-valued trial. But the influences from external factors are controlled, the internal effectiveness is stronger than the one-group pre-test–post-test self-controlled trial described above.

(3) Interrupted time series study: Before and after intervention, multiple measurements are to be made for the outcome variable (at least four times, respectively). This is another expanded form of one-group pre-test–post-test self-controlled trial. The effects of intervention can be evaluated through comparison between time trends before and after interventions. In order to control the possible interference it is better to add a control series. In this way, the study becomes a paralleled double time series study.

18.9. Screening[5,12,13]

Screening is the early detection and presumptive identification of an unrevealed disease or deficit by application of examinations or tests which can be applied rapidly and conveniently to large populations. The purpose of screening is to detect as early as possible, amongst apparently well people, those who actually have a disease and those who do not. Persons with a positive or indeterminate screening test result should be referred for diagnostic follow-up and then necessary treatment. Thus, early detection through screening will enhance the success of preventive or treatment interventions and prolong life and/or increase the quality of life. The validity of a screening test is assessed by comparing the results obtained via the screening test with those obtained via the so-called "gold standard" diagnostic test in the same population screened, as shown in Table 18.9.1.

A = true positives, B = false positives, C = false negatives, D = true negatives

Table 18.9.1. Comparison of classification results by screening test with "Gold standard" in diagnosis of a disease.

Screening test	Disease detected by gold standard test +	−	Total
+	A	B	R_1
−	C	D	R_2
Total	G_1	G_2	N

There are many evaluation indicators to evaluate the merits of a screening test. The main indicators are:

1. Sensitivity: It is also known as true positive rate, which reflects the ability of a test to correctly measure those persons who truly have the disease. It is calculated by expressing the true positives found by the test as a proportion of the sum of the true positives and the false negatives. i.e. Sensitivity $= (A/G_1) \times 100\%$; on the contrary, False negative $= (C/G_1) \times 100\%$. The higher the sensitivity, the lower the false negatives rate.

2. Specificity: Also known as true negatives rate, it reflects the ability of the test to correctly identify those who are disease-free. It is calculated by expressing the true negatives found by the test as a proportion of the sum of the true negatives and the false positives, i.e. Specificity $= (D/G_2) \times 100\%$; on the contrary, False positives $= (B/G_2) \times 100\%$. The higher the specificity, the lower the false positives rate.

3. Youden's index: It equals (sensitivity + specificity −1) or $(A/G_1 + D/G_2) - 1$. It is the ability of the test to correctly measure those who truly have the disease or are disease-free. The higher the Youden's index, the greater the correctness of a diagnosis.

4. Likelihood Ratio (LR): It is divided into positive LR^+ and negative LR^-. The two indices are calculated as:

$$\boldsymbol{LR}^+ = \text{true positives/false positives},$$

$$\boldsymbol{LR}^- = \text{false negatives/true negatives}.$$

The larger the LR^+ or the smaller the LR^-, the higher the diagnostic merit of the screening test.

5. Kappa value: It shows the random consistency ratio of two judgments from two inspectors for the same samples tested. Its value is calculated by

$$\text{Kappa} = \frac{N(A+D) - (R_1G_1 + R_2G_2)}{N^2 - (R_1G_1 + R_2G_2)}.$$

The Kappa value ≤ 0.40 shows poor consistency. The value in 0.4–0.75 means a medium to high consistency. The value above 0.75 shows very good consistency.

There are many methods to determine the cut-off value (critical point) for positive results of a screening test, such as (1) Biostatistical Method. It contains normal distribution method, percentile method, etc; (2) Receiver Operator Characteristic Curve also named ROC Curve Method, which can be used to compare the diagnostic value of two or more screening tests.

18.10. Epidemiologic Compartment Models[14,15]

Epidemic models use the mathematical method to describe propagation law, identify the role of related factors in disease spread among people, and provide guidelines of strategies for disease control. Epidemic models are divided into two categories: deterministic models and random models. Here we introduce compartment models as a kind of typical deterministic models. In 1927, Kermark and Mckendrick studied the Great Plague of London, which took place in 1665–1666, and contributed their landmark paper of susceptible-infectious-recovered (SIR) model. Their work laid the foundation of mathematical modeling for infectious diseases. In the classical compartment modeling, the target population is divided into three statuses called compartments: (1) Susceptible hosts, S, (2) Infectious hosts, I, and (3) Recovered/Removed hosts, R. In the whole epidemic period, the target population, N, keeps unchanged. Let $S(t), I(t)$ and $R(t)$ are the numbers at time t in each compartment, respectively, and $S(t) + I(t) + R(t) = N$. The development of the disease is unidirectional as $S \rightarrow I \rightarrow R$, like measles and chicken pox. Let β be the contact rate, that is, the probability when an infectious person contacts a susceptible person and causes infection. The number infected by an infectious patient is proportional to the number of susceptible hosts, S. And let γ be the recovered rate of an infectious patient in a time unit. The number of recovered patients is proportional to the number of infectious patients. Therefore, the new infected number is expressed as $\beta S(t)I(t)$. The number of individuals with infectious status that changed to recovered (or removed) status is $\gamma I(t)$. The ordinary derivative equations

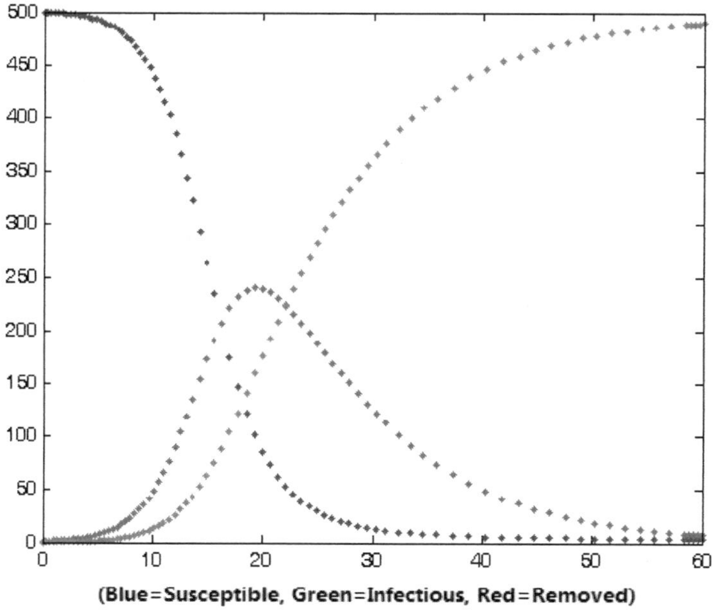

Fig. 18.10.1. Relation among the numbers of susceptables, infectious, and removed. (from wikipedia, the free encyclopedia)

of the SIR model are:

$$\begin{cases} dS/dt = -\beta S(t)I(t) \\ dI/dt = \beta S(t) - \gamma I(t) \\ dR/dt = \gamma I(t) \end{cases}.$$

Under the compartment model, the disease spreads only when the number of susceptible hosts arrives at a certain level. Epidemic ends when the number of recovered individuals arrives at a certain level. The relationship among the number of infected individuals, the number of susceptible individuals, and the number of recovered individuals is shown in Figure 18.10.1.

Figure 18.10.1 shows that in the early period of an epidemic, the number of the susceptible individuals is large. Along with the spread of the infectious disease, the number of the susceptible individuals decreases, and the number of the recovered individuals increases. The epidemic curve goes up in the early period, and goes down later.

When the vital dynamics of the target population is taken into account, the disease process is described as follows:

$$\begin{array}{ccccccc} \alpha N \longrightarrow & S & \xrightarrow{\beta SI} & I & \xrightarrow{\gamma I} & R, \\ & \downarrow & & \downarrow & & \downarrow \\ & \delta s & & \delta I & & \delta R \end{array}$$

where α is the birth rate, δ is the death rate. αN is the number of newborns who participate in the susceptible compartment, δs, δI and δR are the death number removed from corresponding compartment. The ordinary derivative equations of the SIR model now become

$$\begin{cases} dS/dt = \alpha N(t) - \beta S(t)I(t) - \delta S(t) \\ dI/dt = \beta S(t)I(t) - \gamma I(t) - \delta I(t) \\ dR/dt = \gamma I(t) - \delta R(t) \end{cases}.$$

To arrive at the solution of the equations, for simplifying calculation, usually let the birth rate equal the death rate, that is, $\alpha = \delta$. The more factors that are to be considered, the more complex the model structure will be. But all the further models can be developed based on the basic compartment model SIR.

18.11. Herd Immunity[14,16]

An infectious disease can only become epidemic in a population when the number of the susceptible hosts exceeds a critical value. If some part of the target population could be vaccinated that causes the number of susceptible hosts decrease below the critical quantity, the transmission could be blocked and the epidemic can be stopped. The key is how to obtain the critical value which is the proportion of vaccination in a target population needed to avoid the epidemic. With δs compartment model and under the condition of fixed population the needed critical value is estimated below.

1. Epidemic threshold: Conditioned on a fixed population, the structure of differential equations of the compartment model SIR(see term 18.10: Epidemiologic compartment model) is

$$\begin{cases} dS/dt = -\beta SI \\ dI/dt = \beta SI - \gamma I \\ dR/dt = \gamma I \end{cases},$$

where $S(t)$, $I(t)$ and $R(t)$ are the numbers of the susceptible, the infectious and the recovered/removed hosts at time t in each compartment, respectively, parameter β is an average contact rate per unit time, and parameter γ is an average recovery/remove rate per unit time. From the first two equations of the model expression above, βSI is the number of newly effected persons in a unit of time and they moved from the susceptible compartment to the infectious compartment. From the second equation of the structure, γI is the number of the recovered/removed hosts. When $\beta SI > \gamma I$ (or expressed as $\beta S > \gamma$ equivalently), spread occurs. If $\beta S < \gamma$, spread decays. So $\beta S = \gamma$ is an epidemic turning point, or it is called the epidemic threshold value.

2. Basic reproductive number: The basic reproductive rate is defined as

$$R_0 = \beta SI/\gamma I = \beta ST,$$

where $T = 1/\gamma$ is the average time interval during which an infected individual remains contagious. If $R_0 > 1$, each infected host will transmit the disease to at least one other susceptible host during the infectious period, and the model predicts that the disease will spread through the population. If $R_0 < 1$, the disease is expected to decline in the population. Thus, $R_0 = 1$ is the epidemical threshold value, a critical epidemiological quantity that measures if the infectious disease spreads or not in a population.

3. Herd immunity: The herd immunity is defined as the protection of an entire population via artificial immunization of a fraction of susceptible hosts to block the spread of the infectious disease in a population. That plague, smallpox have been wiped out all over the world is the most successful examples.

Let S_T be the threshold population and is substituted into the equation of $R_0 = \beta S/\gamma$ for S. The new equation becomes $R_0 = \beta S_T/\gamma$. Then it is rewritten as follows:

$$R_0\gamma/\beta = S_T \overset{R_0=1}{\Rightarrow} \gamma/\beta = S_T.$$

When $R_0 = 1$, we have $S_T = \gamma/\beta$. If the susceptible number of the population S exceeds the threshold number ST, that is, $S > ST$, the basic reproductive number can be rewritten as $R_0 = S/S_T$. Immunization decreases the number of susceptible hosts of the population, and this lowers the basic reproductive number. Let p be the immunized part of the population, then p and the basic reproductive number have the relation as

$$R_0^p = \frac{(1-p)S}{S_T}.$$

If the basic reproductive number R_0^p can be reduced being less than 1.0 by means of artificial immunization, the contamination will end. In this way, the proportion of critical immunization, p_c can be calculated by the following equation:

$$p_c = 1 - \frac{1}{R_0}.$$

18.12. Relative Risk, RR[2,8]

It is supposed that in a prospective study there are two groups of people, say exposed group A and unexposed group B. The numbers of subjects observed are N_A and N_B, respectively. During the observed period, the numbers of cases, D_A and D_B are recorded, respectively. The data layout is shown in Table 18.12.1, where M_+ and M_- are the totals of the cases and the non-cases summed up by disease category.

The incidences of the two groups are calculated by $F_A = a/N_A$, $F_B = c/N_B$, and the ratio of the two incidences is F_A/F_B. The ratio is called relative risk or risk ratio, RR. That is, $\text{RR}(A : B) = F_A/F_B$. The RR shows the times of the incidence of the exposed group compared to the incidence of the unexposed group. It is a relative index with relative feature, taking value between 0 and ∞. $RR = 1$ shows that the incidences of the two groups are similar. $RR > 1$ shows that the incidence of the exposed group is higher than that of the unexposed group, and the exposed factor is a risk one. $RR < 1$ shows that the incidence of the exposed group is lower than that of the unexposed group and the exposed factor is a protective one. $RR - 1$ expresses the pure incremental or reduced times. RR is also suitable to compare between incidence rates, prevalences that have probabilistic property in statistics. Because the observed RR is an estimate of true value of the variable, it is necessary to take a hypothesis testing before making a conclusion. Its null hypothesis is H_0: RR = 1, and its alterative hypothesis is H_a: RR $\neq$ 1. The formula of the hypothesis testing is varied according to the incidence index used. The Mantel–Haenszel χ^2 statistic

$$\chi^2_{\text{MH}} = \frac{(N-1)(ad-bc)^2}{(N_A N_B M_+ M_-)}.$$

is used for the incidence type data. It follows χ^2 distribution with one degree of freedom when H_0 is true.

Table 18.12.1. Data layout of disease occurrence from prospective study, two exposed groups.

Exposure of risk factor	Number of subjects observed	Disease category: Case	Disease category: Non-case
Exposed group (A)	N_A	a	b
Unexposed group (B)	N_B	c	d
Total	N	M_+	M_-

The estimate of 95% CI of RR takes two steps. At first, the RR is logarithmically transformed as $\ln \text{RR} = \log(\text{RR})$, and $\ln \text{RR}$ distributes symmetrically. Secondly, the variance of the $\ln \text{RR}$ is calculated by

$$\text{Var}(\ln \text{RR}) = \text{Var}(\ln F_A) + \text{Var}(\ln F_B) \approx \frac{(1 - F_A)}{(N_A F_A)} + \frac{(1 - F_B)}{(N_B F_B)}.$$

Finally, the estimate of 95% CI of RR is calculated by

$$(\text{RR}) \exp[\pm 1.96\sqrt{\text{Var}(\ln \text{RR})}].$$

In the above formula, the upper limit is obtained when + sign is taken, and the lower limit obtained when − sign is taken.

The hypothesis testing takes different statistics if RR is calculated by using incidence rates. Let the incidence rates of the two groups to be compared be $f_i = D_i/W_i$, where D_i, W_i, and $f_i (i = 1, 2)$ are observed numbers of cases, person-years, and incidence rates for group i, respectively. The statistic to be used is

$$\chi^2_{(1)} = \frac{(D_1 - E_1)^2}{E_1} + \frac{(D_2 - E_2)^2}{E_2},$$

where $E_1 = (D_1 + D_2)W_1/(W_I + W_2)$ and $E_2 = (D_1 + D_2)W_2/(W_I + W_2)$. Under the null hypothesis, $\chi^2_{(1)}$ follows χ^2 distribution with 1 degree of freedom.

18.13. OR[17,18]

Odds is defined as the ratio of the probability p of an event to the probability of its complementary event $q = 1 - p$, namely odds $= p/q$. People often consider the ratio of two odds' under a different situation where $(p_1/q_1)/(p_0/q_0)$ is called OR. For example, the odds of suffering lung cancer among cigarette smoking people with the odds of suffering the same disease among non-smoking people helps in exploring the risk of cigarette smoking. Like the relative risk for prospective study, OR is another index to measure the association between disease and exposure for retrospective study. When the probability of an event is rather low, the incidence probability p is close to the ratio p/q and so OR is close to RR.

There are two types of retrospective studies: grouping design and matching design (see 18.6) so that there are two formulas for the calculation of OR accordingly.

1. Calculation of OR for data with grouping design: In a case-control study with grouping design, N_A, N_B and a, c are observed total numbers

Table 18.13.1. Data layout of case-control study with grouping design.

Disease group	Exposure category: Exposed	Exposure category: Unexposed	Observed total	Odds of exposure
Case group A	a	b	N_A	$\text{odds}_A = a/b$
Control group B	c	d	N_B	$\text{odds}_B = c/d$
Total	M_e	M_u	N	

and exposed numbers in case group A and control group B, respectively. Table 18.13.1 shows the data layout.

Odds of exposure in group A (Case group) is: $\text{odds}_A = p_A/(1-p_A) = a/b$,

Odds of exposure in group B (Control group) is: $\text{odds}_B = p_B/(1-p_B) = c/d$.

The OR is

$$\text{OR}(A:B) = \frac{\text{odds}_A}{\text{odds}_B} = \frac{a/b}{c/d} = \frac{ad}{bc}.$$

It can be proved theoretically that the OR in terms of exposure for case group to the non-case group is equal to the OR in terms of diseased for exposed group to unexposed group. There are several methods to calculate the variance of the OR. The Woolf's method (1955) is:

$$\text{Var}[\ln(\text{OR})] \cong \left(\frac{1}{a} + \frac{1}{b} + \frac{1}{c} + \frac{1}{d}\right),$$

where ln is the natural logarithm. Under the assumption of log-normal distribution, the 95% confidence limits of the OR are

$$\text{OR}_L = \text{OR} \times e^{-1.96\sqrt{\text{Var}[\ln(\text{OR})]}},$$

$$\text{OR}_U = \text{OR} \times e^{+1.96\sqrt{\text{Var}[\ln(\text{OR})]}}.$$

To test the null hypothesis $H_0\colon OR = 1$, the testing statistic is:

$$\chi^2 = \frac{(ad - bc)^2 N}{(N_A \times N_B \times M_e \times M_n)}.$$

Under the null hypothesis, the statistic χ^2 follows χ^2 distribution with 1 degree of freedom.

2. Calculation of OR for data from case-control study with 1:1 pair matching design: The data layout of this kind of design has been shown in Table 18.6.2. The formula of OR is OR $= b/c$. When both b and c are relatively large, the approximate variance of ln OR is as: $\text{Var}[\ln(OR)] \cong 1/b + 1/c$. The 95% confidence limits of OR are calculated by using the formulas of Woolf's method above. For testing of the null hypothesis OR $= 1$, the McNemar test is used with the statistic

$$\chi^2_{\text{Mc}} = \frac{(|b-c|-1)^2}{(b+c)}.$$

Under the null hypothesis, follows χ^2 distribution with 1 degree of freedom.

18.14. Bias[16,17]

Bias means that the estimated result deviates from the true value. It is also known as systematic error. Bias has directionality, which can be less than or greater than the true value. Let θ be the true value of the effect in the population of interest, γ be the estimated value from a sample. If the expectation of the difference between them equals zero, i.e. $E(\theta-\gamma) = 0$, the difference between the estimate and the true value is resulted from sampling error, there is no bias between them. However, if the expectation of the difference between them does not equal zero, i.e. $E(\theta-\gamma) \neq 0$, the estimated value γ has bias. Because θ is usually unknown, it is difficult to determine the size of the bias in practice. But it is possible to estimate the direction of the bias, whether $E(\theta - \gamma)$ is less than or larger than 0.

Non-differential bias: It refers to the bias that indistinguishably occurs in both exposed and unexposed groups. This causes bias to each of the parameter estimates. But there is no bias in ratio between them. For example, if the incidences of a disease in the exposed group and unexposed group were 8% and 6%, respectively, then the difference between them is $8\% - 6\% = 2\%$, RR $= 8\%/6\% = 1.33$. If the detection rate of a device is lower than the standard rate, it leads to the result that the incidences of exposed and unexposed groups were 6% and 4.5%, respectively with a difference of 1.5% between the two incidences, but the RR $= 1.33$ remains unchanged.

Bias can come from various stages of a research. According to its source, bias can be divided into the following categories mainly:

1. Selection bias: It might occur when choosing subjects. It is resulted when the measurement distribution in the sample does not match with the population, and the estimate of the parameter systemically deviates from the true value of it. The most common selection bias occurs in the controlled trial design, in which the subjects in control group and intervention group distributed unbalanced factors related to exposure and/or disease. Therefore, it results in lack of comparability. In the study of occupational diseases, for example, if comparison is made between morbidities or mortalities suffered by workers holding specific posts and the ones suffered by general population, it may be found that the morbidity or mortality of workers often are obviously lower than that of the general population. This is due to the better health conditions of workers when entering the specific post than that of general population. This kind of selection bias is called Health Worker Effect or HWE.

Berkson's fallacy: Berkson's fallacy is a special type of selection bias that occurs in hospital-based case-control studies. It is generally used to describe the bias caused by the systematic differences between hospital controls and the general population.

There are many ways for controlling selection bias like controlling of each link in object selection, paying attention to the representativeness of subject selection and the way of choice, controlling the eligible criterion strictly in subject selection, etc.

2. Information bias: It refers to a bias occurring in the process of data collection so that the data collected provide incorrect information. Information bias arises in the situation such as when data collection method or measurement standard is not unified, including errors and omissions of information from subjects of the study, etc. Information bias causes the estimation of exposure–response correlation different from the true value. It can occur in any type of study. The method of controlling information bias is to establish a strict supervisory system of data collection, such as the objective index or records, blindness.

3. Confounding bias: Confounding bias refers to the distortion of independent effect of an exposure factor on outcome by the effects of confounding factors, leading to the biased estimation of exposure effect on outcome. (see item 18.15).

18.15. Confounding[4,19]

In evaluating an association between exposure and disease, it is necessary to pay some attention to the possible interference from certain extraneous factors that may affect the relationship. If the potential effect is ignored, bias may result in estimating the strength of the relationship. The bias introduced by ignoring the role of extraneous factor(s) is called confounding bias. The factor that causes the bias in estimating the strength of the relationship is called confounding factor.

As a confounding factor, the variable must associate with both the exposure and the disease. Confounding bias exists when the confounding factor distributes unbalanced in the exposure–disease subgroup level. If a variable associates with disease, but not with exposure, or vice versa, it cannot influence the relationship between the exposure and the disease, then it is not a confounding factor. For example, drinking and smoking has association (the correlation coefficient is about 0.60). In exploring the relationship of smoking and lung cancer, smoking is a risk factor of lung cancer, but drinking is not. However, in exploring the relationship of drinking and lung cancer, smoking is a confounding factor; if ignoring the effect of smoking, it may result in a false relation. The risks of suffering both hypertension and coronary heart disease increase with aging. Therefore, age is a confounding factor in the relationship between hypertension and coronary heart disease. In order to present the effect of risk factor on disease occurrence correctly, it is necessary to eliminate the confounding effect resulted from the confounding factor on the relationship between exposure and disease. Otherwise, the analytical conclusion is not reliable. On how to identify the confounding factor, it is necessary to calculate the risk ratios of the exposure and the disease under two different conditions. One is calculated ignoring the extraneous variable and the other is calculated with the subgroup under certain level of the extraneous variable. If the two risk ratios are not similar, there is some evidence of confounding.

Confounding bias can be controlled both in design stage and in data analysis stage.

In the design stage, the following measures can be taken: (1) Restriction: Individuals with the similar exposed level of confounding factor are eligible subjects and are allowed to be recruited into the program. (2) Randomization: Subjects with confounding factors are assigned to experimental or control group randomly. In this way, the systematic effects of confounding factors can be balanced. (3) Matching: Two or more subjects with the same level of confounding factor are matched as a pair or a (matched set). Then randomization is performed within each matched set. In this way, the effects of confounding factors can be eliminated.

In the data analysis stage, the following measures can be taken: (1) Standardization: Standardization is aimed at adjusting confounding factor to the same level. If the two observed populations have different age structure, age is a confounding factor. In occupational medicine, if the two populations have different occupational exposure history, exposure history is a confounding factor. These differences can be calibrated by using standardization (see 18.16 Standardization Methods). (2) Stratified analysis: At first, the confounding factor is stratified according to its level; then the relation between exposure and disease is analyzed by the stratified group. Within each stratum, the effect of the confounding factor is eliminated. But the more the strata are divided, the more subjects are needed. Therefore, the usage of stratification is restricted in practice. (3) Multivariate analysis; With multivariate regression models, the effects of the confounding factor can be separated and the "pure" (partial) relation between exposure and disease can be revealed. For example, the logistic regression models are available for binomial response data.

18.16. Standardization Methods[8,20]

One purpose of standardization is the control of confounding. Disease incidence or mortality varies with age, sex, etc; the population incidence in a region is influenced by its demography, especially age structure. For convenience, we would take age structure as example hereafter. If two observed population incidences which come from different regions are to be compared, it is necessary to eliminate the confounding bias caused by different age structure. The incidence or rate, adjusted by age structure is called standardized incidence or rate, respectively. Two methods which are applicable to the standardization procedure, the "direct" and "indirect" methods, will be discussed.

1. Direct standardization: A common age-structure is chosen from a so-called standard or theoretical population; the expected incidences are calculated for each age group of the two observed populations based on the common age-structure of the standard population; these standardized age-specific incidences are summed up by population to get two new population incidences called age-adjusted or standardized incidences. The original population incidences before age adjustment are called the crude population incidence or, simply, crude incidence. The precondition for this method is that the crude age-specific incidences must be known. If the comparison is between regions within a country, the nationwide age distribution from census can serve as common age-structure. If the comparison is between different countries or regions worldwide, the age-structures recommended by World Health Organization (WHO) can be used.

Let the incidence of age group $x(x = 1, 2, \ldots, g)$ in region $i(i = 1, 2)$ be $m_{x(i)} = D_{x(i)}/W_{x(i)}$, where $D_{x(i)}$ and $W_{x(i)}$ are numbers of cases and observed subjects of age group x and region i respectively. The formula of direct standardization is

$$M_{\text{adj}(i)} = \sum_{x=1}^{g} S_x m_{x(i)},$$

where $M_{\text{adj}(i)}$ is the adjusted incidence of population i, S_x is the fraction (in decimal) of age group x in standard population. The variance of the adjusted incidence $V(M_{\text{adj}(i)})$ is calculated by the formula

$$V(M_{\text{adj}(i)}) = \sum_{x=1}^{g} S_x^2 \text{Var}(m_{x(i)}) = \sum_{x=1}^{g} S_x^2 \left(\frac{D_{x(i)}}{W_{x(i)}^2} \right).$$

For hypothesis testing between the two standardized population incidences (adjusted incidences) of the two regions, say A and B, under the null hypothesis, the statistic

$$Z = \frac{(M_{\text{adj}(A)} - M_{\text{adj}(B)})}{\sqrt{V(M_{\text{adj}(A)} - M_{\text{adj}(B)})}}$$

approximately follows standard normal distribution under the null hypothesis where $V(\cdot)$ in denominator is the common variance of the two adjusted incidences as

$$V(M_{\text{adj}(A)} - M_{\text{adj}(B)}) = \frac{W_{(A)} \times M_{\text{adj}(A)} + W_{(B)} \times M_{\text{adj}(B)}}{W_{(A)} \times W_{(B)}}.$$

2. Indirect standardization: This method is used in the situation where the total number of cases D and the age-grouped numbers of persons (or person-years) under study are known. But the age-grouped number of cases and the corresponding age-grouped incidence are not known. It is not possible to use direct standardization method for adjusting incidence. Instead, an external age-specific incidence (λ_x) can be used in age group x as standard incidence. And the number of the age-specific expected cases can be calculated as $E_x = W_x \times \lambda_x$, and the total number of expected cases is $E = E_1 + \cdots + E_g$. Finally, the index called standardized incidence ratio, SIR, (or called standardized mortality ratio, SMR, if death is used to replace the case) can be calculated as SIR $= D/E$, where D is the observed total number of cases. Under the assumption that D follows a Poisson distribution, the variance of SIR, Var(SIR) is estimated as Var(SIR) $= D/E^2$. Accordingly, the 95% confidence interval can be calculated. In order to test if there is significant difference of incidences between the standard area and the observed area, under the null hypothesis, the test statistic $\chi^2 = \frac{(D-E)^2}{E}$ follows a χ^2 distribution with 1 degree of freedom.

18.17. Age–period–cohort (APC) Models[21,22]

The time at which an event (disease or death) occurs on a subject can be measured from three time dimensions. They are subject's age, calendar period and subject's date of birth (birth cohort). The imprinting of historical events on health status can be discerned through the three time dimensions. The three types of time imprinting are called age effects, period effects and cohort effects respectively. APC analysis aims at describing and estimating the independent effects of age, period and cohort on the health outcome under study. The APC model is applied for data from multiple cross-sectional observations and it has been used in demography, sociology and epidemiology for a long time. Data for APC model are organized as a two-way structure, i.e. age by observation time as shown in Table 18.17.1.

Early in the development of the model, graphics were used to describe these effects. Later, parameter estimations were developed to describe these effects in order to quantitatively analyze the effects from different time dimensions. Let λ_{ijk} be the expected death rate of age group $i (i = 1, \ldots, A)$, period group $j (j = 1, \ldots, P)$, and cohort group $k (k = 1, \ldots, C), C = A + P - 1$. The APC model is expressed as

$$\lambda_{\text{ijk}} = \exp(\mu + \alpha_i + \beta_j + \gamma_k),$$

where μ is the intercept, α_i, β_j, and γ_k represent the effect of age group i, the effect of time period j, and the effect of birth cohort k, respectively. The

Table 18.17.1. Data of cases/personal-years from multiple cross-sectional studies.

Age group (i)	Observational year (j)			
	1943	1948	1953	1958
15	2/773812 (0.2585)	3/744217 (0.4031)	4/794123 (0.5037)	1/972853 (0.5037)
20	7/813022 (0.8610)	7/744706 (0.9400)	17/721810 (2.3552)	8/770859 (1.0378)
25	28/790501 (3.5421)	23/781827 (2.9418)	26/722968 (3.5963)	35/698612 (5.0099)
30	28/799293 (3.5031)	43/774542 (5.5517)	49/769298 (6.3694)	51/711596 (7.1670)
35	36/769356 (4.6792)	42/782893 (5.3647)	39/760213 (5.1301)	44/760452 (5.7660)
40	24/694073 (3.4578)	32/754322 (4.2422)	46/768471 (5.9859)	53/749912 (7.0675)

Note: Value in parenthesis is the rate × 10^5

logarithmic transformation of the model above becomes

$$\ln \lambda_{\text{ijk}} = \mu + \alpha_i + \beta_j + \gamma_k.$$

The logarithmic transformed form can be used to calculate parameter estimates with Poisson distribution. But because of the exact linear dependence among age, period, and cohort (Period – Age = Cohort), that is, given the calendar year and age, one can determine the cohort (birth year) exactly, the model has no unique solution. For this, several solutions have been developed like (1) Constrained solution: This is an early version of the solution. The model above is essentially a variance type model. In addition to the usually restriction condition where $\alpha_1 = \beta_1 = \gamma_1 = 0$, it needs an additional constrain that one additional parameter among age, period or cohort should be set to 0 when unique solution is obtained. In this way, the parameter estimates are instable with the subjectively chosen constraints. (2) Nonlinear solution: The linear relationship among age, period, and cohort is changed to a nonlinear relationship in order to solve the estimation problem. (3) Multi-step modeling: Cohort effect is defined as interaction of age by period. Based on this assumption two fitting procedures have been developed. (a) The method of two-step fitting: In the first step, a linear model is used to fit the relationship between response with age and period. In the second step, the residuals from the linear model are used as response to fit the interaction of age by period. (b) Median polish model: Its principle is the same as the two-step fitting method, but other than residuals, the median is used to represent the interaction of age by cohort. (4) Intrinsic estimator method: It is also called the IE method. A group of eigenvectors of non-zero eigenvalues is obtained by using principal component analysis. Then, the matrix of eigenvectors is used to fit a principal regression and a series of parameters are obtained. Finally, these parameter estimates from principal regression are reversely transformed to obtain the estimates with originally scaled measures of age, period and cohort in order to obtain intuitive explanation.

18.18. Environmental Exposure Model[23,24]

Environmental epidemiology is defined as the study of influence of environmental pollution on human health, to estimate the adverse health effects of environmental pollution, to establish the dose–response relationship between pollutant and human health. In the environmental model, the independent variable is the strength of the environmental pollutant, which is measured with concentration of the pollutant in external environment, and the

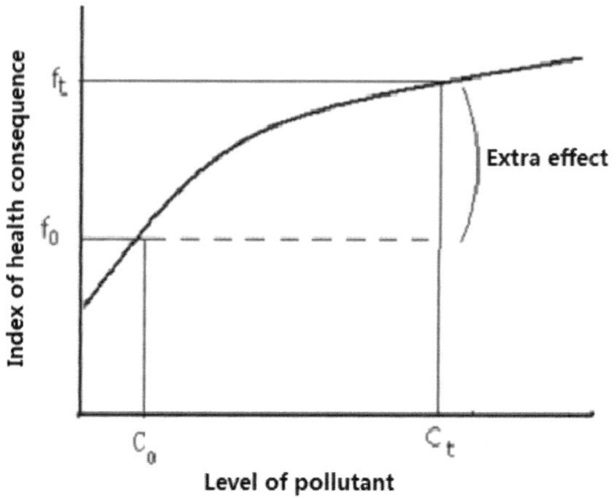

Fig. 18.18.1. Dose–response relationship of environmental pollutant and health consequence.

response is the health response of people on the pollutant. The dose accepted by an individual is dependent both on the concentration of the environmental pollutant and on the exposed time length. The response may be some disease status or abnormal bio-chemical indices. The response variable is categorized into four types in statistics: (1) Proportion or rate such as incidence, incidence rate, prevalence, etc. This type of entry belongs to binomial distribution; (2) Counting number such as the number of skin papilloma; (3) Ordinal value such as grade of disease severity and (4) Continuous measurements, such as bio-chemical values. Different types of measures of the response variable are suitable for different statistical models.

As an example of the continuous response variable, the simplest model is the linear regression model expressed as $f = a_i + bC$. The model shows that the health response f is positively proportional to the dose of pollutant C. The parameter b in the model is the change of response when pollutant changes per unit. But the relation of health response and the environmental pollutant is usually nonlinear as shown in Figure 18.18.1.

This kind of curve can be modeled with exponential regression model as follows:

$$f_t = f_0 \times \exp[\beta(C_t - C_0)],$$

where C_t is the concentration of pollutant at time t, C_0 is the threshold concentration (dose) or referential concentration of pollutant at which the health effect is the lowest, f_t is the predicted value of health response at the level C_t of the pollutant, f_0 is the health response at the level C_0 of the pollutant, β is the regression coefficient which shows the effect of strength of pollutant on health. The threshold concentration C_0 can be referred to the national standard. For example, the (Standard of Ambient Air Quality) (GB3095-1996) of China specifies the concentration of airborne particulate matter PM_{10} as $40.0\,mg/m^3$ for the first level, $100.0\,mg/m^3$ for the second level and $150.0\,mg/m^3$ for the third level. Other variables like age, etc., can be added into the model. The curvilinear model can be transformed as a linear one through logarithmic transformation. The exponentialized value of parameter estimate from the model, $\exp(\beta)$ indicates the health effect caused by per unit change of the pollutant.

When the base incidence f_0, the current incidence f_t and the number of the population of the contaminated area are known, the extra number of new patients, E, can be estimated as $E = (f_t - f_0) \times P_t$.

18.19. Disease Surveillance[11,25]

Disease surveillance is the main source of information for disease control agencies. The system of disease surveillance is the organizational guarantee for disease surveillance, and a platform for accurate and timely transfer and analysis of disease information. It is the infrastructure for disease control strategy. The People's Republic of China Act of Infectious Disease Control is a nationwide infectious disease surveillance system in China. There are many regional registration and report systems of health events, cases and deaths including communicable diseases, occupational diseases, cancer, pregnancy, childbirth, neonatal, injury, and outbreak of environmental events, etc. in China too. Correct diagnosis of diseases, reliability of data, and timeliness of report is required. In doing so, the disease surveillance system can play an important role in disease control program. Disease outbreak is usually associated with infectious diseases, which can spread very quickly and bring tremendous disaster to the people. Clustering is associated with non-infectious diseases, which usually appear with some limitation in space, time and person.

1. **Outbreak pattern with common source**: A group of people are all contaminated by an infectious factor from the same source. For this kind of disease, its epidemic curve rises steeply and declines gradually in continuous time axis.
2. **Propagated pattern**: Disease transmits from one person to another. For this kind disease, its epidemic curve rises slowly and declines steeply. It may have several epidemic peaks.

3. **Mixed spread pattern**: At the early time of this kind of spread, the cases come from a single etiologic source. Then the disease spreads quickly through person to person. Therefore, this epidemic curve shows mixed characteristics.

Disease surveillance is aimed at monitoring if a disease occurs abnormally. For communicable diseases, this high incidence is specially called spread or outbreak. In statistics, it is necessary to check if a disease is randomly distributed or "clustering". The clustering shapes can be further classified into four types: (a) Place clustering: Cases tend to be close to each other in spatial distance. (b) Temporal clustering: Cases tend to be close to each other in time. (c) Space-time interaction: Cases occur closely both in short-time period and in short special distance and (d) Time-cohort cluster. Cases are located in a special population and a special time period. Because in clustering analysis the available cases are usually less than specialized research, descriptive statistics based on large samples like incidence frequency, incidence rate, may not be practical. Statisticians provide several methods which are available for clustering analysis. Most of these methods are based on Poisson distribution theoretically. For example, Knox (1960) provides a method to test if there exists a time-space interaction.

Suppose that n cases had occurred at a special time period in a region, and detailed date and place for each case were recorded. The n cases can be organized an $n(n-1)/2$ pairs. Given a time cut-point $= \alpha$ in advance, the $n(n-1)/2$ pairs can be divided into two groups. Further, given a spatial distance cut-point $= \beta$, the $n(n-1)/2$ pairs can be sub-divided into four groups. In this way, the data can be formed in a 2×2 table. For example, $n = 96$ cases are organized $96 \times (96-1)/2 = 4560$ pairs. With $\alpha = 60$ days as time cut-off point (<60 days, $\geq$60 days) and spatial distance $\beta = 1.0$ kilometer as cut-off point ($<$ 1km, $\geq$ 1km), the total number of 4,560 pairs is reorganized a in 2×2 form as shown in Table 18.19.1.

Table 18.19.1. Time-space category of 96 cases suffering from childhood.

Time-interval (day)	Spatial-distance		Total
	<1 km	≥ 1 km	
<60 days	5	147	152
≥60 days	20	4388	4408
Total	25	4535	4560

Under the null hypothesis, the expectation of observed pairs 5 in cell (1, 1) is calculated as $\lambda = (25 \times \times 152)/4560 = 0.8333$. Based on the theory of Poisson distribution, the probability that the number equal or larger than 5 in cell (1, 1) is $\Pr(X \geq 5) = 0.0017$. The probability is less than the significant level $\alpha = 0.05$ in statistics.

18.20. STROBE Statement[26,27]

The initial STROBE group was established in 2004. A workshop was held in September the same year. Then the group published its first statement, "Assessing the quality of research". Latter, the group formed the STROBE Statement, "Strengthening the reporting quality of observational studies in epidemiology (STROBE) statement: guidelines for reporting observational studies". The STROBE Statement has a checklist of items that should be addressed in articles reported from the three main study designs of analytical epidemiology: cohort, case-control and cross-sectional studies aimed to strengthen the quality of articles from observation researches. The checklist contains 22 items that are considered essential for good reporting of an observational study. These items relate to the article's title and abstract (item 1), the introduction (items 2 and 3), methods (items 4–12), results (items 13–21) and other information (item 22). In each item, a list of necessary elements (recommendations) were also provided. The following is the checklist of items:

1. **Title and abstract**: (a) Indicate the study's design with a commonly used term in the title or in the abstract. (b) Provide in the abstract an informative and balanced summary of what was done and what was found.
2. **Background/rationale**: Explain the scientific background and rationale for the investigation being reported.
3. **Objectives**: State specific objectives, including any prespecified hypotheses.
4. **Study Design**: Present key elements of study design early in the chapter.
5. **Setting**: Describe the setting, locations, and relevant dates, including periods of recruitment, exposure, follow-up, and data collection.
6. **Participants**: (a) Cohort study — Give the eligibility criteria, and the sources and methods of selection of participants. Describe methods of follow-up. Case-control study — Give the eligibility criteria, and the sources and methods of case ascertainment and control selection. Give

the rational for the choice of cases and controls. Cross-sectional study — Give the eligibility criteria, and the sources and methods of selection participants.
(b) Cohort study — For matched studies, give matching criteria and number of exposed and unexposed. Case-control study — For matched studies, give matching criteria and the number of controls per case.

7. **Variables**: Clearly define all outcomes, exposures, predictors, potential confounders and effect modifiers. Give diagnostic criteria, if applicable.
8. **Data sources/measurement**: For each variable of interest, give sources of data and details of methods of assessment (measurement). Describe comparability of assessment methods if there is more than one group.
9. **Bias**: Describe any efforts to address potential sources of bias.
10. **Study Size**: Explain how the study size was arrived at.
11. **Quantitative Variables**: Explain how quantitative variables were handled in the analyses. If applicable, describe which groupings were chosen, and why.
12. **Statistical Methods**: (a) Describe all statistical methods, including those used to control for confounding. (b) Describe any methods used to examine subgroups and interactions. (c) Explain how missing data were addressed. (d) Cohort study — If applicable, explain how the failure loss to follow-up was addressed. Case-control study — If applicable, explain how matching of cases and controls was addressed. Cross-sectional study — If applicable, describe analytical methods taking account of sampling strategy. (e) Describe any sensitivity analyses.
13. **Participants**: (a) Report the numbers of individuals at each stage of the study, e.g. potentially eligible numbers, examining them for eligibility, confirmation eligibility, inclusion in the study, completion of follow-up proven, and analysis. (b) Give reasons for non-participation at each stage. (c) Consider use of a flow diagram.
14. **Descriptive Data**: (a) Give characteristics of study participants and information on exposures and potential confounders. (b) Indicate the number of participants with missing data for each variable of interest. (c) Cohort study — summarize follow-up time (e.g. average and total amount).
15. **Outcome Data**: Report numbers of outcome events or summary measures over time.
16. **Main Results**: (a) Give unadjusted estimates and, if applicable, confounder-adjusted estimates and their precision (e.g. 95% CI). Make

clear which confounders were adjusted for and why they were included. (b) Report category boundaries when continuous variables were categorized. (c) If relevant, consider translating estimates of relative risk into absolute risk for a meaningful time period.

17. **Other Analyses**: Report other analyses done, e.g. analyses of subgroups and interactions, and sensitivity analyses.
18. **Key Results**: Summarize key results with reference to study objectives.
19. **Limitations**: Discuss limitations of the study, taking into account sources of potential bias or imprecision. Discuss both direction and magnitude of any potential bias.
20. **Interpretation**: Give a cautious overall interpretation of results considering objectives, limitations, multiplicity of analyses, results from similar studies and other relevant evidence.
21. **Generalizability**: Other Information: Discuss the generalizability (external validity) of the study results.
22. **Funding**: Give the source of funding and the role of the funders for the present study and, if applicable, for the original study on which the present chapter is based.

References

1. Breslow, NE, Day, NE. *Statistical Methods in Cancer Research.* Lyon France: IARC Scientific Publications, No. 32, 1980.
2. Esteve, J, Benhamou, E, Raymond, L. *Descriptive Epidemiology.* Lyon France: IARC Scientific Publications, No. 128, 1994.
3. Bütherp, P, Mullerr, R. *Epidemiology: An Introduction.* New York, NY: Oxford University Press, 2012.
4. Kleinbaum, DG, Kupper, LL, Morgensternh. *Epidemiologic Research: Principles and Quantitative Methods.* Belmont California: Lifetime Learning Publications, 1982.
5. Oleckno, WA. *Epidemiology: Concept and Methods.* Long Grove, Illinois: Waveland Press Inc. 2008.
6. Song, C, Kulldorff, M. Power evaluation of disease clustering tests. *Int. J. Health. Geogr*, 2003, 2(1): 9–16.
7. Tangot. *Statistical Methods for Disease Clustering.* New York: Springer, 2010.
8. Szklo, M, Nieto, EJ. *Epidemiology: Beyond the Basics*, (3rd edn.). Burtington MA: Jones & Bartlett Learning, 2014.
9. Zheng, T, Boffetta, P, Boyle, P. *Epidemiology and Biostatistics.* Lyon France: IPRI (International Prevention Research Institute), 2011.
10. Maclure, M. The case-cross over design: A method for studying transient effects on the risk of acute events. *Ame. J. Epidem.*, 1991, 133: 144–153.
11. Brownson, RC, Petitti, DB. (eds). *Applied Epidemiology: Theory to Practice.* Oxford, New York: Oxford University Press, 2006.
12. Khoury, MJ, Newill, CA,Chase, GA. Epidemiologic evaluation of screening for risk factors: Application to genetic screening. *Ame. J. Pub. Health*, 1985, 75(10): 1204–1208.

13. Peishan Wang. *Epidemiology.* Beijing: Tsinghua University Press, 2014: 152–165, 166–181.
14. Brauer, F, Driessche, PVD, Wu, J (eds). *Mathematical Epidemiology.* Berlin, Heidelberg: Springer-Verlag, 2008.
15. Ma, ZE, Zhou, YL, Wang, WD. *Mathematical Modeling and Research of Dynamics for Infectious Diseases.* Beijing: Scientific Publication. 2004. (in Chinese)
16. Gail, MH, Benichou, J, (eds). *Encyclopedia of Epidemiologic Methods.* Chichester England: John Wiley & Sons, Ltd, 2000.
17. Schlesselman, JJ, Stolley, PD. *Case — Control Studies: Design, Contact, Analysis.* New York: Oxford, 1982.
18. Armitage, P, Berry, G, Mathews, JNS. *Statistical Methods in Medical Research.* (4th edn.). Oxford, Blackwell Scientific Publications, 2002.
19. Bonita, R, Beaglehole, RK. Jellstrom, T. *Basic Epidemiology.* (2nd edn.). Geneva, Switzerland: WHO Press, 2006.
20. Ahmad, OB, Boschi-Pinto, C, Lopez, AD, Christopher, JL, Lozano, MR, Inoue, M. Age standardization of rates: A new WHO standard. GPE Discussion Paper Series: No. 31, EIP/GPE/EBD, World Health Organization, 2001.
21. Hold, TR. The estimation of age, period and cohort effects for vital rates. *Biometrics,* 1983, 39: 311–24.
22. Yang, Y, L and, KC. *Age–Period–Cohort Analysis: New Models, Methods, and Empirical Applications.* Boca Raton, FL: CRC Press, 2013.
23. International Programme on Chemical Safety (IPCS). *Environmental Health Criteria on Principles for Modelling Dose–Response for the Risk Assessment of Chemicals.* Geneva: WHO, 2009.
24. Peng, XW, Wang, JC, Yu, SL. *R and its Applications in Environmental Epidemiology.* Beijing, China Environmental Science Press, 2013. (in Chinese)
25. David, FN, Barton, DE. Two space-time interaction tests for epidemiology. *Brit. J. Prev. Soc. Med.*, 1966, 20: 44–48.
26. Elm, EV, Altman, DG, Egger, M, *et al.* The Strengthening the Reporting of Observational Studies in Epidemiology (STROBE) statement: Guidelines for reporting observational studies. *Int. J. Surg.*, 2014, 12: 1495–1499.
27. Vandenbroucke, JP, Elm, EV, Altman, DG, *et al.* Strengthening the Reporting of Observational Studies in Epidemiology (STROBE): Explanation and elaboration. *Int. J. Surg.*, 2014, 12: 1500–1524.

---

*For the introduction of the corresponding author, see the front matter.

CHAPTER 19

EVIDENCE-BASED MEDICINE

Yi Wan*, Changsheng Chen and Xuyu Zhou

19.1. Evidence-Based Medicine (EBM)[1]

EBM is the conscientious, explicit, and judicious use of current best evidence in making decisions about the care of individual patients. EBM is the integration of best research evidence with clinical expertise and patient values, and is part into practice under specific circumstances. The core conception of EBM is that the clinical decision making should be based on objective evidence. All medical treatment schedule or guidelines developed by doctors and health policies developed by government institutions should be based on the best evidence available currently.

Since 1980s, David Sackett, Gordon Guyatt and many pioneers on EBM began to explore evidence-based practice. In November 1992, they published a paper on behalf of the working group on EBM in the *JAMA* named "Evidence-Based Medicine: A New Approach to Teaching the Practice of Medicine", which marked the birth of EBM. After 20 years of development, the concepts, methods, practice patterns and findings of EBM have penetrated deep into all areas of healthcare, which dramatically changed the practice mode of clinical medicine in the 21st century. It produces far-reaching impact on the development of medical science and relevant disciplines, and a number of branches of domains are formed including evidence-based health care, evidence-based health policy, evidence-based pharmacy, evidence-based nursing care, etc.

There are five steps for practice of EBM: (1) translation of uncertainty to an answerable question; (2) systematic retrieval of the best evidence

*Corresponding author: wanyi@fmmu.edu.cn

available; (3) critical appraisal of evidence for validity, reliability and applicability to find the best evidence; (4) application of results in practice and guidance of decision making; (5) evaluation of application performance. The five steps are also named as 5A, that is, Ask, Acquire, Appraise, Apply and Act.

The first step in the practice of EBM is to ask an answerable question, which can be developed in accordance with the PICOS elements. Taking intervention study as example, PICOS elements are:

P: patient or population, the type and characteristics of study participants, type of disease, etc.;

I: intervention, the interventions intended to be used for patients;

C: comparison, the interventions for comparison (control is not required for every question);

O: outcome, important outcome measures or clinical results concerned;

S: study design, the design of study, such as randomized controlled trials (RCTs), cohort studies, case-control studies, diagnostic testing.

Evidence and its quality is the basis for decision making in the practice of EBM. Evidence has various types, different grades and levels, and they need to be constantly updated. Carrying out high-quality clinical research on the problem to obtain precise and reliable scientific evidence, or carrying out quantitative or qualitative systematic review on a particular issue, and providing high-quality evidence to solve the problem are the processes of evidence creation and evidence-based practice in EBM.

19.2. Cochran Library[2,3]

Cochrane Library (ISSN 1465-1858) is a collection of six databases that contain different types of high-quality, independent evidence to inform healthcare decision making, and a seventh database that provides information about Cochrane groups.

Cochrane Library is an electronic library serving health staff, providing an important database for EBM. Cochrane Library is the major product of Cochrane Collaboration. Among clinical medical databases, reasons for taking Cochrane Library as an important database for EBM include: it is the most comprehensive database on systematic review which achieves sustainable attention; it is an electronic journal with easily available updates and comments to revise mistakes and ensures the quality to guarantee the reliability of the conclusion. Cochrane Library is suitable for clinical doctors, clinical researchers and education providers, and medical and health administration related staff. The seven databases of Cochrane Library are

(1) Cochrane Database of Systematic Reviews (CDSR)
(2) Cochrane Central Register of Controlled Trials (CENTRAL)
(3) Cochrane Methodology Register (CMR)
(4) Database of Abstracts of Reviews of Effects (DARE)
(5) Health Technology Assessment Database (HTA)
(6) NHS Economic Evaluation Database (EED)
(7) About the Cochrane Collaboration

Cochrane Library is published by Wiley. CDSR is built throughout the month with new and updated reviews and protocols being continuously published when ready. CENTRAL and the "About the Cochrane Collaboration" databases are published monthly. HTA is published quarterly according to a schedule. DARE and NHS EED were published on a quarterly schedule up to April 2015, when updating stopped. CMR was publishing up to July 2012, when updating stopped.

The "About the Cochrane Collaboration" database includes contacts and information on the aims and scope of the Cochrane Review Groups, Methods Groups, Fields, and Networks along with information about Cochrane Centers and the Cochrane Editorial Unit.

19.3. Levels of Evidence[4–6]

The levels of evidence refer to using the principles and methods of clinical epidemiology and related quality evaluation criteria to evaluate the validity, reliability and clinical application value of evidence.

There are a variety of evaluation methods on levels of evidence. The most frequently used standard for levels of evidence is the evaluation criteria for levels of evidence developed by Oxford Center for Evidence-Based Medicine in May 2001. On the basis of evidence grading, for the first time, the criteria proposed the classification concept, which involves seven aspects including treatment, prevention, causes, harm, prognosis, diagnosis, and economics analysis. It has more pertinence and applicability, and becomes a classic standard in teaching of EBM and evidence-based clinical practice. Based on the different levels of causal relationship among different study designs, evidences are divided into five levels, and recommendations are divided into four grades: A (excellent), B (good), C (satisfied), and D (poor) according to the quality, consistency, clinical significance, universality and applicability of the evidence. The grade A recommendation should come from the evidence of the first level, which shows consistentcy among conclusions of all studies, has clinical significance, and the sample of the study is consistent with the target population. Therefore, this recommendation can be directly applied to various medical practices. However, the evidence with grades B and C recommendations might have certain problems in the above aspects, which limits their applicability. And that with grade D recommendation cannot be applied to medical practice.

In 2004, a set of evidence quality and grading of recommendation system was proposed by the grading of recommendation assessment, development and evaluation working group (GRADE) which was established by guideline developers, authors of systematic reviews and clinical epidemiologists. The grading system overcomes the limitation in evaluation of quality of evidence only from the aspect of study design. On the basis of whether future research will change the confidence on the evaluation of current treatment efficacy and the possibility of changing, it classifies the quality of evidence into four grades: high, medium, low, and very low. The RCTs are still considered as high-quality evidence, but the grade of evidence will be downgraded if the study has limitations, findings are inconsistent, direct evidences are not provided, inaccurate results are reported and reporting bias is presented. The quality grade of evidence of observational study will be enhanced with rigorous design and good implementation with great efficacy or a dose–response relationship. The strength of recommendation provided by the GRADE evidence evaluation system only includes two levels: "strong" and "weak". When the evidence clearly shows benefit of intervention outweighs disadvantage (or disadvantage outweighs benefit), it is strongly recommended (or not recommended). When the quality of evidence is low, or the evidence suggests uncertain or equal advantage and disadvantage, the recommendation is subject to weak intensity. In addition, selection of participants and availability of resources will also affect the recommendation intensity. The system is simple and easy to use with wide application, which can be used to develop various clinical recommendations by medical professionals and clinical nursing care. The Cochrane Collaboration, World Health Organization (WHO) and other international organizations have supported and widely used the GRADE system.

19.4. Systematic Review[1]

Systematic review is a new literature review method, which refers to systematic and comprehensive collection of published and unpublished studies for a specific problem, using the principles and methods of critical appraisal to select studies in line with the quality criteria, and performing qualitative or quantitative synthesis (Meta-analysis) to draw reliable conclusion. Systematic review can be used not only for clinical research, but also for basic research, policy study, economics and other fields.

Early in 1979, Archie Cochrane, the late renowned British epidemiologist, proposed the basic idea of system review. In 1989, Iain Chalmers carried out a quantitative synthesis of RCTs of using short course and low price steroid on tendency of preterm birth in pregnant women, which was considered as the prototype of systematic review. In 1993, with the rapid spread of the conception of EBM, the British Cochrane Center formally proposed the term of systematic review. As a new method of generating high-quality evidence, the concepts and methods of systematic review received wide promotion, recognition and acceptance.

Systematic review can be qualitative (qualitative systematic review) or quantitative (quantitative systematic review, which contains Meta-analysis). If the included studies lack data or quantitative synthesis is impossible because of large heterogeneity, only qualitative description can be performed. Therefore, it is not mandatory to include and perform Meta-analysis in a systematic, review because it is essentially a statistical method.

Cochrane systematic reviews (CSRs) are systematic reviews completed by the Cochrane Collaboration reviewers according to unified work manual under the guidance and assistance of the editorial team of corresponding Cochrane review group. Because there is strict Cochrane Collaboration organization management and quality control system, using a fixed format and unified system review software "RevMan" to enter and analyze data, to write proposal and full text, to regularly update after publication, its quality is often higher than that of non-CSRs, and it is considered as the most reliable evidence to evaluate the efficacy of interventions. Currently, CSRs are mainly evaluation of intervention from RCTs.

The traditional literature review is narrative, which does not need rigorous evaluation of the quality of the literatures, and might have some limitations. High quality systematic review requires clear research questions and hypotheses, strives to collect all published and unpublished studies to reduce publication bias and other biases, has clear inclusion and exclusion criteria to reduce selection bias, and all included studies should be rigorously appraised individually, and potential sources of bias and heterogeneity of findings need to be explored.

The basic steps of systematic review include (1) formulating questions, (2) developing study protocol and determination of inclusion and exclusion criteria, (3) systematically and comprehensively retrieving the literatures, (4) screening the literatures with the inclusion criteria, (5) quality appraisal of the studies, (6) extracting data, (7) analysis and report of results, (8) interpretation of results and report writing, (9) updating systematic review.

19.5. Meta-analysis[7,8]

Traditional medical literature review mainly relies on the authorities to summarize and evaluate according to their understanding of the basic theory of a field and knowledge on related disciplines. Collection of information and data depend on the researcher's experience and subjective desire, and different reviewers studying on the same field often come to very different conclusions. Obviously, the traditional literature review method lacks objectivity, and cannot quantitatively synthesize total effect. In 1955, Beecher took a comprehensive quantitative study on the results of 15 studies in the medical field, which showed that placebo had 35% treatment effect. In 1976, G. V. Glass firstly named the comprehensive literature research method of merger statistics for "Meta-analysis", which was developed into a comprehensive quantitative method. Meanwhile, application of Meta-analysis also expanded from education, psychology and other social sciences to biomedicine, and had been widely used in the late 1980s.

There are different opinions on the definition of Meta-analysis, which can be divided into narrow and broad.

Narrow — "The Cochrane Library" defined it as: Meta-analysis is statistical technique for assembling the results of several studies in a single numerical estimate.

Broad — the definition in the "Evidence-Based Medicine" book is: A systematic review that uses quantitative methods to summarize the results.

Meta-analysis is a kind of systematic review, and systematic review can be Meta-analysis or cannot be Meta-analysis.

Meta-analysis is a research method for systematic and quantitative statistical analysis and comprehensive evaluation on the results of several independent studies with the same study objective. Initially, a sufficient number of research results (such as P-value) were collected from the literatures, which was combined as a quality qualitative result by using statistical analysis. Currently, Meta-analysis has become a necessary statistical method in EBM for quantitative systematic review on the literatures, and the commonly used software for Meta-analysis include RevMan, STATA, etc. Because the data used in Meta-analysis is mainly the statistical analysis results reported in the literatures, such as the P-value of hypothesis testing, correlation coefficient of two variables, rate or mean difference between the test group and the control group, odds ratio (OR) exposed to the risk factor between the case group and the control group, etc., so it is also called "reanalysis" of the statistical results of the literatures.

The most important role of Meta-analysis is to more objectively and comprehensively reflect previous findings in order to make it a more comprehensive understanding of the discovery (or hypothesis), and to provide a basis for further research. Specifically, Meta-analysis is intended to address (1) increasing the statistical power to improve the estimate of the effect size (ES) of the study factor, (2) identifying the differences among individual study and solving contradictions and uncertainties caused by these differences, (3) looking for new hypothesis to answer the question not mentioned or cannot be answered in individual study.

19.6. ES[7,9]

Meta-analysis focuses on the merger of ES to obtain a quantitative merger result. The ES, also called effect magnitude, is a dimensionless statistic reflecting the size of association between treatment factor (level) and response variable of each study, such as logarithm of OR or relative risk (RR) of two rates, the difference between the two rates (rate difference, RD), standardized mean difference (SMD) between experimental group and control group (the difference between the two means divided by the standard deviation of the control group or merge standard deviation), correlation coefficient, etc. The common ES in Meta-analysis includes difference between two groups and correlation between two variables. ES eliminates the effects of different units of measurement results, therefore, the ES of each study can be compared or merged. The basic idea of Meta-analysis is to weightedly merge the collected outcome variables or statistical indicators from various studies (such as mean difference, RD, OR, RR, correlation coefficient, etc.), calculate the merged statistics (merged ES) to get more reliable conclusion.

1. RD, RR and OR

Assuming k-studies included in a Meta-analysis, for dichotomous variables, taking fourfold table as an example, a_i, b_i, c_i, d_i represent the number of cases in each grid of the fourfold table of the i-study. In clinical trials and cohort studies, n_{1i}, n_{2i} represent the sample sizes in the interventional group (exposure group) and the control group of the i-study, p_{1i}, p_{2i} represent the ratios of positive events in the interventional group (exposure group) and the control group. In case-control studies, n_{1i}, n_{2i} represent the sample sizes in the case group and the control group of the i-study, p_{1i}, p_{2i} represent the proportions of cases exposed to a risk factor in the case group and the control group. Therefore, the statistics can be calculated: RD, RR and OR. In order to meet the requirements of normality, general natural logarithm will be performed in the calculation of RR and OR, calculated 95% confidence internal (CI) of log(OR) or log(RR) then can be converted to 95% CI of RR or OR.

2. Mean difference and SMD

If various studies reported means as outcome variables, mean difference can be used for merger. n_{1i}, n_{2i} represent the sample sizes in the interventional group and the control group of the i study in Meta-analysis, $\bar{x}_{1i}, \bar{x}_{2i}$ represent the means of the interventional group and the control group of the i study, then the mean difference between the two groups is $\bar{x}_{1i} - \bar{x}_{2i}$.

Due to the potential different dimension of means in studies in Meta-analysis, outcome variables can be standardized to eliminate the effect of dimension. The standardized dimensionless statistic is the ES.

3. Other statistics

If the ES related outcome variables (statistical indicators) are not directly provided in original studies included in the Meta-analysis, and only the statistical test results (such as t-value, u-value, F-value, χ^2-value, P-value, etc.) are reported, sometimes these test statistics can be converted into ESs. For example, the u-statistic, comparison of two means of measurement data, can be converted into ES:

$$\hat{\delta} = u\sqrt{\left(\frac{1}{n_{1i}} + \frac{1}{n_{2i}}\right)}.$$

In addition, if the study only reports P-value of hypothesis test or test statistic, simple qualitative integrated approach can also be used, such as merging P-value method (Fisher method), merging u-value method (Stouffer method), etc.

19.7. Heterogeneity Test[7,9,10]

Variation among studies included in Meta-analysis is called heterogeneity. Before the merging of effect in meta-analysis, heterogeneity test needs to be conducted, also known as homogeneity test.

The Q-statistic or I^2-statistic are generally used to identify and investigate heterogeneity and its sources among studies.

The heterogeneity test uses Q-statistic for chi-square test (θ_i is the "real effect" of the i study):

H_0: $\theta_1 = \theta_2 = \cdots = \theta_k$.

H_1: not all $\theta_1, \theta_2, \ldots, \theta_k$ are the same.

Significant level α (e.g. $\alpha = 0.05$).

If H_0 is true, under the condition of a large sample study, the test statistic is

$$Q_w = \sum_i^k W_i(Y_i - \hat{\theta})^2 \sim \chi^2_{k-1},$$

in which W_i is the weighting coefficient. Y_i is the ES of each individual study, its overall parameter is θ. k-represents k-independent studies included in Meta-analysis. $\hat{\theta}$ can be obtained by maximum likelihood estimation or weighted least squares estimation:

$$\hat{\theta} = \sum W_i Y_i / \sum W_i, \quad W_i = 1/s_i^2.$$

If Q_w is greater than the critical value of χ^2 distribution with degrees of freedom of $k-1$, H_0 will be rejected, which means heterogeneity exists among the included studies in the Meta-analysis, the "real effect" of k-studies are not identical. The combined effect size in Meta-analysis should reflect the average (or aggregate level) of the "true effect", and random effects model should be used.

If Q_w is not greater than the critical value of χ^2 distribution with degrees of freedom of $k-1$, H_0 will not be rejected, which means not enough heterogeneity exists among the included studies in the Meta-analysis. Then the k-studies might come from the same population, which means the "real effect" of k-studies are identical, and fixed-effects model could be used.

As can be seen, Q-statistic is actually a weighted sum of squares of the ES. However, the power of the Q-test is low, and factors influencing the power of the Q-test include the number of studies included, total amount of information (i.e. total weight or inverse of variance), distribution of different studies' weight (that is, degree of dispersion of ES), etc. When the number of studies included in the Meta-analysis is small, rejection of H_0 does not necessarily mean no heterogeneity among studies, which probably is because of Type II error due to low-test power.

In 2003, on the basis of Q-statistic, JPT Higgins *et al.* adopted I^2 statistic (see 19.8 I^2 statistic) as an evaluation index for heterogeneity analysis in Meta-analysis.

19.8. I^2-statistic[3,10,11,12]

In homogeneity test (heterogeneity test) of Meta-analysis, its Q-statistic is vulnerably affected by the quantity of research literatures. If many research literatures are included, pooled variance is small, then its contribution to the Q-value is large when the weight is large, which easily obtains false positives (that is, reject H_0, heterogeneity) result; conversely, if small number of research literatures is included, the weight will also be small, and the test power is often too low, which is easy to obtain false negatives (that is, not rejecting H_0, homogeneity) result. Therefore, it easily leads to choosing the wrong model, in particular choosing the wrong fixed-effects model instead of the random effects model, which may make the results differ very far, or even get the opposite conclusion. To solve this problem, Higgins,[10] corrected Q-statistic with degrees of freedom, and proposed I^2-statistic as indicator for evaluating heterogeneity to reduce the impact of the number of research literatures on the heterogeneity test results. The I^2-statistic is commonly used as another heterogeneity test method based on the Q-statistic, which is calculated as

$$I^2 = \begin{cases} \frac{Q-(k-1)}{Q} \times 100\%, & Q > k-1, \\ 0 & Q \leq k-1, \end{cases}$$

wherein Q is the chi-squared statistic of heterogeneity test, k is the number of studies included in Meta-analysis, and $k-1$ is the degrees of freedom.

I^2 reflects the proportion of heterogeneity part in the total variation of the ES, and its value range is 0–100%. If I^2 is 0, then no heterogeneity was observed among studies, and the larger the I^2, the greater the heterogeneity. According to the size of the I^2-statistic, Higgins[10] divided heterogeneity into three levels: low, medium, and high, corresponding I^2 of 25%, 50%, and 75%, respectively. Wang[13] showed that in general, if I^2 is greater than 50%, then there is obvious heterogeneity. However, in practice, He[11] reported that $I^2 <$ 56% suggests the presence of heterogeneity among studies, and $I^2 < 31\%$ suggests homogeneity among studies. Thresholds for the interpretation of I^2 can be misleading, since the importance of inconsistency depends on several factors. In *Cochrane Handbook for Systematic Reviews of Interventions* a rough guide to interpretation of I^2 is as follows:

0–40%: might not be important;

30–60%: may represent moderate heterogeneity;

50–90%: may represent substantial heterogeneity;

75–100%: considerable heterogeneity.

Generally, $I^2 > 40\%$ suggests the presence of heterogeneity among studies.

Compared with the Q-statistic, I^2 is a relative rate, which does not depend on the number of included studies, and also has nothing to do with the category of the ES. Therefore, it can better reflect the proportion of non-sampling error (heterogeneity among studies) in the total variation. In practice, Q- and I^2-statistics are provided at the same time for a comprehensive understanding of heterogeneity.

19.9. Mathematical Model for Merging of ES[7,9]

Meta-analysis includes point estimation and interval estimation of the combined ES, and the analysis of the sources of variation is crucial on model selection in ES estimation. The sources of variation in estimation of the combined ES in Meta-analysis have at least two parts: inner-study variation and inter-study variation. The inner-study variation refers to the different sample size and sampling error for each independent studies in Meta-analysis. In general, study with large sample size has relatively small sampling error, high precision, and large weight in combined analysis of ES. The inter-study variation refers to the differences of individual studies in many aspects, including study design, study participants, bias control, etc., and the quality of the studies are diverse. If the inter-study variation is small, that is, the difference among the studies is only because of sampling, each individual study included in the Meta-analysis is from the same population, and the effect of each independent study is only an estimate of the parameter of overall effect, then fixed-effects model can be used. If the inter-study variation is large, that is, variation is not caused only by sampling, each independent study is from different and related population, and each study has its corresponding overall parameter, then random-effects model can be used. Therefore, the mathematical models for combined effect estimation in Meta-analysis include fixed-effects model and random-effects model.

(1) Fixed-effects model

Fixed-effects model assumes that the effect index statistic of the studies is homogeneous, which are independent random samples from the same population. The difference among effect index statistics of studies is only from sampling error, variation among different studies is very small, and the difference between the effect index statistics for each study and the population parameter is due to sampling error. Assuming ES for each independent study is Y_i, the overall parameter is θ, that is, $E(Y_i) = \theta$, $s_i^2 = \text{var}(Y_i)$ represents the variance of the i-study. When the sample size is large, according to the central limit theorem, Y_i approximately obeys normal distribution with population mean of θ. The s_i^2 is assumed known, in the fixed-effects model, $Y_i \overset{\text{indep}}{\sim} N(\theta, s_i^2), i = 1, 2, \ldots, K$ represents the K-independent studies included in the Meta-analysis, and θ is the combined effect size of the Meta-analysis. Therefore, the combined ES given by the fixed-effects model is the point estimate and its 95% CI for the same population parameter of each study.

(2) Random-effects model

Random-effects model assumes that the effect index statistic of the studies is heterogeneous, which are independent random samples from different populations. The difference of effect index statistic among studies cannot be explained by sampling error. The variation among studies varied greatly, the effect index statistics for each study is corresponding to its population parameters θ_i $(i = 1, 2, \ldots, k)$, but $\theta_1, \theta_2, \ldots, \theta_k$ can be assumed approximately obeying $N(\theta, \tau_\theta^2)$, where θ is the overall mean of $\theta_1, \theta_2, \ldots, \theta_k$. Assuming Y_i is the ES of the included i-study in Meta-analysis, Y_i is from the normal distribution with mean of θ_i and variance of s_i^2, that is, θ_i is the "real effect" of the i-study. $\theta_1, \theta_2, \ldots, \theta_k$ is independent of each other. θ is the combined effect (average or overall level of effect) of Meta-analysis, τ_θ^2 is inter-study variation, namely random effect. In the random-effects model, there is $Y_i|\theta_i, s_i^2 \overset{\text{indep}}{\sim} N(\theta_i, s_i^2)$, $\theta_i|\theta, \tau_\theta^2 \overset{\text{indep}}{\sim} N(\theta, \tau_\theta^2)$. Therefore, the combined effect size given by the random-effects model is the point estimate and its 95% CI for the population mean θ of population parameters $\theta_1, \theta_2, \ldots, \theta_k$.

19.10. Merging of OR[7,14,15]

It aims to merge the logarithm of OR (or RR) of the two rates in relative studies. It assumes that there are k-case — control studies, and the results for the i-study are

	Exposure factor		
	+	−	$\mathrm{OR}_i = \frac{a_i d_i}{b_i c_i}$
Case	a_i	b_i	
Control	c_i	d_i	$\mathrm{ES} = y_i = \ln(\mathrm{OR}_i)$

The steps for combining of OR values are as follows:

(1) Homogeneity test

H_0: Population means of ES y of studies are equal.

H_1: Population means of ES y of studies are not all equal.

Significant level (e.g. $\alpha = 0.05$).

Calculating the standard error $SE_{\ln(\mathrm{OR}_i)}$ (if the value in a_i, b_i, c_i and d_i is "0", then it is set to "0.5" for calculation) and weighting coefficients w_i:

$$\mathrm{SE}_{\ln(\mathrm{OR}_i)} = \sqrt{\frac{1}{a_i} + \frac{1}{b_i} + \frac{1}{c_i} + \frac{1}{d_i}},$$

$$w_i = \frac{1}{\mathrm{SE}^2_{\ln(\mathrm{OR}_i)}} = \left(\frac{1}{a_i} + \frac{1}{b_i} + \frac{1}{c_i} + \frac{1}{d_i}\right)^{-1}.$$

Then the test statistic $Q = \sum w_i y_i^2 - \frac{(\sum w_i y_i)^2}{\sum w_i}$, Q obeys chi-square distribution with $\nu = k-1$. If the result of chi-square test refuses H_0, random-effects model will be used for weighted merger; otherwise, fixed-effects model is used for weighted merger.

(2) Weighted merger by fixed-effects model

The weighted mean $\bar{y}$ and the variance of $\bar{y}$ for the study y_i are

$$\bar{y} = \frac{\sum w_i y_i}{\sum w_i}, \quad S_{\bar{y}}^2 = \left(\sum w_i\right)^{-1}.$$

The combined OR value and 95% confidence intervals (95% CI) are

$$\mathrm{OR} = \exp(\bar{y}), \quad \text{and} \quad 95\%\ \mathrm{CI}: \exp(\bar{y} \pm 1.96 S_{\bar{y}}).$$

(3) Weighted merger by random effects model

In Meta-analysis, if homogeneity test rejects the null hypothesis, the random-effects model should be used for weighted merger of OR_i. When the homogeneity test statistic $Q < k-1$, it is similar with the fixed-effects model; when $Q \geq k-1$, the random-effects model mainly corrects w_i from the fixed-effects model, which changes the weighting coefficient w_i into $w_i^* = (w_i^{-1} + h)^{-1}$, in which

$$h = \frac{Q - k + 1}{\Sigma w_i - \Sigma w_i^2 / \Sigma w_i}.$$

Other calculations are the same as the fixed-effects model.

In addition to dealing with homogeneity test and weighted merger of OR values in case-controlled studies, the above methods can also be used for RR values in RCTs and cohort studies. For example, a_i and b_i are the positive number and negative number in the experimental group, respectively, and c_i and d_i are the positive number and negative number in the control group, respectively. When both positive rates (or negative rates) of the two groups are small, $\frac{a_i d_i}{b_i c_i}$ can be used to approximately estimate the RR, followed by homogeneity test and weighted merger.

19.11. Merging of RD[7,14,15]

It aims to merge the difference between two rates (RD) of the relevant studies. It assumes that in k-studies reports, the observational results of the experimental group and the control group of the i-study are as shown in Table 19.11.1.

The positive rates of the experimental group and the control group of the i-study are $p_{1i} = \frac{m_{1i}}{n_{1i}}$ and $p_{2i} = \frac{m_{2i}}{n_{2i}} (i = 1, 2, \ldots, k)$, respectively, and the combined rate is $p_i = \frac{m_{1i}+m_{2i}}{n_{1i}+n_{2i}}$. The ES of the i-study is the rate difference, $RD_i = p_{1i} - p_{2i}$. Furthermore, the related ES can also be presented as $\mathrm{OR}_i = \frac{a_i d_i}{b_i c_i}$ in order to use the above OR values merge method to perform Meta-analysis. The steps are as follows:

(1) Homogeneity test

H_0: Population means of ES RD_i of studies are equal.

H_1: Population means of ES RD_i of studies are not all equal.

Significant level (e.g. $\alpha = 0.05$).

Calculation:

$$u_i = \frac{p_{1i} - p_{2i}}{\sqrt{p_i(1-p_i)(\frac{1}{n_{1i}} + \frac{1}{n_{2i}})}},$$

$$\chi^2 = \sum u_i^2 - \frac{(\sum u_i)^2}{k}, \quad \nu = k - 1.$$

If $P > \alpha$, fixed-effects model is used for weighted merger. Otherwise, random-effects model is used.

(2) Weighted merger by fixed-effects model

As weighting coefficient $w_i = n_{1i}n_{2i}/(n_{1i} + n_{2i})$, the weighted mean $\overline{\mathrm{RD}}$ and variance of $\overline{\mathrm{RD}}$ of ES RD_i of each study are

$$\overline{\mathrm{RD}} = \frac{\sum w_i \mathrm{RD}_i}{\sum w_i},$$

$$S^2_{\overline{\mathrm{RD}}} = \frac{\sum w_i p_i(1-p_i)}{(\sum w_i)^2}.$$

Table 19.11.1. Observational results of the two groups of the i-study.

Experimental group				Control group			
Sample size	Positive number	Negative number	Positive rate	Sample size	Positive number	Negative number	Positive rate
n_{1i}	$m_{1i}(a_i)$	b_i	p_{1i}	n_{2i}	$m_{2i}(c_i)$	d_i	p_{2i}

And the 95% CI is $\overline{\text{RD}} \pm 1.96 S_{\overline{\text{RD}}}$

(3) Weighted merger by random-effects model

If the result of homogeneity test rejects H_0, the random-effects model should be used for weighted merging of the difference between two rates, the weighting coefficient w_i should be changed to

$$w_i^* = \left[\frac{1}{n_{1i}} p_{1i}(1-p_{1i}) + \frac{1}{n_{2i}} p_{2i}(1-p_{2i})\right]^{-1}.$$

The 95% CI of population mean of $\text{RD}_i = p_{1i} - p_{2i}$ should be changed to $\overline{\text{RD}} \pm \frac{1.96}{\sqrt{\sum w_i^*}}$, and other calculations are the same as in fixed-effects model.

19.12. Merging of Mean Difference[7,14,15]

It aims to merge the SMD between the experimental and control groups (the difference between the two means divided by the standard deviation of the control group or merge standard deviation). The means of the experimental group and the control group in the i-study of the k ($k \geq 2$) studies are referred as $\bar{X}_{1i}$ and $\bar{X}_{2i}$, respectively, and their variances are S_{1i}^2 and S_{2i}^2, then the combined variance S_i^2 is

$$S_i^2 = \frac{(n_{1i}-1)s_{1i}^2 + (n_{2i}-1)s_{2i}^2}{n_{1i}+n_{2i}-2}.$$

Sometimes, the S_i^2 can be substituted by the variance of the control group, then the ES of the i-study is $d_i = (\bar{X}_{1i} - \bar{X}_{2i})/S_i, i = 1, 2, 3, \ldots, k$. The merging steps are as follows:

(1) Calculating the weighted average ES and the estimation error: the weighted mean of ES d_i of each study (average effect size) is

$$\bar{d} = \frac{\sum w_i d_i}{\sum w_i},$$

where w_i, is the weight coefficient, and it can be the total number of cases of each study.

The variance of ES d_i of each study is

$$S_d^2 = \frac{\sum w_i (d_i - \bar{d})}{\sum w_i} = \frac{\sum w_i d_i^2 - \bar{d}^2 \sum w_i}{\sum w_i}.$$

The variance of the random error is

$$S_e^2 = \frac{4k}{\sum w_i}\left(1 + \frac{\bar{d}^2}{8}\right).$$

(2) Homogeneity test

H_0: Population means of ES d_i of studies are equal.

H_1: Population means of ES d_i of studies are not all equal.

Significant level (e.g. $\alpha = 0.05$).

$$\chi^2 = \frac{kS_d^2}{S_e^2}, \quad \nu = k - 1.$$

If the H_0 is rejected and H_1 is accepted at $\alpha = 0.05$ level, each study has inconsistent results, the merging of d_i (95% CI) should adopt random-effects model. If the homogeneity test does not reject H_0, the fixed-effects model should be adopted.

(3) The 95% CI of the overall mean ES

Fixed-effects model:

$$\bar{d} \pm 1.96 S_{\bar{d}} = \bar{d} \pm 1.96 S_e/\sqrt{k}.$$

Random-effects model:

$$\bar{d} \pm 1.96 S_\delta = \bar{d} \pm 1.96\sqrt{S_d^2 - S_e^2}.$$

19.13. Forest Plot[16]

Forest plot is a necessary part of a Meta-analysis report, which can simply and intuitively describe the statistical analysis results of Meta-analysis.

In plane rectangular coordinate system, forest plot takes a vertical line as the center, a horizontal axis at the bottom as ES scale, and a number of segments paralleling to the horizontal axis represents the ES of each study included in Meta-analysis and its 95% CI. The combined ES and 95% CI is represented by a diamond located at the bottom of forest plot (Figure 19.13.1).

The vertical line representing no effect is also named as invalid line. When the ES is RR or OR, the corresponding horizontal scale of the invalid line is 1, and when the ES is RD, weighted mean difference (WMD) or SMD, the corresponding horizontal scale of the invalid line is 0.

In forest plot, each segment represents a study, the square on the segment represents the point estimate of the ES of the study, and the area of each square is proportional to the study's weight (that is, sample size) in the Meta-analysis. The length of the segment directly represents 95% CI of the ES of the study, short segment means a narrow 95% CI and its weight is also relatively large in combined effect size. If the confidence intervals for

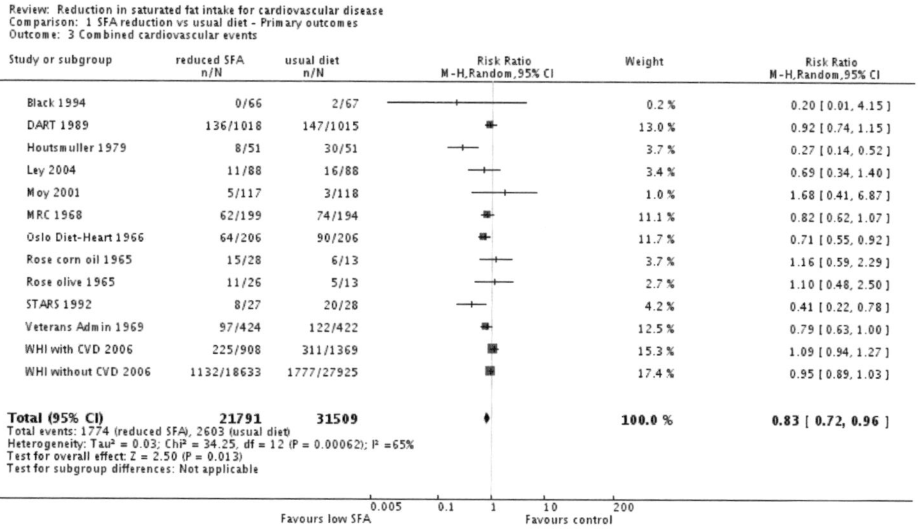

Fig. 19.13.1. Forest plot in Meta-analysis.

individual studies overlap with the invalid line, that is, the 95% CI of ES RR or OR containing 1, or the 95% CI of ES RD, WMD or SMD containing 0, it demonstrates that at the given level of confidence, their ESs do not differ from no effect for the individual study.

The point estimate of the combined effect size located at the widest points of the upper and lower ends of the diamond (diamond center of gravity), and the length of the ends of the diamond represents the 95% CI of the combined effect size. If the diamond overlaps with the invalid line, which represents the combined effect size of the Meta-analysis is not statistically significant.

Forest plot can be used for investigation of heterogeneity among studies by the level of overlap of the ESs and its 95% CIs among included studies, but it has low accuracy.

The forest plot in Figure 19.13.1 is from a CSR, which displays whether reduction in saturated fat intake reduces the risk of cardiovascular events. Forest plot shows the basic data of the included studies (including the sample size of each study, weight, point estimate and 95% CI of the ES RR, etc.). Among nine studies with RR < 1 (square located on left side of the invalid line), six studies are not statistically significant (segment overlapping with the invalid line). The combined RR by random-effects model is 0.83, with 95% CI of [0.72, 0.96], which was statistically significant (diamond at the bottom of forest plot not overlapping with the invalid line) The Meta-analysis shows, compared with normal diet, dietary intervention with reduction in saturated fat intake can reduce the risk of cardiovascular events by 17%. In the lower left of the forest plot, results of heterogeneity test and Z-test results of combined effect size are also given. The test result for heterogeneity shows $P = 0.00062 < 0.1$ and $I^2 = 65\%$, which indicates significant heterogeneity among included studies. And $P = 0.013 < 0.05$ for Z-test shows that the results of the Meta-analysis is statistically significant.

19.14. Bias in Meta-analysis[17]

Bias refers to the results of a study systematically deviating from the true value. Meta-analysis is natural as an observational study, and bias is inevitable. DT Felson reported that bias in Meta-analysis can be divided into three categories: sampling bias, selection bias and bias within the research. To reduce bias, a clear and strict unity of literature inclusion and exclusion criteria should be developed; all related literatures should be systematically, comprehensively and unbiasedly retrieved; in the process of selecting studies and extracting data, at least two persons should be involved independently with blind method, furthermore, specialized data extraction form should be designed and quality evaluation criteria should be cleared.

Cochrane Systematic Review Handbook suggests measuring the integrity of the included studies in Meta-analysis mainly through report bias, including seven categories: publication bias, time lag bias, multiple publication bias, geographical bias, citing bias, language bias and result reporting bias.

In the above different bias, publication bias is the most studied, which is caused because statistically significant results are more easily published in comparision to results without statistical significance. Publication bias has great impact on the validity and reliability of the Meta-analysis results. However, control of publication bias is difficult to practice, and some existing methods can only roughly investigate and identify publication bias, including funnel plot, Egger linear regression test, Begg rank correlation test, trim and fill method, fail–safe number, etc.

Funnel plot (Figure 19.14.1) is a common method for qualitative judgment of publication bias, the basic assumption is that the accuracy of the included studies with ES increases with sample size. In small studies with ES as the abscissa, the sample size (or ES of standard error) for the vertical axis is a scatter plot, if there is no publication bias, scatter should form a symmetrical inverted funnel-shaped, that is, low precision spread at the bottom of the funnel, and high precision large sample studies are distributed on top of the funnel and focus narrows. If the funnel plot asymmetry exists

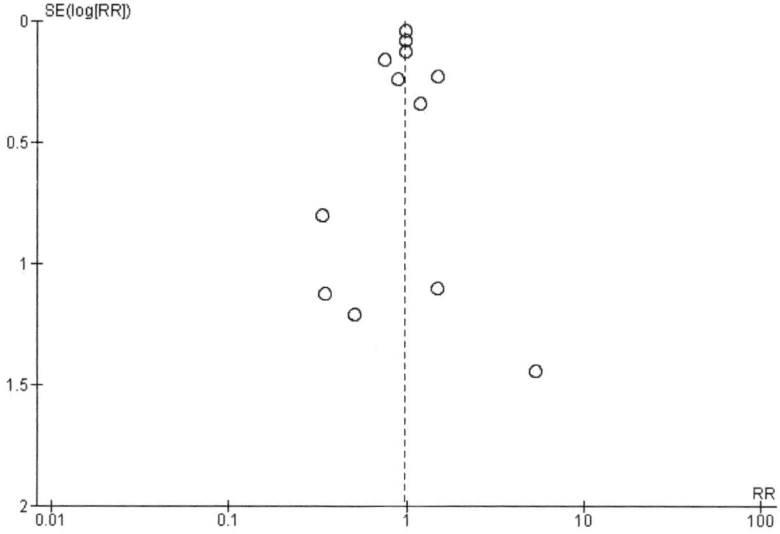

Fig. 19.14.1. Funnel plot in Meta-analysis.

or is incomplete, it will prompt publication bias. It should be noted that, in addition to publication bias, heterogeneity among studies and small studies of low quality can also affect the symmetry of the funnel plot, especially when the Meta-analysis included only in a few small studies, the use do funnel plot is difficult to judge whether there is publication bias. Funnel plot in Figure 19.14.1 shows a basic symmetry, which is less likely to suggest the presence of publication bias.

In Meta-analysis, sensitivity analysis can also be used to examine the soundness of the conclusion, potential bias and heterogeneity. Commonly used methods for sensitivity analysis include the difference of the point and interval estimation of combined effect size among selection of different models; the change of the results of the Meta-analysis after excluding studies with abnormal results (such as study with low quality, too large or too small sample size). If the results of the Meta-analysis do not substantially change before and after the sensitivity analysis, the results of the combined effect is relatively reliable.

19.15. Meta-analysis of Diagnostic Test Accuracy[18,19]

In medicine, a diagnostic test is any kind of medical test performed to aid in the diagnosis or detection of disease, using application of laboratory test, equipment and other means, and identifying the patient with some kinds of disease from patients with other diseases or conditions. Generalized diagnostic methods include a variety of laboratory tests (biochemistry, immunology, microbiology, pathology, etc.), diagnostic imaging (ultrasound, CT, X-ray, magnetic resonance, etc.), instrument examination (ECG, EEG, nuclear scan, endoscopy, etc.) and also enquiry of medical history, physical examination, etc.

For a particular diagnostic test, it may have been a number of studies, but because these studies have different random errors, and the diagnostic values of studies are often different, the obtained accuracy evaluation index of the diagnostic tests are not the same. Because of differences in regions, individuals, diagnostic methods and conditions, published findings on the same diagnostic method might be different or even contradictory; and with the continued improvement in new technologies, more and more choices are available. In order to undertake a comprehensive analysis of the results of different studies to obtain a comprehensive conclusion, Meta-analysis of diagnostic test accuracy is needed. Meta-analysis of diagnostic test accuracy emerged in recent years, and is recommended by the working group on diagnostic test accuracy study report specification (STARD) and the Cochrane Collaboration.

Meta-analysis of diagnostic test accuracy is mainly to evaluate the accuracy of a diagnostic measure on the target disease, mostly evaluation of the sensibility and specificity on target disease, and reporting likelihood ratio, diagnostic OR, etc. For evaluation of the diagnostic value of a certain diagnostic measure on target disease, case-control studies are generally included and the control group are healthy people. Furthermore, in order to evaluate the therapeutic effect or improvement on the prognosis of patients after the use of diagnostic measure, RCTs should be included. In both cases, the Meta-analysis is the same as the Meta-analysis of intervention studies.

The key of evaluation of diagnostic tests is to obtain the diagnostic accuracy results. By accuracy evaluation index, the degree of coincidence between the test result and the reference standard result is obtained. Commonly used effect index in Meta-analysis of diagnostic test accuracy includes sensitivity (Sen), specificity (Spe), likelihood ratio (LR), diagnostic odds ratio (DOR) and symmetric receiver operating characteristic (SROC) curve, etc.

The results in Meta-analysis of diagnostic test accuracy include summarized sen and spe of diagnostic test, a summary ROC curve and related parameters, the summary results of diagnostic relative accuracy, etc.

The clinical significance of the Meta-analysis of diagnostic test accuracy includes providing the best current clinical diagnostic methods, being conducive to early correct diagnosis and early treatment to enhance clinical benefit, its results having the benefits of reducing length of stay and saving health resources, thus increasing health economic benefits, furthermore, promoting the development of clinical diagnostic tests-related conditions.

19.16. Meta-regression[20–22]

Meta-regression is the use of regression analysis to explore the impact of covariates including certain experiments or patient characteristics on the combined ES of Meta-analysis. Its purpose is to make clear the sources of heterogeneity among studies, and to investigate the effect of covariates on the combined effects. Meta-regression is an expansion of subgroup analysis, which can analyze the effect of continuous characteristics and classification features, and in principle, it can simultaneously analyze the effect of a number of factors. In nature, Meta-regression is similar with general linear regression. In general linear regression analysis, outcome variables can be estimated or predicted in accordance with one or more explanatory variables. In Meta-regression, the outcome variable is an estimate of ES (e.g. mean difference MD, RD, logOR or logRR, etc.). Explanatory variables are study characteristics affecting the ES of the intervention, which is commonly referred to as "potential effect modifiers" or covariates. Meta-regression and general linear regression usually differ in two ways. Firstly, because each study is being assigned with weight according to the estimated value of its effect, study with large sample size has relatively bigger impact on correlation than study with small sample size. Secondly, it is wise to retain residual heterogeneity between intervention effects by the explanatory variables. This comes to the term "random effect Meta-regression" because additional variability is not treated in the same way as in random-effects Meta-analysis.

Meta-regression is essentially an observational study. There may be a large variation in the characteristic variable of the participants in test, but it can only be aggregated for analysis as study or test level covariate, and sometimes, summary covariate does not represent the true level of the individual which produces the "aggregation bias". False positive conclusion might occur in data mining, especially when small number of included studies with many experimental features, if multiple analyses are performed on each test feature, false positive results might possibly occur. Meta-regression analysis cannot fully explain all heterogeneity, allowing the existence of remaining heterogeneity. Therefore, in Meta-regression analysis, it should pay special attention to (1) ensuring an adequate number of studies included in the regression analysis, (2) presetting covariates to be analyzed in research process, (3) selecting appropriate number of covariates, and the exploration of each covariate must comply with scientific principles, (4) effects of each covariate cannot often be identified, (5) there should be no interaction among covariates. In short, it must fully understand the limitations of Meta-regression and their countermeasures in order to correctly use Meta-regression and interpret the obtained results.

Commonly used statistical methods for Meta-regression analysis include fixed effects Meta-regression model and random-effects Meta-regression model. In the random-effects model, there are several methods which can be used to estimate the regression equation coefficients and variation among studies, including maximum likelihood method, moment method, limiting maximum likelihood method, Bayes method, etc.

19.17. Network Meta-analysis (NMA)[23]

When comparing multiple interventions, evidence network may have both direct evidence based on head-to-head comparison in classic Meta-analysis and indirect evidence. A set of methods extending Meta-analysis with direct comparison of two groups to simultaneous comparison among a series of different treatments on a number of treatment factors is called network Meta-analysis.

Network Meta-analysis includes adjusted indirect comparison and mixed treatment comparison.

(1) Adjusted indirect comparison

To compare the effectiveness of intervention measures B and C, if there is no evidence of direct comparison, a common control A can be based on, Indirect evidence of B versus C can be obtained by A versus B and A versus C (Figure 19.17.1(a)). In Figure 19.17.1(b), through the common control A, it can also get six different indirect evidence for intervention comparison: B versus C, B versus D, B versus E, C versus D, C versus E, D versus E.

(2) Mixed treatment comparison

The results of direct comparison and indirect comparison can be combined, and it can simultaneously analyze comparison of treatment effects among multiple interventions, as shown in Figure 19.17.1(c) and 19.17.1(d). In Figure 19.17.1(c), the interventions A, B and C form a closed loop, which represents both direct and indirect comparison. Figure 19.17.1(d) is more complex, there is at least one closed loop, which can combine the indirect comparison evidence on the basis of direct comparison. The difference

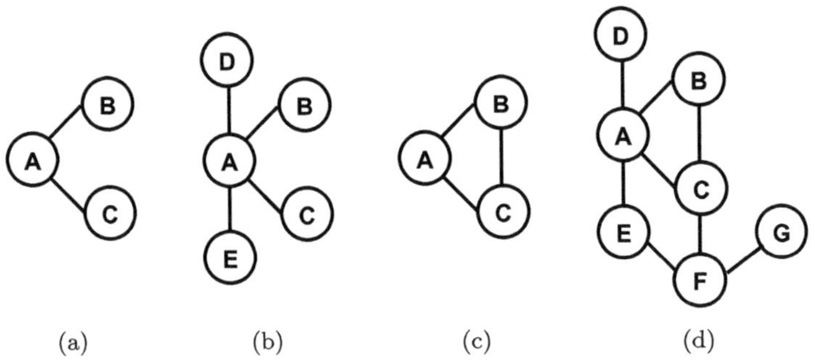

Fig. 19.17.1. Types of network Meta-Analysis.

between Figure 19.17.1(a), (b) and Figure 19.17.1(c), (d) is that the former is an open-loop network, and the latter has at least one closed loop.

Network Meta-analysis involves three basic hypotheses: homogeneity, similarity and consistency. Test of homogeneity is the same as classic Meta-analysis. Adjusted indirect comparison needs to consider similarity assumption, and currently, there are no clear test methods, which can be judged from two aspects of clinical similarity and methodology similarity. Mixed treatment comparison needs to merge direct evidence and indirect evidence which should perform consistency test, and commonly used methods include Bucher method, Lumley method, etc. Furthermore, network Meta-analysis also needs to carry out validity analysis to examine the validity of the results and the interpretation of bias.

Network Meta-analysis with open-loop network can use Bucher adjusted indirect comparison method in classical frequentist framework, merge with the inverse variance method by stepwise approach. It can also use generalized linear model and Meta-regression model, etc.

Mixed treatment comparison is based on closed-loop network, which generally uses the Bayesian method for Meta-analysis and is realized by "WinBUGS" software. Advantage of Bayesian Meta-analysis is that the posterior probability can be used to sort all interventions involved in the comparison, and to a certain extent, it overcomes the limitation of unstable iterative maximum likelihood function in parameter estimation in frequentist method which might lead to biased result, it is more flexible in modeling. Currently, most network Meta-analysis analyzes the literature by using Bayesian method.

The report specification of network Meta-analysis can adopt "The PRISMA Extension Statement for Reporting of Systematic Reviews Incorporating Network Meta-analyses of Health Care Interventions", which revises and supplements based on the PRISMA statement, and adds five entries.

19.18. Software for Meta-analysis[24]

Over the past decade, with rapid development of Meta-analysis methodology, Meta-analysis software emerged, and the software can be divided into two categories: Meta-analysis specific software and general-purpose software with Meta-analysis function. Currently, commonly used software for Meta-analysis are the following:

(1) Review Manager (RevMan)

It is a Meta-analysis specific software for preparing and maintaining CSR for international Cochrane Collaboration, which is developed and maintained by the Nordic Cochrane Centre, and can be downloaded for free. The current latest version is RevMan 5.3.5, and it is available for different operating system including Windows, Linux, and Mac. RevMan has four built-in types of CSR production format including intervention systematic review, systematic reviews of diagnostic test accuracy, methodology system review and summary evaluation of system review, which is simple in operation, without programming, and with intuitive and reliable results. It is the most widely used and mature Meta-analysis software. With RevMan, it can easily complete merger of ES, test for merger of ES, combining confidence intervals, test for heterogeneity, and subgroup analysis, draw forest plot and funnel plot, can also create the risk of bias assessment tool, evidence results summary table, PRISMA literature retrieve flowchart, and can import data from each other with GRADE classification software GRADEprofiler.

(2) STATA

STATA has powerful features and is a small sized statistical analysis software. It is the most respected general purpose software for Meta-analysis. Command of Meta-analysis is not the official Stata command, which is a set of procedures with extremely well functions written by a number of statisticians and Stata users, and can be integrated into STATA. STATA can complete almost all types of Meta-analysis including Meta-analysis of dichotomous variables, continuous variables, diagnostic tests, simple P-value, single rate, dose–response relationship, and survival data, as well as Meta-regression analysis, cumulative Meta-analysis, and network Meta-analysis, etc. Furthermore, it can draw high quality forest plot and funnel plot, and can also provide a variety of qualitative and quantitative tests for test of publication bias and methods for heterogeneity evaluation.

(3) R

R is a free and open source software belonging to GNU system, and it is a complete data processing, computing and mapping software system. Part of statistical functions of R is integrated in the bottom of R environment, but most functions are provided in the form of expansion packs. Statisticians provide a lot of excellent expansion packs for Meta-analysis in R with characteristics of full-featured and fine mapping, etc., and it can do almost all types of Meta-analysis. R is also known as an all-rounder for Meta-analysis.

(4) WinBUGS

WinBUGS is a software used for Bayesian Meta-analysis. Based on MCMC method, WinBUGS carries out Gibbs sampling for a number of complex models and distributions, and the mean, standard deviation and 95% CI of posterior distribution of the parameters can easily be obtained, and other information as well. STATA and R can invoke WinBUGS through respective expansion packs to complete Bayesian Meta-analysis.

Furthermore, there are also Comprehensive Meta-Analysis (CMA, commercial software), OpenMeta [Analyst] (free software), Meta-DiSc (free software for Meta-analysis of diagnostic test accuracy), as well as general purpose statistical software SAS, MIX plug-in for Microsoft Excel, which all can implement Meta-analysis.

19.19. PRISMA Statement[12,25]

In order to improve the reporting of systematic review and Meta-analysis, "Preferred Reporting Items for Systematic Reviews and Meta-Analyses: The PRISMA Statement" was published simultaneously in several important international medical journals by PRISMA working group led by David Moher from University of Ottawa, Canada in 2009, including *British Medical Journal, Journal of Clinical Epidemiology, Annals of Internal Medicine*, PLoS Medicine, etc.

PRISMA statement is the revision and summary guide of the Quality of Reporting of Meta-Analysis (QUOROM) issued in 1996, which was first published in 2009 in *PLoS Medicine.* One of the reasons to rename the QUOROM to PRISMA is that medical researchers need to focus not only on Meta-analysis, but also on systematic review. The development of the statement plays an important role in improving and enhancing the quality of reporting of systematic reviews and Meta-analysis.

PRISMA statement consists of a checklist of 27 entries and a four-phase flow diagram. The purpose of this statement is to help authors improve writing and reporting of systematic reviews and meta-analysis. It is mainly for the systematic review of RCTs, but PRISMA is also suitable for other types of systematic reviews as a basis for standardized reporting of systematic reviews, especially for studies with evaluation of interventions. PRISMA can also be used for critical appraisal of published systematic reviews. However, PRISMA statement is not a tool to evaluate the quality of systematic reviews.

Many methods have been applied in systematic review to explore a wider range of research questions. For example, currently systematic review can be used to study cost-effectiveness issues, diagnosis or prognosis, genetic-related studies and policy development issues. Entry and aspects covered by PRISMA are suitable for all of the above systematic reviews, and it is not just for studies on evaluation of treatment effect and safety. Of course, in some cases, appropriate modifications on some of the entries or chart are necessary. For example, to assess the risk of bias is critical, however, for assessing the systematic review of diagnostic test accuracy, the entry often tends to verify the representation and disease state of the participants, etc., which is different from the systematic review on interventions. The flowchart may also need to make appropriate adjustments when it is used for Meta-analysis with single sample data.

In order to increase the applicability of PRISMA, an explanation and elaboration document is also developed. For each entry, this document contains a standardized reporting instance, indicating the underlying causes, support evidence and references. The document is also a valuable resource for learning methodology of systematic review. Like other publications of EBM, PRISMA also updated and further improved.

References

1. Li, YP. *Evidence Based Medicine*. Beijing: People's Medical Publishing House, 2014. p. 4.
2. About the Cochran Library. http://www.cochranelibrary.com/about/about-the-cochrane-library.html.
3. Higgins, JPT, Green, S (eds.). Cochrane Handbook for Systematic Reviews of Interventions Version 5.1.0 [updated March 2011]. The Cochrane Collaboration, 2011. www.cochrane-handbook.org.
4. Atkins, D, Best, D, Briss, PA, *et al.* Grading quality of evidence and strength of recommendations. *BMJ*, 2004, 328: 1490–1494.

5. cOCEBM Levels of Evidence Working Group. "The Oxford 2011 Levels of Evidence. Oxford Centre for Evidence-Based Medicine. http://www.cebm.net/index.aspx?o=5653.
6. Guyatt, GH, Oxman, AD, Vist, GE, *et al.* GRADE: An emerging consensus on rating quality of evidence and strength of recommendations. *BMJ*, 2008, 336: 924–926.
7. Sackett, DL, Richardson, WS, Rosenberg, W, *et al. Evidence-Based Medicine: How to Practice and Teach EBM.* London, Churchill Livingstone, 2000.
8. Fleiss, JL, Gross, AJ. Meta-analysis in epidemiology. *J. Clin. Epidemiology*, 1991, 44(2): 127–139.
9. Higgins, JPT, Thompson, SG, Deeks, JJ, *et al.* Measuring inconsistency in meta-analyses. *BMJ*, 2003, 327: 557–560.
10. He, H, Chen, K. Heterogeneity test methods in meta-analysis. *China Health Stat.*, 2006, 23(6): 486–490.
11. Moher, D, Liberati, A, Tetzlaff, J, Altman, DG, The PRISMA Group. Preferred reporting items for systematic reviews and meta-analyses: The PRISMA statement. *PLoS Med.*, 2009, 6(6): e1000097.
12. Chen, C, Xu, Y. How to conduct a meta-analysis. *Chi. J. Prev. Medi.*, 2003, 37(2): 138–140.
13. Wang, J. *Evidence-Based Medicine.* (2nd edn.). Beijing: People's Medical Publishing House, 2006, pp. 81, 84–85, 87–88, 89–90.
14. Hedges, LV, Olkin, I. *Statistical Methods for Meta-Analysis.* New York: Academic Press Inc., 1985.
15. Hunter, JE, Schmidt, FL. *Methods of meta-analysis: Correcting error and bias in research findings.* London: Sage Publication Inc, 1990.
16. Hooper, L, Martin, N, Abdelhamid, A, *et al.* Reduction in saturated fat intake for cardiovascular disease. *Cochrane Database Syst. Rev.*, 2015, (6): CD011737.
17. Felson, D. Bias in meta-analytic research. *J. Clin. Epidemiol.*, 1992, 45: 885–892.
18. Bossuyt, PM, Reitsma, JB, Bruns, DE, *et al.* The STARD Statement for reporting studies of diagnostic accuracy: Explanation and elaboration. *Clin. Chem.* 2003; 49: 7–18.
19. Deeks, JJ, Bossuyt, PM, Gatsonis, C. Cochrane Handbook for Systematic Reviews of Diagnostic Test Accuracy Version 0.9. The Cochrane Collaboration, 2013. http://srdta.cochrane.org/.
20. Deeks, JJ, Higgins, JPT, Altman, DG (eds.). Analysing data and undertaking Meta-analyses. In: Higgins, JPT, Green, S (eds.). *Cochrane Handbook for Systematic Reviews of Interventions.* Version 5.1.0 [updated March 2011]. The Cochrane Collaboration, 2011. www.cochrane-handbook.org.
21. Liu, XB. *Clinical Epidemiology and Evidence-Based Medicine.* (4th edn.). Beijing: People's Medical Publishing House, 2013. p. 03.
22. Zhang, TS, Zhong, WZ. *Practical Evidence-Based Medicine Methodology.* (1st edn.). Changsha: Central South University Press, 2012, p. 7.
23. Higgins, JPT, Jackson, D, Barrett, JK, *et al.* Consistency and inconsistency in network meta-analysis: Concepts and models for multi-arm studies. *Res. Synth. Methods*, 2012, 3(2): 98–110.
24. Zhang, TS, Zhong, WZ, Li, B. *Practical Evidence-Based Medicine Methodology.* (2nd edn.). Changsha: Central South University Press, 2014.
25. The PRISMA Statement website. http://www.prisma-statement.org/.

About the Author

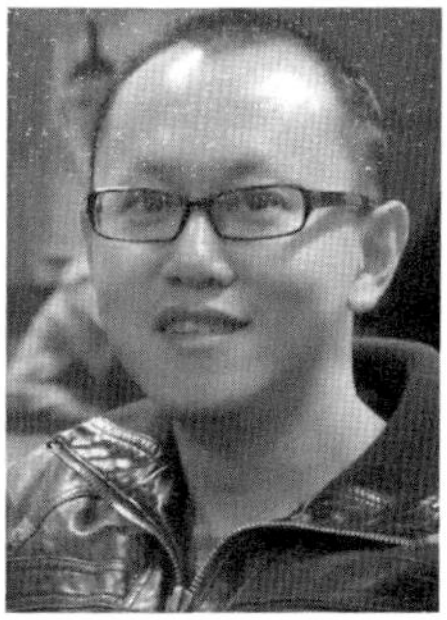

Yi Wan is working as an Associate Professor at School of Public Health where he is a lecturer of Epidemiology and Health Statistics. He has a Medical Degree from China, and he has done his PhD at Fourth Military Medical University in Xi'an. As a visiting scholar, he has been to Department of Primary Health Care, University of Oxford between 2007 and 2008, and received a scholarship from the Center for Evidence-Based Medicine, University of Oxford. In 2011–2013, he served as medical logistics officer in the United Nations mission in Liberia. Over the last 18 years, he has focused his scientific interests on the topics related to health management, biostatistical methodology and evidence-based medicine including monitoring of chronic diseases. With his expertise in biostatistics, evidence-based practice and clinical epidemiology, he has published numerous SCI journal papers and book chapters, served as an editorial member of several academic journals, reviewed for many reputed journals, coordinated/participated in several national projects, and received several academic honors including the first-class of the Scientific and Technological Progress Award of People's Liberation Army (2006), the National Award for Excellence in Statistical Research (2010), and Excellence in Teaching and Education, etc. Innovative, translational and longstanding research has always been his pursuit in his academic career.

CHAPTER 20

QUALITY OF LIFE AND RELEVANT SCALES

Fengbin Liu*, Xinlin Chen and Zhengkun Hou

20.1. Health Status[1–3]

Since the 18th century, people have considered being healthy as the absence of disease or infirmity. Guided by this concept, people have been accustomed to evaluating the health status of individuals and populations according to concepts of illness such as applying morbidity, prevalence or survival rates to evaluate the effectiveness of preventing and treating a disease and applying "well-healed", "effective", "improved", "non-effective" and so on to evaluate the treatment of the individual.

In 1946, the World Health Organization (WHO) proposed the idea that "Health is a state of complete physical, mental and social well-being and not merely the absence of disease or infirmity". The concept of health thus developed from a traditional physical health to a more comprehensive health, including physiological health, mental health, social health and even moral health and environmental health among others. This development of the concept of health has helped the biomedical mode develop into a biological–psychological–social medicine mode.

Physiological health refers to the overall health status of the body's physiological function including the intactness of the body structure and normal physiological functioning, which is mainly manifested as normal height, weight, body temperature, pulse, breath and fecal and urinary functioning; healthy complexion and hair; and bright eyes, a reddish tongue, a non-coated tongue, a good appetite, resistance to illness, sufficient tolerance against epidemic disease, etc. Mental health refers to a positive mental status that is

*Corresponding author: liufb163@163.com

continuous. In this state, an individual is full of vitality; he or she can adapt well to the environment and capitalize on the potentials of mind and body. The ideal state of mental status is the maintenance of normality of character and intelligence, correct cognition, proper emotions, rational will, positive attitudes, and appropriate behavior as well as good adaptability. Social health, or social adaptation, refers to an individual having good interactions with his or her social environment and good interpersonal relationships, as well as having the ability to realize his or her own social role, which is the optimal status for social men to fulfill their personal role and tasks.

Health Measurement is the process of quantifying the concept of health and constructs or phenomena that are related to health, namely using instruments to reflect health in terms of the properties and characteristics of the measured object. The measurement of physiological health includes physique, function and physical strength, and the evaluation of functional status. The evaluation of mental health is mainly accomplished by measuring personality, intelligence, emotions, feelings, cognitive mentality and the overall mental state. It usually includes disharmony in behavioral functioning, the frequency and intensity of mental tension, the fulfillment of mental and life satisfaction, etc. The measurement of social health often includes social resources and interpersonal relationships and is accomplished by measuring interpersonal relationships, social support, social adaptation and behavioral modes.

20.2. Psychological Assessment[4–6]

Psychological assessment measures, evaluates and analyzes people's mental characteristics through different scientific, objective and standard methods. It is a testing program that applies a particular operational paradigm to quantify people's mental characteristics such as their capability, personality and mental health on the basis of certain theories of psychology. The generalized psychological assessment contains not only measures that apply psychological tests but also those that use observations, interviews, questionnaires, experiments, etc.

The major methods of psychological assessment include traditional tests (paper and pencil), the use of scales, projective tests and instrument measurements. The main features of psychological assessment are indirectness and relativity. Indirectness refers to the fact that psychological traits cannot be measured directly and that they manifest themselves as a series of overt behaviors that have an internal connection; accordingly, they can only be measured indirectly. Relativity refers to the fact that psychological traits have no absolute standard.

The content of psychological tests mainly covers some individual characteristics such as perceptions, skills, capability, temperament, character, interests and motives. According to the function of the test, psychological assessment can be divided into cognitive testing, intelligence testing, personality testing and behavioral testing.

Cognitive testing, or capability testing, refers to the evaluation of one's or a group's capability in some way. This capability can be current practical capability, potential capability in the future, general capability, or some kind of specific capability regarding a certain topic such as music, art or physical education.

Intelligence testing is a scientific test of intelligence that mainly tests one's ability to think critically, learn and adjust to the environment. Modern psychology generally considers intelligence as human's ability to learn as well as to adjust to the environment. Intelligence includes one's ability to observe, memorize and imagine as well as to think. Frequently used intelligence scales include the Binet–Simon Intelligence Scale, Wechsler Adult Intelligence Scale, Stanford–Binet Intelligence Scale and Raven Intelligence Test.

Personality testing measures an individual's behavioral independence and tendencies, mainly focusing on character, interests, temperament, attitude, morality, emotion and motives. Questionnaires and projective tests are two major methods used in personality testing. Some frequently used scales for personality testing are the Minnesota Multiphasic personality inventory, the Eysenck personality questionnaire, the 16 personality factor questionnaire (Cattell), the temperament sorter and mood projective tests.

Behavior is the range of human actions in daily life. Behavior testing is a psychological assessment that tests all human activities.

20.3. Quality of Life (QOL)[7–9]

The study of quality of life (QOL) originated in the United States of America in the 1930s, when QOL was used as a sociological indicator by sociological researchers. At the time, QOL was used to indicate the development of society and people's living standards, and it was thus restricted to objective indicators such as birth rate, mortality, resident's income and consumption level, employment status, living conditions and environmental conditions. In the 1950s, the field of subjective research on QOL emerged. These researchers emphasized the idea that QOL was a subjective indicator, and they noted the subjective feelings of an individual towards society and his or her environment. Subsequently, QOL was gradually applied in other subjects, especially in the medical sciences. At the end of the 1970s, the study of QOL was widely prevalent in the medical sciences. Moreover, many QOL instruments for cancer and other chronic diseases emerged at the end of the 1980s. As an indispensable indicator and instrument, QOL has been widely applied to every domain of society.

QOL is generally based on living standards, but given its complexity and universality, it also places particular emphasis on the degree of satisfaction of high-level requirements such as an individual's spirit, culture and the evaluation of one's environmental conditions. QOL is generally believed to be a comprehensive indicator of one's happiness towards all aspects of life. It typically contains domains such as physical status, psychological status, mental health, social activities, economic happiness, social participation and self-perception of happiness and satisfaction.

There continues to be controversy over the meaning of QOL. However, it is generally accepted that (1) QOL is measurable, and it can be measured by methods of psychological assessment, (2) QOL is a subjective evaluation index that focuses on the subjective experience of the subject, (3) QOL is a multi-dimensional concept that mainly includes physical function, mental function and social function, and (4) QOL is culture-dependent, and it must be established in a particular culture.

It is widely accepted that health is not merely the absence of disease or infirmity but a state of complete physical, mental and social well-being due to the change in disease spectrum and the development of medical science. As the traditional health assessment indicator did not adequately cover the concept of health, medical specialists proposed the idea of health-related quality of life (HRQOL). It is generally acknowledged that measures of HRQOL began in 1949 when Karnofsky and Burchenal used a performance index (Karnofsky scale) to measure the body function of patients undergoing chemotherapy.

Since the beginning of the 1990s, the WHO has brought together a group of experts from different cultures (the WHOQOL Group) to discuss the concept of QOL. In the process, the WHOQOL Group defined HRQOL as the individual's perception of their position in life in the context of the culture and value systems in which they live and in relation to their goals, expectations, standards and concerns. HRQOL is a concept that has broad connotations, including an individual's physiological health, mental status, independence, social relationships, personal convictions and relationship with the surroundings. According to this definition, HRQOL is part of an individual's subjective evaluation, which is rooted in the context of culture and social environment.

20.4. Clinical Outcomes Assessment (COA)[10–12]

Clinical outcomes assessment (COA) refers to the assessment of a study's object in terms of the events, variables or experiences caused by clinical interventions. Clinical outcomes include many aspects such as patient's symptoms and mental state and the efficacy of prevention and treatment of a disease. Each outcome supports important and reliable evidence regarding the efficacy of a clinical intervention.

Based on the source of assessment, COAs can be classified into those using a patient-reported outcome (PRO), clinician-reported outcome (CRO) and observer-reported outcome (ObsRO).

In 2009, the United States Department of Health and Human Services (HHS) and the U.S. Food and Drug Administration (FDA) defined a PRO as "Any report of the status of a patient's health condition that comes directly from the patient, without interpretation of the patient's response by a clinician or anyone else". As an endpoint indicator, PROs not only cover health status, physical and psychosocial functioning and HRQOL but also patient's satisfaction with care, compliance related to treatment and any information on the outcomes from the patient's point of view through interviews, questionnaires or daily records, among others.

A CRO refers to the patient's health status and therapeutic outcomes as evaluated by the clinician and assesses the human body's reaction to interventions from the clinician's perspective. CROs mainly include (1) clinician's observations and reports of the symptoms and signs that reflect a therapeutic effect, such as hydrothorax, hydroperitoneum, and lesion area for dermatosis, or symptoms and signs that clinicians investigate such as thirst and dryness for sicca syndrome, (2) clinician's explanations based on the outcomes of laboratory testing and measures of medical instruments such as routine blood examination, electrocardiogram and results of a CT scan, and (3) scales completed by clinicians, for example, the Ashworth spasticity scale, which measures the level of patient's spasms and must be conducted by a clinician, or the brief psychiatric rating scale, which must be completed based on the real situation.

An ObsRO refers to the patient's health status and therapeutic outcomes as evaluated by observers, and it assesses the human body's reaction to interventions from the observer's perspective. For example, the health status of patients with cerebral palsy should be reported by their caregivers due to impairments in consciousness.

20.5. Quality of Life Scales[9,13,14]

Quality of life scales refer to the instruments used to measure QOL, which are developed on the basis of programmed methods of generic instruments.

According to the measurement object, QOL scales can be divided into general scales and specific scales. General scales such as the MOS item short from health survey (the SF-36), the WHOQOL and the Chinese quality of life (ChQOL) are applied to the general population, while specific scales such as the EORTC questionnaire QLQ-C30 and the Functional Assessment of Cancer Therapy-General (FACT-G) scale are applied to cancer patients. In terms of the administration methods, QOL scales can be divided into self-administered scales and rater-administered scales.

Generally, QOL scales comprise many domains. The conceptual structure of QOL is shown in Figure 20.5.1.

A domain, or dimension, is a part of the overall concept of QOL and constitutes a major framework of theoretical models. General scales usually contain the domains of physiological, psychological and social function. For example, the FACT-G contains four domains: physical health status, societal or family situation, relationship status and functional status. Based on the characteristics and unique manifestations of a disease, researchers can also develop other domains.

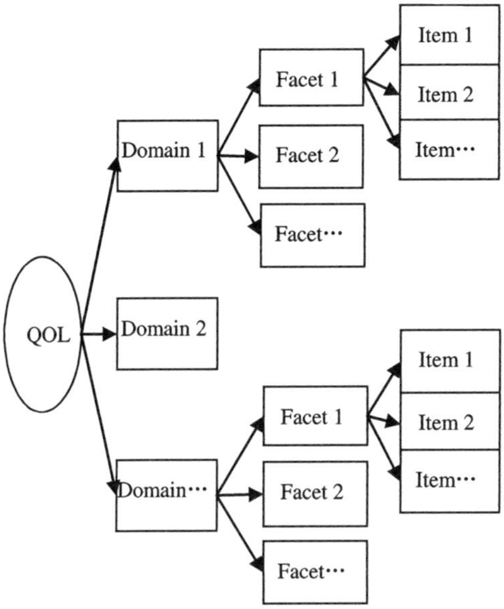

Fig. 20.5.1. Conceptual QOL structure.

A facet, which is a component of a domain, comprises a number of items within the same domain. There are some scales that do not contain facets; rather, their domains are composed of items directly.

An item is a single question or statement as well as its standard response options that is used when assessing a patient, and it targets a particular concept. Items are the most elemental component of a scale. Generally, a Likert Scale or Visual Analogue Scale (VAS) are applied as response options for an item. For example, for the question: Are you in pain? The options (1) No, (2) Occasionally and (3) Often compose a Likert-type Scale. Alternatively, a line that is drawn 10 cm long with one end marked as 0 to signify no pain and the other end as 10 to signify sharp pain is an example of a VAS; the middle part of the line suggests different pain intensities.

20.6. Scale Development[14–16]

Scale development refers to the entire process of developing a scale. The process of developing a scale is repetitive and includes the development of the conceptual framework, creation of the preliminary scale, revision of the conceptual framework, assessment of the measurement properties, identification of the conceptual framework, data-gathering, data analysis, data-interpreting and modification of the scale.

In 2009, the HHS and FDA summarized five steps in the development of PROs to provide guidance for the industry: hypothesize the conceptual framework; adjust the conceptual framework and draft instrument; confirm the conceptual framework and assess other measurement properties; collect, analyze and interpret data; and modify the instrument (Figure 20.6.1).

Cited from U.S. Department of HHS, *et al.* Guidance for Industry Patient-Reported Outcome Measures: Use in Medical Product Development to Support Labeling Claims. http://www.fda.gov/downloads/drugs/guidancecomplianceregulatoryinformation/guidances/ucm193282.pdf.

(1) Hypothesize the conceptual framework: This step includes listing theoretical theories and potential assessment criteria, determining the intended population and characteristics of the scale (scoring type, model and measuring frequency), carrying out literature reviews or expert reviews, refining the theoretical hypothesis of the conceptual framework, collecting plenty of alternative items based on the conceptual framework to form an item pool in which the appropriate items are selected and transformed into feasible question-and-answer items in the preliminary scale.

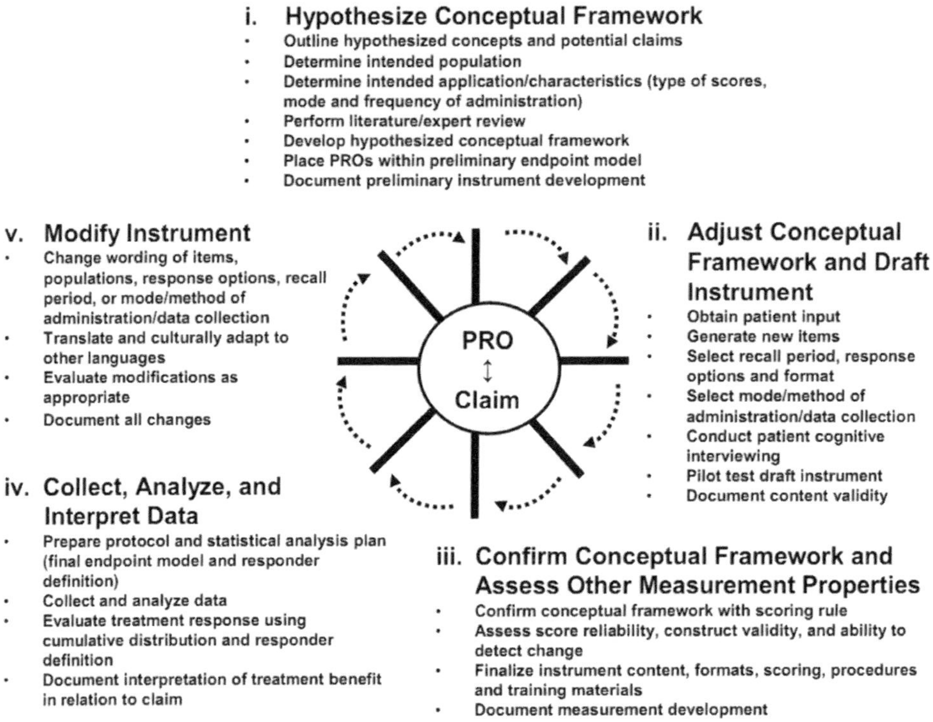

Fig. 20.6.1. The PRO instrument development and modification process.

(2) Adjust the conceptual framework and draft instrument: This step includes collecting patient information, generating new items, choosing the response options and format, determining how to collect and manage data, carrying out cognitive interviews with patients, testing the preliminary scale and assessing the instrument's content validity.
(3) Confirm the conceptual framework and assess other measurement properties: This step includes understanding the conceptual framework and scoring rules, evaluating the reliability, validity and distinction of the scale, designing the content, format and scoring of the scale, and completing the operating steps and training material.
(4) Collect, analyze and interpret data: This step includes preparing the project and statistical analysis plan (defining the final model and response model), collecting and analyzing data, and evaluating and explaining the treatment response.
(5) Modify the instrument: This step includes modifying the wording of items, the intended population, the response options, period for return visits, method of collecting and managing the data, translation of the

scale and cultural adaptation, reviewing the adequacy of the scale and documenting the changes.

Item Selection applies the principles and methods of statistics to select important, sensitive and typical items from different domains. Item selection is a vital procedure in scale development. The selected items should be of much interest, have a strong sensitivity, be representative, and have the feasibility and acceptability. Some common methods used in item selection are measures of dispersion, correlation coefficients, factor analysis, discriminant validity analysis, Cronbach's alpha, test-retest reliability, clustering methodology, stepwise regression analysis and item response theory (IRT).

20.7. Reliability[17,18]

The classical test theory (CTT) considers reliability to be the ratio of the variance of the true score to the variance of the measured score. Reliability is defined as the overall consistency of repeated measures, or the consistency of the measured score of two parallel tests. The most commonly used forms of reliability include test–retest reliability, split–half reliability, internal consistency reliability and inter–rater agreement.

Test–retest reliability refers to the consistency of repeated measures (two measures). The interval between the repeated measures should be determined based on the properties of the participants. Moreover, the sample size should be between 20 and 30 individuals. Generally, the Kappa coefficient and intra-class correlation coefficient (ICC) are applied to measure test–retest reliability. The criteria for the Kappa coefficient and ICC are the following: very good (>0.75), good (>0.4 and ≤0.75) and poor (≤0.4).

When a measure or a test is divided in two, the corrected correlation coefficient of the scores of each half represent the split-half reliability. The measure is split into two parallel halves based on the item's numbers, and the correlation coefficient (r_{hh}) of each half is calculated. The correlation coefficient is corrected by the Spearman–Brown formula to obtain the split-half reliability (r).

$$r = \frac{2r_{hh}}{1 + r_{hh}}.$$

We can also apply two other formulas, see below.

(1) Flanagan formula

$$r = 2\left(1 - \frac{S_a^2 + S_b^2}{S_t^2}\right),$$

S_a^2 and S_b^2 refer to the variances of the scores of the two half scales; S_t^2 is the variance of the whole scale.

(2) Rulon formula

$$r = 1 - \frac{S_d^2}{S_t^2},$$

S_d^2 refers to the difference between the scores of the two half scales; S_t^2 is the variance of the whole scale.

The hypothesis tested for split-half reliability is the equivalence of the variance of the two half scales. However, it is difficult to meet that condition in real situations. Cronbach proposed the use of internal consistency reliability (Cronbach's α, or α for short).

$$\alpha = \frac{n}{n-1}\left(1 - \frac{\sum_{i=1}^{n} S_i^2}{S_t^2}\right),$$

n refers to the number of the item; s_i^2 refers to the variance of the i item; and s_t^2 refers to the variance of the total score of all items. Cronbach's α is the most commonly used reliability coefficient, and it is related to the number of items. The fewer the items, the smaller the α. Generally, $\alpha > 0.8, 0.8 \geq \alpha > 0.6$ and $\alpha \leq 0.6$ are considered very good, good and poor reliability, respectively.

Finally, inter–rater agreement is applied to show the consistency of different raters in assessing the same participant at the same time point. Its formula is the same as that of the α coefficient, but n refers to the number of raters, s_i^2 is the variance of the i rater, and s_t^2 is the variance of the total raters.

20.8. Validity[18–20]

Validity refers to the degree to which the measure matches the actual situation of the participants; that is to say, whether the measure can measure the true concept. Validity is the most important property of a scientific measure. The most commonly used forms of validity include content validity, criterion validity, construct validity and discriminant validity.

Content validity examines the extent to which the item concepts are comprehensively represented by the results. The determination of good content validity meets two requirements: (1) the scope of the contents is identified when developing the scale and (2) all the items fall within the scope. The items are a representative sample of the identified concept.

The methods used to assess content validity mainly include the expert method, duplicate method and test–retest method. The expert method invites subject matter experts to estimate the consistency of the items and the intended content and includes (1) identifying specifically and in detail the scope of the content in the measure, (2) identifying the intended content of each item, and (3) comparing the established content with the intended content to determine whether there is a difference. The coverage of the identified content and the number of the items should be investigated.

Criterion validity refers to the degree of agreement between a particular scale and the criterion scale (gold standard). We can obtain criterion validity by calculating the correlation coefficient between the measured scale and the criterion scale. QOL lacks a gold standard; therefore, the "quasi-gold standard" of a homogeneous group is usually applied as the standard. For example, the SF-36 Health Survey can be applied as the standard when developing a generic scale, and the QLQ-C30 or FACT-G can be applied as the standard when developing a cancer-related scale.

Construct validity refers to the extent to which a particular instrument is consistent with theoretically derived hypotheses concerning the concepts that are being measured. Construct validity is the highest validity index and is assessed using exploratory factor analysis and confirmatory factor analysis. The research procedures of construct validity are described below:

(1) Propose the theoretical framework of the scale and explain the meaning of the scale, its structure, or its relationship with other scales.
(2) Subdivide the hypothesis into smaller outlines based on the theoretical framework, including the domains and items; then, propose a theoretical structure such as the one in Figure 20.5.1.
(3) Finally, test the hypothesis using factor analysis.

Discriminant validity refers to how well the scale can discriminate between different features of the participants. For example, if patients in different conditions (or different groups of people such as patients and healthy individuals) score differently on a scale, this indicates that the scale can discriminate between patients in different conditions (different groups of people), namely, the scale has good discriminant validity.

20.9. Responsiveness[21,22]

Responsiveness is defined as the ability of a scale to detect clinically important changes over time, even if these changes are small. That is to say, if the participants' conditions change as the environment changes, the results will also respond to the changes. For example, if the scores of the scale increase as the patient's condition improves (by comparing the scores of the patients before and after treatment), this indicates that the scale has good responsiveness.

Interpretation refers to the explanation of changes in a patient's QOL. Generally, the minimal clinically important difference (MCID) is applied to interpret the QOL.

The MCID, or minimal important difference (MID), is defined as the smallest change in treatment effectiveness that a patient would identify as important (e.g. no side effects and benefits to the patient). It was first proposed by Jaeschke *et al.* The MCID is the threshold value of clinical significance. Only when the score surpasses this value are the changes considered of clinical significance. Hence, we not only need to measure the changes before and after treatment, but we also need to determine whether the MCID is of clinical significance when the scale is applied to evaluating the clinical effectiveness.

There is no standard method for identifying the MCID. Commonly used methods include the anchor-based method, distribution-based method, expert method and literature review method.

(1) Anchor-based methods compare the score changes with an "anchor" (criterion) to interpret the changes. Anchor-based methods can provide the identified MCID with a professional interpretation of the relationship between the measured scale and the anchor. The shortcoming of this method is that it is hard to find a suitable anchor because different anchors may yield different MCIDs.
(2) Distribution-based methods identify the MCID on the basis of characteristics of the sample and scale from the perspective of statistics. The method is easy to perform because it has an explicit formula, and the measuring error is also taken into account. However, the method is affected by the sample (such as those from different regions) as well as the sample size, and it is difficult to interpret.
(3) The expert method identifies the MCID through expert's advice, which usually applies the Delphi method. However, this method is subjective, empirical and full of uncertainty.
(4) The literature review method identifies the MCID according to a meta-analysis of the existing literature. The expert method and literature review method are basically used as auxiliary methods.

20.10. Language and Cultural Adaptation[23,24]

Language and cultural adaptation refers to the process of introducing the foreign scale (source scale) into the target scale and inspecting the equivalence of the two versions of the scale. Given the differences in language and cultural background, the introduction of the foreign scale should obey the principles of cultural adaptation. The fundamental processes to introduce a foreign scale are shown below.

(1) It is important to contact the original author(s) to gain permission to use/modify their scale. Researchers can do this by letter or email.
(2) Forward translation: after receiving permission to use the foreign scale, invite two bilingual translators, called the first translator (T1) and the second translator (T2), to translate it into the target scale independently. Then, conduct a synthesis of the two translations, termed T-12, with a written report carefully documenting the synthesis process. Disagreements between T1 and T2 should be resolved by a third party coordinator after group discussion.
(3) Back translation: two bilingual translators (native speakers of the source language) with at least 5 years of experience in the target language can then be invited to back translate the new draft scale into the source language. After comparing the source scale and the back translated version, disagreements between them should be carefully analyzed.
(4) Expert committee: the expert committee usually includes experts on methodology and healthcare, linguists and the aforementioned translator (including the coordinator). The tasks of the committee include (1) collecting all the versions of the scale (including the translated versions and the back translated versions) and contacting the author and (2) examining the concepts, semantics and operational equivalence of the items. The committee should ensure the clarity of the instructions and the integrity of the basic information. The items and their wording should be in agreement with the local language and cultural background. The items that are appropriate for the local culture should be included, and the items that do not adhere to the local culture should be removed. The committee should reach a consensus on each item. If needed, the process of forward translation and back translation can be repeated.
(5) Pre-testing: after the committee approves the translated scale, recruit 30 to 40 participants to pre-test it, i.e. to test how well the participants interact with the scale. Update the scale after identifying potential and technical problems. Then, send all related materials to the original

author for further audit and cultural adaption, which can be followed by determination of the final version.

(6) Evaluation of the final version: the reliability, validity and discriminant validity of the survey used in the field should be evaluated. In addition, IRT can be applied to examine whether there was differential item functioning (DIF) of the items. The translation and application of the foreign scale can lead to an instrument that assesses the target population in a short period of time. Moreover, comparing the QOL of people from different cultures benefits international communication and cooperation.

20.11. Measurement Equivalence[25,26]

Measurement equivalence refers to people from different nationalities or races who have the same QOL to obtain similar QOL results when using the same scale that has been translated into their corresponding language, i.e. the scale has good applicability in different nations or races.

Measurement equivalence mainly includes the following concepts:

(1) Conceptual equivalence: This mainly investigates the definitions and understandings of health and QOL of people from different cultures as well as their attention to different domains of health and QOL. Literature reviews and expert consultations are applied to evaluate conceptual equivalence.
(2) Item equivalence: This refers to whether the item's validity is the same across different languages and cultural backgrounds. It includes response equivalence. Item equivalence indicates that the item measures the same latent variables and that the correlations among the items are uniform in different cultures. Literature reviews, the Delphi method, focus groups and the Rasch model are applied to evaluate item equivalence.
(3) Semantic equivalence: To reach semantic equivalence, the key concepts and words must be understood exactly before the translation, and the translation of the scale must obey the rules of forward translation and back translation mentioned above.
(4) Operational equivalence: This refers to having a similar format, explanation, mode, measuring method and time framework for scales in different languages. Expert consultation is used to estimate the operational equivalence.
(5) Measurement equivalence: When the observed score and latent trait (the true score) of the scale are the same even when the respondents are in different groups, we can claim that the scale has measurement equivalence.

For example, if individuals from different groups have the same scores on a latent trait, then their observed scores are equivalent. The objective of measurement equivalence is to ensure that people from different groups share similar psychological characteristics when using different language scales (similar reliability, validity, and responsiveness and lack of DIF). Structural equation modeling and IRT are major methods used to assess measurement equivalence.

(6) Functional equivalence: This refers to the degree to which the scales match each other when applied in two or more cultures. The objective of functional equivalence is to highlight the importance of the aforementioned equivalences when obtaining scales with cross-cultural equivalence.

20.12. CTT[27–29]

CTT is a body of related psychometric theory that predicts the outcomes of psychological testing such as the difficulty of the items or the ability of the test-takers. Generally, the aim of CTT is to understand and improve the reliability of psychological tests. CTT may be regarded as roughly synonymous with true score theory.

CTT assumes that each person has a true score (τ) that would be obtained if there were no errors in measurement. A true score is defined as the expected number-correct score over an infinite number of independent administrations of the test. Unfortunately, test users never obtain the true score instead of the observed score (x). It is assumed that

$$x = c + s + e = \tau + e,$$

x is the observed score; τ is the true score; and e is the measurement error. The operational definition of the true score is as an average of repeated measures when there is no measurement error.

The basic hypotheses of CTT are (1) the invariance of the true score, i.e. the individual's latent trait (true score) is consistent and does not change during a specific period of time, (2) the average measurement error is 0, namely $\mathrm{E}(e) = 0$, (3) the true score and measurement error are independent, namely the correlation coefficient between the true score and measurement error is 0, (4) measurement errors are independent, namely the correlation coefficient between measurement errors is 0, and (5) equivalent variance, i.e. two scales are applied to measure the same latent trait, and equivalent variances of measurement error are obtained.

Reliability is defined as the proportion of the variance of the true score to that of the observed one. The formula is $r_{xx} = 1 - \frac{\sigma_e^2}{\sigma_x^2}$.

σ_e^2 is the variance of the measurement error; σ_x^2 is the variance of the observed score. If the ratio of the measurement error is small, then the scale is more reliable.

Validity is the proportion of the variance of the true score for the population to that of the observed score. The formula is $Val = \frac{\sigma_c^2}{\sigma_x^2} = 1 - \frac{\sigma_s^2+\sigma_e^2}{\sigma_x^2}$

σ_c^2 is the variance of the true and valid score; σ_s^2 is the variance of systematic error. QOL is a latent trait that is shown only by individual's behaviors. Validity is a relative concept because it is not exactly accurate. Validity reflects random and systematic errors. A scale is considered to have high reliability when the random and systematic error variances account for a small proportion of the overall variance. Reducing random and systematic error can ensure improved validity of the measure. Additionally, a suitable criterion should be chosen.

Discriminant validity refers to the ability of the scale to discriminate between the characteristics of different population and is related to validity. Also see "20.8 validity".

20.13. IRT[30–32]

IRT, also known as latent trait theory or modern test theory, is a paradigm for the design, analysis and scoring of tests, questionnaires and similar instruments that measure abilities, attitudes or other variables. IRT is based on the idea that the probability of a correct/keyed response to an item is a mathematical function of person and item parameters. It applies a nonlinear model to investigate the nonlinear relationship between the subject's response (observable variable) to the item and the latent trait.

The hypotheses of IRT are unidimensionality and local independence. Unidimensionality suggests that only one latent trait determines the response to the item for the participant. That is to say, all the items in the same domain measure the same latent trait. Local independence states that no other traits affect the subject's response to the item except the intended latent trait that is being measured.

An item characteristic curve (ICC) refers to a curve that reflects the relationship between the latent trait of the participant and the probability of the response to the item. ICCs apply the latent trait and the probability as the X-axis and Y-axis, respectively. The curve is usually an "S" shape (see Figure 20.13.1).

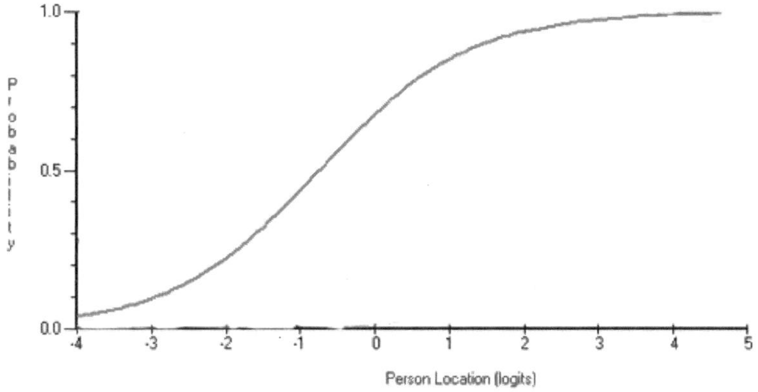

Fig. 20.13.1. An example of an ICC curve.

Item information function reflects the effective information of the item for the participant with latent trait θ. The formula is $I_i(\theta) = \frac{[P_i'(\theta)]^2}{P_i'(\theta)*Q_i(\theta)}$.

θ is the latent trait; $P_i(\theta)$ refers to the probability of the participant's (with latent trait θ) response to item $i; Q_i(\theta) = 1 - P_i(\theta)$; and $P_i'(\theta)$ refers to the ICC's first-order derivative of level θ.

Test information function reflects the accuracy of the test for participants in all ranges of the latent trait and equals the sum of all item information functions.

$$I(\theta) = \sum_{i=1}^{n} \frac{[P_i'(\theta)]^2}{P_i'(\theta) * Q_i(\theta)}.$$

An item is considered to have (DIF) if participants from different groups with the same latent trait have different response probabilities. DIF can be divided into uniform and non-uniform DIF. An item is considered to have uniform DIF if the average response probability of a group is higher than that of the other group regardless of the level of latent trait. However, an item is considered to have non-uniform DIF if the response probability of a group is higher than that of the other group in one level of the latent trait but lower than that of the other group in other levels.

20.14. Item Response Model[33–35]

An item response model is a formula that describes the relationship between a subject's response to an item and their latent trait. Some common models are:

(1) The normal ogive model, which was established by Lord in 1952.

$$P_i(\theta) = \int_{-\infty}^{a_i(\theta-b_i)} \frac{1}{\sqrt{2\pi}} e^{-z^2/2} dz.$$

θ refers to the latent trait; $P_i(\theta)$ refers to the subject's (of θ ability level) probability of choosing the correct answer on the item i. b_i is the threshold parameter for the item i, and a_i is the discriminant parameter. The shortcomings of this model are not easy to calculate.

(2) The Rasch model, which was proposed by Rasch in the 1950s.

$$P_i(\theta) = \frac{1}{1+\exp[-(\theta-b_i)]}.$$

This model has only one parameter (b_i) and is also called a single parameter model.

(3) The Birnbaum model (with a_i), which was introduced by Birnbaum based on the Rasch model from 1957–1958.
$P_i(\theta) = 1/\{1 + \exp[-1.7 * a_i(\theta - b_i)]\}$ is a double parameter model. After introducing a guessing parameter, it is transformed into a three-parameter model. The models described above are used for binary variables.

(4) Graded response model, which is used for ordinal data and was first reported by Smaejima in 1969. The model is:

$$P(X_i = k|\theta) = P_k^*(\theta) - P_{k+1}^*(\theta),$$

$$P_k^*(\theta) = \frac{1}{1+\exp[-a_k D(\theta - b_k)]}.$$

$P_k^*(\theta)$ refers to the probability of the participant scoring k and above. $P_0^*(\theta) = 1$.

(5) Nominal response model, which is used for multinomial variables and was first proposed by Bock in 1972. The model is:

$$P_{ik}(\theta) = \frac{\exp(b_{ik} + a_{ik}\theta)}{\sum_{i=1}^{m} \exp(b_{ik} + a_{ik}\theta)} \quad k = 1, \dots, m.$$

(6) The Masters model, which was proposed by Masters in 1982. The model is:

$$P_{ijx}(\theta) = \frac{\exp(\sum_{k=1}^{x} (\theta_j - b_{ik}))}{\sum_{h=1}^{m} \exp(\sum_{k=1}^{h} (\theta_j - b_{ik}))} \quad x = 1, \dots, m.$$

Muraki proposed an extended Masters model in 1992. The model is:

$$P_{ih}(\theta) = \frac{\exp(\sum_{h=1}^{k} D^* a_i(\theta - b_{ih}))}{\sum_{c=1}^{m_i} \exp(\sum_{h=1}^{c} D^* a_i(\theta - b_{ih}))}.$$

In addition, there are multidimensional item response theories that have been proposed such as the Logistic MIRT by Reckase and Mckinley in 1982 and the MGRM by Mukira and Carlson in 1993.

20.15. Generalizability Theory (GT)[36–38]

Generalizability theory (GT) is a theory that introduces irrelevant factors or variables that interfere with the score of the model and then uses statistical techniques to estimate how much the score is affected by those factors or the interaction of the factors to reduce measurement error and improve reliability.

The book "Theory of generalizability: A liberalization of reliability theory" was published by Cronbach, Nageswari and Gleser in 1963 and marked the birth of GT. The book "Elements of generalizability theory", published by RL Brennan, and the software GENOVA were developed in 1983. The two events together indicated that GT had begun to mature.

GT was improved by the introduction of a research design and analysis method based on classical test theory (CTT). The superiorities of GT are that it (1) is easy to meet the assumption of randomly parallel tests, (2) is easy to determine the cause of the error through variance of analysis, and (3) guides practical application by identifying an optimized design through determining the measurement situation and changing the situation within a limited range in advance.

GT includes generalized research and decision research. (1) Generalized research refers to research in which the researcher estimates the variances of all the measures and their interactions on the basis of the universe of admissible observations. The universe of admissible observations refers to a collection of the entire conditional universe during actual measurement. Generalized research is related to the universe of admissible observations in that the entire error source can be determined. (2) Decision research refers to research in which variance estimations are carried out for all the measures and their interactions on the basis of the universe of generalization. The universe of generalization refers to a set that contains all side conditions and is involved in the decision-making when generalizing results. Decision research is applied to establish a universe of generalization based on the results of generalized research and is used to measure all types of error as well as the accuracy indicator.

Common designs of GT include random single crossover designs and random double-sided crossover designs. Random single crossover design is a design that has only one measurement facet and in which there is a crossover relationship between the measured facet and the target; moreover, the measured facet and target are randomly sampled, and the population and universe are infinite. For random crossover double-sided designs, the universe of admissible observations comprises two facets and the levels between the facets and the target.

GT can be applied to not only norm-referenced tests but also to criterion-referenced tests.

20.16. Computer-adaptive Testing (CAT)[39,40]

Computer-adaptive testing (CAT), which was established on the basis of IRT, is a new test that automatically chooses items according to the subject's ability. CAT evaluates the subject's ability according to the difficulty (threshold) of the items rather than the number of items the subject can answer correctly.

CAT is a successful application of IRT because it can build item banks, introduce computer techniques to choose items automatically and evaluate the tested ability accurately. Generally, CAT applies a double-parameter model or a three-parameter logistic model.

Major steps of CAT:

(1) Setting up an item bank: the item bank is crucial for conducting CAT, and it needs to have a wide range of threshold values and to be representative. The item bank includes numbers, subject, content, options, threshold value and discriminant parameters, frequency of items used and answer time.
(2) Process of testing: (1) Identify the initial estimated value. We have usually applied the average ability of all participants or a homogeneous population as the initial estimated value. (2) Then, choose the items and begin testing. The choice of item must consider the threshold parameter (near to or higher than the ability parameter). (3) Estimate ability. A maximum likelihood method is used to estimate the ability parameter in accordance with the test results. (4) Identify the end condition. There are three strategies used to end the test, which include fixing the length of the test, applying an information function $I(\theta) \leq \varepsilon$ and reaching

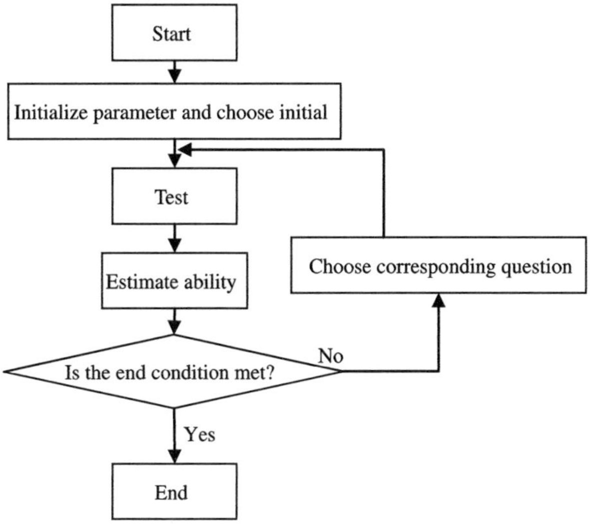

Fig. 20.16.1. CAT flowchart.

an estimated ability parameter that is less than a preset value. If any of the aforementioned conditions are met, the test ends or it chooses another item to test and repeats the process mentioned above until the end condition is met. For a flowchart, please see Figure 20.16.1.

CAT uses the fewest items and gives the nearest score to actual latent trait. CAT can reduce expenses, manpower and material resources, makes it easier for the subject to complete the questionnaire and reflects the subject's health accurately.

20.17. The SF-36 (Short-Form Health Survey Scale)[41,42]

The SF-36 (Short-Form Health Survey Scale) is a generic outcome measure designed to assess a person's perceived health status. The SF-36 was used to assess the QOL of the general population over 14 years old and was developed by the RAND Corporation, Boston, USA. The original SF-36 originated from the Medical Outcomes Study (MOS) in 1992. Since then, a group of researchers from the original study has released a commercial version of the SF-36, while the original version is available in the public domain license-free from RAND. The SF-12 and SF-8 were first released as shorter versions in 1996 and 2001, respectively.

The SF-36 evaluates health from many perspectives such as physiology, psychology and sociology. It contains eight domains: physical functioning

Table 20.17.1. Domains, content, and item numbers of the SF-36.

Domain	Content	Item number
PF	Physical limitation	3a, 3b, 3c, 3d, 3e, 3f, 3g, 3h, 3i, 3j
RP	Influence of physical health on work and daily life	4a, 4b, 4c, 4d
BP	Influence of pain on work and daily life	7, 8
GH	Self-estimation of health status	1, 11a, 11b, 11c, 11d
VT	Degree of energy or exhaustion	9a, 9e, 9g, 9i
SF	Influence of physical health and emotional problem on social activities	6, 10
RE	Influence of emotional changes on work and daily life	5a, 5b, 5c
MH	Common mental health problems (depression, anxiety, etc.)	9b, 9c, 9d, 9f, 9h
HT	Compared to health status 1 year ago	2

Note: The SF-36 is widely used across the world with at least 95 versions in 53 languages.

(PF), role physical (RP), bodily pain (BP), general health (GH), vitality (VT), social role functioning (SF), role emotional (RE) and mental health (MH), and it also consists of 36 items. The eight domains can be classified into the physical component summary (PCS) and the mental component summary (MCS); of these, the PCS includes PF, RP, BP and GH, and the MCS includes VT, SF, RE and MH. The SF-36 also includes a single-item measure that is used to evaluate the subject's health transition or changes in the past 1 year.

The SF-36 is a self-assessment scale that assesses people's health status in the past 4 weeks. The items apply Likert scales. Each scale is directly transformed into a 0–100 scale on the assumption that each question carries equal weight. A higher score indicates a better QOL of the subject. The corresponding content and items of the domains are shown in Table 20.17.1.

20.18. WHO Quality of Life Assessment (WHOQOL)[43–45]

The World Health Organization Quality of Life assessment (WHOQOL) is a general scale developed by the cooperation of 37 regions and centers (organized by the WHO) with 15 different cultural backgrounds and was designed according to health concepts related to QOL. The WHOQOL scales include the WHOQOL-100 and the WHOQOL-BREF.

The WHOQOL-100 contains six domains, within which there are a total number of 24 facets, and each facet has four items. There are 4 other items that are related to the evaluation of GH status and QOL

Table 20.18.1. Structure of WHOOQOL-100.

I. Physical domain	**IV. Social domain**
13. Personal relationship	
1. Pain and discomfort	14. Degree of satisfaction with social support
2. Energetic or wearied	15. Sexual life
3. Sleep and rest	
	V. Environment
II. Psychological domain	16. Social security
4. Positive feelings	17. Living environment
5. Thinking, learning, memory and concentration	18. Financial conditions
	19. Medical service and society
6. Self-esteem	20. Opportunity to obtain new information, knowledge and techniques
7. Figure and appearance	
8. Passive feelings	21. Opportunity for and participation in entertainment
III. Level of independence	
9. Action competence	22. Environmental conditions (pollution/noise/traffic/climate)
10. Activity of daily living	23. Transportation
11. Dependence on medication	
12. Work competence	**VI. Spirituality/Religion/Personal beliefs**
	24. Spirituality/religion/personal beliefs

score. The six domains are the physical domain, psychological domain, level of independence, social domain, environmental domain and spirituality/religion/personal beliefs (spirit) domain. The structure of the WHOOQOL-100 is shown in Table 20.18.1.

The WHOQOL-BREF is a brief version of the WHOQOL-100. It contains four domains, namely a physical domain, psychological domain, social domain and environmental domain, within which there are 24 facets, each with 1 item. There are 2 other items that are related to general health and QOL. The WHOQOL-BREF integrates the independence domain of the WHOQOL into the physical domain, while the spirit domain is integrated into the psychological domain.

In addition, the Chinese version of the WHOQOL-100 and WHOQOL-BREF introduces two more items: family friction and appetite.

The WHOQOL-100 and WHOQOL-BREF are self-assessment scales that assess people's health status and daily life in the past 2 weeks. Likert scales are applied to all items, and the score of each domain is converted to a score of 0–100 points; the higher the score, the better the health status of the subject. The WHOQOL is widely used across the world, with at least 43 translated versions in 34 languages. The WHOQOL-100 and WHOQOL-BREF have been shown to be reliable, valid and responsive.

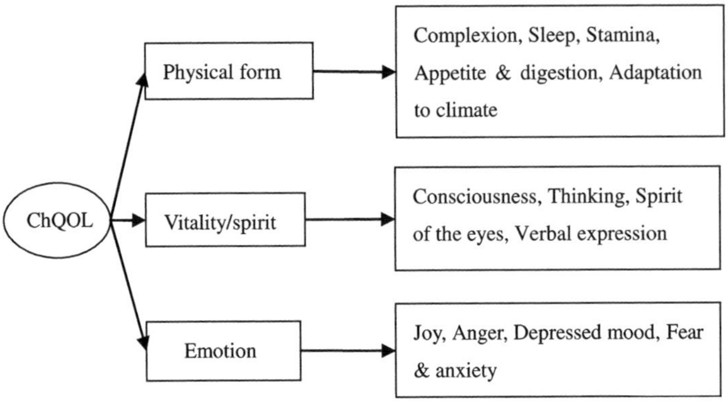

Fig. 20.19.1. Structure of the ChQOL.

20.19. ChQOL[46,47]

ChQOL is a general scale developed by Liu *et al.* on the basis of international scale-development methods according to the concepts of traditional Chinese medicine and QOL. The scale contains 50 items covering 3 domains: a physical form domain, vitality/spirit domain and emotion domain. The physical form domain includes five facets, namely complexion, sleep, stamina, appetite and digestion, and adaptation to climate. The vitality/spirit domain includes four facets, consciousness, thinking, spirit of the eyes, and verbal expression. The emotion domain includes four facets, joy, anger, depressed mood, and fear and anxiety. The structure of the ChQOL is shown in Figure 20.19.1.

The ChQOL is a self-assessment scale that assesses people's QOL in the past 2 weeks on Likert scales. The scores of all items in each domain are summed to yield a single score for the domain. The scores of all domains are summed to yield the total score. A higher score indicates a better QOL.

The ChQOL has several versions in different languages, including a simplified Chinese version (used in mainland China), a traditional Chinese version (used in Hong Kong), an English version and an Italian version. Moreover, the scale is included in the Canadian complementary and alternative medicine (INCAM) Health Outcomes Database. The results showed that both the Chinese version and the other versions have good reliability and validity.

The Chinese health status scale (ChHSS) is a general scale developed by Liu *et al.* on the basis of international scale-development methods, and the development was also guided by the concepts of traditional Chinese medicine and QOL.

The ChHSS includes 31 items covering 8 facets: energy, pain, diet, defecation, urination, sleep, body constitution and emotion. There are 6 items for energy, 2 for pain, 5 for diet, 5 for defecation, 2 for urination, 3 for sleep, 3 for body constitution and 4 for emotion. There is another item that reflects general health.

The ChHSS applies a Likert scale to estimate people's health status in the past 2 weeks. It is a reliable and valid instrument when applied in the patients receiving traditional Chinese medicine as well as in those receiving integrated Chinese medicine and Western medicine.

20.20. Patient Reported Outcomes Measurement Information System[48,49]

The Patient Reported Outcomes Measurement Information System (PROMIS) is a measurement tool system that contains various reliable and precise patient–reported outcomes for physical, mental and social well-being. PROMIS tools measure what patients are able to do and how they feel by asking questions. PROMIS measures can be used as primary or secondary endpoints in clinical studies of the effectiveness of treatment.[1]

PROMIS measures allow the assessment of many PRO domains, including pain, fatigue, emotional distress, PF and social role participation, based on common metrics that allow for comparisons across domains, across chronic diseases, and with the general population. Furthermore, PROMIS tools allow for computer adaptive testing, which can efficiently achieve precise measurements of health status domains with only a few items. There are PROMIS measures for both adults and children.

PROMIS was established in 2004 with funding from the National Institutes of Health (NIH) of the United States of America as one of the initiatives of the NIH Roadmap for Medical Research. The main work includes establishing the framework of the domains, developing and proofreading candidate items for adults and children, administering the candidate items to a large sample of individuals, building web-based computerized adaptive tests (CATs), conducting feasibility studies to evaluate the utility of PROMIS, promoting widespread use of the instrument in scientific research and clinical practice, and contacting external scientists to share the methodology, scales and software of PROMIS.

The theoretical framework of PROMIS is divided into three parts for adults: physical health, mental health and social health. The self-reported health domains contain profile domains and additional domains (Table 20.20.1).

Table 20.20.1. Adult self-reported health domains.

	Profile domains	Additional domains
Physical Health	Physical function; Pain intensity; Pain interference; Fatigue; Sleep disturbance	Pain behavior; sleep-related (daytime) impairment; sexual function
Mental Health	Depression; Anxiety	Anger; applied cognition; alcohol use, consequences, and expectations; psychosocial illness impact
Social Health	Satisfaction with participation in social roles	Satisfaction with social roles and activities; Ability to participate in social roles and activities; Social support; Social isolation; Companionship

The development procedures of PROMIS include: (1) Defining the concept and the framework. A modified Delphi method and analysis methods were used to determine the main domains (Table 20.20.1). The sub-domains and their concepts were also identified through discussion and modification. (2) Establishing and correcting the item pool. The item pool was established through quantitative and qualitative methods. The steps include screening, classifying, choosing, evaluating and modifying the items through focus groups. Subsequently, PROMIS version 1.0 was established. (3) Testing PROMIS version 1.0 with a large sample. A survey of the general American population and people with chronic disease were investigated from July 2006 to March 2007. The data were analyzed using IRT, and 11 item banks were established for the CAT and were used to develop a brief scale.

Previously, most health scales had been developed based on CTT, which could not compare people with different diseases. However, PROMIS was developed based on IRT and CAT, and thus this comparison was feasible. The PROMIS domains are believed to be important aspects of evaluating health and clinical treatment efficacy.

References

1. World Health Organization. *Constitution of the World Health Organization — Basic Documents*, (45th edn.). Supplement. Geneva: WHO, 2006.
2. Callahan, D. The WHO definition of "health". *Stud. Hastings Cent.*, 1973, 1(3): 77–88.
3. Huber, M, Knottnerus, JA, Green, L, *et al.* How should we define health?. *BMJ*, 2011, 343: d4163.
4. WHO. *The World Health Report 2001: Mental Health — New Understanding, New Hope.* Geneva: World Health Organization, 2001.

5. Bertolote, J. The roots of the concept of mental health, *World Psychiatry*, 2008, 7(2): 113–116.
6. Patel, V, Prince, M. Global mental health — a new global health field comes of age. *JAMA*, 2010, 303: 1976–1977.
7. Nordenfelt, L. *Concepts and Measurement of Quality of Life in Health Care*. Berlin: Springer, 1994.
8. WHO. The Development of the WHO Quality of Life Assessment Instrument. Geneva: WHO, 1993.
9. Fang, JQ. *Measurement of Quality of Life and Its Applications*. Beijing: Beijing Medical University Press, 2000. (In Chinese)
10. U.S. Department of Health and Human Services *et al.* Patient-reported outcome measures: Use in medical product development to support labeling claims: Draft guidance. *Health Qual. Life Outcomes*, 2006, 4: 79.
11. Patient Reported Outcomes Harmonization Group. Harmonizing patient reported outcomes issues used in drug development and evaluation [R/OL]. http://www.eriqa-project.com/pro-harmo/home.html.
12. Acquadro, C, Berzon, R, Dubois D, *et al.* Incorporating the patient's perspective into drug development and communication: An ad hoc task force report of the Patient-Reported Outcomes (PRO) Harmonization Group meeting at the Food and Drug Administration, February 16, 2001. *Value Health*, 2003, 6(5): 522–531.
13. Mesbah, M, Col, BF, Lee, MLT. *Statistical Methods for Quality of Life Studies*. Boston: Kluwer Academic, 2002.
14. Liu, BY. *Measurement of Patient Reported Outcomes — Principles, Methods and Applications*. Beijing: People's Medical Publishing House, 2011. (In Chinese)
15. U.S. Department of Health and Human Services *et al.* Guidance for Industry Patient-Reported Outcome Measures: Use in Medical Product Development to Support Labeling Claims. http://www.fda.gov/downloads/drugs/ guidancecomplianceregulatoryin formation/guidances/ucm193282.pdf.
16. Mesbah, M, Col, BF, Lee, MLT. *Statistical Methods for Quality of Life Studies*. Boston: Kluwer Academic, 2002.
17. Fang, JQ. *Medical Statistics and Computer Testing* (4th edn.). Shanghai: Shanghai Scientific and Technical Publishers, 2012. (In Chinese)
18. Terwee, C, Bot, S, de Boer, M, *et al.* Quality criteria were proposed for measurement properties of health status questionnaires. *J. Clin. Epidemiol.*, 2007, 60(1): 34–42.
19. Wan, CH, Jiang, WF. *China Medical Statistics Encyclopedia: Health Measurement Division*. Beijing: China Statistics Press, 2013. (In Chinese)
20. Gu, HG. *Psychological and Educational Measurement*. Beijing: Peking University Press, 2008. (In Chinese)
21. Jaeschke, R, Singer, J, Guyatt, GH, Measurement of health status: Ascertaining the minimal clinically important difference. *Controll. Clin. Trials*, 1989, 10: 407–415.
22. Brozek, JL, Guyatt, GH, Schtlnemann, HJ. How a well-grounded minimal important difference can enhance transparency of labelling claims and improve interpretation of a patient reported outcome measure. *Health Qual Life Outcomes*, 2006, 4(69): 1–7.
23. Mapi Research Institute. Linguistic validation of a patient reported outcomes measure [EB/OL]. http://www.pedsql.org/translution/html.
24. Beaton, DE, Bombardier, C, Guillemin, F, *et al.* Guidelines for the process of cross-cultural adaptation of self-report measures. *Spine*, 2000, 25(24): 3186–3191.
25. Spilker, B. Quality of Life and Pharmacoeconomics in Clinical Trials. Hagerstown, MD: Lippincott-Raven, 1995.

26. Drasgow, F. Scrutinizing psychological tests: Measurement equivalence and equivalent relations with external variables are the central issues. *Psychol. Bull.*, 1984, 95: 34–135.
27. Allen, MJ, Yen, WM. *Introduction to Measurement Theory.* Long Grove, IL: Waveland Press, 2002.
28. Alagumalai, S, Curtis, DD, Hungi, N. *Applied Rasch Measurement: A Book of Exemplars. Dordrecht,* The Netherlands: Springer, 2005.
29. Dai, HQ, Zhang, F, Chen, XF. *Psychological and Educational Measurement.* Guangzhou: Jinan University Press, 2007. (In Chinese)
30. Hambleton, RK, Swaminathan, H, Rogers, HJ. *Fundamentals of Item Response Theory.* Newbury Park, CA: Sage Press, 1991.
31. Holland, PW, Wainer, H. *Differential Item Functioning.* Hillsdale, NJ: Lawrence Erlbaum, 1993.
32. Du, WJ. *Higher Item Response Theory.* Beijing: Science Press, 2014. (In Chinese)
33. Hambleton, RK, Swaminathan, H, Rogers, HJ. *Fundamentals of Item Response Theory.* Newbury Park, CA: Sage Press, 1991.
34. Ostini, R, Nering, ML. *Handbook of Polytomous Item Response Theory Models.* SAGE Publications, Inc, 2005.
35. Van der Linden, WJ, Hambleton, RK. *Handbook of Modern Item Response Theory.* New York: Springer, 1997.
36. Brennan, RL. *Generalizability Theory.* New York: Springer-Verlag, 2001.
37. Chiu, CWC. *Scoring Performance Assessments Based on Judgements: Generalizability Theory.* New York: Kluwer, 2001.
38. Yang, ZM, Zhang, L. *Generalizability Theory and Its Applications.* Beijing: Educational Science Publishing House, 2003. (In Chinese)
39. Weiss, DJ, Kingsbury, GG. Application of computerized adaptive testing to educational problems. *J. edu. meas.*, 1984, 21: 361–375.
40. Wainer, H, Dorans, NJ, Flaugher, R, *et al. Computerized Adaptive Testing: A Primer.* Mahwah, NJ: Routledge, 2000.
41. http://www.sf-36.org/.
42. McHorney, CA, Ware, JE Jr, Raczek, AE. The MOS 36-Item Short-Form Health Survey (SF-36): II. Psychometric and clinical tests of validity in measuring physical and mental health constructs. *Med Care.* 1993, 31(3): 247–63.
43. http://www.who.int/mental_health/publications/whoqol/en/.
44. World Health Organization. *WHOQOL User Manual.* Geneva: WHO, 1998.
45. The WHOQOL Group. The world health organization quality of life assessment (WHOQOL): Development and general psychometric properties. *Soc. Sci. Medi.*, 1998, 46: 1569–1585.
46. Leung, KF, Liu, FB, Zhao, L, *et al.* Development and validation of the Chinese quality of life instrument. *Health Qual. Life Outcomes*, 2005, 3: 26.
47. Liu, FBL, Lang, JY, Zhao, L, *et al.* Development of health status scale of traditional chinese medicine (TCM-HSS). *J. Sun Yat-Sen University* (Medical Sciences), 2008, 29(3): 332–336.
48. National Institutes of Health. PROMIS domain framework [EB/OL]. http://www.nihpromis.org/Documents/PROMIS_Full_Framework.pdf.
49. http://www.nihpromis.org/.

About the Author

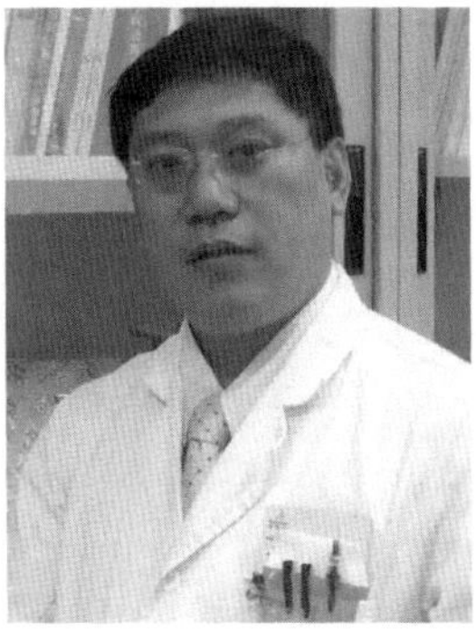

Fengbin Liu is Director and Professor, Department of Internal Medicine in the First Affiliated Hospital of Guangzhou University of Chinese Medicine, Vice Chief, the World Association for Chinese Quality of Life (WACQOL) Vice Chief, the Gastrointestinal Disease chapter, China Association of Chinese Medicine, Editorial board member of *World Journal of Integrated Medicine World Journal of Gastroenterology*, *Guangzhou University Journal of Chinese Medicine*, and Contributing Reviewer of *Health and Quality of Life Outcomes.*

Professor Liu's research interests include Clinical Outcomes and Efficiency Evaluation of Chinese Medicine and Clinical Research on Integrated Medicine for Gastroenterology. He has developed the Chinese Quality of life Scale (ChQoL), the Chinese health status scale (ChHS), the Chinese gastrointestinal disease PRO Scale (ChGePRO), the Chinese chronic liver disease PRO Scale (ChCL-PRO), the Chinese myasthenia gravis PRO Scale (ChMG-PRO). He has translated the English edition of the quality of life scale for functional dyspepsia (FDDQOL) into Chinese edition.

CHAPTER 21

PHARMACOMETRICS

Qingshan Zheng*, Ling Xu, Lunjin Li, Kun Wang, Juan Yang,
Chen Wang, Jihan Huang and Shuiyu Zhao

21.1. Pharmacokinetics (PK)[1,2]

PK is the study of drug absorption, distribution, metabolism and excretion (ADME) based on the dynamic principles. It is a practical tool for the drug research and development, rational use and quality control.

Pharmacokinetic study covers a wide scope, including single/multiple-dose study, drug metabolite study, comparative pharmacokinetic study (e.g. food effect and drug interaction), as well as toxicokinetics. The test subjects are generally animals or human such as the healthy individuals, patients with renal and hepatic impairment, or patients whom the drug product is intended.

21.1.1. *Compartment model*

Compartment model, a classic means to illustrate pharmacokinetics, is a type of mathematical model used to describe the transmission of drugs among the compartments in human body. Each compartment does not represent a real tissue or an organ in anatomy. Common compartment models consist of one-, two- and three-compartment models.

The parameters of compartment model are constants that describe the relation of time and drug concentration in the body.

(1) Apparent volume of distribution (V) is a proportionality constant describing the relation between total drug dose and blood drug rather than a physiological volume. It can be defined as the apparent volume

*Corresponding author: qingshan.zheng@drugchina.net

into which a drug distributes. In the one-compartment model, V is given by the following equation:

$$V = \text{Amount of drug in the body}/\text{Concentration of drug in the plasma}.$$

(2) Total clearance (CL) refers to the elimination of apparent volume of distribution from the body per unit time. The relationship of CL with the elimination rate constant (k) and the distribution volume is: $CL = k \cdot V$.
(3) Elimination half-life ($t_{1/2}$), the time required for the plasma concentration to fall to half of its initial concentration, is a constant used to reflect the elimination rate in the body. For drugs fitting the first-order elimination, the relationship of $t_{1/2}$ and the k is as follows: $t_{1/2} = 0.693/k$.

21.1.2. *Non-compartment model*

Non-compartment model is a method of moment to calculate the pharmacokinetic parameters. According to this model, the relationship of plasma concentration (C) and time (T) fits a randomly distributed curve suitable to any compartment model. Some of the commonly used parameters are listed as follows:

(1) Area under the concentration-time curve (AUC) is the integral of the concentration-time curve.

$$AUC = \int c \cdot dt.$$

(2) Mean residual time (MRT) reflects the average residence time of drug molecules in the body.

$$MRT = \frac{\int t \cdot c \cdot dt}{AUC}.$$

(3) Variance of mean residence time (VRT) reflects the differences of the average residence times of drug molecules in the body.

$$VRT = \int (t - MRT)^2 \cdot c \cdot dt/AUC.$$

21.2. Dose Proportionality Response[3,4]

Dose proportionality response characterizes the proportional relationship between dosage and drug exposure parameters *in vivo*. The exposure parameter is usually illustrated by the maximum plasma concentration ($C_{\max}$)

or area under the plasma concentration-time curve (AUC). In presence of n-fold increase in drug dosage, the dose proportionality response is still recommended upon an n-fold increase in the $C_{\max}$ and AUC, implying that the kinetic of drug is linear. Otherwise, saturable absorption (less than n-fold) or saturable metabolism (more than n-fold) may present in absence of n-fold increase in $C_{\max}$ and AUC, suggesting that the kinetic of the drug is nonlinear. The linear kinetics can be used to predict the medication effects and safety within a certain dosage range, while the nonlinear PK may undergo loss of predictability in dosage change.

Exposure parameters, a group of dose-dependent pharmacokinetic parameters including AUC, $C_{\max}$, steady-state plasma concentrations (C_{ss}), are the key points for the estimated relationship of dose proportionality response. The other dose-independent parameters, such as peak time ($T_{\max}$), half-time ($t_{1/2}$), CL, volume of distribution at steady state (V_{ss}) and rate constant (K_e), are not necessary for the analysis.

Dose proportionality response of a new drug is determined in multidose pharmacokinetic trial, which is usually performed simultaneously with clinical tolerance trial.

Evaluation model: The parameters commonly used for the evaluation of dose proportionality include (1) linear model, such as $PK = \alpha + \beta \cdot Dose$, where PK is the pharmacokinetic parameter (AUC or $C_{\max}$), (2) dose-adjusted PK parameter followed by analysis of variance (ANOVA) testing: $PK/Dose = \mu + a_i$, (3) power model: $PK = \alpha \cdot Dose^{\beta}$.

Evaluation method (1) The hypothesis test: the conditions of the test are $\alpha = 0, \beta > 0$ for linear model, $a_i = 0$ for ANOVA, and $\beta = 1$ for power model; (2) Confidence Intervals (CIs): establish the relationship between the discriminant interval of dose proportionality response and the statistical model by using the following steps: $r = h/l$, where PK_h and PK_l represent parameters for the highest dose (h) and the lowest dose (l), respectively. (i) $PK_h/PK_l = r$, dose proportionality is recommended; (ii) If the ratio of the PK parameters of standardized dose to the geometric mean (R_{dnm}) equal to 1 after dividing by r on both sides of the equation, the dose response relationship is recommended; (iii) According to the safety and efficacy, the low (q_L) and high (q_H) limit of R_{dnm} serve as the critical values of the two sides of the inequation; (iv) To estimate the predictive value and the corresponding confidence interval of R_{dnm} according to the statistical models; (v) Calculation of inequality and model parameters. This method can be used in the analysis of parameters and calculation of CI for variance model, linear regression model and power function model. If the parameters of the $(1 - \alpha)\%$ CI are completely within the discriminant interval, the dose proportionality is recommended.

21.3. Population PK[5]

It is a calculating method for the PK parameter covering various factors that combines the classic PK model with population approach.

Population PK provide abundant information, including: (1) the parameters of typical values, which refer to the description of drugs disposition in typical patients, and characterize the PK parameters of a population or the subpopulation; (2) fixed effects, as the parameters of observed covariates, such as gender, body weight, liver and kidney function, diet, drug combination, environment, and genetic traits; (3) the random effect parameter, also called random variations, including, intra-individual variability and inter-individual variability (residual), which is represented by the standard deviation.

Characteristics of population PK: (1) Compared with classic method, its data sampling point and time of population PK is more flexible. It shows better performance in analyzing sparse data, which could maximize the use of data. (2) It could introduce the impact of various covariates as fixed effect to the model, and test whether the covariates have a significant effect on model parameters, so as to estimate PK parameters individually. It contributes to the designing of individual treatment plan. (3) Also, it involves the simultaneous estimation of typical value, intra- and inter-individual variability of observed population, which provides useful information for the simulation study. The simulated results could indicate the plasma concentration of the drug and PK behavior in different individuals with different dosage and dosing intervals, which could guide the reasonable usage in clinical application.

The nonlinear mixed effects model (NONMEM) was initially proposed by Sheiner *et al.* in 1977. The final model is obtained according to the principle of minimal optimization of the objective function. The change of the objective function values fits the chi-square distribution. The necessity of a parameter or a fixed effect depends on the significance of the changes of objective function value.

The parameter estimation in NONMEM is based on the extended least squares method. The original algorithm is first-order approximation (FO), and then some algorithms are available, such as a first-order approximation (FOCE), Laplace and EM algorithm.

The commonly used software include NONMEM, ADAPT, S-plus, DAS and Monolix.

The general process of modeling: Firstly, the structure model is established, including linear compartments, and Michaelis–Menten nonlinear model. Secondly, statistical model is established to describe intra- and inter-individual variability. The evaluation of intra-individual variability is commonly based on additive error, proportional error and proportional combined additive error model, while those for the inter-individual variation evaluation usually involves additive error or exponential error model. Finally, covariate model is established by gradually introducing the covariates in linear, exponential or classification to determine the effects of covariate on PK parameters.

Two methods have been commonly used for the model validation, including internal and external validation methods. The former includes data split method, cross-validation method, Jackknife method and Bootstrap method, while the latter focuses on the extrapolative prediction ability of candidate model on other data. In addition, the application of standard diagnostic plot method is of prime importance.

Population PK is labor-intensive and time-consuming. Meanwhile, special training should be given to the analysts.

21.4. Pharmacodynamics (PD)[6,7]

Pharmacodynamics focuses on the relationship between drug dosage (the same concentration, thereafter) and drug reaction, namely dose–response relationship. It is called the quantitative dose–effect relationship if drug reaction is a continuous variable. If the drug reaction is a time variable, it is called the time dose–effect relationship. For the drug reaction shows two categorical data of "appear" or "not appear", it is called the quality reactive dose–effect relationship.

The concentration–response relationships above mentioned can be described by three types of dose response curves. Mathematical models can be used to describe the curves containing adequate data points. In clinical trials, the process of identifying the optimal therapeutic dose among multiple doses is called dose finding. Based on the concentration–response curves, pharmacodynamics models presented in various forms are established, and the common models are as follows:

21.4.1. *Fixed-effects model*

Fixed-effects model, also called quantitative effect model, is fixed based on Logistic regression method of statistics. Usually, the drug concentration is associated with a certain fixed effect. The simplest fixed-effects model is the threshold effect model, which generates the fixed effect (E_{fixed}) when reaching or surpassing the threshold concentration ($C_{\text{threshold}}$). For example, patients may present with deafness in the presence of trough concentration of $>4\ \mu$g/mL for more than 10 days during the medication of gentamicin. This means is the drug concentration (C) reaches or surpasses the threshold concentration (i.e. $C \geq C_{\text{threshold}}$), and then the drug reaction (E) reaches or is superior to the fixed effect (i.e. $E \geq E_{\text{fixed}}$).

21.4.2. *Linear model*

In this model, a proportion is hypothesized to be available between drug concentration and drug effect directly.

$$E = m \times C + E_0,$$

where E_0 represents the baseline effect, m represents the scale factor (the slope of a straight line of E to C).

21.4.3. *Logarithmic linear model*

Its formula is

$$E = m \times \log C + b,$$

where m and b represent the slope and intercept of semi-log straight-line made by E to C. Logarithmic linear model is a special case of the maximum effect model. A linear relationship is presented between E and C upon the maximum effect model is within a scope of 20–80%.

21.4.4. *E_{max} model*

Its form is

$$E = \frac{E_{\text{max}} \times C}{ED_{50} + C},$$

where E_{max} represents the probably maximum effect, and ED_{50} is the drug concentration to achieve 50% of E_{max}. If the baseline effect (E_0) is available, the following formula can be used:

$$E = E_0 + \frac{E_{\text{max}} \times C}{ED_{50} + C}.$$

21.4.5. *Sigmoidal E_{max} model*

It is the expansion of the maximum effect model, and the relationship between effect and concentration is

$$E = E_0 + \frac{E_{\text{max}} \times C^{\gamma}}{ED_{50} + C^{\gamma}},$$

where γ represents the shape factor. In cases of larger γ, a steeper linear relation is observed in the effect-concentration diagram.

21.5. Pharmacokinetic–pharmacodynamic Model (PK–PD model)[7,8]

Such model connects PK to PD, and establishes the relationship between drug dosage, time, concentration (or exposure) and response. It is widely used in optimal dose finding, individual therapy decision, drug mechanisms illustration, and the quantitative expression of drug characteristics.

PK–PD models can be divided into empirical model, mechanism model and semi-mechanism model. In addition, the study on the relationship between PK exposure parameters and response also belongs to the scope of PK–PD model essentially.

21.5.1. *Empirical model*

The empirical model is established based on the relationship between concentration in plasma/action sites and time. Such model can be divided into direct and indirect link models. Direct link model means the equilibrium of the plasma and the site of action occurs quickly without time lag in non-steady states. In indirect link model, a separation is noted between concentration-time and response-time processes, which leads to a hysteresis loops in the concentration–response curve. For indirect link model, such lag is commonly described through a hypothetical compartment or an effect-compartment.

Direct response model is defined as a model with direct PD changes after the combination of drug and action site. An indirect response model is defined in cases of other physiological factors producing efficacy after the combination. For indirect response models, the structures of specific model will be different according to the inhibiting or stimulating effects of drugs on the physiological processes. Upon understanding of drug mechanisms, the indirect process can be decomposed into a number of parts with physiological significance, which could further derivate as a mechanism model.

21.5.2. *Mechanism model*

In recent years, extensive studies have been carried out to investigate the intermediate mechanisms of plasma concentration to efficacy in some drugs. Besides, increasing studies are apt to focus on the mechanism model, which leads to the formation of a materialized network model of "single dose-time-concentration-intermediate-efficacy". Its prediction is more accurate and reliable than empirical model.

21.5.3. *Semi-mechanism model*

This model is generally utilized when the mechanism of action is only partial known. It can be considered as a combination of empirical model and mechanism model.

21.5.4. *Exposure-response model*

Exposure-response model, also been known as E-R model, is a special type of PK–PD model that is used more extensively. On many occasions, the multidoses-PK exposure parameters–response relationship is much easier to be obtained. The PK exposure parameters include AUC, $C_{\max}$, and C_{ss}. E-R model has largely extended the application scope of PK–PD model.

The increasing emerge of the new methods has promoted the development of PK–PD models. For instance, the introduction of population approach contributes to the studies on the population PK–PD model, which could evaluate the effects of covariates on parameters. Meanwhile, the physiology factors using as predictive correction factors are introduced to establish the physiology based PK model (PBPK). It can actually provide an analyzing method for physiological PK–PD model, and facilitate to PK and PD prediction among different populations or different species, which provides possibility for the bridging study.

21.6. Accumulation Index[9,10]

Drug accumulation will be induced if the second dose is given before the complete elimination of the previous one. Accumulation index (R_{ac}), describing the degree of accumulation of the drug quantitatively, is an important parameter for the evaluation of drug safety. Moderate drug accumulation is the basis for maintenance of drug efficacy, however, for a drug with narrow therapeutic window and large toxic side effects (e.g. digitalis drugs), cautious attention should be paid to the dosing regimen in order to prevent the toxic side effects due to the accumulation effects.

As revealed in the previous literatures, four common R_{ac} calculation methods are available (Table 21.6.1). As significant differences are noticed in the results from different calculation methods, an appropriate method should be selected based on the actual situation. Formula 1 is most widely

Table 21.6.1. Summary of accumulation index calculation method.

Number	Formula	Explanation
Formula 1	$\frac{AUC_{0-\tau,ss}}{AUC_{0-\tau,1}}$	$AUC_{0-\tau,ss}$: the steady-state areas under the plasma concentration-time curves during a dosing interval $(0-\tau)$ $AUC_{0-\tau,1}$: the areas under the plasma concentration-time curves after the first dose during a dosing interval $(0-\tau)$
Formula 2	$\frac{C_{\max,ss}}{C_{\max,1}}$	$C_{\max,ss}$: maximum plasma concentration at steady-state $C_{\max,1}$: maximum plasma concentration after the first dose
Formula 3	$\frac{C_{\text{trough},ss}}{C_{\text{trough},1}}$	$C_{\text{trough},ss}$: trough concentration at steady-state $C_{\text{trough},1}$: trough concentration after the first dose
Formula 4	$(1-e^{-\lambda\tau})^{-1}$	λ: elimination rate constant; τ: dosing interval

recommended to calculate the R_{ac} if the efficacy or safety of drugs is significantly related to AUC, such as β-lactam and quinolone antibiotics. In formula 2, $C_{\max}$ reflects the maximum exposure of drugs in body. Formula 2 is most appropriate for the calculation of R_{ac} when drugs' efficacy or safety is related to $C_{\max}$, such as aminoglycoside antibiotics. Formula 3, usually with a low C_{trough}, can be greatly influenced by detection error and individual variation, which hampers the accuracy of the calculation. Equation 4 can predict the accumulation index of steady-state under the single dose on the premise that the drug is in line with the characteristic of a linear pharmacokinetic profile. This is mainly associated with the fact that drug elimination rate constant (λ) is a constant only under linear conditions.

The extent of drug accumulation can be classified according to the threshold proposed by FDA for drug interactions. Four types of drug accumulation are defined, including non-accumulation (R_{ac} of <1.2), weak accumulation ($1.2 \leq R_{ac} < 2$), moderate accumulation ($2 \leq R_{ac} < 5$) and strong accumulation ($R_{ac} \geq 5$). Notably, the threshold value can only be used to determine whether the drug exposure in steady state is significantly higher than that under a single dose, rather than a parameter to judge the side effects. This is mainly related to the fact that the drug with large therapeutic window is still safe in spite of its high R_{ac}. Furthermore, it is meaningless to simply evaluate the value of R_{ac} without considering the dose level. Nevertheless, it won't produce side effects even if the R_{ac} is large in presence of low initial dose.

21.7. Bioavailability (BA)[7,11]

BA is the fraction of an administered dose of absorbed drug dose that reaches the systemic circulation. Another relevant concept is bioequivalence (BE), which refers to a comparison of the absorption rate and extent of the active ingredient of test formulation and a reference drug of the same dose under the same experimental conditions. Usually, BE studies take BA results as destination indicators. On this basis, a comparison is carried out according to the predetermined equivalent criteria.

Three main PK parameters are involved in the BE analysis: (1) AUC, reflecting the drug absorption; (2) $C_{\max}$; (3) time of maximum observed plasma concentration ($T_{\max}$). $C_{\max}$ and $T_{\max}$ reflect the absorption, distribution, excretion and metabolism of drugs synthetically by the observed measurements.

BA analysis is mainly dependent on the AUC. AUC_{0-t} (the plasma concentration-time area under the curve with time from 0 to t) can be calculated by linear or logarithmic trapezoidal method. t refers to the sampling time of the last measurable concentration. The linear trapezoidal method is illustrated as follows:

$$AUC_{0-t} = \sum_{i=0}^{t} (C_i + C_{i-1}) \cdot (t_i - t_{i-1})/2.$$

The calculation method of $AUC_{0-\infty}$ (the plasma concentration-time area under the curve with time from 0 to ∞ with extrapolation of the terminal phase):

$$AUC_{0-\infty} = AUC_{0-t} + C_t/\lambda_z.$$

C_t, the concentration of the last measurable sample; λ_z, elimination rate constant at the end of the drug-time curve, obtained from the slope of the terminal linear portion of the logarithmic plasma concentration-time curve.

BA and BE studies are mostly executed by crossover design or parallel design.

BA includes absolute bioavailability and relative bioavailability. Absolute bioavailability is the proportion of the dose absorbed into the systemic circulation to the total dosage. Drugs administrated via extravascular (exe) route are compared to the reference drug of intravenous (iv) formulation. Absolute bioavailability F:

$$F = \frac{AUC_{exe} \cdot Dose_{iv}}{AUC_{iv} \cdot Dose_{exe}} \cdot 100\%.$$

Relative bioavailability is a comparison of absorption fraction of test formulation (T) and reference formulation (R) of the same drug (e.g. tablet versus capsule). The relative bioavailability F:

$$F = \frac{AUC_T \cdot Dose_R}{AUC_R \cdot Dose_T} \cdot 100\%.$$

BE analysis mainly involves the evaluation of the AUC and $C_{\max}$ of test preparation and reference preparation after logarithmic transformation by multivariate analysis of variance (ANOVA), two one-sided t-tests and $(1-2\alpha)\%$ CI. ANOVA could indicate the mean squared error (MSE) for the two one-sided t-tests. Equivalence criteria are usually determined in accordance with relevant regulations. If necessary, non-parametric test for $T_{\max}$ should also be carried out.

21.8. Synergism[12,13]

Synergism, a concept of drug interaction, refers to the additional benefit just like $1+1>2$. Such type of benefit could be presented as unchanged efficiency with a decreased dose after drug combination (applicable to isobologram and median-effect principle), or an enhanced potency of drug combination (applicable to weighed modification model). Another concept, opposite to synergism, is antagonism, refers to the effect like $1+1<2$.

21.8.1. *Isobologram*

It is a classical method only utilized in the experimental studies of two drugs:

$$Q = d_1/D_1 + d_2/D_2.$$

$Q = 1$, additive drug interaction; $Q > 1$, antagonism; $Q < 1$, synergism. Dose combination $d_1 + d_2$, single-item dose D_1 and D_2 are all equivalent dosages. At the effect level x, mark the points of equivalent dose in abscissa of drug A and ordinate of drug B when using a combination of drug A and drug B. The equivalent line can be obtained by linking the two points. When $Q = 1$, the intersection point of d_1 and d_2 falls exactly on the equivalent line; when $Q < 1$, the intersection point of d_1 and d_2 falls below the equivalent line; when $Q > 1$, the intersection falls above the equivalent line.

21.8.2. *Median-effect principle*

TC Chou *et al.* proposed that the cell experiments of n the cytotoxic anti-tumor drugs can be analyzed at any effect level (x).

$$\text{CI} = \frac{\sum d_i}{D_{x,i}}.$$

CI $= 1$, additive drug interaction; CI > 1, antagonism; CI < 1, synergism. At the x effect level, $D_{x,i}$ refers to the equivalent dose when the drugs are used individually, and $d_i(i = 1, 2 \ldots, n)$ is the equivalent dose of drug combination.

21.8.3. *Weighed modification model*

Take combination of two drugs as example, the combined effect (E_{obs}) of component term (X_i), exponent term (X_i^2), interaction term (X_iX_j) and stochastic effect terms (η and ε) are:

$$E_{\text{obs}} = E_0 + \frac{E_{\max}}{\gamma} \cdot \frac{\rho}{X_{50} + \rho} + \eta + \varepsilon.$$

$E_{\max}$, maximum effect value; E_0, baseline effect (0 is adopted in the absence of baseline); γ, dose-effect curve flatness of combination (fluctuate around 1). ρ is calculated according to the formula: $\rho = B_1X_1 + B_2X_2 + B_3X_1^2 + B_4X_2^2 + B_{12}X_1X_2$, where $X_i(i = 1, 2)$ is the dose of the ith term; B_i is the dose–effect relationship index of the ith term, called weighted index. To make the B_i of different components comparable, the original dose should be normalized, which means to divide the doses of different combination groups by the average dose of the corresponding component. Inter-group variation (η) is assumed to be distributed with $N(0, \omega^2)$, while the residual effect with $N(0, \sigma^2)$. If interaction term (X_1X_2) and exponential term (X_i^2) are included in the model, the decrease of objective function value should meet the statistical requirements. Weighted index B_{12} can be used to determine the nature of the interaction. In cases of greater value and stronger efficacy, $B_{12} > 0$ represents a synergistic effect between X_1 and X_2, while $B_{12} < 0$ represents antagonism. Meanwhile, $B_{12} = 0$ indicates no interaction or additive effect. This rule can be extended to multidrug analysis.

21.9. Drug-drug Interaction (DDI)[14]

DDI includes PK and PD interactions. For clinical trials performed in human, PK interaction is widely adopted in the new drug research as PD interaction evaluation is expensive, time-consuming and usually troublesome. This kind of research is limited to comparison of two drugs so as to form a relatively normative DDI evaluation method, which aims to estimate whether the clinical combination of drugs is safe and the necessity of dosage adjustment. Calculation of a variety of special parameters is involved in this process.

DDI trial is usually divided into two categories (i.e. *in vitro* experiment and the clinical trial). At terms of study order: (1) Initially, attention should be paid to the obvious interaction between test drugs and inhibitors and inducers of transfer protein and metabolic enzyme. (2) In presence of obvious drug interaction, a tool medicine will be selected at the early phase of clinical research to investigate its effects on PK parameters of the tested drug with an aim to identify the availability of drug interaction. (3) Upon availability of a significant interaction, further confirmatory clinical trials will be conducted for dosage adjustment.

FDA has issued many research guidelines for *in vitro* and *in vivo* experiments of DDI, and the key points are:

1. If *in vitro* experiment suggests the test drug is degraded by a certain CYP enzyme or unknown degradation pathway, or the test drug is a CYP enzyme inhibitor ($[I]/K_i > 0.1$) or inducer (increase of enzyme activity of at least 40% compared with positive control group, or no *in vitro* data), it is necessary to conduct clinical trials at early research stage to judge the availability of obvious interaction. Further, clinical experiments are needed for dosage adjustment upon the effect is clear. In addition, $[I]$ means the concentration of tested drug at the active sites of enzymes, which approximately equals the average steady-state concentration $\bar{C}$ after taking the highest dosage clinically; K_i means inhibition constant.
2. For *in vitro* experiments in which tested drug acts as P-glycoprotein substrate that reacts with its inhibitor, bi-directional transmission quantitative measurement values of tested drugs that could permeate Caco-2 or MDR1 epithelial cells membrane serve as the indices. For example, clinical trials are needed in cases of a flow rate ratio of ≥ 2, in combination with significant inhibition of flow rate using P-glycoprotein inhibitor. If tested drug acts as P-glycoprotein inhibitor and its agent, the relationship between the decrease of flow rate ratio of P-glycoprotein substrate and the increase of tested drug concentration is investigated. Then the half of inhibition concentration (IC_{50}) is measured. It is necessary to conduct clinical trials if $[I]/IC_{50}$ (or K_i) of >0.1.
3. The primary purpose of early clinical trials is to determine the presence of interaction, most of which are carried out as independent trials. To evaluate the effects of an enzyme inhibitor or inducer (I) on tested drug (S), unidirectional-acting design (I, S+I) could be used. As for evaluation of interaction between tested drug and combined drug, bidirectional-acting

design (S, I, S+I) must be employed. U.S. FDA advocates crossover design, but parallel design is more commonly used. BE analysis is adopted for the data analysis, also known as comparative pharmacokinetic analysis, but the conclusions are "interaction" and "no interaction". The presence of interaction is judged according to 80–125% of standard.

4. Confirmatory clinical trials for dosage adjustment could be carried out in the latter stages (IIb–IV phases), and population PK analysis is still an option.

21.10. First-in-Human Study[15–17]

It is the first human trial of a drug and its security risk is relatively high. During this process, initial dose calculating and dose escalation extending are necessary. Drug tolerance is also primarily investigated to provides reference for the future trials.

Trial population: Healthy subjects are selected for most of the indications. However, in some specific areas, such as cytotoxic drug for antitumor therapy, patients of certain disease are selected for the trials. Furthermore, for some drugs, expected results cannot be achieved from healthy subjects, such as testing the addiction and tolerance of psychotropic drugs.

Initial dose: Maximum recommended starting dose (MRSD) is typically used as the initial dose which will not produce toxic effect normally. The U.S., European Union and China have issued their own guidelines for MRSD calculation, among which NOAEL method and MABEL method are commonly used.

NOAEL method is calculated based on no observed adverse effect level (NOAEL)g on animal toxicological test, which is mainly used to (1) determine NOAEL; (2) calculate human equivalent dose (HED); (3) select most suitable animal species and reckon the MRSD using the safety index (SI).

Minimal anticipated biological effect level (MABEL) is used as a starting dose in human trials. Researchers need to predict the minimum biological activity exposure in human according to the characteristics of receptor bonding features or its functions from pharmacological experiments, and then integrate exposure, PK and PD features to calculate MABEL by using different models according to specific situations.

Dosage escalation: Dose can be escalated gradually to determine maximum tolerated dose (MTD) in absence of adverse reaction after the starting dose. It is also called dose escalation trial or tolerance trial. Below are the two most common methods for the dose escalation designs:

1. Modified Fibonacci method: The initial dose is set as n (g/m^2), and the doses followed sequentially are $2n$, $3.3n$, $5n$ and $7n$, respectively. Since then, the escalated dose is 1/3 of the previous one.
2. PGDE method: As many initial doses of first-in-human study are relatively low, most of escalation process is situated in the conservative part of improved Fibonacci method, which leads to an overlong trial period. On this occasion, pharmacologically guided dose escalation should be used. A goal blood drug concentration is set in advance according to pre-clinical pharmacological data, and then to determine subsequent dose level on the basis of each subject's pharmacokinetic data at the real time. This method can reduce the number of subjects at risk.

21.11. Physiologically-Based-Pharmacokinetics (PBPK) Model[18,19]

In PBPK model, each important issue and organ is regarded as a separate compartment linked by perfusing blood. Abided by mass balance principle, PK parameters are predicted by using mathematic models which combines demographic data, drug enzyme metabolic parameters with physical and chemical properties of the drug. Theoretically, PBPK is able to predict drug concentration and metabolic process in any tissues and organs, providing quantitative prediction of drug disposition at physiological and pathological views, especially in extrapolation between different species and populations. Therefore, PBPK can guide research and development of new drugs, and contribute to the prediction of drug interactions and clinical trial design and population selection. Also, it could be used as a tool to study the PK mechanism.

Modeling parameters include empirical models parameters, body's physiological parameters and drug property parameters such as the volume or weight of various tissues and organs, perfusion rate and filtration rate, enzyme activity, drug lipid-solubility, ionizing activity, membrane permeability, plasma-protein binding affinity, tissue affinity and demographic characteristics.

There are two types of modeling patterns in PBPK modeling: top-down approach and bottom-up approach. The former one, which is based on observed trial data, uses classical compartmental models, while the latter one constructs mechanism model based on system's prior recognition.

Modeling process: (1) Framework of PBPK model is established according to the physiological and anatomical arrangement of the tissues and organs linked by perfusing blood. (2) To establish the rule of drug disposition in tissue. It is common for perfusion limited model that a single well-stirred compartment represents a tissue or an organ. Permeability limited model contains two or three well-stirred compartments between which rate-limited membrane permeation occurs. Dispersion model uses partition coefficient to describe the degree of mixing, which is equal to well-stirred model approximately when partition coefficient is infinite. (3) The setting of parameters for PBPK modeling related with physiology and compound. (4) Simulation, assessment and verification.

Allometric scaling is an empirical model method which is used in PBPK or used alone. Prediction of the animal's PK parameters can be achieved by using information of other animals. It is assumed that the anatomical structure, physiological and biochemical features between different species are similar, and are related with the body weight of the species. The PK parameters of different species abide by allometric scaling relationships: $Y = a \cdot BW^b$, where Ymeans PK parameters; a and b are coefficient and exponential of the equation; BW means body weight. The establishment of allometric scaling equation often requires three or more species, and for small molecule compound, allometric scaling can be adjusted by using brain weight, maximum lives and unbound fraction in plasma. Rule of exponents is used for exponential selection as well.

As PBPK is merely a theoretical prediction, it is particularly important to validate the theoretical prediction from PBPK model.

21.12. Disease Progression Model[20,21]

It is a mathematical model to describe disease evolution over time without effective intervention. An effective disease progress model is a powerful tool for the research and development of new drugs, which provides a reference for no treatment state. It is advocated by FDA to enable researchers to obtain information whether the tested drug is effective or not in cases of small patient number and short study time. Disease progression model can also be used in clinical trials simulation to distinguish disease progression, placebo effect and drug efficacy, that is,

$$\text{Clinical efficacy} = \text{disease progress} + \text{drug action} + \text{placebo effect}.$$

Common disease progression models are:

21.12.1. *Linear progress model*

The feature of linear progress model is that it assumes the change rate of disease is constant, and the formula is

$$S(t) = S_0 + E_{\text{off}}(Ce_A) + (E_{\text{prog}}(t) + \alpha) \cdot t,$$

where S_0 means baseline level; $S(t)$ represents the status of disease at time t; slope α represents the rate of disease change over time. Two types of drug interventions are added in this model. One is an "effect compartment" $E_{off}(Ce_A)$ which is considered as a drug effect to attenuate the disease status at baseline level. $E_{prog}(t)$ represents the improvement of the entire course of the disease after drug administration, in other words, that is to slow down the speed of the disease progress. Drug effect is at least one of the intervention ways above mentioned.

21.12.2. *Exponential model*

It is commonly used to describe a temporary disease states, such as recovering from a trauma

$$S(t) = S_0 \cdot e^{-(K_{\text{prog}} + E_1(t))} - E_2(t),$$

where S_0 means baseline, $S(t)$ represents the status of disease at time t, K_{prog} represents recovery rate constant. Drug effect causes improvements of conditions and changes of recovery rate constant, which means addition of $E_1(t)$ can change recovery rate constant. Drug effect can also be used to attenuate the disease status, which means introduction of drug effect $E_2(t)$ into linear disease progression model.

21.12.3. E_{max} *model*

As for describing the natural limit value for severity scores, E_{max} model is commonly used in disease modeling.

$$S(t) = S_0 + \frac{S_{\text{max}} \cdot [1 + E_1(t)] \cdot t}{S_{50} \cdot [1 + E_2(t)] + t}.$$

S_0 means baseline level, $S(t)$ represents the status of disease at t moment, S_{max} is maximum recovery parameter, S_{50} means the time to half of the maximum recovery value; Efficacy term $E_1(t)$ represents the effects of drug intervention on maximum recovery parameter, which contributes to the disease recovery. Efficacy term $E_2(t)$ represents the effect of drug intervention on half of the maximum recovery parameter, which contributes to the disease recovery and slows down the speed of disease deterioration.

The advantage of disease progression model is that it can well describe the evolution of biomarkers in the disease progression and variation within/between individuals, which introduces individual covariant as well. As a new trend in modeling base drug development, it rapidly serves as an important tool to investigate the effects of drugs on disease.

21.13. Model-Based Meta-Analysis (MBMA)[22,23]

MBMA is a newly developed meta-analysis method that can generate quantitative data by modeling. It can be used to test the impact on efficacy of different factors, including dose, duration, patient's conditions and other variables. It can also distinguish inter-trial, inter-treatment arm and residual error. Compared with the conventional meta-analysis, MBMA could use the data more thoroughly and bring more abundant information, implying it is a powerful tool to identify the safety and efficacy of drugs. Therefore, MBMA can provide the evidence for decision making and developing dosage regimen during the drug development.

Steps: Firstly, a suitable search strategy and inclusion/exclusion criteria should be established according to the purpose, and then data extraction is performed from the included articles. Secondly, the suitable structural and statistical models are selected based on the type and characteristics of data. Finally, the covariates should be tested on the model parameters.

Models: In MBMA method, structural model should be built according to the study purpose or professional requirements. The structural model usually consists of placebo effect and drug effect, while the statistical model consists of inter-study variability, inter-arm variability and residual error. The typical model of MBMA is as follows

$$E_{ik}(t) = E_0 \cdot \exp^{-kt} + \frac{E_{\max} \cdot \mathrm{DOSE}_{ik}}{ED_{50} + \mathrm{DOSE}_{ik}} + \eta_i^{\mathrm{study}} + \frac{1}{\sqrt{n_{ik}}}\eta_{ik}^{\mathrm{arm}} + \frac{1}{\sqrt{n_{ik}}}\delta_{ik}(t).$$

$E_{ik}(t)$ is the observed effect in the kth group of ith study; $E_0 \cdot \exp^{-kt}$ represents the placebo effect; η_i^{study} is the inter-study variability; η_{ik}^{arm} and $\delta_{ik}(t)$ represent the inter-arm variability and residual error, respectively, and both of which need to be corrected by sample size$(1/\sqrt{n_{ik}})$. Due to the limitation of data conditions, it is not possible to evaluate all the variabilities at the same time. On this basis, simplification should be performed to the variability.

In this model, efficacy is presented as this formula:

$$\frac{E_{max} \cdot DOSE_{ik}}{ED_{50} + DOSE_{ik}}.$$

$DOSE_{ik}$ is dosage; $E_{\max}$ represents the maximal efficacy; ED_{50} stands for the dosage when efficacy reaches 50% of $E_{\max}$.

Before testing the covariates of the model parameters, we should collect potential factors as many as possible. The common factors mainly include race, genotype, age, gender, weight, preparation formulation, baseline, patient condition, duration of disease as well as drug combination. These factors could be introduced into the structural model step by step in order to obtain the PD parameters under different factors, which can guide individualized drug administration.

The reliability of final model must be evaluated by graphing method, model validation, and sensitivity analysis.

As the calculation in the MBMA is quite complicated, it is necessary to use professional software, and NONMEM is the mostly recognized software.

21.14. Clinical Trial Simulation (CTS)[24,25]

CTS is a simulation method which approximately describes trial design, human behavior, disease progression and drug behavior by using mathematical model method and numerical computation method. Its purpose is to simulate the clinical reaction of virtual objects. In this simulation method, trial design provides dosage selection algorithm, inclusion criteria and demographic information. Human behavior involves trial compliance such as medication compliance of objects and data loss by researchers. As the disease state may change in the progress of trial, it is necessary to build disease progress model. The drug behavior *in vivo* can be described by PK model and PD model.

With the help of CTS, researchers form a profound comprehension on all the information and hypothesis of new compound, which sequentially reduces the uncertainty of drug research and development. The success rates of trials can be increased through answering a series of "what if" questions. For example, what if these situations occur, how about the trial results: What if non-compliance rate increases 10%? What if maximum of effect lower than expected? What if the inclusion criterion has a change?

The model of CTS should approximate to the estimation of clinical efficacy. Thus, it is recommended to build model based on dosage–concentration–effect relationship. One simulation model mainly consist of three parts as below.

21.14.1. *Input–output model (IO)*

Input–output model includes (1) structural model: PK model, PD model, disease state and progress model and placebo effect model; (2) covariate model, which is used to predict the individual model parameters in combination with patients characteristics (e.g. age and weight) related to inter-individual variability; (3) pharmacoeconomic model, which predicts response (e.g. expense) as a function of trial design and execution; (4) stochastic model, including population parameter variation, inter-individual and intra-individual variations of model parameter and residual error variation, which is used to explain modeling error and measuring error.

21.14.2. *Covariate distribution model*

Unlike covariate model mainly used to connect covariates and IO parameters, covariate distribution model is mainly used to obtain the distribution of demographic covariates of samples, which reflects the expected frequency distribution of different covariates according to covariate distribution model of trial population. What is more, such model can describe the relationship among covariates such as the relationship between age and renal function.

21.14.3. *Trial execution model*

The protocol cannot be executed perfectly, and sometimes departure occurs in the clinical progress, such as withdrawal, dosage record missing, and observation missing. Trial execution model includes original protocol model and deflective execution model.

Nowadays, many software are available for CTS, among which commercial software providing systematic functions for professional simulation is user-friendly. As the whole trial is realized by simulation method, it is necessary for staff with different professional background to work together.

21.15. Therapeutic Index (TI)[26,27]

TI a parameter used to evaluate drug safety, is widely used to screen and evaluate chemotherapeutic agents such as antibacterial and anticarcinogen. Thus, it is also termed chemotherapeutic index.

$$TI = LD_{50}/ED_{50}.$$

LD_{50} is median lethal dose, and ED_{50} is median effective dose. Generally, drugs with a higher *TI* will be more safe, which means a lower probability of toxicity under the therapeutic dose. For the drugs with a lower *TI*, higher possibility of toxic reaction may present as their therapeutic doses are similar to toxic doses, together with the influence of individual variation and drug interactions. Therefore, the drug concentration should be monitored to adjust dosage timely. Notably, drugs with higher *TI* values do not always reflect the safety precisely.

21.15.1. Safety Margin (SM)

SM is another parameter to evaluate drug safety, and it is defined as

$$SM = (LD_1/ED_{99} - 1) \times 100\%.$$

LD_1 is 1% lethal dose, and ED_{99} stands for 99% effective dose. Comparing to *TI*, *SM* contains greater clinical significance. As LD_1 and ED_{99} are localized at the flat end of sigmoid curve, large determinate errors may present, which may hamper the accuracy of the determination. When LD_1 is larger than ED_{99}, the value of *SM* is larger than 0, which indicates that drug safety is quite high. Or else, the value of *SM* is smaller than 0 in cases of LD_1 smaller than ED_{99}, which indicates the drug safety is quite low.

There are differences between *TI* and *SM*:

Drug A: $TI = 400/100 = 4$
Drug A: $SM = 200/260 - 1 = -0.3$
Drug B: $TI = 260/100 = 2.6$
Drug B: $SM = 160/120 - 1 = 0.33$

Only evaluated by *TI* value, it seems that drug A is superior to drug B in safety. However, at the terms of *SM* value, *SM* of drug A is smaller than 0, which indicates quite a lot patients show toxicity despite 99% of patients with response. For drug B, the *SM* is larger than 0, which indicates there are not even one patients in toxic yet when 99% of patients with response. In a word, the safety of drug B is superior to that of drug A.

The similar safety parameters are certain safety factor (*CSF*) and *SI*:

$$CSF = LD_1/ED_{99}.$$

$$SI = LD_5/ED_{95}$$

The relationship between safety parameters is shown in Figure 21.15.1, where *ED* curve is the sigmoid curve of efficacy and *LD* curve is the sigmoid curve of toxic reaction, and *P* is positive percentage.

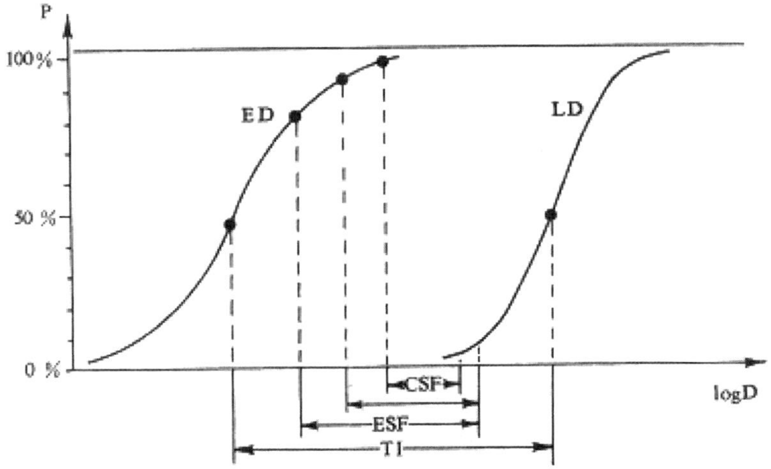

Fig. 21.15.1. The relationship between safety parameters.

21.16. *In Vitro–In Vivo* Correlation (IVIVC)[28]

IVIVC is used to describe the relationship between *in vitro* properties and *in vivo* characteristics of drug. The relationship between drug's dissolution rate (or degree) and plasma concentration (or absorbed dose) is a typical example. Using this method, we can predict intracorporal process of drugs according to experimentation *in vitro*. Furthermore, we can optimize formulation designs, set advantageous dissolution specifications, adjust manufacturing changes, and even replace an *in vitro* BE study by a reasonable study of *in vitro* dissolution rate.

There are three types of analysis models in IVIVC:

21.16.1. *Level A model*

In this model, correlation analysis is performed between the data at each corresponding time point of *in vitro* dissolution curve and those of *in vivo* input rate curve, which is called point-to-point correlation. In a linear correlation, the *in vitro* dissolution and *in vivo* input curves may be directly superimposable or may be made to be superimposable by using a scaling factor. Nonlinear correlations, while uncommon, may also be appropriate. This analysis involves all the data *in vitro* and *in vivo*, and can reflect the complete shape of the curves.

There are two specific algorithms: (1) Two-stage procedure is established based on deconvolution method. The first stage is to calculate the *in vivo* cumulative absorption percent (F_a) of the drug at each time point. The second stage is to analyze the correlation between *in vitro* dissolution data [*in vitro* cumulative dissolution percent (F_d) of the drug at each time point] and *in vivo* absorption data (corresponding F_a at the same time point). (2) Single-step method is an algorithm based on a convolution procedure that models the relationship between *in vitro* dissolution and plasma concentration in a single step. On this basis, a comparison was performed to the plasma concentrations predicted from the model and the observed values directly.

21.16.2. *Level B model*

The Level B IVIVC model involves the correlation between mean *in vitro* dissolution rate and the mean *in vivo* absorption rate. The Level B correlation, like a Level A, uses all of the *in vitro* and *in vivo* data, but is not considered to be a point-to-point correlation. The *in vivo* parameters include mean residence time (MRT), mean absorption time (MAT) or mean dissolution time (MDT). The *in vitro* parameter includes mean dissolution time *in vitro* (MDT *in vitro*).

21.16.3. *Level C model*

The Level C IVIVC establishes the single-point relationship between one dissolution point (e.g. $T_{50}\%$ and $T_{90}\%$ calculated by Weibull function) and a certain PK parameter (e.g. AUC, $C_{\max}, T_{\max}$). This kind of correlation is classified as partial correlation, and the obtained parameters cannot reflect character of the whole dissolution and absorption progress. Level C model may often be used to select preparations and to formulate quality standards. Being similar with Level C IVIVC model, multiple Level C IVIVC model is a multiple-point correlation model between dissolution at different time points and single or several PK parameters.

Among these models, Level A IVIVC is considered to be the most informative, and it can provide significant basis on predicting results *in vivo* from *in vitro* experiments. Thus, it is mostly recommended. Multiple Level C correlations can be as useful as Level A correlations. Level C correlations can be useful at the early stages of formulation development when pilot formulations are being selected. By the way, Level B correlations are least useful for regulatory purposes.

21.17. Potency[15,29]

It is a drug parameter based on the concentration–response relationship. It can be used to compare the properties of drugs with the same pharmacological effects. The potency, a comparative term, shows certain drug dose when it comes to required effect, which reflects the sensitivity of target organs or tissues to the drug. It is the main index of bioassay to connect the needed dose of one drug producing expected curative efficacy with those of different drugs producing the same efficacy. The research design and statistical analysis of bioassay is detailed in many national pharmacopoeias. In semi-log quantitative response dose-efficacy diagram, the curve of high potency drug is at the left side and its EC_{50} is lower. The potency of drug is related to the affinity of receptor. The determination of potency is important to ensure equivalence of clinical application, and potency ratios are commonly used to compare potencies of different drugs.

Potency ratio is the ratio of the potencies of two drugs, which means the inverse ratio of the equivalent amount of the two drugs. It is especially important in the evaluation of biological agents.

$$\text{Potency ratio} = \frac{\text{potency of the certain drug}}{\text{potency of standard drug}} = \frac{\text{a dose of standard drug}}{\text{equivalent dose of certain drug}}.$$

Potency of standard is usually considered as 1. The following two points are worth noting: (1) Potency ratio can be computed when the dose-effect curves of two drugs are almost parallel. On this basis, the ratio of the equivalent amount of the two drugs is a constant, regardless of a high or low efficacy. If two dose-efficacy curves are not parallel, the equivalent ratio and different intensity differs, and in this case, the potency ratio cannot be calculated. (2) The discretion of potency and potency ratio only refers to the equivalent potency, not the ratio of the intensity of drugs.

Another index for the comparison between drugs is efficacy. It is an ability of the drug to produce maximum effect activity or the effect of "peak". Generally, efficacy is a pharmacodynamical index produced by the combination of drug and receptor, which has certain correlation with the intrinsic activity of a drug. Efficacy is often seen as the most important PD characteristics of drug, and is usually represented by C_{50} of drug. The lower the C_{50} is, the greater the efficacy of the drug is. In addition, we can also get the relative efficacy of two drugs with equal function through comparing the maximum effects.

One way to increase the efficacy is to improve the lipophilicity of drug, which can be achieved by increasing the number of lipophilic groups to promote the combination of drugs and targets. Nevertheless, such procedure will also increase the combination of drugs and targets in other parts of body, which may finally lead to increase or decrease of overall specificity due to elevation of drugs non-specificity.

No matter how much dose of the low efficacy drugs is, it cannot produce the efficiency as that of high efficacy drugs. For the drugs with equal pharmacological effects, their potencies and efficacy can be different. It is clinically significant to compare the efficacies between different drugs.

The scopes and indications of high efficacy drugs and inefficient ones are clinically different. Moreover, their clinical status varies widely. In clinical practice, drugs with higher efficiency are preferred by the clinicians under similar circumstances.

21.18. Median Lethal Dose[27,30]

Median lethal dose (LD_{50}), a dose leads to a death rate of 50% in animal studies, is an important parameter reflecting the acute toxicity test. The smaller LD_{50} is, the greater drug toxicity is. Numerous methods have been developed for the calculation of LD_{50}, and Bliss method is the most recognized and accepted one by national regulators. Its calculation process is as follows:

1. Assume that the relation between the logarithm of dose and animal mortality fits a normal accumulation curve: using the dose as the abscissa and animal mortality as the ordinate, a bell curve not identical with normal curve is obtained with a long tail only at the side of high dose. If the logarithm of doses is used as the abscissa, the curve will be a symmetric normal curve.

2. The relation between the logarithm of dose and cumulative mortality is S curve: Clark and Gaddum assume that the relation between the logarithm of dose and the cumulative percentage of qualitative response fits a symmetric S curve, namely the normal accumulation curve, which shows the following characteristics: (1) μ serves as the mean and σ as the standard deviation, and then the curve can be described according to the formula of $\Phi(\frac{X_K-\mu}{\sigma})$; (2) The curve is centripetal symmetry, and the ordinate values and abscissa values of its symmetry center are 50% cumulative mortality rates and $\log LD_{50}$, respectively; (3) The curve is flat at both ends and sharply oblique at the middle. As middle dose slightly changes, the mortality nearby LD_{50} is remarkably changed, unlike both ends (nearby LD_5 or LD_{95}) with very small changes. This shows that LD_{50} is more sensitive and accurate than the LD_5 and LD_{95} in expressing virulence. The points nearby 50% mortality rate in the middle segment of the curve are more important than those nearby LD_5 and LD_{95}; (4) According to the characteristics of the normal cumulative curve, Bliss lists weight coefficient of each mortality point to weigh the importance of each point; (5) In theory, the S curve is close to but will not reach 0% and 100%. Nevertheless, in practical, how to deal

with zero death and all death since the number of animals (n) in the group is limited? In general, we estimate n/n to $(n-0.25)/n$ and $0/n$ to $0.25/n$.

In order to facilitate the regression analysis, we need to transform the S curve into straight line. Bliss put forward the concept of "probability unit" (probit, probability unit) of mortality K, which is defined as

$$Y_K = 5 + \Phi\left(\frac{X_K - \mu}{\sigma}\right).$$

$X_K = log(LD_K)$, and a linear relationship is assumed between the probability unit and dose logarithm ($Y_K = a + b \cdot X_K$). This is the so-called "probit conversion" principle. The estimate values of a and b are obtained by regression, and then we can calculate

$$LD_K = log^{-1}\left(\frac{Y_k - a}{b}\right).$$

Besides the estimation of LD_{50} point, more information is required to submit to the regulators: (1) 95% CI for LD_{50}, X_{50} [the estimated value of $\log(LD_{50})$] and its standard error (S_{X50}). (2) Calculation of LD_{10}, LD_{20} and LD_{90} using the parameters a and b of regression equation. (3) Experiment quality and reliability, such as whether the distance between each point on the concentration–response relationship and linear is too big, whether the $Y-X$ relationship basically is linear, and whether individual differences are in line with normal distribution.

21.19. Dose Conversion Among Different Kinds of Animal[31,32]

It means that there exists a certain regulation among different kinds of animal (or human) on the equivalent dose, which can be obtained through mutual conversion. According to the HED principle issued by FDA, equivalent dose conversion among different kinds of animal (including human) can be achieved via properly derivation and calculation, introduction of animal shape coefficient, as well as compiling the conversion formula.

Dose conversion among different kinds of animal principle

The body coefficient (k) is approximately calculated according to the weight and animal shape coefficient as follows:

$$k = A/W^{2/3}.$$

A is the surface area (m^2), and W is weight (kg). The k value of sphere was 0.04836. The more the animal's shape is close to a sphere, the smaller the k value is. Once the body coefficient is obtained, it could be used the equation of $A = k \cdot W^{2/3}$ to estimate the surface area.

Classic formula of dose conversion among different kinds of animal:

As animal dose is roughly proportional to the surface area, the surface area could be estimated via the equation $A = k \cdot W^{2/3}$.

$$D_{(a)}: D_{(b)} \approx A_a: A_b \approx k_a \cdot W_a^{2/3}: k_b \cdot W_b^{2/3}.$$

Thus, the dose of each animal is

$$D_{(b)} = D_{(a)} \cdot (k_b/k_a) \cdot (W_b/W_a)^{2/3}.$$

The dose of one kilogram is

$$D_b = D_a \cdot (k_b/k_a) \cdot (W_a/W_b)^{1/3}.$$

Those formulas above are general formulas suitable for any animals and any weight. In the formulas, $D_{(a)}$ is the known dose of the animal a (mg per animal), while $D_{(b)}$ is the dose of the animal b (mg per animal) to be estimated. $D_{(a)}$ and $D_{(b)}$ are presented in a unit of mg/kg. A_a and A_b are the body surface area (m^2). k_a and k_b are the shape coefficient, W_a and W_b are the weight (kg) (Subscript a and b represents the known animal and required animal, respectively, thereafter).

Dose conversion table among different kinds of animals: The animal shape coefficient and standard weight are introduced in those formulas. The conversion factor (R_{ab}) can be calculated in advance and two correction coefficients (S_a, S_b) can be looked-up in the table.

$$R_{ab} = (K_a/K_b) \cdot (W_b/W_a)^{1/3},$$

$$s = (W_{\text{standard}}/W_a)^{1/3}.$$

Thus, we can design dose (mg/kg) conversion table of animals from a to b. D_a and D_b are the doses of standard weight (mg/kg), and D'_a and D'_b are the doses of non-standard weight. The values of R_{ab}, S_a and S_b can be found in the table.

To get the standard weight via standard weight, we use the following formula:

$$D_b = D_a \cdot R_{ab}.$$

The following formula is used to get non-standard weight via standard weight:

$$D_b' = D_a \cdot R_{ab} \cdot S_b.$$

To get the non-standard weight via non-standard weight, we use the following formula:

$$D_b' = D_a' \cdot S_a \cdot R_{ab} \cdot S_b.$$

When the animal is presented in standard weight, S_a and S_b are equal to 1, and the above formulas can be mutual transformed.

21.20. Receptor Kinetics[7,33]

It is the quantitative study of the interaction between the drugs and the receptors, such as combination, dissociation and internal activity. Receptor theory plays an important role in illustrating how endogenous ligands and drug work. Simultaneously, it provides important basis for drug design, screening, searching for endogenous ligands, protocol design and the observation of drug effect. Receptor kinetics involves a large number of quantitative analysis, such as affinity constant (K_A), dissociation constant (K_D), various rate constants, Hill coefficient, and receptor density ($B_{\max}$).

Clark occupation theory is the most basic theory of receptor kinetics which states that the interaction of receptor and ligand follows the combination and dissociation equilibrium principle. According to this theory, $[R]$, $[L]$ and $[RL]$ represent the concentrations of free receptor, free ligand and combined ligand, respectively. When the reaction reaches equilibrium, equilibrium dissociation constants (K_D) and affinity constant (K_A) are calculated as follows:

$$K_D = \frac{[R][L]}{[RL]},$$

$$K_A = 1/K_D.$$

In cases of a single receptor with no other receptors, Clark equation can be used upon the reaction of receptor and ligand reaching the equilibrium

$$B = \frac{B_{\max}L}{K_D + L}.$$

K_D is the dissociation constant, $B_{\max}$ is the biggest number of single combining site, and L is the concentration of free marked ligand.

Hill equation is used to analyze the combination and dissociation between multiple loci receptor and the ligand. If Hill coefficient (n) is equal to 1, it is equal to Clark equation. This model can be used for the saturation analysis about the combination of a receptor with multiple loci (equally binding sites) and ligand. Assume that (1) free receptors and n combined ligand receptors are in an equilibrium state; (2) there are strong synergistic effects among those loci. This means the combination of one locus with the ligand would facilitate the combination of the other loci and their ligands, which contributes to the combination of loci and n ligands. Therefore, the concentration of receptor combined with less than n ligands can be neglected. In this given circumstances, Hill equation is listed as follows:

$$B = \frac{B_{\max} L^n}{K_D + L^n}.$$

In cases of absence of equilibrium in the reaction, dynamic experiments should be carried out. It is used to analyze the breeding time of equilibrium binding experiment, and estimate the reversibility of ligand-receptor reaction. It keeps the total ligand concentration $[L_T]$ unchanged, and then the concentrations of specific combination $[RL]$ are measured at different times.

$$d[RL]/dt = k_1[R][L] - k_{-2}[RL].$$

In this equation, k_1 and k_2 represent the association rate constant and dissociation rate constant, respectively.

As the biological reaction intensity depends not only on the affinity of the drug and receptor, but also on a variety of factors such as the diffusion of the drug, enzyme degradation and reuptake, the results of marked ligand binding test *in vitro* and the drug effect intensity *in vivo* or *in vitro* organ are not generally the same. Therefore, Ariens intrinsic activity, Stephenson spare receptors, Paton rate theory and the Theory of receptor allosteric are complement and further development of receptor kinetics quantitative analysis method.

References

1. Rowland, M, Tozer, NT. *Clinical Pharmacokinetics and Pharmacodynamics: Concepts and Applications.* (4th edn.). Philadelphia: Lippincott Williams & Wilkins, 2011: 56–62.
2. Wang, GJ. *Pharmacokinetics.* Beijing: Chemical Industry Press, 2005: 97.
3. Sheng, Y, He, Y, Huang, X, *et al.* Systematic evaluation of dose proportionality studies in clinical pharmacokinetics. *Curr. Drug. Metab.*, 2010, 11: 526–537.
4. Sheng, YC, He, YC, Yang, J, *et al.* The research methods and linear evaluation of pharmacokinetic scaled dose-response relationship. *Chin. J. Clin. Pharmacol.*, 2010, 26: 376–381.
5. Sheiner, LB, Beal, SL. Pharmacokinetic parameter estimates from several least squares procedures: Superiority of extended least squares. *J. Pharmacokinet. Biopharm.*, 1985, 13: 185–201.
6. Meibohm, B, Derendorf, H. Basic concepts of pharmacokinetic/pharmacodynamic (PK/PD) modelling. *Int. J. Clin. Pharmacol. Ther.*, 1997; 35: 401–413.
7. Sun, RY, Zheng, QS. *The New Theory of Mathematical Pharmacology.* Beijing: People's Medical Publishing House, 2004.
8. Ette, E, Williams, P. *Pharmacometrics — The Science of Quantitative Pharmacology.* Hoboken, New Jersey: John Wiley & Sons Inc, 2007: 583–633.

9. Li, L, Li, X, Xu, L, *et al.* Systematic evaluation of dose accumulation studies in clinical pharma-cokinetics. *Curr. Drug. Metab.*, 2013, 14: 605–615.
10. Li, XX, Li, LJ, Xu, L, *et al.* The calculation methods and evaluations of accumulation index in clinical pharmacokinetics. *Chinese J. Clin. Pharmacol. Ther.*, 2013, 18: 34–38.
11. FDA. Bioavailability and Bioequivalence Studies for Orally Administered Drug Products — General Considerations [EB/OL]. (2003-03). http://www.fda.gov/ohrms/dockets/ac/03/briefing/3995B1_07_GFI-BioAvail-BioEquiv.pdf. Accessed on July, 2015.
12. Chou, TC. Theoretical basis, experimental design, and computerized simulation of synergism and antagonism in drug combination studies. *Pharmacol. Rev.*, 2006, 58: 621–681.
13. Zheng, QS, Sun, RY. Quantitative analysis of drug compatibility by weighed modification method. *Acta. Pharmacol. Sin.*, 1999, 20, 1043–1051.
14. FDA. Drug Interaction Studies Study Design, Data Analysis, Implications for Dosing, and Labeling Recommendations [EB/OL]. (2012-02). http://www.fda.gov/ downloads/drugs/guidancecomplianceregulatoryinformation/guidances/ucm292362.pdf. Accessed on July 2015.
15. Atkinson, AJ, Abernethy, DR, Charles, E, *et al.* *Principles of Clinical Pharmacology.* (2nd edn.). London: Elsevier Inc, 2007: 293–294.
16. EMEA. Guideline on strategies to identify and mitigate risks for first-in-human clinical trials with investigational medicinal products [EB/OL]. (2007-07-19). http://www.ema.europa.eu/docs/en_GB/document_library/Scientific_guideline/2009/09/WC500-002988.pdf. Accessed on Auguset 1, 2015.
17. FDA. Guidance for Industry Estimating the Maximum Safe Starting Dose in Initial Clinical Trials for Therapeutics in Adult Healthy Volunteers [EB/OL]. (2005-07). http://www.fda.gov/downloads/drugs/guidancecomplianceregulatoryinformation/gui dances/ucm078932.pdf. Accessed on August 1, 2015.
18. Jin, YW, Ma, YM. The research progress of physiological pharmacokinetic model building methods. *Acta. Pharm. Sin.*, 2014, 49: 16–22.
19. Nestorov, I. Whole body pharmacokinetic models. *Clin. Pharmacokinet.* 2003; 42: 883–908.
20. Holford, NH. Drug treatment effects on disease progression. *Annu. Rev. Pharmacol. Toxicol.*, 2001, 41: 625–659.
21. Mould, GR. *Developing Models of Disease Progression. Pharmacometrics: The Science of Quantitative Pharmacology.* Hoboken, New Jersey: John Wiley & Sons, Inc. 2007: 547–581.
22. Li, L, Lv, Y, Xu, L, *et al.* Quantitative efficacy of soy isoflavones on menopausal hot flashes. *Br. J. Clin. Pharmacol.*, 2015, 79: 593–604.
23. Mandema, JW, Gibbs, M, Boyd, RA, *et al.* Model-based meta-analysis for comparative efficacy and safety: Application in drug development and beyond. *Clin. Pharmacol. Ther.*, 2011, 90: 766–769.
24. Holford, NH, Kimko, HC, Monteleone, JP, *et al.* Simulation of clinical trials. *Annu. Rev. Pharmacol. Toxicol.*, 2000, 40: 209–234.
25. Huang, JH, Huang, XH, Li, LJ, *et al.* Computer simulation of new drugs clinical trials. *Chinese J. Clin. Pharmacol. Ther.*, 2010, 15: 691–699.
26. Muller, PY, Milton, MN. The determination and interpretation of the therapeutic index in drug development. *Nat. Rev. Drug Discov.*, 2012, 11: 751–761.
27. Sun, RY. *Pharmacometrics.* Beijing: People's Medical Publishing House, 1987: 214–215.

28. FDA. Extended Release Oral Dosage Forms: Development, Evaluation and Application of *In Vitro/In Vivo* Correlations [EB/OL]. (1997-09). http://www.fda.gov/downloads/drugs/guidancecomplianceregulatoryinformation/guidances/ucm070239.pdf. Accessed on August 4, 2015.
29. Li, J. Clinical pharmacology. 4th. Beijing: People's Medical Publishing House, 2008: 41–43.
30. Bliss, CI. The method of probits. *Science*, 1934, 79: 38–39.
31. FDA. Estimating the safe starting dose in clinical trials for therapeutics in adult healthy volunteers [EB/OL]. (2002-12). http://www.fda.gov/OHRMS/DOCKETS/98fr/02d-0492-gdl0001-vol1.pdf. Accessed on July 29, 2015.
32. Huang, JH, Huang, XH, Chen, ZY, *et al.* Equivalent dose conversion of animal-to-animal and animal-to-human in pharmacological experiments. *Chinese Clin. Pharmacol. Ther.*, 2004, 9: 1069–1072.
33. Sara, R. *Basic Pharmacokinetics and Pharmacodynamics.* New Jersey: John Wiley & Sons, Inc., 2011: 299–307.

About the Author

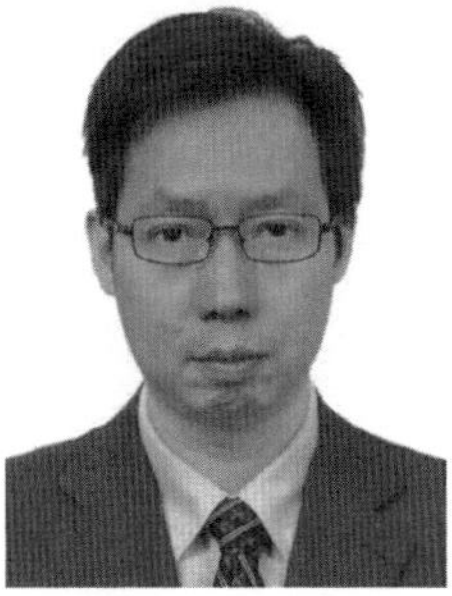

Dr. Qingshan Zheng is Director and Professor at the Center for Drug Clinical Research, Shanghai University of Traditional Chinese Medicine, the President of Professional Committee of Pharmacometrics of Chinese Pharmacological Society and an editorial board member of nine important academic journals. He has been working in academic institutes and hospitals in the field of biostatistics and pharmacometrics, and has extensive experience in designing, management and execution of clinical trials. He has published more than 250 papers.

CHAPTER 22

STATISTICAL GENETICS

Guimin Gao* and Caixia Li

22.1. Genome, Chromosome, DNA and Gene[1]

The normal human genome is composed of 23 chromosomes: 22 autosomes (numbered 1–22) and 1 sex chromosome (an X or a Y). Cells that contain one copy of the genome, such as sperm or unfertilized egg cells, are said to be haploid. Fertilized eggs and most body cells derived from them contain two copies of the genome and are said to be diploid. A diploid cell contains 46 chromosomes: 22 homologous pairs of autosomes and a pair of fully homologous (XX) or partially homologous (XY) sex chromosomes (see Figure 22.1.1).

A chromosome is composed of deoxyribonucleic acid (DNA) and proteins. The DNA is the carrier of genetic information and is a large molecule consisting of two strands that are complementary. It is a double helix formed by base pairs attached to a sugar-phosphate backbone. The information in DNA is stored as a code made up of four chemical bases: adenine (A), guanine (G), cytosine (C), and thymine (T). DNA bases pair up with each other, A with T and C with G, to form units called base pairs. Human DNA consists of about three billion base pairs, and more than 99% of those base pairs are the same in all people (Figure 22.1.2).

A gene is the basic physical and functional unit of heredity, which is a segment of DNA needed to contribute to a phenotype/function (Figure 22.1.3). In humans, genes vary in size from a few hundred DNA base pairs to more than two million base pairs.

*Corresponding author: ggao@health.bsd.uchicago.edu

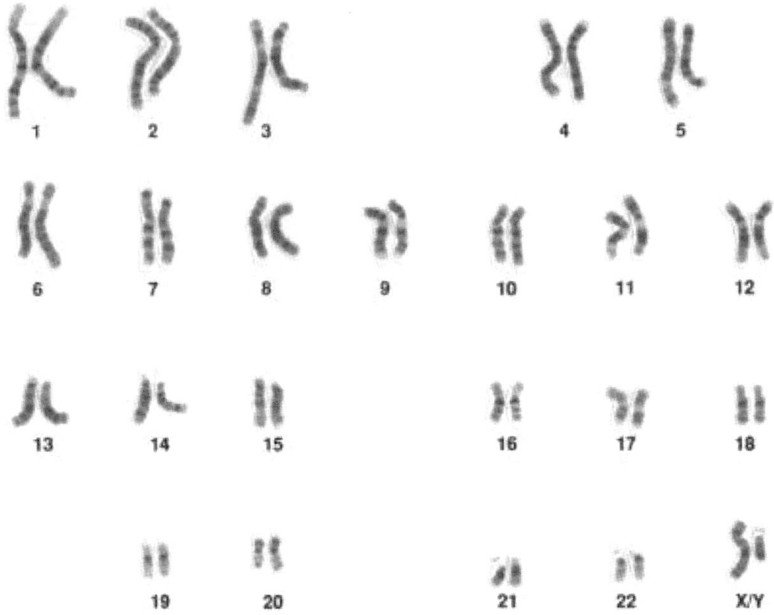

Fig. 22.1.1. Diploid genome of a human male (http://en.wikipedia.org/wiki/Genome).

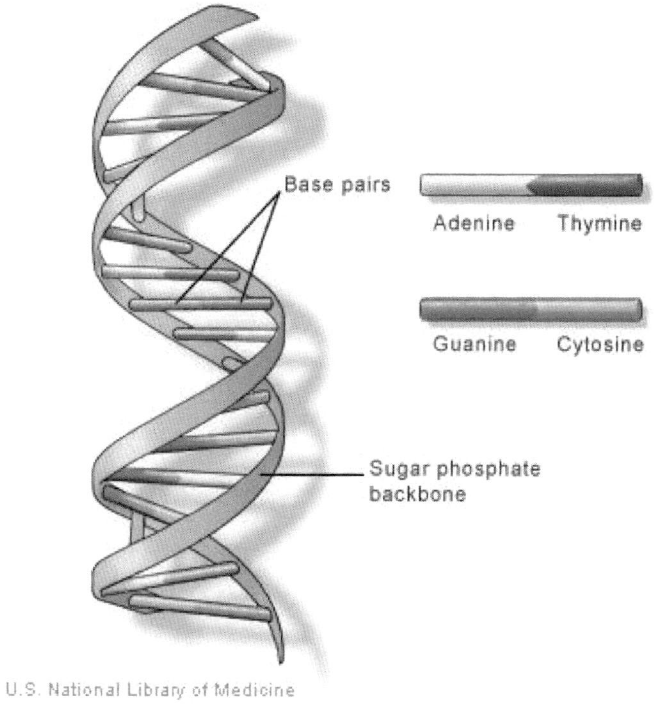

Fig. 22.1.2. DNA structure (U.S. National Library of Medicine).

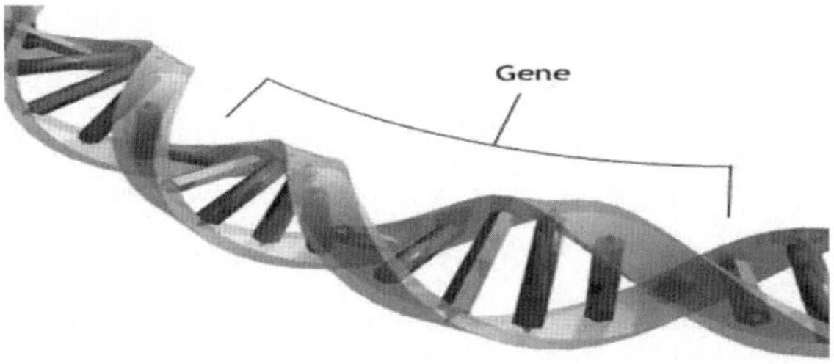

Fig. 22.1.3. A gene structure (http://www.councilforresponsiblegenetics.org/ geneticprivacy/DNA_sci_2.html)

22.2. Mitosis, Meiosis, Crossing Over, and Genetic Recombination[1,2]

Mitosis is a process of cell duplication, or reproduction, during which one cell gives rise to two genetically identical daughter cells (see Figure 22.2.1). Mitosis is the usual form of cell division seen in somatic cells (cells other than germ cells).

Meiosis is a division of a germ cell involving two fissions of the nucleus and giving rise to four gametes, or sex cells (sperm and ova), each possessing half the number of chromosomes of the original cell (see Figure 22.2.2). These sex cells are haploids.

Chromosomal crossover (or crossing over) is the exchange of genetic material between homologous chromosomes that results in recombinant chromosomes. It occurs during meiosis (from meiotic division 1 to 2, see Figures 22.2.2 and 22.2.3).

When the alleles in an offspring haplotype at two markers derive from different parental chromosomes, the event is called a recombination. For example, there is a recombination between x and z in the most right haplotype in Figure 22.2.3. A recombination between two points in the

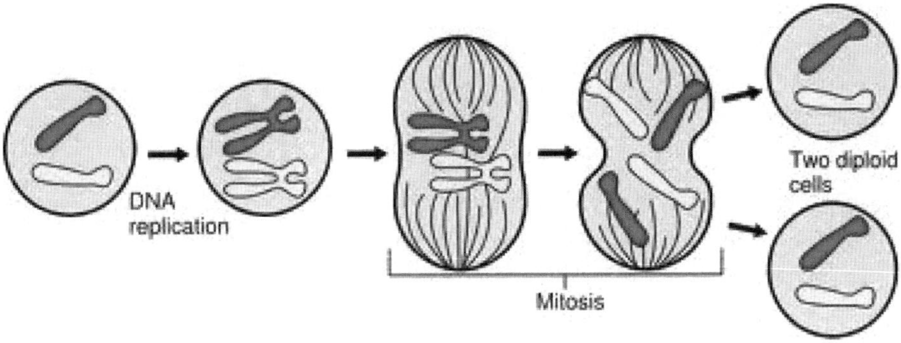

Fig. 22.2.1. Mitosis (http://en.wikipedia.org/wiki).

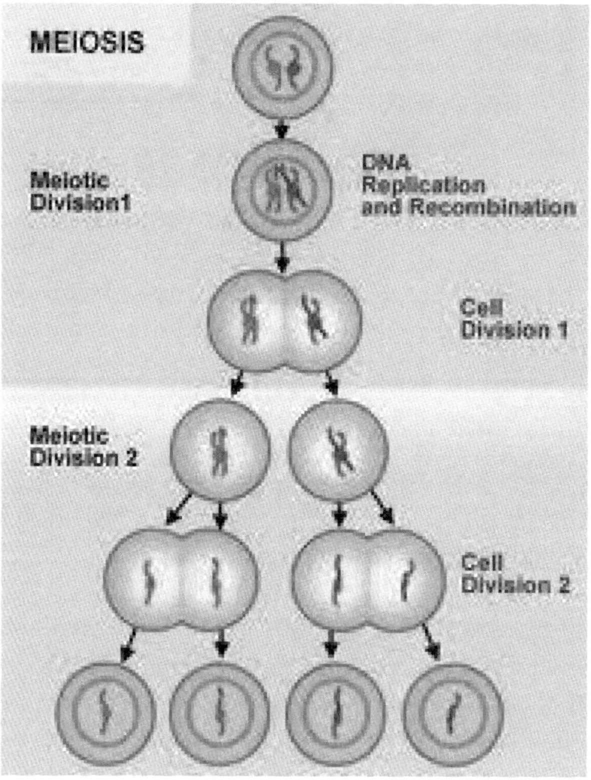

Fig. 22.2.2. Meiosis overview (http://rationalwiki.org/wiki/Meiosis).

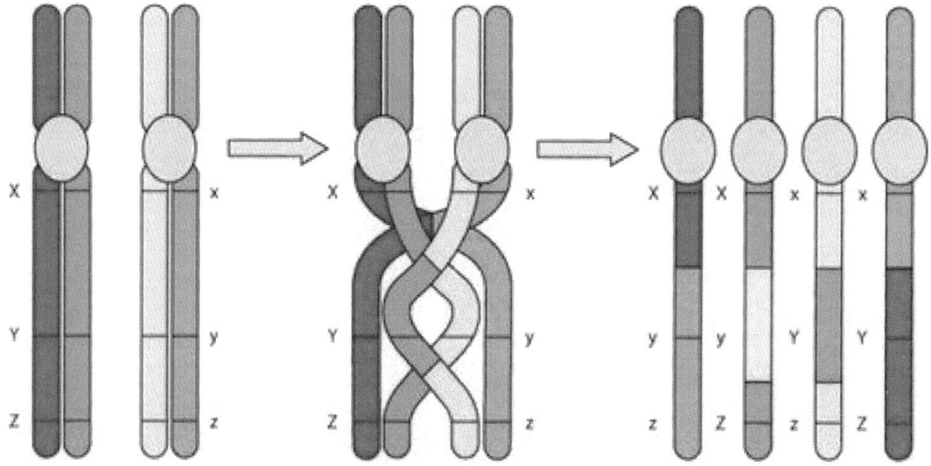

Fig. 22.2.3. Chromosomes crossing over (The New Zealand Biotechnology Hub).

chromosome occurs whenever there is an odd number of crossing over between them. The further apart two points on the chromosome are, the greater probability that a crossover occurs, and higher probability that a recombination happens. Recombination probability termed recombination fraction θ, can be estimated by distance between two points.

22.3. DNA Locus, Allele, Genetic Marker, Single-Nucleotide Polymorphism (SNP), Genotype, and Phenotype[1]

In genetics, a locus (plural loci) is the specific location of a gene, DNA sequence, or position on a chromosome. A variant of the similar DNA sequence located at a given locus is called an allele. The ordered list of loci known for a particular genome is called a genetic map. A genetic marker is a special DNA locus with at least one base being different between at least two individuals in the population. For a locus to serve as a marker, there is a list of qualities that are especially desirable, such as a marker needs to be heritable in a simple Mendelian fashion. A genetic marker can be described as a variation (which may arise due to mutation or alteration in the genomic loci) that can be observed. It may be a short DNA sequence or a long one. Commonly used types of genetic markers include: Simple sequence repeat (or SSR), SNP, and Short tandem repeat (or STR) (see Figure 22.3.1).

An SNP is a DNA sequence variation occurring when a single nucleotide — A, T, C, or G — in the genome differs between members of a species (or between paired chromosomes in an individual). Almost all common SNPs have only two alleles. SNPs are the most common type of genetic variation among people. Each SNP represents a difference in a single DNA building block, called a nucleotide. SNPs occur once in every 300 nucleotides on average, which means there are roughly 10 million SNPs in the human genome.

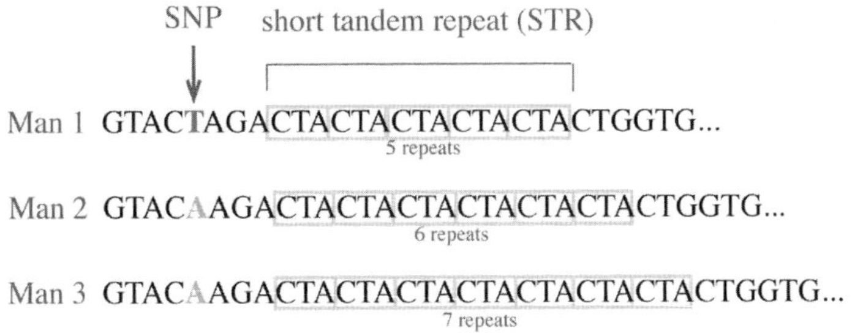

Fig. 22.3.1. An SNP (with two alleles T and A) and a STR (with three alleles: 3, 6, and 7) (http://www.le.ac.uk/ge/maj4/NewWebSurnames041008.html).

SNPs may fall within coding sequences of genes, non-coding regions of genes, or in the intergenic regions (regions between genes). SNPs in the protein-coding region are of two types, synonymous and non-synonymous SNPs. Synonymous SNPs do not affect the protein sequence while non-synonymous SNPs change the amino acid sequence of protein. The non-synonymous SNPs are of two types: missense and nonsense. SNPs that are not in protein-coding regions may still affect gene splicing, transcription factor binding, messenger RNA degradation, or the sequence of non-coding RNA. Gene expression affected by this type of SNP is referred to as an eSNP (expression SNP) and may be upstream or downstream from the gene.

In a diploid cell of an individual, the two alleles at one locus are a genotype, which determines a specific characteristic (phenotype) of that cell/individual. For an SNP with allele A and a, three possible genotypes for an individual are AA, Aa, and aa. If two alleles at a locus in an individual are different (such as in the genotype Aa), the individual is heterozygous at that locus, otherwise, the individual is homozygous. In contrast, phenotype is the observable trait (such as height and eye color) or disease status that may be influenced by a genotype.

22.4. Mendelian Inheritance, and Penetrance Function[1]

Mendelian inheritance is inheritance of biological features that follows the laws proposed by Gregor Johann Mendel in 1865 and 1866 and re-discovered in 1900. Mendel hypothesized that allele pairs separate randomly, or segregate, from each other during the production of gametes: egg and sperm; alleles at any given gene are transmitted randomly and with equal probability; each individual carries two copies of each gene, one inherited from each parent. This is called the Law of Segregation.

Mendel also postulated that the alleles of different genes are transmitted independently. This is known as the Law of Independent Assortment. Now we know that this does not apply when loci are located near each other on the same chromosome (linked). This law is true only for loci that are located on different chromosomes.

If the two alleles of an inherited pair differ (the heterozygous condition), then one determines the organism's appearance (or phenotype) and is called the dominant allele; the other has no noticeable effect on the organism's appearance and is called the recessive allele. This is known as the Law of Dominance. An organism with at least one dominant allele will display the effect of the dominant allele (https://en.wikipedia.org/wiki/Mendelian_inheritance).

The penetrance function is the set of probability distribution functions for the phenotype given the genotype (s). Letting Y denote the phenotype and G the genotype, we write the penetrance as $\Pr(Y|G)$. For binary disease trait Y (with $Y = 1$ indicating affected and 0 unaffected), we write the penetrance or risk of disease as function of genotype $\Pr(Y = 1|G)$, simply as $\Pr(Y|G)$.

Suppose we know that a disease is caused by a single major gene that exists within the population in two distinct forms (alleles): d, the wild type or normal allele, and D, the mutant or disease susceptibility allele. Genotype dd would thus represent the normal genotype. If $\Pr(Y|Dd) = \Pr(Y|DD)$, i.e. a single copy of the mutant allele D is sufficient to produce an increase in risk, we say that the allele D is dominant over allele d. If $\Pr(Y|Dd) = \Pr(Y|dd)$, i.e. two copies of the mutant allele are necessary to produce an increase in risk, or equivalently, one copy of the normal allele is sufficient to provide protection; we say that D is recessive to d (or equivalently, d is dominant over D).

If the probability of disease give genotype dd, $\Pr(Y|dd) = 0$, there no phenocopies; that is, all cases of the disease are caused by the allele D. If $\Pr(Y|DD) = 1$ [or $\Pr(Y|Dd) = 1$ in the case of a dominant allele] we say the genotype is fully penetrant, which often happens in a Mendelian disease, which is controlled by a single locus. However, most complex diseases (traits) involve genes that have phenocopies and are not fully penetrant; thus, $0 < \Pr(Y|G) < 1$ for all G. For example, in an additive model, $\Pr(Y|dD)$ is midway between $\Pr(Y|dd)$ and $\Pr(Y|DD)$.

22.5. Hardy–Weinberg Equilibrium (HWE) Principle[1]

In a large random-mating population with no selection, no mutation and no migration, the gene (allele) and genotype frequencies are constant from generation to generation. The population with constant gene and genotype frequencies is said to be in HWE (https://en.wikipedia.org/wiki/Hardy%E2%80%93Weinberg_principle).

In the simplest case of a single locus with two alleles denoted A and a with frequencies $f(A) = p$ and $f(a) = q$, respectively, where $p+q = 1$. The expected genotype frequencies are $f(AA) = p^2$ for the AA homozygotes, $f(aa) = q^2$ for the aa homozygotes, and $f(Aa) = 2pq$ for the heterozygotes. The genotype proportions p^2, $2pq$, and q^2 are called the HW proportions. Note that the sum of all genotype frequencies of this case is the binomial expansion of the square of the sum of p and q, i.e. $(p + q)^2 = p^2 + 2pq + q^2 = 1$. Assumption of HWE is widely used in simulation studies to generation data sets.

Deviations from HWE: The seven assumptions underlying HWE are as follows: (1) organisms are diploid, (2) only sexual reproduction occurs, (3) generations are non-overlapping, (4) mating is random, (5) population size is infinitely large, (6) allele frequencies are equal in the sexes, and (7) there is no migration, mutation or selection.

Violations of the HW assumptions can cause deviations from expected genotype proportions (i.e. the HW proportions).

Testing for HWE: A goodness-of-fit test (or Pearson's chi-squared test) can be used to determine if genotypes at a marker in a population follow HWE. If we have a series of genotype counts at the marker from a population, then we can compare these counts to the ones predicted by the HW model and test HWE by using a test statistic of a "chi-square" distribution with $v = 1$ degrees of freedom.

For small sample, Fisher's exact test can be applied to testing for HW proportions. Since the test is conditional on the allele frequencies, p and q, the problem can be viewed as testing for the proper number of heterozygotes. In this way, the hypothesis of HW proportions is rejected if the number of heterozygotes is too large or too small.

In simulation studies, HWE is often assumed to generate genotype data at a marker. In addition, HWE tests have been applied to quality control in GWAS. If the genotypes at a marker do not follow HWE, it is possible that a genotyping error occurred at the marker.

22.6. Gene Mapping, Physical Distance, Genetic Map Distance, Haldane Map Function[2]

Gene mapping, describes the methods used to identify the locus of a gene and the distances between genes. There are two distinctive types of "Maps" used in the field of genome mapping: genetic maps and physical maps. While both maps are a collection of genetic markers and gene loci, genetic maps' distances are based on the genetic linkage information measured in centimorgans, while physical maps use actual physical distances usually measured in number of base pairs. The physical map could be a more "accurate" representation of the genome; genetic maps often offer insights into the nature of different regions of the chromosome.

In physical mapping, there are no direct ways of marking up a specific gene since the mapping does not include any information that concern traits and functions. Therefore, in genetic study, such as linkage analysis, genetic distance are preferable because it adequately reflects either the probability of a crossing over in an interval between two loci or the probability of observing a recombination between the markers at the two loci (https://en.wikipedia.org/wiki/Gene_mapping).

Genetic map distance, or map length of a chromosomal segment is defined as the expected number of crossing overs taking place in the segment. The unit of genetic distance is Morgan (M), or centiMorgan (cM), where 1 M = 100 cM. A segment of length 1 M exhibits on average one crossing over per meiosis. A basic assumption for genetic map distance is that the probability of a crossing over is proportional to the length of the chromosomal region.

Haldane map function expresses the relationship between genetic distance (x) and recombination fraction (θ): $x = -\ln(1 - 2\theta)/2$, or $\theta = (1 - e^{-2x})/2$. In these equations, the distances of x are expressed in units Morgan (M). Recombination fractions are usually expressed in percent. An assumption for Haldane map function is no interaction between crossing overs.

Physical distance is the most natural measure of genetic distance between two genetic loci. The unit of physical distance is basepair (bp), kilobases (Kb), or megabases (Mb), where 1 Kb = 1000 bp, and 1 Mb = 1000 Kb.

Relationship between physical distance and genetic map distance: On average, 1 cM corresponds to 0.88 Mb. However, the actual correspondence varies for different chromosome regions. The reason for this is that the occurrence of crossing overs is not equally distributed across the genome. There are recombination hot spots and cold spots in the genome that show greatly increased and decreased recombination activities, respectively. In addition, chiasmata are more frequent in female than in male meiosis. Hence, the total map length is different between genders. Useful rules of thumb regarding the autosomal genome are that 1 male cM averages 1.05 Mb and 1 female cM averages 0.70 Mb. The total length of the human genome can be assumed to be approximately 3,300 cM.

22.7. Heritability[3]

Heritability measures the fraction of phenotype variability that can be attributed to genetic variation. Any particular phenotype (P) can be modeled as the sum of genetic and environmental effects:

$$P = \text{Genotype}(G) + \text{Environment}(E).$$

Likewise the variance in the trait — Var (P) — is the sum of effects as follows:

$$\text{Var}(P) = \text{Var}(G) + \text{Var}(E) + 2\text{Cov}(G, E).$$

In a planned experiment $\mathrm{Cov}(G, E)$ can be controlled and held at 0. In this case, heritability is defined as

$$H^2 = \frac{\mathrm{Var}(G)}{\mathrm{Var}(P)}.$$

H^2 is the broad-sense heritability. This reflects all the genetic contributions to a population's phenotypic variance including additive, dominant, and epistatic (multi-genic interactions) as well as maternal and paternal effects.

A particularly important component of the genetic variance is the additive variance, $\mathrm{Var}(A)$, which is the variance due to the average effects (additive effects) of the alleles. The additive genetic portion of the phenotypic variance is known as narrow-sense heritability and is defined as

$$h^2 = \frac{\mathrm{Var}(A)}{\mathrm{Var}(P)}.$$

An upper case H^2 is used to denote broad sense, and lower case h^2 for narrow sense.

Estimating heritability: Since only P can be observed or measured directly, heritability must be estimated from the similarities observed in subjects varying in their level of genetic or environmental similarity. Briefly, better estimates are obtained using data from individuals with widely varying levels of genetic relationship — such as twins, siblings, parents and offspring, rather than from more distantly related (and therefore less similar) subjects.

There are essentially two schools of thought regarding estimation of heritability. The first school of estimation uses regression and correlation to estimate heritability. For example, heritability may be estimated by comparing parent and offspring traits. The slope of the line approximates the heritability of the trait when offspring values are regressed against the average trait in the parents.

The second set of methods of estimation of heritability involves analysis of variance (ANOVA) and estimation of variance components. A basic model for the quantitative trait (y) is

$$y = \mu + g + e,$$

where g is the genetic effect and e is the environmental effect (https://en.wikipedia.org/wiki/Heritability).

Common misunderstandings of heritability estimates: Heritability estimates are often misinterpreted if it is not understood that they refer to the *proportion of variation between individuals* on a trait that is due to genetic factors. It does not indicate the degree of genetic influence on the development of a trait of an individual. For example, it is incorrect to say that since the heritability of personality traits is about 0.6, which means that 60% of your personality is inherited from your parents and 40% comes from the environment.

22.8. Aggregation and Segregation[1,2]

Aggregation and segregation studies are generally the first step when studying the genetics of a human trait. Aggregation studies evaluate the evidence for whether there is a genetic component to a study by examining whether there is familial aggregation of the trait. The questions of interest include: (1) Are relatives of diseased individuals more likely to be diseased than the general population? (2) Is the clustering of disease in families different from what you'd expect based on the prevalence in the general population?

Segregation analysis refers to the process of fitting genetic models to data on phenotypes of family members. For this purpose, no marker data are used. The aim is to test hypotheses about whether one or more major genes and/or polygenes can account for observed pattern of familial aggregation, the mode of inheritance, and estimate the parameters of the best-fitting genetic model. The technique can be applied to various types of traits, including continuous and dichotomous traits and censored survival times. However, the basic techniques are essentially the same, involving only appropriate specification of the penetrance function $\Pr(Y|G)$ and ascertainment model.

Families are usually identified through a single individual, called the proband, and the family structure around that person is then discovered.

Likelihood methods for pedigree analysis: The likelihood for a pedigree is the probability of observing the phenotypes, $\mathbf{Y}$, given the model parameters $\Theta = (\mathbf{f}, q)$ and the method of ascertainment A, that is, $\Pr(\mathbf{Y}|\Theta, A)$, where $\mathbf{f} = (f_0, f_1, f_2)$ are the penetrance parameters for genotypes with 0, 1, 2 disease alleles, respectively; q is allele frequency. If we ignore A and assume that conditional on genotypes, individuals' phenotypes are independent, then we have

$$\Pr(\mathbf{Y}|\Theta) = \sum_{\mathbf{g}} \Pr(\mathbf{Y}|\mathbf{G} = \mathbf{g}; f) \Pr(\mathbf{G} = \mathbf{g}|q),$$

where $\mathbf{G}$ is the vector of genotypes of all individuals. Since we do not observe the genotypes $\mathbf{G}$, the likelihood must be computed by summing over all possible combinations of genotypes $\mathbf{g}$. This can entail a very large number of terms — 3^N for a single diallelic major gene in the pedigree with N individuals. The Elston–Stewart peeling algorithm (implemented in the software S.A.G.E) can be used to estimate the parameters $\Theta = (\mathbf{f}, q)$ and efficiently calculate likelihood L by representing it as a telescopic sum and eliminating the right-most sum in each step. For the peeling algorithm the computational demand increases linearly with the number of pedigree members but exponentially with the number of loci. For larger pedigrees or complex loops, exact peeling (even at a single locus) can become computationally demanding or infeasible. Thus, approximation peeling methods were proposed.

22.9. Linkage Analysis, LOD Score, Two-Point Linkage Analysis, Multipoint Linkage Analysis[1]

Genetic linkage is the tendency of alleles that are located close together on a chromosome to be inherited together during the meiosis phase of sexual reproduction. Genes whose loci are nearer to each other are less likely to be separated onto different chromatids during chromosomal crossover, and are therefore said to be genetically *linked*. In other words, the nearer two genes are on a chromosome, the lower is the chance of a swap occurring between them, and the more likely they are to be inherited together (https://en.wikipedia.org/wiki/Genetic_linkage).

Linkage analysis is the process of determining the approximate chromosomal location of a gene by looking for evidence of cosegregation with other genes whose locations are already known (i.e. marker gene). Cosegregation is a tendency for two or more genes to be inherited together, and hence for individuals with similar phenotypes to share alleles at the marker locus. If a genetic marker (with known location) is found to have a low recombiantion rate (θ) with a disease gene, one can infer that the disease gene may be close to that marker. Linkage analysis may be either parametric (assuming a specific inheritance model) or non-parametric.

LOD score (logarithm (base 10) of odds), is often used as a test statistic for parametric linkage analysis. The LOD score compares the likelihood of obtaining the test data if the two loci are indeed linked, to the likelihood of observing the same data purely by chance. By convention, a LOD score greater than 3.0 is considered evidence for linkage, as it indicates 1,000 to 1 odds that the linkage being observed did not occur by chance. On the other hand, a LOD score less than -2.0 is considered evidence to exclude linkage. Although it is very unlikely that a LOD score of 3 would be obtained from a single pedigree, the mathematical properties of the test allow data from a number of pedigrees to be combined by summing their LOD scores.

Two-point analysis: Two-point analysis is also called single-marker analysis. To test if a maker locus is linked to an unknown disease-causing locus, we can test the hypothesis H_0: $\theta = 0.5$ versus H_0: $\theta < 0.5$, where θ is the recombination fraction between the marker and the disease locus. By a parametric method, we often assume a mode of inheritance such as a dominant or recessive model. Let $L(\theta)$ is the likelihood function and $\hat{\theta}$ is the maximum likelihood estimate, then the corresponding LOD score $= \log_{10} \frac{L(\hat{\theta})}{L(\theta)|_{\theta=0.5}}$.

Multipoint linkage analysis: In multipoint linkage analysis, the location of a disease gene is considered in combination with many linked loci. Given a series of markers of known location, order, and spacing, the likelihood of the pedigree data is sequentially calculated for the disease gene to be at any position within the known map of markers. The software MORGAN (https://www.stat.washington.edu/thompson/Genepi/MORGAN/Morgan.shtml) and SOLAR (http://www.txbiomed.org/departments/genetics/genetics-detail?r=37) can be used for multipoint linkage analysis.

22.10. Elston–Stewart and Lander–Green Algorithms[4,5]

Multipoint linkage analysis is the analysis of linkage data involving three or more linked loci, which can be more powerful than two-point linkage analysis. For multipoint linkage analysis in pedigrees with large sizes or large numbers of markers, it is challenging to calculate likelihood of the observed data. Below we describe three well-known algorithms for linkage analysis.

Elston–Stewart algorithm: For a large pedigree, Elston and Stewart (1971) introduced a recursive approach, referred to as peeling, to simplify the calculation of the likelihood of observed phenotype vector $\mathbf{x} = (x_1, \dots, x_n), L = P(\mathbf{x}) = \sum_{\mathbf{g}} P(\mathbf{x}|\mathbf{g})P(\mathbf{g})$, where $\mathbf{g} = (g_1, \dots, g_n)$ is the genotype vector, n is pedigree size, and g_k is an specific genotype of individual k at a single locus or at multiple loci ($k = 1, \dots, n$); When pedigree size n is *large*, the number of possible assignments of $\mathbf{g}$ becomes too large to enumerate all possible assignments and calculate their likelihood values. The Elston–Stewart algorithm calculate likelihood L efficiently by representing it as a telescopic sum and eliminating the right-most sum in each step. The Elston–Stewart algorithm was extended to evaluate the likelihood of complex pedigrees but can be computationally intensive for a large number of markers.

Lander–Green algorithm: To handle large numbers of markers in pedigrees, Lander and Green (1987) proposed an algorithm based on an a hidden Markov model (HMM). The Lander–Green algorithm considers the inheritance pattern across a set of loci, $\mathbf{S} = (v_1, \dots, v_L)$, which is not explicitly observable, as the state sequence in the HMM, with recombination causing state transitions between two adjacent loci. The space of hidden states is the set of possible realizations of the inheritance vector at a locus. The genotypes of all pedigree members at a single locus are treated as an observation, and the observed marker data at all loci $\mathbf{M} = (M_{\cdot,1}, \ldots, M_{\cdot,L})$ are treated as the observation sequence in the HMM, where $M_{\cdot,j}$ denotes the observed marker data of all pedigree members at locus j. For a pedigree of small or moderate size, the likelihood of the observed marker data $\mathbf{M}, P(\mathbf{M}) = \sum_{\mathbf{S}} P(\mathbf{S}, \mathbf{M})$, can be calculated efficiently by using the HMM.

Markov Chain Monte Carlo (MCMC) sampler: For large and complex pedigrees with large numbers of loci and in particular with substantial amounts of missing marker data, exact methods become infeasible. Therefore, MCMC methods were developed to calculate likelihood by sampling haplotype configurations from their distribution conditional on the observed data. For example, LM-sampler implemented in the software M is an efficient MCMC method that combines an L-sampler and an M-sampler. The L-sampler updates jointly the meiosis indicators in $S_{\cdot,j}$ at a single locus j; the M-sampler updates jointly the components of $S_{i,\cdot}$, the meiosis indicators for all loci at a single meiosis i, by local reverse (chromosome) peeling.

22.11. Identical by Descent (IBD) and Quantitative Trait Locus (QTL) Mapping[2,6]

Two alleles are IBD if they are derived from a common ancestor in a pedigree. Two alleles are identical by state if they are identical in terms of their DNA composition and function but do not necessarily come from a common ancestor in a pedigree. In pedigree studies, many quantitative traits (such as BMI, height) are available. Linkage analysis of quantitative traits involve identifying quantitative trait loci (QTLs) that influence the phenotypes.

Haseman–Elston (HE) method: HE is a simple non-parametric approach for linkage analysis of quantitative traits, which was originally developed for sib-pairs and extended later for multiple siblings and for general pedigrees. If a sib-pair is genetically similar at a trait locus, then the sib-pair should also be phenotypically similar. The HE method measures genetic similarity by IBD sharing proportion τ at a locus and measures phenotypic similarity by squared phenotypic difference y. The HE method tests hypothesis H_0: $\beta = 0$ versus $H_1 : \beta < 0$ based on the linear regression model: $y = \alpha + \beta\tau + e_{\cdot}$.

Variance component analysis: For linkage analysis of quantitative traits in large pedigrees, a popular method is variance component analysis using linear mixed models. For a pedigree with n individuals, if we assume one putative QTL position, the phenotypes can be modeled by

$$\mathbf{y} = \mathbf{Xb} + \mathbf{Zu} + \mathbf{Zv} + \mathbf{e}, \tag{22.11.1}$$

where $\mathbf{y}$ is a vector of phenotypes, $\mathbf{b}$ is a vector of fixed effects, $\mathbf{u}$ is a vector of random polygenic effects, $\mathbf{v}$ is a vector of random QTL effects at the putative QTL position, $\mathbf{e}$ is a vector of residuals, $\mathbf{X}$ and $\mathbf{Z}$ are known incidence/covariate matrices for the effects in $\mathbf{b}$ and in $\mathbf{u}$ and $\mathbf{v}$, respectively. The covariance matrix of the phenotypes under model (1) is

$$\mathbf{V} = \text{Var}(\mathbf{y}) = \mathbf{Z}(\mathbf{A}\sigma_u^2 + \mathbf{G}\sigma_v^2)\mathbf{Z}' + \mathbf{I}\sigma_e^2,$$

where $\mathbf{A}$ is the numerator relationship matrix, σ_u^2, σ_v^2, and σ_e^2 are variance components associated with vectors $\mathbf{u}$, $\mathbf{v}$, and $\mathbf{e}$, respectively, and $\mathbf{G} = \{g_{\text{ij}}\}$ is the IBD matrix (for n individuals) at a specific QTL position conditional on the marker information.

Assuming multivariate normality, or $\mathbf{y} \sim N(\mathbf{Xb}, \mathbf{V})$, the restricted log-likelihood of the data can be calculated as $L \propto -0.5[\ln(|\mathbf{V}|) + \ln(|\mathbf{X}'\mathbf{V}^{-1}\mathbf{X}|) + (\mathbf{y} - \mathbf{X}\hat{\mathbf{b}})'\mathbf{V}^{-1}(\mathbf{y} - \mathbf{X}\hat{\mathbf{b}})]$, where $\hat{\mathbf{b}}$ is the generalized least-square estimator of $\mathbf{b}$.

When no QTL is assumed to be segregating in the pedigree, the mixed linear model (1) reduces to the null hypothesis model with no QTL, or

$$\mathbf{y} = \mathbf{Xb} + \mathbf{Zu} + \mathbf{e}, \tag{22.11.2}$$

$$\mathbf{V} = \text{Var}(\mathbf{y}) = \mathbf{ZA}\ \mathbf{Z}'\sigma_u^2 + \mathbf{I}\sigma_e^2.$$

Let L_1 and L_0 denote the maximized log-likelihoods pertaining to models (22.11.1) and (22.11.2), respectively. The log-likelihood ratio statistic $\text{LogLR} = -2(L_0 - L_1)$ can be calculated to test $H_0\colon \sigma_v^2 = 0$ versus $H_A\colon \sigma_v^2 > 0$ at a putative QTL position. Under the null hypothesis H_0, LogLR is asymptotically distributed as a 0.5:0.5 mixture of a χ^2 variable and a point mass at zero.

22.12. Linkage Disequilibrium and Genetic Association Tests[2]

In population genetics, LD is the non-random association of alleles at different loci, i.e. the presence of statistical associations between alleles at different loci that are different from what would be expected if alleles were independently, randomly sampled based on their individual allele frequencies. If there is no LD between alleles at different loci they are said to be in *linkage equilibrium* (https://en.wikipedia.org/wiki/Linkage_disequilibrium,171: 365–376)

Suppose that in a population, allele A occurs with frequency p_A at one locus, while at a different locus allele B occurs with frequency p_B. Similarly, let p_{AB} be the frequency of A and B occurring together in the same gamete (i.e. p_{AB} is the frequency of the AB haplotype). The level of LD between A and B can be quantified by the coefficient of LD D_{AB}, which is defined as $D_{AB} = p_{AB} - p_A p_B$. LD corresponds to $D_{AB} \neq 0$.

Measures of LD derived from D: The coefficient of LD D is not always a convenient measure of LD because its range of possible values depends on the frequencies of the alleles it refers to. This makes it difficult to compare the level of LD between different pairs of alleles. Lewontin suggested normalizing D by dividing it by the theoretical maximum for the observed allele frequencies as follows: $D' = D/D_{\max}$, where

$$D_{\max} = \begin{cases} \min\{p_A p_B, (1-p_A)(1-p_B)\} & \text{when } D < 0 \\ \min\{p_A(1-p_B), (1-p_A)p_B\} & \text{when } D > 0 \end{cases}.$$

D' $= 1$ or D' $= -1$ means no evidence for recombination between the markers. If allele frequencies are similar, high D' means the two markers are good surrogates for each other. On the other hand, the estimate of D' can be inflated in small samples or when one allele is rare.

An alternative to D' is the correlation coefficient between pairs of loci, expressed as

$$r = \frac{D}{\sqrt{p_A(1-P_A)P_B(1-P_B)}}.$$

$r^2 = 1$ implies the two markers provide exactly the same information. The measure r^2 is preferred by population geneticists.

Genetic association tests for case-control designs: For case-control designs, to test if a marker is associated with the disease status (i.e. if the marker is in LD with the disease locus), one of the most popular tests is the Cochran–Armitage trend test, which is equivalent to a score test based on a logistic regression model. However, the Cochran–Armitage trend test cannot account for covariates such as age and sex. Therefore, tests based on logistic regression models are widely used in genome-wide association studies. For example, we can test the hypothesis H_0: $\beta = 0$ using the following model:

logit $\Pr(Y_i = 1) = \alpha_0 + \alpha_1 x_i + \beta G_i$, where x_i denotes the vector of covariates, $G_i = 0, 1$, or 2 is the count of minor alleles in the genotype at a marker of individual i.

22.13. Genome-Wide Association Studies (GWAS), Population Stratification, and Genomic Inflation Factor[2]

GWAS are studies of common genetic variation across the entire human genome designed to identify genetic associations with observed traits. GWAS were made possible by the availability of chip-based microarray technology for assaying one million or more SNPs.

Corrections for multiple testing: In a GWAS analysis, each SNP is tested for association with the phenotype. Therefore, hundreds of thousands to millions of tests are conducted, each one with its own false positive probability. The cumulative likelihood of finding one or more false positives over the entire GWAS analysis is therefore much higher. One of the simplest approaches to correct for multiple testing is the Bonferroni correction. The Bonferroni correction adjusts the alpha value from $\alpha = 0.05$ to $\alpha = (0.05/K)$ where K is the number of statistical tests conducted. This correction is very conservative, as it assumes that each of the k-association tests is independent of all other tests — an assumption that is generally untrue due to LD among GWAS markers. An alternative to Bonferroni correction is to control the false discovery rate (FDR). The FDR is the expected proportion of false positives among all discoveries (or significant results, the rejected null hypotheses). The Benjamini and Hochberg method has been widely used to control FDR.

Population stratification is the presence of a systematic difference in allele frequencies between subpopulations in a population. Population stratification can cause spurious associations in GWAS. To control population stratification, a popular method is to adjust the 10 top principal components (PCs) of genome-wide genotype scores in the logistic regression models used in association tests.

Principal Components Analysis is a tool that has been used to infer population structure in genetic data for several decades, long before the GWAS era. It should be noted that top PCs do not always reflect population structure: they may reflect family relatedness, long-range LD (for example, due to inversion polymorphisms), or assay artifacts; these effects can often be eliminated by removing related samples, regions of long-range LD, or low-quality data, respectively, from the data used to compute PCs. In addition, PCA can highlight effects of differential bias that require additional quality control.

A limitation of the above methods is that they do not model family structure or cryptic relatedness. These factors may lead to inflation in test statistics if not explicitly modeled because samples that are correlated are assumed to be uncorrelated. Association statistics that explicitly account for family structure or cryptic relatedness are likely to achieve higher power, due to improved weighting of the data.

The Genomic inflation factor (λ) is defined as the ratio of the median of the empirically observed distribution of the test statistic to the expected median. Under the null hypothesis of no population stratification, suppose the association test is asymptotic χ^2 distribution with one degree of freedom. If the observed statistics are χ_j^2 $(j = 1, \ldots, K)$, then $\lambda = median(\chi_1^2, \ldots, \chi_K^2)/0.456$. The genomic inflation factor λ has been widely used to measure the inflation and the excess false positive rate caused by population stratification.

22.14. Haplotye, Haplotype Blocks and Hot Spots, and Genotype Imputation[7]

A haplotype consists of the alleles at multiple linked loci (one allele at each locus) on the same chromosome. Haplotyping refers to the reconstruction of the unknown true haplotype configurations from the observed data (https://en.wikipedia.org/wiki/Imputation_%28genetics%29).

Haplotype blocks and hot spots: the chromosomal regions with strong LD, hence only a few recombinations, were termed haplotype blocks. The length of haplotype blocks was variable, with some extending more than several hundred Kb. The areas with many recombinations are called recombination hot spots.

Genotype imputation: Genotyping arrays used for GWAS are based on tagging SNPs and therefore do not directly genotype all variation in the genome. Sequencing the whole genome of each individual in a study sample is often too costly. Genotype imputation methods are now being widely used in the analysis of GWAS to infer the untyped SNPs.

Genotype imputation is carried out by statistical methods that combine the GWAS data from a study sample together with known haplotypes from a reference panel, for instance from the HapMap and/or the 1,000 Genomes Projects, thereby allowing to infer and test initially-untyped genetic variants for association with a trait of interest. The imputation methods take advantage of sharing of haplotypes between individuals over short stretches of sequence to impute alleles into the study sample. Existing software packages for genotype imputation are IMPUTE2 and MaCH.

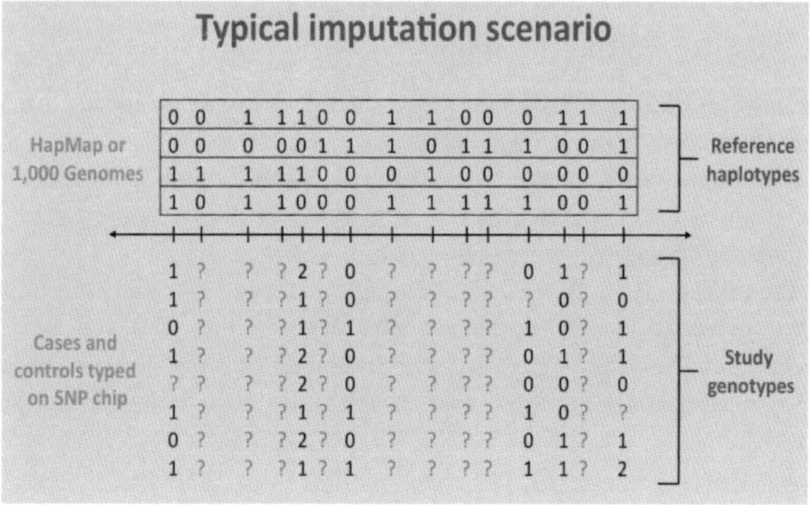

Fig. 22.14.1. Schematic drawing of imputation.

Importantly, imputation has facilitated meta-analysis of datasets that have been genotyped on different arrays, by increasing the overlap of variants available for analysis between arrays. The results of multiple GWAS studies can be pooled together to perform a meta-analysis.

The Figure 22.14.1 shows the most common scenario in which imputation is used: unobserved genotypes (question marks) in a set of study individuals are imputed (or predicted) using a set of reference haplotypes and genotypes from a study sample.

In Figure 22.14.1, haplotypes are represented as horizontal boxes containing 0s and 1s (for alternate SNP alleles), and unphased genotypes are represented as rows of 0s, 1s, 2s, and ?s (where "1" is the heterozygous state and '?' denotes a missing genotype). The SNPs (columns) in the dataset can be partitioned into two disjoint sets: a set T that is genotyped in all individuals and a set U that is genotyped only in the haploid reference panel. The goal of imputation in this scenario is to estimate the genotypes of SNPs in set U in the study sample.

Imputation algorithms often include two steps:

Step 1. Phasing: estimate haplotype at SNPs in T in the study sample.
Step 2. Imputing alleles at SNPs in U conditional on the haplotype guesses from the first step.

These steps are iterated in a MCMC framework to account for phasing uncertainty in the data.

22.15. Admixed Population, Admixture LD, and Admixture Mapping[8,9]

Admixed populations are populations formed by the recent admixture of two or more ancestral populations. For example, African Americans often have ancestries from West Africans and Europeans. The global ancestry of an admixed individual is defined as the proportion of his/her genome inherited from a specific ancestral population. The local ancestry of an individual at a specific marker is the proportion of alleles at the marker that are inherited from the given ancestral population with a true value of 0, 0.5, or 1. The difference between the local ancestry at a specific marker and the global ancestry of an individual is referred to as the local deviation of ancestry at the marker.

Admixture LD is formed in local chromosome regions as a result of admixture over the past several hundred years when large chromosomal segments were inherited from a particular ancestral population, resulting in the temporary generation of long haplotype blocks (usually several megabases (Mbs) or longer), in which the local ancestry at two markers may be correlated.

Background LD is another type of LD, which is inherited by admixed populations from ancestral populations. The background LD is the traditional LD that exists in much shorter haplotype blocks (usually less than a few hundred kilobases (Kbs)) in homogeneous ancestral populations and is the result of recombination over hundreds to thousands of generations. To illustrate admixture LD and background LD, we show a special case in Figure 22.14.1 where a large chromosomal region with admixture LD contains a small region with background LD and a causal variant is located inside the small background LD region. For association studies, we hope to identify SNPs that are in background LD with causal variants.

Admixture mapping: Admixture LD has been exploited to locate causal variants that have different allele frequencies among different ancestral populations. Mapping by admixture LD is also called admixture mapping. Admixture mapping can only map a causal variant into a wide region of 4–10 cM. Roughly speaking, most admixture mapping tests are based on testing the association between a trait and the local ancestry deviation at a marker. A main advantage of admixture mapping is that only ancestry informative markers (AIMs) are required to be genotyped and tested. An AIM is a marker that has a substantial allele frequency difference between two ancestral populations.

Fine mapping in admixed populations: Identifying a region that contains a disease gene by admixture mapping is only the first step in the gene-discovery process. This would then be followed by fine-mapping: a targeted (case-control) association study for the disease phenotype using dense markers from the implicated chromosomal segment. Fine-mapping studies in admixed populations must account for the fact that, when not adjusting for local ancestry, admixture LD can produce associations involving variants that are distant from the causal variant. On the other hand, admixture association can actually be used to improve fine-mapping resolution by checking whether the level of admixture association that would be expected based on the population differentiation of a putatively causal SNP is actually observed.

22.16. Family-Based Association Tests (FBATs) and the Transmission Disequilibrium Test[2,10]

For genetic association studies, tests which are based on data from unrelated individuals are very popular, but can be biased if the sample contains individuals with different genetic ancestries. FBATs avoid the problem of bias due to mixed ancestry by using within family comparisons. Many different family designs are possible, the most popular using parents and offspring, but others use just sibships. Dichotomous, measured and time-to-onset phenotypes can be accommodated. FBATs are generally less powerful than tests based on a sample of unrelated individuals, but special settings exist, for example, testing for rare variants with affected offspring and their parents, where the family design has a power advantage.

The transmission disequilibrium test (TDT): The simplest family-based design for testing association uses genotype data from trios, which consist of an affected offspring and his or her two parents. The idea behind the TDT is intuitive: under the null hypothesis, Mendel's laws determine which marker alleles are transmitted to the affected offspring. The TDT compares the observed number of alleles that are transmitted with those expected in Mendelian transmissions. The assumption of Mendelian transmissions is all that is needed to ensure valid results of the TDT and the FBAT approach. An excess of alleles of one type among the affected indicates that a disease-susceptibility locus (DSL) for a trait of interest is linked and associated with the marker locus.

FBAT statistic: The TDT test was extended to family-based association approach, which is widely used in association studies. Let X denote the coded offspring genotype. Let P denote the genotype of the offspring's parents, and $T = Y - \mu$ denote the coded offspring trait, where Y is the phenotypic variable and μ is a fixed, pre-specified value that depends on the nature of the sample and phenotype. Y can be a measured binary or continuous variable. The covariance statistic used in the FBAT test is $U = \Sigma T * (X - E(X|P))$, where U is the covariance, $E(X|P)$ is the expected value of X computed under the null hypothesis, and summation is over all offspring in the sample. Mendel's laws underlie the calculation of $E(X|P)$ for any null hypothesis. Centering X by its expected value conditional on parental genotypes has the effect of removing contributions from homozygous parents and protecting against population stratification.

The FBAT is defined by dividing U^2 by its variance, which is computed under the appropriate null hypothesis by conditioning on T and P for each offspring. Given a sufficiently large sample, that is, at least 10 informative families, the FBAT statistic has a χ^2-distribution with 1 degree of freedom.

22.17. Gene-Environment Interaction and Gene-Gene Interaction (Epistasis)[1,2]

Gene–environment ($G \times E$) interaction is defined as "a different effect of an environmental exposure on disease risk in persons with different genotypes" or, alternatively, "a different effect of different environmental exposures." Interactions are often analyzed by statistical models such as multiplicative or additive model. Statistical interaction means a departure of the observed risks from some model for the main effects. Statistical interaction does not necessarily imply biological interaction and vice versa. Nevertheless, such interactions are often interpreted as having biological significance about underlying mechanisms.

Case-control studies for $G \times E$ interactions: Let $p(D) = \Pr(\text{affected})$ denote the disease risk of an individual. The log odds of disease can be modeled as

$$\text{logit}(p(D)) = \beta_0 + \beta_G G + \beta_E E + \beta_{GE} G \times E,$$

where G and E are the genotypic and environmental scores, respectively; β_{GE} is the log odds ratio (OR) of the interaction effect. A test can be constructed to test the hypothesis H_0: $\beta_{GE} = 0$.

Case-only studies for $G \times E$ interactions: Another design that can be used to examine $G \times E$ interactions is the case-only design, where controls are not needed. Under the assumption that the gene and environmental risk factor are independently distributed in the population, then one can detect

$G \times E$ interactions simply by looking for association between the two factors (G and E) among cases. In the following logistic regression model for case-only studies, we use the exposure probability $p(E)$ instead of disease risk $p(D)$ as used in case-control designs.

$$\text{logit}P(E) = \log[\text{P}(E)/(1 - \text{P}(E)] = \beta_0 + \beta_{GE}G.$$

Gene by gene $(G - G)$ interaction analysis: For a case-control design, let X_A and X_B denote the genotype scores at two markers based on two assumed genetic models (such as additive by additive, or additive by dominant). Let y denote the disease status. The $(G–G)$ interaction model can be given by

$$\text{logitp}(y) = \mu_0 + \alpha X_A + \beta X_B + \gamma X_A \times X_B,$$

where γ is the coefficient of $G - G$ interaction. A statistic can be constructed to test the hypothesis $H_0\colon \gamma = 0$.

An alternative approach to test $G–G$ interaction is using ANOVA method. For example, to test dominant-by-dominant interaction at two markers, we can treat the genotypic value at each marker as a categorical variable and each marker has two levels of genotype values. Then, we can conduct ANOVA based on a 2×2 contingent table.

22.18. Multiple Hypothesis Testing, Family-wise Error Rate (FWER), the Bonferroni Procedure and FDR[11]

Multiple hypothesis testing involves testing multiple hypotheses simultaneously; each hypothesis is associated with a test statistic. For multiple hypothesis testing, a traditional criterion for (Type I) error control is the FWER, which is the probability of rejecting one or more true null hypotheses. A multiple testing procedure is said to control the FWER at a significance level α if FWER $\leq \alpha$.

The Bonferroni procedure is a well-known method for controlling FWER with computational simplicity and wide applicability. Consider testing m (null) hypotheses $(H_1, H_2, \ldots, H_m)$. Let $(p_1, p_2, \ldots, p_m)$ denote the corresponding p-values. In the Bonferroni procedure, if $p_j \leq \alpha/m$, then reject the null hypothesis H_j; otherwise, it fails to reject H_j $(j = 1, \ldots, m)$. Controlling FWER is practical when very few features are expected to be truly alternative (e.g. GWAS), because any false positive can lead to a large waste of time.

The power of Bonferroni procedures can be increased by using weighted p-values. The weighted Bonferroni procedure can be described as follows.

Given non-negative weights $(w_1, w_2, \ldots, w_m)$ for the tests associated with the hypotheses $(H_1, H_2, \ldots, H_m)$, where $\frac{1}{m}\sum_{j=1}^{m} w_j = 1$. For hypothesis $H_j (1 \leq j \leq m)$, when $w_j > 0$, reject H_j if $\frac{p_j}{w_j} \leq \frac{\alpha}{m}$ and fail to reject H_j when $w_j = 0$.

The weighted Bonferroni procedure controls FWER at level α. The weights $(w_1, w_2, \ldots, w_m)$ can be specified by using certain prior information. For example, in GWAS, the prior information can be linkage signals or results from gene expression analyses.

The criterion of FWER can be very conservative. An alternative criterion for (Type I) error control is FDR.

FDR is the (unobserved) expected proportion of false discoveries among total rejections. The FDR is particularly useful in exploratory analyses (such as gene expression data analyses), where one is more concerned with having mostly true findings among a set of statistically significant discoveries rather than guarding against one or more false positives. FDR-controlling procedures provide less stringent control of Type I errors compared to FWER controlling procedures (such as the Bonferroni correction). Thus, FDR-controlling procedures have greater power, at the cost of increased rates of Type I errors.

The Benjamini–Hochberg (BH) procedure controls the FDR (at level α). The procedure works as follows:

Step 1. Let $p_{(1)} \leq p_{(2)} \leq \ldots \leq p_{(K)}$ be the ordered P-values from K tests.
Step 2. Calculate $s = \max(j \colon p_{(j)} \leq j\alpha/K)$.
Step 3. If s exists, then reject the null hypotheses corresponding to $p_{(1)} \leq p_{(2)} \leq \ldots \leq p_{(s)}$; otherwise, reject nothing.

The BH procedure is valid when the m tests are independent, and also in various scenarios of dependence (https://en.wikipedia.org/wiki/False_ discovery_rate).

22.19. Next Generation Sequencing Data Analysis[12,13]

Next-generation sequencing (NGS), also known as high-throughput sequencing, is the catch-all term used to describe a number of different modern sequencing technologies including:

- Illumina (Solexa) sequencing
- Roche 454 sequencing
- Ion torrent: Proton/PGM sequencing
- SOLiD sequencing

These recent technologies allow us to sequence DNA and RNA much more quickly and cheaply than the previously used Sanger sequencing, and as such have revolutionized the study of genomics and molecular biology. Massively parallel sequencing technology facilitates high-throughput sequencing, which allows an entire genome to be sequenced in less than one day.

The NGS-related platforms often generate genomic data with very large size, which is called big genomic data. For example, sequencing a single exome (in a single individual) can result in approximately 10 Gigabytes of data and sequencing a single genome can result in approximately 200 Gigabytes. Big data present some challenges for statistical analysis.

DNA sequence data analysis: A major focus of DNA sequence data analysis is to identify rare variants associated with diseases using case-control design and/or using family design.

RNA sequence data analysis: RNA-sequencing (RNA-seq) is a flexible technology for measuring genome-wide expression that is rapidly replacing microarrays as costs become comparable. Current differential expression analysis methods for RNA-seq data fall into two broad classes: (1) methods that quantify expression within the boundaries of genes previously published in databases and (2) methods that attempt to reconstruct full length RNA transcripts.

ChIP-Seq data analysis: Chromatin immunoprecipitation followed by NGS (ChIP-Seq) is a powerful method to characterize DNA-protein interactions and to generate high-resolution profiles of epigenetic modifications. Identification of protein binding sites from ChIP-seq data has required novel computational tools.

Microbiome and Metagenomics: The human microbiome consists of trillions of microorganisms that colonize the human body. Different microbial communities inhabit vaginal, oral, skin, gastrointestinal, nasal, urethral, and other sites of the human body. Currently, there is an international effort underway to describe the human microbiome in relation to health and disease. The development of NGS and the decreasing cost of data generation using these technologies allow us to investigate the complex microbial communities of the human body at unprecedented resolution.

Current microbiome studies extract DNA from a microbiome sample, quantify how many representatives of distinct populations (species, ecological functions or other properties of interest) were observed in the sample, and then estimate a model of the original community.

Large-scale endeavors (for example, the HMP and also the European project, MetaHIT3) are already providing a preliminary understanding of the biology and medical significance of the human microbiome and its collective genes (the metagenome).

22.20. Rare Variants Analysis for DNA Sequence Data[14,15]

Rare genetic variants, defined as alleles with a frequency less than 1–5%, can play key roles in influencing complex disease and traits. However, standard methods used to test for association with single common genetic variants are underpowered for rare variants unless sample sizes or effect sizes are very large. Therefore, SNP set (or gene)-based tests have been developed for rare variants analysis. Below we have described a Sequencing Kernel Association Test (SKAT).

Assume n subjects are sequenced in a region with p variant sites observed. Covariates might include age, gender, and top PCs of genetic variation for controlling population stratification. For the ith subject, y_i denotes the phenotype variable, $\mathbf{X_i} = (X_{i1}, X_{i2}, \ldots, X_{im})$ denotes the covariates, and $\mathbf{G_i} = (G_{i1}, G_{i2}, \ldots, G_{ip})$ denotes the genotypes for the p variants within the region. Typically, we assume an additive genetic model and let $G_{ij} = 0, 1$, or 2 represent the number of copies of the minor allele. To relate the sequence variants in a region to the phenotype, consider the linear model

$$\mathrm{y}_i = \alpha_0 + \boldsymbol{\alpha}'\mathbf{X}_\mathrm{i} + \beta'\mathbf{G}_\mathrm{i} + \varepsilon_i,$$

when the phenotypes are continuous traits, and the logistic model

$$\text{logit P}(\mathrm{y}_i = 1) = \alpha_0 + \boldsymbol{\alpha}'\mathbf{X}_\mathrm{i} + \boldsymbol{\beta}'\mathbf{G}_\mathrm{i},$$

when the phenotypes are dichotomous (e.g. y $= 0/1$ for case or control). Here, α_0 is an intercept term, $\boldsymbol{\alpha} = [\alpha_1, \ldots, \alpha_m]'$ is the vector of regression coefficients for the m covariates, $\boldsymbol{\beta} = [\beta_1, \ldots, \beta_m]'$ is the vector of regression coefficients for the p observed gene variants in the region, and for continuous phenotypes ε_i is an error term with a mean of zero and a variance of σ^2. Under both linear and logistic models, and evaluating whether the gene variants influence the phenotype, adjusting for covariates, corresponds to testing the null hypothesis H_0: $\boldsymbol{\beta} = 0$, that is, $\beta_1 = \beta_2 = \cdots = \beta_{m.} = 0$. The standard p-DF likelihood ratio test has little power, especially for rare variants. To increase the power, SKAT tests H_0 by assuming each β_j follows an arbitrary distribution with a mean of zero and a variance of $w_j\tau$, where τ is a variance component and w_j is a prespecified weight for variant j. One can easily see that H_0: $\beta = 0$ is equivalent to testing H_0: $\tau = 0$, which can be conveniently tested with a variance-component score test in the corresponding mixed model, this is known to be the most powerful test locally. A key advantage of the score test is that it only requires fitting the null model $y_i = \alpha_0 + \boldsymbol{\alpha}'\mathbf{X_i} + \varepsilon_i$ for continuous traits and the logit $\mathrm{P}(y_i = 1) = \alpha_0 + \alpha'\mathbf{X_i}$, for dichotomous traits.

Specifically, the variance-component score statistic is $\boldsymbol{Q} = (\mathbf{y} - \hat{\boldsymbol{\mu}}^2)'\mathbf{K}(\mathbf{y} - \hat{\boldsymbol{\mu}}^2)$, where $\mathbf{K} = \mathbf{GWG}'$, $\hat{\boldsymbol{\mu}}$ is the predicted mean of $\mathbf{y}$ under H_0, that is $\hat{\boldsymbol{\mu}} = \hat{\boldsymbol{\alpha}}_0 + \hat{\boldsymbol{\alpha}}'\mathbf{X_i}$ for continuous traits and $\hat{\boldsymbol{\mu}} = \mathrm{logit}^{-1}(\hat{\boldsymbol{\alpha}}_0 + \hat{\boldsymbol{\alpha}}'\mathbf{X_i})$ for dichotomous traits; and $\hat{\boldsymbol{\alpha}}_0$ and $\hat{\boldsymbol{\alpha}}$ are estimated under the null model by regressing $\mathbf{y}$ on only the covariates X. Here, $\mathbf{G}$ is an $\mathrm{n} \times \mathrm{p}$ matrix with the (i, j)-th element being the genotype of variant j of subject i, and $\mathbf{W} = \mathrm{diag}(w_1, \ldots, w_p)$ contains the weights of the p variants.

Under the null hypothesis, Q follows a mixture of chi-square distributions. The SKAT method has been extended to analyze family sequence data.

References

1. Thomas, DC. *Statistical Methods in Genetic Epidemiology.* Oxford: Oxford University Press, Inc., 2003.
2. Ziegler, A, König, IR. *A Statistical Approach to Genetic Epidemiology: Concepts and Applications.* (2nd edn.). Hoboken: Wiley-VCH Verlag GmbH & Co. KGaA, 2010.
3. Falconer, DS, Mackay, TFC. *Introduction to Quantitative Genetics* (4th edn.). Harlew: Longman, 1996.
4. Ott, J. *Analysis of Human Genetic Linkage.* Baltimore, London: The Johns Hopkins University Press, 1999.
5. Thompson, EA. *Statistical Inference from Genetic Data on Pedigrees. NSF-CBMS Regional Conference Series in Probability and Statistics,* (Vol 6). Beachwood, OH: Institute of Mathematical Statistics.
6. Gao, G, Hoeschele, I. Approximating identity-by-descent matrices using multiple haplotype configurations on pedigrees. *Genet.*, 2005, 171: 365–376.
7. Howie, BN, Donnelly, P, Marchini, J. A flexible and accurate genotype imputation method for the next generation of genome-wide association studies. *PLoS Genetics,* 2009, 5(6): e1000529.
8. Smith, MW, O'Brien, SJ. Mapping by admixture linkage disequilibrium: Advances, limitations and guidelines. *Nat. Rev. Genet.*, 2005, 6: 623–32.
9. Seldin, MF, Pasaniuc, B, Price, AL. New approaches to disease mapping in admixed populations. *Nat. Rev. Genet.*, 2011, 12: 523–528.
10. Laird, NM, Lange, C. Family-based designs in the age of large-scale gene-association studies. *Nat. Rev. Genet.*, 2006, 7: 385–394.
11. Kang, G, Ye, K, Liu, L, Allison, DB, Gao, G. Weighted multiple hypothesis testing procedures. *Stat. Appl. Genet. Molec. Biol.*, 2009, 8(1).
12. Wilbanks, EG, Facciotti, MT. Evaluation of algorithm performance in ChIP-Seq peak detection. *PLoS ONE,* 2010, 5(7): e11471.
13. Rapaport, F, Khanin, R, Liang, Y, Pirun, M, Krek, A, Zumbo, P, Mason, CE, Soccil, ND, Betel, D. 3,4 Comprehensive evaluation of differential gene expression analysis methods for RNA-seq data. *Genome Biology.*, 2013, 14: R95.

14. Chen, H, Meigs, JB, Dupuis, J. Sequence kernel association test for quantitative traits in family samples. *Genet. Epidemiol.*, 2013, 37: 196–204.
15. Wu, M, Lee, S, Cai, T, Li, Y, Boehnke, M, Lin, X. Rare variant association testing for sequencing data using the sequence kernel association test (SKAT). *Am. J. Hum. Genet.* 89: 82–93.

About the Author

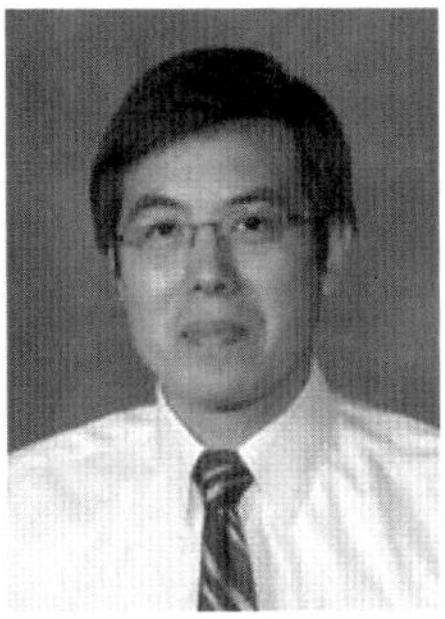

Dr. Guimin Gao is currently a Research Associate Professor in the Department of Public Health Sciences at the University of Chicago. He served as an Associate Professor in the Department of Biostatistics at Virginia Commonwealth University between December 2009 and July 2015 and served as a Research Assistant Professor at the University of Alabama at Birmingham. He completed graduate studies in biostatistics at Sun Yatsen University of Medical Sciences in China (Ph.D. in 2000) and postdoctoral studies in statistical genetics at Creighton University and Virginia Tech (2001–2005). Dr. Gao served as the principal investigator between 2007–2014 for a R01 research grant awarded by the National Institutes of Health (NIH), entitled "Haplotyping and QTL mapping in pedigrees with missing data". He has reviewed manuscripts for 16 journals and reviewed many grant applications for NIH. Dr. Gao has published 45 peer reviewed papers.

CHAPTER 23

BIOINFORMATICS

Dong Yi* and Li Guo

23.1. Bioinformatics[1–3]

Bioinformatics is a scientific field that develops tools to preserve, search and analyze biological information using computers. It is among the most important frontiers and core areas of life science and natural science in the 21st century. The research focuses on genomics and proteomics, and it aims to analyze biological information on expression, structure and function based on nucleotide and protein sequences.

The substance of bioinformatics is to resolve biological problems using computer science and network techniques. Its birth and development were historically timely and necessary, and it has quietly infiltrated each corner of life science. Data resources in life science have expanded rapidly in both quantity and quality, which urges to search powerful instrument to organize, preserve and utilize biological information. These large amounts of diverse data contain many important biological principles that are crucial to reveal riddles of life. Therefore, bioinformatics is necessarily identified as an important set of tools in life science.

The generation of bioinformatics has mainly accompanied the development of molecular biology. Crick revealed the genetic code in 1954, indicating that deoxyribonucleic acid (DNA) is a template to synthesize ribonucleic acid (RNA), and RNA is a template to synthesize protein (Central Dogma) (Figure 23.1.1). The central dogma plays a very important guiding role in later molecular biology and bioinformatics. Bioinformatics has further been rapidly developed with the completion of human genome sequencing

*Corresponding author: yd_house@hotmail.com

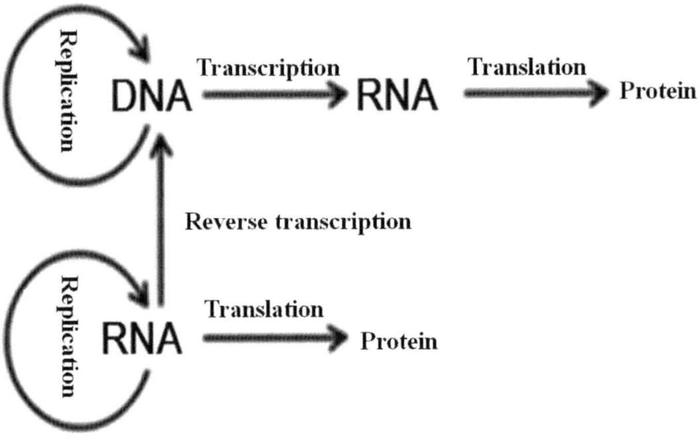

Fig. 23.1.1. Central dogma.

in February 2001. Biological data have rapidly expanded to ocean with the rapid development of DNA automatic sequencing. Unquestionably, the era of accumulating data is changing to an era of explaining data, and bioinformatics has been generated as an interdisciplinary field because these data always contain potential valuable meanings. Therefore, the core content of the field is to study the statistical and computational analysis of DNA sequences to deeply understand the relationships of sequence, structure, evolution and biological function. Relevant fields include molecular biology, molecular evolution, structural biology, statistics and computer science, and more.

As a discipline with abundant interrelationships, bioinformatics aims at the acquisition, management, storage, allocation and interpretation of genome information. The regulatory mechanisms of gene expression are also an important topic in bioinformatics, which contributes to the diagnosis and therapy of human disease based on the roles of molecules in gene expression. The research goal is to reveal fundamental laws regarding the complexity of genome structure and genetic language and to explain the genetic code of life.

23.2. Statistical Methods in Bioinformatics[4,5]

Analytical methods in bioinformatics have been rapidly developed alongside bioinformatics techniques, such as statistical, neural network, Markov chain and fractal methods. Statistical methods are an important subset, including sequence alignment, protein structural analysis and expression analysis based on basic problems in bioinformatics. Here, we will mainly introduce the main statistical methods in bioinformatics.

Statistical methods in sequence alignment: DNA and protein sequences are a basic study objective that can provide important biological information. Basic Local Alignment Search Tool (BLAST) is a tool to analyze similarity in DNA or protein sequence databases, and applying the Poisson distribution. BLAST can provide a statistical description of similarity via rapid similarity comparison with public databases. Some statistical values to indicate the confidence level of the result, including the probability (P) and expected value (e), are provided in BLAST. P indicates the confidence level of the score derived from the alignment result.

Statistical methods in protein structure: Protein structure indicates spatial structure, and the study of structure can contribute to understanding the role and function of proteins. As an example of classification methods, the SWISS-PORI database includes Bayes and multiple Dirichlet mixture equations.

Statistical methods in expression analysis: The analysis of gene expression is a research hotspot and a challenge in bioinformatics. The common method is clustering, with the aim of grouping genes. Frequently used clustering methods include K-means clustering, hierarchical clustering and self-organizing feature maps. Hierarchical clustering is also termed level clustering. K-means clustering is not involved in the hierarchical structure of categories in data partitioning, which leads to the minimum sum of squares of distances between all the vectors and the center of clustering, which is obtained based on a sum-squared error rule. There are many methods to analyze differentially expressed genes. The simplest method is the threshold value method, in which differentially expressed genes are obtained based on fold change. This method is quite arbitrary and not rigorous due to larger human factors. Statistical methods, including the t-test, ANOVA model of variance, Significance Analysis of Microarrays (SAM) and information entropy, can rigorously obtain abnormally expressed genes. Genes with close functional relationships may be correlated with each other (linear correlation or nonlinear correlation), and a statistical correlation coefficient (a linear correlation coefficient or nonlinear correlation coefficient) can also be estimated, especially in the correlation analysis of drug and genes.

Moreover, statistical methods are also widely used in other analyses. For example, classification analysis is involved in linear discriminant analysis (Fisher linear discriminant analysis), k-nearest neighbor, support vector machine (SVM), Bayes classifier, artificial neural network and decision tree methods, among others. Entropy, an important theory in statistics, is also applied to the analysis of nucleotide sequences.

23.3. Bioinformatics Databases[6–8]

More database resources for bioinformatics have been established with more intensive research. In general, there are three predominant types of databases: nucleotide sequence databases, protein sequence databases and protein structure databases (Figure 23.3.1), although there are also bioinformatics knowledge bases, genome databases, bioinformatics tools databases and so on. These online resources provide abundant resources for data integration analysis. Herein, we introduce the three main nucleic acid databases and their features in bioinformatics:

NCBI-GenBank (http://www.ncbi.nlm.nih.gov/genbank) in the National Center for Biotechnology Information (NCBI): NCBI-GenBank is a synthesis database containing catalogues and biological annotations, including more than 300,000 nucleotide sequences from different laboratories and large-scale sequencing projects. The database is built, maintained and managed by NCBI. Entrez Gene provides a convenient retrieval mode, linking classification, genome, atlas, sequence, expression, structure, function, bibliographical index and source data.

European Molecular Biology Laboratory, European Bioinformatics Institute (EMBL-EBI): EMBL-EBI is among the most important bioinformatics websites (http://www.ebi.ac.uk/), located in the Wellcome Trust Genome Campus in England. EBI ensures that molecular and endosome research information is public and free to facilitate further scientific progress. EBI also provides service for establishing/maintaining databases, information services for molecular biology, and bioresearch for molecular biology and

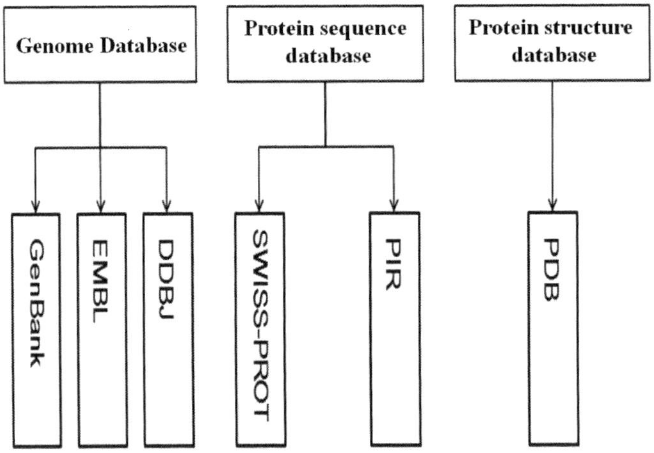

Fig. 23.3.1. Common bioinformatics databases.

computational molecular biology and is intensively involved in many facets, including molecular biology, genosome, medical and agricultural research, and the agriculture, biotechnology, chemical and pharmaceutical industries.

DNA Data Bank of Japan (DDBJ): DDBJ is established in the National Institute of Genetics (NIG) as an international DNA database. It began constructing a DNA database in 1986 and has frequently cooperated internationally with NCBI and EBI. DNA sequences are a vast data resource that plays a more direct role in revealing evolution than other biological data. DDBJ is the only DNA database in Japan, and DNA sequences are collected from researchers who can obtain internationally recognized codes.

These three databases symbiotically constitute the central federated database of international nucleotide sequences, and they exchange data every day to ensure synchronicity.

23.4. Database Retrieval and Analysis[9,10]

Databases such as GenBank must adapt to the information explosion of a large number of sequences due to the human genome project (HGP) and other scientific studies, and it is quite important to efficiently retrieve and analyze data. Herein, we address database retrieval and analysis based on the three large databases.

NCBI-GenBank data retrieval and analysis: The Entrez system is flexible retrieval system that integrates the taxonomy of DNA and protein data, including genome, atlas, protein structure and function, and PubMed, with the medical literature, and it is used to visit GenBank and obtain sequence information. BLAST is the most basic and widely used method in GenBank, a database search procedure based on sequence similarity. BLAST can retrieve sequence similarity in GenBank and other databases. NCBI provides a series of BLAST procedure sets to retrieve sequence similarity, and BLAST can run in NCBI website or as independent procedure sets after download in FTP. BLAST comprises several independent procedures, defined according to different objects and databases (Table 23.4.1).

Table 23.4.1. The main BLAST procedures.

Name	Queried sequence	Database
Blastn	Nucleotide	Nucleotide
Blastp	Protein	Protein
Blastx	Nucleotide	Protein
Tblastn	Protein	Nucleotide
TBlastx	Nucleotide	Nucleotide

EBI protein sequence retrieval and analysis: SRS is the main bioinformatics tool used to integrate the analysis of genomes and related data, and it is an open system. Different databases are installed according to different needs, and SRS has three main retrieval methods: quick retrieval, standard retrieval and batch retrieval. A perpetual project can be created after entry into SRS, and the SRS system allows users to install their own relevant databases. Quick retrieval can retrieve more records in all the databases, but many of them are not relevant. Therefore, users can select standard retrieval to quickly retrieve relevant records, and the SRS system can allow users to save the retrieved results for later analysis.

DDBJ data retrieval and analysis: Data retrieval tools include getentry, SRS, Sfgate & WAIS, TXSearch and Homology. The first four are used to retrieve the original data from DDBJ, and Homology can perform homology analysis of a provided sequence or fragment using FASTA/BLAST retrieval. These retrieval methods can be divided into accession number, keyword and classification retrieval: getentry is accession number retrieval, SRS and Sfgate & WAIS are keyword retrieval, and TXSearch is classification retrieval. For all of these retrieval results, the system can provide processing methods, including link, save, view and launch.

23.5. DNA Sequence Analysis[11,12]

DNA is a molecule with a duplex structure composed of deoxyribonucleotides, storing the genetic instructions to guide biological development and vital function. The main function of DNA is long-term information storage as well as blueprints or recipes for constructing other compounds, such as RNA and protein. A DNA fragment with genetic information is called a gene, and other sequences may play a role via their structure or contribute to a regulatory network. The main components of DNA analysis include the following:

Determination of open reading frames (ORFs): A gene can be translated into six reading frames, and it is quite important to determine which is the correct ORF. Generally, we select the maximum ORF without a termination codon (TGA, TAA or TAG) as a correct result. The ending of an ORF is easier to estimate than the beginning: the general initiation site of a coding sequence is a methionine codon (ATG), but methionine also frequently appears within a sequence, so not every ATG marks the beginning of a sequence. Certain rules can help us to search for protein coding regions in DNA: for example, ORF length (based on the fact that the probability of a longer ORF is very small), the recognition of a Kozak sequence to determine the initiation site of a coding region, and different statistical rules between coding sequences and non-coding sequences.

Intron and exon: Eukaryotic genes include introns and exons, where an exon consists of a coding region, while an intron consists of a non-coding region. The phenomenon of introns and exons leads to products with different lengths, as not all exons are included in the final mRNA product. Due to mRNA editing, an mRNA can generate different polypeptides that further form different proteins, which are named splice variants or alternatively spliced forms. Therefore, mapping the results of a query of cDNA or mRNA (transcriptional level) may have deficiencies due to alternative splicing.

DNA sequence assembly: Another important task in DNA sequence analysis is the DNA sequence assembly of fragments generated by automatic sequencing to assemble complete nucleotide sequences, especially in the case of the small fragments generated by high-throughput sequencing platforms. Some biochemical analysis requires highly accurate sequencing, and it is important to verify the consistency of a cloned sequence with a known gene sequence. If the results are not consistent, the experiment must be designed to correct the discrepancy. The reasons for inaccurate clone sequences are various, for example, inappropriate primers and low-efficiency enzymes in Polymerase Chain Reaction (PCR). Obtaining a high confidence level in sequencing requires time and patience, and the analyst should be familiar with the defects of experiment, GC enrichment regions (which lead to strong DNA secondary structure and can influence sequencing results), and repetitive sequences. All of these factors make sequence assembly a highly technical process.

The primary structure of DNA determines the function of a gene, and DNA sequence analysis is an important and basic problem project in molecular genetics.

23.6. RNA Sequence Analysis[13,14]

RNA is a carrier of genetic information in biological cells, as well as some viruses and viroids. It is a chain molecule constructed via phosphate ester bond condensation. RNA is transcribed from a DNA template (one chain) according to base complementarity, and its function is to serve as a bridge to transmit and realize the expression of genetic information in protein. RNA mainly includes mRNA, tRNA, rRNA, and miRNA among others (Table 23.6.1).

RNA structure includes the primary sequence, secondary structure and tertiary structure. Complementary RNA sequences are the basis of secondary

Table 23.6.1. Main RNA species and functions.

Species	Function
Messenger RNA (mRNA)	Template for protein synthesis
Ribosome RNA (rRNA)	Ribosome component
Transfer RNA (tRNA)	Transport of amino acids
Heterogeneous nuclear RNA (hnRNA)	Precursor of mature mRNA
Small nuclear RNA (snRNA)	Shearing and transfer of hnRNA
Small nucleolar RNA (snoRNA)	Processing and modification of rRNA
Small cytoplasmic RNA	Composed of synthetic signal of directed synthesis protein in endoplasmic reticulum
Small interfering RNA (siRNA)	Always exogenous, degrades complementary mRNA
microRNA (miRNA)	Always endogenous, degrades mRNA or hinders translation

structure, and the formation of conserved secondary structures via complementary nucleotides is more important than sequence. Prediction methods for RNA secondary structure mainly include sequence comparative analysis and predictive analysis. They are divided into the largest number of base pairing algorithm and the minimum free energy algorithm based on different scoring functions, and they are divided into the dot matrix method and dynamic programming method based on the calculation method.

Herein, we simply introduce some database and analysis software for RNA structure and function:

tRNAscan-SE(http://lowelab.ucsc.edu/tRNAscan-SE/): a tRNA data base;

Rfam(http://rfam.sanger.ac.uk/ and in the US at http://rfam.janelia.org/): an RNA family database;

NONCODE(http://www.noncode.org): a non-coding RNA database;

PNRD(http://structuralbiology.cau.edu.cn/PNRD): a database of non-coding RNA in plants;

PLncDB(http://chualab.rockefeller.edu/gbrowse2/homepage.html): a data base of long non-coding RNA in plants;

RNAmmer1.2: predictive rRNA;

RNAdraw: software for RNA secondary structure;

RNAstructure: software for RNA secondary structure;

RnaViz: drawing program for RNA secondary structure;

Pattern Search and Discovery: the common online RNA tools provided by Institute Pasteur;

Ridom: bacterial rRNA analysis;

ARWEN: detection of tRNA in mtDNA;

LocARNA: multiple sequence alignment of RNA;

CARNA: multiple sequence alignment of RNA sequences;

CONTRAfold: prediction of secondary structure.

23.7. Protein Sequence Analysis[15,16]

Protein sequence analysis, also called feature analysis or physicochemical property analysis, mainly includes the molecular weight of proteins, amino acid composition, isoelectric point, extinction coefficient, hydrophilicity and hydrophobicity, transmembrane domains, signal peptides, and modification sites after translation, among other information. Expert Protein Analysis System (ExPASy) can be used to retrieve the physicochemical property features of an unknown protein to identify its category, which can serve as a reference for further experiments.

Hydrophilicity or hydrophobicity is analyzed using the ProtScale web in ExPASy. There are three types of amino acids in proteins: hydrophobic amino acids, polar amino acids and charged amino acids. Hydrophilicity and hydrophobicity provide the main driving force for protein folding, and the hydropathy profile can thus reflect protein folding. ProtScale provides 57 scales, including molecular mass, number of codons, swelling capacity, polarity, coefficient of refraction and recognition factor.

A protein in a biological membrane is called a membrane protein, and such proteins perform the main functions of biological membranes. The difficulty of protein isolation and distributed location are used to classify membrane proteins into extrinsic membrane proteins and intrinsic membrane proteins. An extrinsic membrane protein spans throughout the entire double lipid layer, and both ends are exposed inside and outside the membrane. The percentages of membrane proteins are similar in different species, and approximately a quarter of known human proteins are identified as membrane proteins. It is difficult to identify their structures because membrane proteins are insoluble, difficult to isolate and difficult to crystallize. Therefore, the prediction of transmembrane helices in membrane proteins

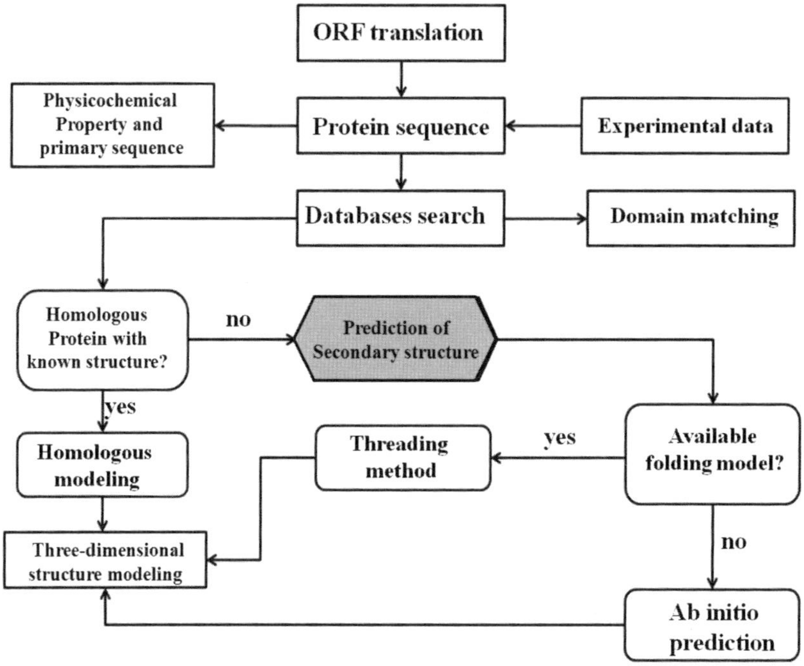

Fig. 23.7.1. Process of protein structure prediction.

is an important application of bioinformatics. Based on the current transmembrane helical TMbase database (TMbase is derived from Swiss-Prot with additional information, including the number of transmembrane structures, location of membrane spanning domain, and flanking sequences), the TMHMM and DNAMAN software programs can be used to predict transmembrane helices.

TMHMM integrates various characteristics, including the hydrophobicity of the transmembrane domain, bias of charge, length of helix, and limitation of membrane protein topology, and Hidden Markov Models are used to integrally predict the transmembrane domains and the inside and outside membrane area. TMHMM is the best available software to predict transmembrane domains, especially to distinguish soluble proteins and membrane proteins, and therefore, it can be used to predict whether an unknown protein is a membrane protein. DNAMAN, developed by the Lynnon Biosoft company, can perform almost all common analyses of nucleotide and protein sequences, including multiple sequence alignment, PCR primer design, restriction enzyme analysis, protein analysis and plasmid drawing. Furthermore, the TMpred webserver developed by EMBnet also predicts transmembrane domains and the transmembrane direction based on statistical analysis in the TMbase database.

The overall accuracy of prediction software programs is not above 52%, but more than 86% of transmembrane domains can be predicted using various software. Integrating the prediction results and hydrophobic profiles from different tools can contribute to higher prediction accuracies.

23.8. Protein Structure Analysis[17,18]

Protein structure is the spatial structure of a protein. All proteins are polymers containing 20 types of L-type α-amino acids, which are also called residues after proteins are formed. When proteins are folded into specific configurations via plentiful non-covalent interactions (such as hydrogen bonds, ionic bonds, Van der Waals forces and the hydrophobic effect), they can perform biological function. Moreover, in the folding of specific proteins, especially secretory proteins, disulfide bonds also play a pivotal role. To understand the mechanisms of proteins at the molecular level, their three-dimensional structures are determined.

The molecular structures of proteins are divided into four levels to describe different aspects: primary structure, the linear amino acid sequence of the polypeptide chain; secondary structure: the stable structures formed via hydrogen bonding of C=O and N–H between different amino acids, mainly including α helix and β sheet; tertiary structure, the three-dimensional structure of the protein in space formed via the interaction of secondary structure elements; and quaternary structure, functional protein complex molecule formed via the interactions of different polypeptide chains (subunits).

Primary structure is the basis of protein structure, while the spatial structure includes secondary structure, three-dimensional structure and quaternary structure. Specifically, secondary structure indicates the local spatial configuration of the main chain and does not address the conformation of side chains. Super-secondary structure indicates proximate interacting secondary structures in the polypeptide chain, which form regular aggregations in folding. The domain is another level of protein conformation between secondary structure and three-dimensional structure, and tertiary structure is defined as the regular three-dimensional spatial structure produced via further folding of secondary structures. Quarternary structure is the spatial structure formed by secondary bonds between two or more independent tertiary structures.

The prediction of protein structures mainly involves theoretical analysis and statistical analysis (Figure 23.7.1). Special software programs include Predict Protein, which can be used to predict secondary structure; InterProScan, which can predict structural domains; and SWISS-MODEL/SWISS-PdbViewer, which can be used to analyze tertiary structure.

Structural biology is developed based on protein structure research and aims to analyze protein structures using X-ray crystallography, nuclear magnetic resonance, and other techniques.

23.9. Molecular Evolution Analysis[19,20]

Evolution has been examined at the molecular evolution level since the mid-20th century with the development of molecular biology, and a set of theories and methods have been established based on nucleotides and proteins. The huge amount of genomic information now available provides strong assistance in addressing significant problems in biological fields. With the whole-genome sequencing project, molecular evolution has become one of the most remarkable fields in life science. These significant issues include the origin of genetic codes, formation and evolution of the genome structure, evolution drivers, biological evolution, and more. At present, the study of molecular evolution is mainly focused on molecular sequences, and studies at the genome level to explore the secrets of evolution will create a new frontier.

Molecular evolution analysis aims to study biological evolution through constructing evolutionary trees based on the similarities and differences of the same gene sequences in different species. These gene sequences may be DNA sequences, amino acid sequences, or comparisons of protein structures, based on the hypothesis of the similarity of genes in similar organisms. The similarities and differences can be obtained through comparison between different species. In the early stages, extrinsic factors are collected as markers in evolution, including size, color and number of limbs. With the completion of genome sequencing in more model organisms, molecular evolution can be studied at the genome level. In mapping to genes in different species, there are three conditions: orthologous, genes in different species with the same function; paralogous: genes in the same species with different functions; and xenologs: genes transiting between organisms via other methods, such as genes injected by a virus. The most commonly used method is to construct an evolutionary tree based on a feature (special region in DNA or protein sequence), distance (alignment score) and traditional clustering method (such as UPGMA).

The methods used to construct evolutionary trees mainly include distance matrix methods, where distances are estimated between pairwise species. The quality of the tree depends on the quality of the distance scale, and calculation is direct and always depends on the genetic model. Maximum parsimony, which is rarely involved in genetic hypotheses, is performed by seeking the smallest alteration between species. Maximum likelihood (ML) is highly dependent on the model and provides a basis for statistical inference but is computationally complex. The methods used to construct trees based on evolutionary distances include the unweighted pair-group method with arithmetic means (UPGMA), Neighbor-Joining method (NJ), maximum parsimony (MP), ML, and others. Some software programs can be used to construct trees, such as MEGA, PAUP, PHYLIP, PHYML, PAML and BioEdit. The types of tree mainly include rooted tree and unrooted tree, gene tree and species tree, expected tree and reality tree, and topological distance. Currently, with the rapid development of genomics, genomic methods and results are being used to study issues of biological evolution, attracting increased attention from biological researchers.

23.10. Analysis of Expressed Sequences[21,22]

Expressed sequences refer to RNA sequences that are expressed by genes, mostly mRNA. Expressed sequence tags (ESTs) are obtained from sequenced cDNA in tissues or cells via large-scale random picking, and their lengths are always from dozens of bp to 500 bp. Most of them are incomplete gene sequences, but they carry parts of genetic sequences. EST has been the most useful type of marker in studying gene expression because it is simple and cheap and can be rapidly obtained. In 1993, database of ESTs (dbEST) was specifically established by NCBI to collect and conserve EST sequences and detailed annotations, and it has been among the most useful EST databases. Other EST databases have been developed, including UniGene, Gene Indices, REDB, Mendel-ESTS and MAGEST, and dbEST. The UniGene and Gene Indices databases have been frequently used because of their abundant data.

ESTs are called a window for genes and can reflect a specific expressed gene in a specific time and tissue in an organism. ESTs have wide application: for example, they can be used to draw physical profiles, recognize genes, establish gene expression profiles, discover novel genes, perform silico PCR cloning, and discover SNPs. The quality of ESTs should be preprocessed and reviewed before clustering and splicing, and EST analysis mainly includes data preprocessing, clustering, splicing and annotation of splicing results. The first three of these steps are the precondition and basis for annotation.

The preprocessing of ESTs includes fetching sequences, deleting sequences with low quality, screening out artifactual sequences that are not expressed genes using BLAST, Repeat Masker or Crossmatch, deleting embedded cloned sequences, and deleting shorter sequences (less than 100 bp). Clustering analysis of ESTs is a method to simplify a large-scale dataset via partitioning specific groups (categories) based on similarity or correlation, and EST sequences with overlap belonging to the same gene can be clustered together. EST clustering analysis includes loose clustering and stringent clustering, and clustering and assembly are a continuous process, also termed EST sequence assembly. The same types of sequences can be assembled into longer contigs after clustering. The common clustering and assembly software programs include Phrap, which can assemble the whole reads with higher accuracy based on a swat algorithm and can be used to assemble shotgun sequencing sequences; CAP3, which is used to perform clustering and assembly analysis of DNA sequences and can eliminate regions with low quality at the 3' and 5' ends; TIGR Assembler, a tool used to assemble contigs using mass DNA fragments from shotgun sequencing; and Staden Package, an integrated package used in sequencing project management, including sequence assembly, mutation detection, sequence analysis, peak sequence diagramming and processing of reads.

23.11. Gene Regulation Network[23,24]

With the completion of the HGP and rapid development of bioinformatics, studies on complex diseases have been performed at the molecular level and examining systematic aspects, and research models have changed from "sequence-structure-function" to "interaction-network-function". Because complex diseases always involve many intrinsic and extrinsic factors, research at multiple levels that integrates the genes and proteins associated with diseases and the combined transcriptional regulatory network and metabolic pathways can contribute to revealing the occurrence of regularity in complex diseases.

There are many networks of different levels and forms in biological systems. The most common biomolecular networks include genetic transcriptional regulatory networks, biological metabolism and signaling networks, and protein-protein interaction networks. Gene expression regulation can occur at each level in the genetic information transmission process, and the regulation of transcription is the most important and complex step and the important research topic. A gene regulatory network is a network containing gene interactions within cells (or a specific genome), and in many cases, it also particularly refers to gene interaction based on gene regulation.

Currently, there are many software programs designed to visually represent and analyze biomolecular networks.

CytoScape: This software program can not only represent a network but also further analyze and edit the network with abundant annotation. It can be used to perform in-depth analysis on the network using its own or other functional plug-in tools developed by third parties.

CFinder software: This software program is used to search and visualize based on overall collection methods and network modules, and it can search connected sets of specific sizes to further construct larger node groups via the shared nodes and edges.

mfinder and MAVisto software: These two software programs are used to search network motifs: mfinder is used by entering commands, while MAVisto contains a graphical interface.

BGL software package and Matlabbgl software: The BGL software can be used to analyze network topology properties, which can rapidly estimate the distance of nodes, the shortest path, many topological properties and the prior ergodicity of width and depth. Matlabbgl is developed based on BGL and can be used to perform network analysis and computation based on the Matlab platform.

Pathway Studio software: This program is business bioinformatics software, and the visualization software can be used to draw and analyze biological pathways in different models.

GeneGO software and database: GeneGO is a supplier that can provide software solutions for chemoinformatics and bioinformatics data mining in systems biology, and the main products include MetaBase, MetaCore, and MetaDrug among others.

Most studies are performed on two levels, such as disease and gene, disease and pathway, disease and SNP, disease and miRNA, drug and target protein, or SNP and gene expression. A bipartite network is constructed to integrate information at both levels and to analyze the characteristics of the network or reconstructed network. Information from multiple disciplines can then be integrated, studied and analyzed, as the integration of multiple dimensions is an important method in studying complex diseases.

23.12. High-throughput Detection Techniques[8,25]

Currently, widely applied high-throughput detection techniques mainly include gene chip and high-throughput sequencing techniques. The gene chip, also termed the DNA chip or biochip, is a method for detecting unknown nucleotides via hybridization with a series of known nucleic acid probes, and

Table 23.12.1. Mainstream sequencing platforms.

Company	Technical principle	Technology developers
Applied Biosystems (ABI)	Massively parallel cloning connect DNA sequencing method based on beads	Agencourt Bioscience Corp. in America
Illumina	Sequencing by synthesis	David Bentley, a chief scientist in Solexa in England
Roche	Massively parallel pyrophosphate synthesis sequencing method	Jonathan Rothber, originator of 454 Life Sciences in America
Helicos	Massively parallel single molecule synthesis sequencing method	Stephen Quake, bioengineer at Stanford University in America

its theory is based on hybridization sequencing methods. Some known target probes are fixed on the surface of a chip. When fluorescently labeled nucleotide sequences are complementary to the probes, the set of complementary sequences can be obtained based on determination of the strongest fluorescence intensity. Thus, the target nucleotide sequences can be recombined.

The gene chip was ranked among the top 10 advances in natural science in 1998 by the American Association for the Advancement of Science, and it has been widely applied in many fields in life science. It has enormous power to simultaneously analyze genomes with speed and accuracy, and it is used to detect gene expression, mutation detection, genome polymorphism analysis, gene library construction and sequencing by hybridization.

DNA sequencing techniques are used to determine DNA sequences. The new generation sequencing products include the 454 genome sequencing system from Roche Applied Science, Illumina sequencers developed by the Illumina company in America and the Solexa technology company in England, the SOLiD sequencer from Applied Biosystems, the Polonator sequencer from Dover/Harvard and the HeliScope Single Molecule Sequencer from the Helicos company. DNA sequencing techniques have been widely applied throughout every field of biological studies, and many biological problems can be solved by applying high-throughput sequencing techniques (Table 23.12.1).

The rapid development of DNA sequencing methods has prompted research such as screening for disease-susceptible populations, the identification of pathogenic or disease suppression genes, high-throughput drug design and testing, and personalized medicine, and revealing the biological significance of sequences has become a new aim for scientists. High-throughput methods can be applied to many types of sequencing, including whole genome, transcriptome and metagenome, and further provide new methods of post-genomic analysis. Moreover, sequencing techniques provide various data at reasonable costs to allow deep and comprehensive analysis of the interactions among the genome, transcriptome and metagenome. Sequencing will soon become a widespread normal experimental method, which will bring revolutionary changes to biological and biomedical research, especially contributing to the solution of many biological and medical mysteries.

23.13. Analysis of Expression Profile[26,27]

One of the most important features of expression profiles is that the number of detected genes is always in the thousands or even tens of thousands, but there may be only dozens or hundreds of corresponding samples due to cost and sample source. Sample sizes are far smaller than gene numbers; there are more random interference factors and larger detection errors, and expression profiles have typical problems of high dimensionality and high noise. Simultaneously, from the perspective of taxonomy, many genes are insignificant because genes with similar functions always have highly related expression levels. Therefore, dimension reduction processing is highly important for expression data. These methods mainly include feature selection and feature extraction.

There are three levels of expression data analysis: single gene analysis aims to obtain differentially expressed genes; multiple gene analysis aims to analyze common functions and interactions; and system level analysis aims to establish gene regulatory networks to analyze and understand biological phenomena. The common categories of research methods include non-supervised methods and supervised methods: the former are used to cluster similar modes according to a distance matrix without additional class information, such as clustering analysis; and the latter require class information on objects other than gene expression data, including the functional classification of genes and pathological classification of samples.

Frequently used software programs for expression profile analysis mainly include (in the case of microarray expression data):

ArrayTools: BRB-ArrayTools is an integrated software package for analyzing gene chip data. It can handle expression data from different microarray platforms and two-channel methods and is used for data visualization, standard processing, screening of differentially expressed genes, clustering analysis, categorical forecasting, survival analysis and gene enrichment analysis. The ArrayTools software provides user-friendly presentation through Excel, and computation is performed by external analysis tools.

DChip (DNA-Chip Analyzer): This software aims to analyze gene expression profiles and SNPs at the probe level from microarrays and can also analyze relevant data from other chip analysis platforms.

SAM: SAM is a statistical method of screening differentially expressed genes. The input is a gene expression matrix and corresponding response variable, and the output is a differential gene table (up-regulated and down-regulated genes), δ values and evaluation of the sample size.

Cluster and TreeView: Cluster is used to perform cluster analysis of data from a DNA chip, and TreeView can be used to interactively visualize clustering results. The clustering functions include data filtering, standard processing, hierarchical clustering, K-means clustering, SOM clustering and principal component analysis (PCA).

BioConductor: This software is mainly used to preprocess data, visualize data, and analyze and annotate gene expression data.

Bioinformatics Toolbox: This software is a tool used to analyze genomes and proteomes, developed based on MATLAB, and its functions include data formatting and database construction, sequence analysis, evolution analysis, statistical analysis and calling other software programs.

23.14. Gene Annotation[28,29]

With the advent of the post-genome era, the research focus of genomics has been changed to functional study at all molecular levels after clarifying all the genetic information, and the most important factor is the generation of functional genomics. The focus of bioinformatics is to study the biological significance of sequences, processes and the result of the transcription and translation of coding sequences, mainly analyzing gene expression regulation information and the functions of genes and their products. Herein, we introduce common annotation systems for genes and their products, tools, and analyses developed based on gene set function analysis and the functional prediction of gene products.

Gene Ontology (GO database): GO mainly establishes the ontology of genes and their products, including cellular components, molecular functions and biological processes, and has been among the most widely used gene annotation systems.

The Kyoto Encyclopedia of Genes and Genomes (KEGG) is a database for the systematic analysis of gene function and genome information, integrating genomics, biochemistry and system functional proteomics, which contributes to performing studies as a whole on genes and their expression.

The characteristic feature of the KEGG database is to integrate the analysis of screened genes with the system functions of higher classes of cells, species and ecological systems. Based on estimated capture and experimental knowledge, this artificially created knowledge base is similar to the computer simulation of biological systems. Compared with other databases, a significant feature of KEGG is that it has strong graphic functions to present multiple metabolic pathways and relationships between different pathways instead of heavy documentation, which can provide an intuitive comprehensive understanding of target metabolic pathways.

Based on consistent prior biological knowledge from published co-expression or biological pathways, gene sets are always first defined using GO or KEGG. Biological pathways are analyzed based on known gene interactions, and gene function is predicted using GO or KEGG, including the functional prediction of differentially expressed genes and protein interaction networks, along with the comparison of gene function.

The common function prediction software programs mainly include software based on GO, such as expressing analysis systematic explorer (EASE), developed by NIH; Onto-Express, developed by the University of Detroit's Wayne; and the Rosetta system, developed by the University of Norway and Uppsala University; and software programs based on KEGG, such as GenMAPP, Pathway Miner, KOBAS, and GEPAT. These software programs developed based on GO and KEGG perform annotation, enrichment analysis and function prediction from different angles.

23.15. Epigenetics Analysis[18,30]

Epigenetics is a branch discipline of genetics that studies heritable changes in gene expression without involving the variation of nucleotide sequences. In biology, epigenetics indicates various changes in gene expression, and the changes are stable in cell division and even atavism but without involving the variation of DNA. That is, the gene is not varied, although environmental factors may lead to differential gene expression. Epigenetics phenomena of are quite abundant, including DNA methylation, genomic imprinting, maternal effects, gene silencing, nucleolar dominance, the activation of dormancy transposons and RNA editing.

Taking DNA methylation as an example, the recognition of CpG mainly includes two strategies: prediction methods based on bioinformatics algorithms and experimental methods, represented by restriction endonucleases. Genome-wide DNA methylation detection has been widely applied, such as in commercial oligonucleotide arrays, including microarray beads developed by Illumina, flat-panel arrays developed by Affymetrix and NimbleGen, and an ink-jet array developed by Agilent. The prediction methods for DNA methylation are mainly integrated models based on discrimination models of sequences and other epigenetic modifications, including cytosine methylation prediction from DNA sequences, prediction based on CpG sites (Methylator), and prediction of CpG islands based on sequence features (HDMFinder, where genomic features contribute to the recognition of CpG methylation).

Some researchers have established databases for storing experimental epigenetics data and have developed relevant algorithms to analyze genome sequences. The frequently used databases and software programs are as follows:

Commonly used databases: The HEP aims to determine, record and interpret genomic DNA methylation patterns in all the human genes in major tissues. HHMD contains the tool HisModView to visualize histone modification, which examines the relationship of histone modification and DNA methylation via understanding the distribution of histone modification against the background of genome annotation. MethyCancer aims to study the interactions of DNA methylation, gene expression and tumors.

Commonly used software programs: EpiGraph is a user-friendly software program used for epigenome analysis and prediction and can be used to perform bioinformatics analysis of complex genome and epigenome datasets. Methylator is a program for predicting the methylation status of dinucleotide cytosine in CpG using SVM and has higher accuracy than other traditional machine learning methods (such as neural network and Bayesian statistics). CpG_MI is a program to identify genomic function based on the recognition of mutual information, which has higher prediction accuracy, and most recognized CpG islands have correlated with histone modification areas. CpG_MI does not depend on limiting the length of CpG islands, in contrast to traditional methods.

Due to epigenetics, acquired heredity has attracted attention again and has become one of the hottest fields in life science in just a few years.

23.16. SNP Analysis[31,32]

Single nucleotide polymorphism (SNP) indicates DNA sequence polymorphism caused by a single nucleotide mutation in the genome. It is the commonest variation among human autogenous variations and accounts for more than 90% of known polymorphisms. SNPs occur widely in the human genome: there is a SNP every 500–1000 bp, and the total number may be

3,000,000 or more. This type of polymorphism involves only in the variation of a single nucleotide, mainly derived from transition or transversion, or insertion or deletion, but generally the SNP is not based on insertion or deletion. SNPs have been studied as tags because the features can be adapted to study complex traits and perform genetic dissection of the disease, as well as gene recognition based on population.

As a new generation of genetic marker, SNPs have characteristics including higher quantity, widespread distribution and high density, and they have been widely applied in genetic research. The important SNP databases include dbSNP and dbGap. To meet the needs of genome-wide variations and large-scale sampling design for association study, gene mapping, function and pharmacogenetics, population genetics, evolutionary biology, positional cloning and physical mapping, NCBI and NHGRI collaboratively created dbSNP. The functions of dbSNP mainly include genetic variation sequence analysis, the cross-annotation of genetic variation based on NCBI, the integration of exterior resources and the functional analysis of genetic variation. Moreover, the dbGap database of genotype and phenotype, established by NCBI, mainly stores and releases data and results on relevant genotype and phenotypes, including genome-wide association study, medical sequencing, diagnostic molecular science, and associations of genotypes and non-clinical features.

The genetic location of SNPs in complex diseases, including sample selection criteria, linkage analysis, association analysis and choice of statistical analysis, will have significant implications for obtaining specific pathogenic factors based on accurate definition or refining the classification levels of diseases.

There are some commonly used integrated software. For example, the Plink software is an open and free tool to analyze genome wide association, and its basis is genotype and phenotype data. The Haploview software developed by the University of Cambridge can recognize TagSNP and infer haplotypes, and its analysis modules include linkage disequilibrium analysis, haplotype analysis, TagSNP analysis, association study and stability of permutation tests. SNPtest is a strong package analyzing genome-wide association studies that can perform association at a genome-wide scale and frequency testing or Bayes testing for single SNP association. The analysis modules in SNPtest include statistical description, Hardy–Weinberg equilibrium testing, basic correlation testing and Bayes test. Merlin is a package for pedigree analysis based on a sparse genetic tree that indicates genes in a pedigree. Merlin can be used to perform parametric or non-parametric linkage analysis, linkage analysis based on regression, association analysis for quantitative character, estimation of IBD and domestic relation, haplotype analysis, error detection and simulation analysis.

23.17. ncRNA and Complex Disease[18,33,34]

Non-coding RNA (ncRNA) indicates RNA that does not encode protein, including many types of RNA with known or unknown function, such as rRNA, tRNA, snRNA, snoRNA, lncRNA and microRNA (miRNA), and ncRNAs can play important roles in complex diseases. Some ncRNA and diseases databases have been reported, including LncRNADisease (association of lncRNA and disease) and miR2Disease (relevant miRNAs in human disease). Herein, taking miRNA as an example due to the larger number of studies, we mainly introduce the relationships of miRNA and complex disease.

miRNA polymorphism and complex disease: Polymorphisms of miRNA can influence miRNA function at different levels, at any stage from the generation of miRNA to its function. There are three types of miRNA polymorphism: (1) polymorphism in miRNA can affect the formation and function of miRNA; (2) polymorphism in target mRNA can affect the regulatory relationships of miRNA and target mRNA; (3) polymorphism can change drug reactions and miRNA gene epigenetic regulation.

miRNA expression profiles and complex disease: Expression profiles of miRNA can be used to identify cancer-related miRNAs. For example, using miRNA expression profiles from a gene chip or sequencing platform, differentially expressed miRNAs after normalization are further experimentally identified. These identified abnormal miRNAs and their dysfunction can contribute to the occurrence of cancers via regulating transcriptional changes to the target mRNAs. Simultaneously, miRNA expression profiles can be used to classify human cancers through hierarchical clustering analysis, using the average link algorithm and Pearson correlation coefficient, of samples and miRNAs, respectively. The integrated analysis of miRNA and mRNA expression profiles contributes to improving accuracy and further revealing the roles of miRNA in the occurrence and development of disease. Thus, miRNA may be a new potential marker for disease diagnosis and prognosis because of its important biological functions, such as the regulation of cell signaling networks, metabolic networks, transcriptional regulatory networks, protein interaction networks and miRNA regulation networks.

Current canonical miRNA databases include TarBase and miRBase: TarBase is a database of the relationships of miRNA and target mRNA, and miRBase contains miRNA sequences and the annotation and prediction of target mRNAs and is one of the main public databases of miRNAs. There are also other relevant databases, including miRGen, MiRNAmap and microRNA.org, and many analysis platforms for miRNA, such as miRDB, DeepBase, miRDeep, SnoSeeker, miRanalyzer and mirTools, all of which provide convenient assistance for miRNA study.

Some scientists predict that ncRNAs have important roles in biological development that are not secondary to proteins. However, the ncRNA world is little understood, and the next main task is to identify more ncRNAs and their biological functions. This task is more difficult than the HGP and requires long-term dedication. If we can clearly understand the ncRNA regulatory network, it will be the final breakthrough for revealing the mysteries of life.

23.18. Drug Design[35]

One of the aims of the HGP is to understand protein structure, function, interaction and association with human diseases, and then to seek treatment and prevention methods, including drug therapy. Drug design based on the structure of biological macromolecules and micromolecules is an important research field in bioinformatics. To inhibit the activities of enzymes or proteins, a molecule inhibitor can be designed as a candidate drug using a molecular alignment algorithm based on the tertiary structure of the protein. The aim of the field is to find new gene-based medicines and has great economic benefits.

DNA sequences are initially analyzed to obtain coding regions, and then the relevant protein spatial structure is predicted and simulated, and the drug is designed according to the protein function (Figure 23.18.1). The main topics are as follows: (1) the design, establishment and optimization of biological databases; (2) the development of algorithms for the effective extraction of information from the database; (3) interface design for user queries; (4) effective methods for data visualization; (5) effective connection of various sources and information; (6) new methods for data analysis; and (7) prediction algorithms for the prediction of new products, new functions, disease diagnosis and therapy.

Software programs for drug design include MOE, developed by CCG Company in Canada, which is an integrated software system for molecular simulation and drug design. It integrates visualization, simulation, application and development. MOE can comprehensively support drug design through molecular simulation, protein structure analysis, small molecular

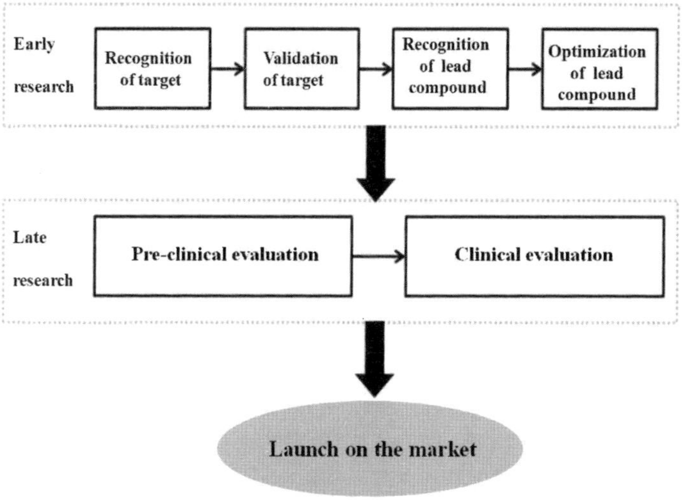

Fig. 23.18.1. Study and development of drug.

processing, and docking of protein and micromolecule under the unified operating environment. The InsightII3D package developed by Accelrys Company integrates sets of tools from functional research on biological molecules to target-based drug design and assists the performance of theoretical research and specific experimental design. InsightII can provide modeling and visualization of biological molecules and small organic molecules, functional analysis tools, structure transformation tools and dynamics simulation tools, helping to understand the structure and function of molecules to specifically design experimental schemes, improve experimental efficiency and reduce research costs. MolegroVirtualDocker, another drug design software program, can predict the docking of a protein and small molecule, and the software provides all the functions needed during molecular docking. It produces docking results with high accuracy and has a simple and user-friendly window interface. SYBYL contributes to understanding the structure and properties of molecules, especially the properties of new chemical entities, through combining computational chemistry and molecular simulation. Therefore, SYBYL can provide the user with solutions to molecular simulations and drug design.

Bioinformatics is highly necessary for the research and development of modern drugs and for the correlation of bioinformatics data and tools with biochemistry, pharmacology, medicine and combinatorial chemical libraries, which can provide more convenient and rapid methods to improve quality, efficiency, and prediction accuracy in drug research and development.

23.19. Bioinformatics Software[36–38]

Bioinformatics can be considered as a combination of molecular biology and information technology (especially internet technology). The research materials and results of bioinformatics are various biological data, the research tool is the computer, and the research method is search (collection and screening) and processing (editing, reduction, management and visualization). Herein, we introduce some commonly used software programs for data analysis at different levels:

Conventional data processing:

(1) Assembly of small DNA fragments: Phredphrap, velvet, and others;
(2) Sequence similarity search: BLAST, BLAT, and others;
(3) Multiple sequence alignment: Clustalx and others;
(4) Primer design: Primer, oligo, and others;
(5) Analysis of enzyme site: restrict and others;
(6) Processing of DNA sequences: extractseq, seqret, and others.

Feature analysis of sequences:

(1) Feature analysis of DNA sequences: GENSCAN can recognize ORFs, POLYAH can predict transcription termination signals, PromoterScan predicts promoter regions, and CodonW analyzes codon usage bias;
(2) Feature analysis of protein sequences: ProtParam analyzes the physical and chemical properties, ProtScale analyzes hydrophilicity or hydrophobicity, TMpred analyzes transmembrane domains, and Antheprot analyzes protein sequence;
(3) Integrated analysis of sequences: EMBOSS, DNAStar, Omiga 2.0, VectorNTI, and others.

Expression profile analysis from gene chip (please see Sec. 23.13).

High throughput sequencing data analysis:

(1) Sequence alignment and assembly (please see Table 23.19.1).
(2) SNP analysis in resequencing data: MAQ, SNP calling, and others;
(3) CNV analysis: CBS, CMDS, CnvHMM, and others;
(4) RNA-seq analysis: HISAT, StringTie, Ballgown, and others;
(5) miRNA-seq analysis: miRDeep, miRNAkey, miRExpress, DSAP, and others;

Table 23.19.1. Tools to analyze small DNA fragments.

Name of software	Function
Cross_match	Sequence alignment
ELAND	Sequence alignment
Exonerate	Sequence alignment
MAQ	Sequence alignment and detection of variation
ALLPATHS	Sequence assembly
Edena	Sequence assembly
Euler-SR	Sequence assembly
SHARCGS	Sequence assembly
SHRAP	Sequence assembly

(6) Annotation: ANNOVAR, BreakSeq, Seattle Seq, and others;
(7) Data visualization: Avadis, CIRCOS, IGV, and others;
(8) Detection of fusion genes: BreakFusion, Chimerascan, Comrad, and others.

Molecular evolution:

(1) The MEGA software is used to test and analyze the evolution of DNA and protein sequences; (2) the Phylip package is used to perform phylogenetic tree analysis of nucleotides and proteins; (3) PAUP* is used to construct evolutionary trees (phylogenetic trees) and to perform relevant testing.

23.20. Systems Biology[36–38]

Systems biology is the subject studying all of the components (gene, mRNA, protein, and others) in biological systems and the interactions of these components in specific conditions. Unlike previous experimental biology concerning only selected genes and proteins, systems biology studies all the interactions of all the genes, proteins and components (Figure 23.20.1). The subject is a huge topic based on its integrality, a newly arising subject in life science, and a central driver of medicine and biology in the 21st century.

As a large integrative field of science, systems biology characteristics indicate new properties that occur via the interaction of different components and levels, and the analysis of components or lower levels does not

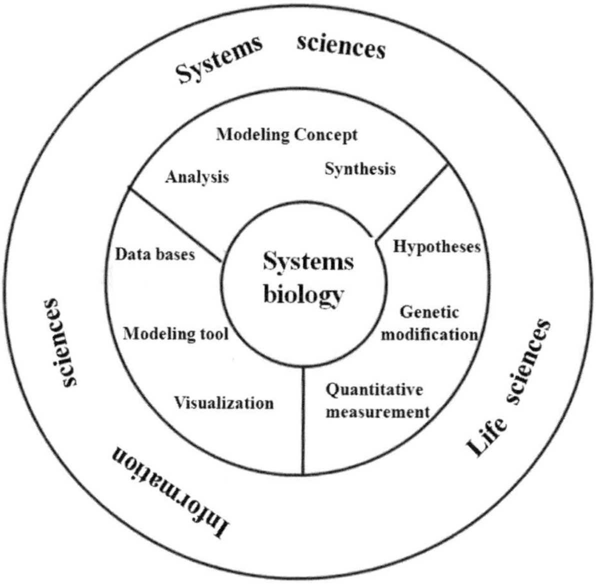

Fig. 23.20.1. Research methods in systems biology.

really predict higher levels of behavior. It is an essential challenge in systems biology to study and integrate analyses to find and understand these emergent properties. The typical molecular biology study is of the vertical type, which studies an individual gene and protein using multiple methods. Genomics, proteomics and other "omics" are studies of the horizontal type, simultaneously studying thousands of genes or proteins using a single method. Systems biology aims to become a "three-dimensional" study via combining horizontal and vertical research. Moreover, systems biology is also a typical multidisciplinary research field and can interact with other disciplines, such as life science, information science, statistics, mathematics and computer science.

Along with the deepening of research, comprehensive databases of multiple omics have been reported: protein–protein interaction databases, such as BOND, DIP and MINT; protein–DNA interaction databases, such as BIND and Transfac; databases of metabolic pathways, such as BioCyc and KEGG; and the starBase database, containing miRNA–mRNA, miRNA–lncRNA, miRNA–circRNA, miRNA–ceRNA and RNA-protein interactions in regulatory relationships.

According to different research purposes, there are many software programs and platforms integrating different molecular levels. Cytoscape, an open source analysis software program, aims to perform integrative analysis of data at multiple different levels using plug-ins. The CFinder software can be used to search network modules and perform visualization analysis based on the Clique Percolation Method (CPM), and its algorithm mainly focuses on undirected networks but it also contains processing functions of directed networks. The GeneGO software and database are commonly used data mining tools in systems biology.

The soul of systems biology is integration, but research levels have high variation in different biological molecules, as these different molecules have various difficulties and degrees of technology development. For example, genome and gene expression studies have been perfected, but the study of protein remains difficult, and the study of metabolism components involving small biological molecules is more immature. Therefore, it is a great challenge to truly integrate different molecular levels.

References

1. Pevsner, J. *Bioinformatics and Functional Genomics.* Hoboken: Wiley-Blackwell, 2009.
2. Xia, Li *et al. Bioinformatics* (1st edn.). Beijing: People's Medical Publishing House, 2010.
3. Xiao, Sun, Zuhong Lu, Jianming Xie. *Basics for Bioinformatics.* Tsinghua: Tsinghua University Press, 2005.
4. Fua, WJ, Stromberg, AJ, Viele, K, *et al.* Statistics and bioinformatics in nutritional sciences: Analysis of complex data in the era of systems biology. *J. Nutr. Biochem.* 2010, 21(7): 561–572.
5. Yi, D. An active teaching of statistical methods in bioinformatics analysis. *Medi. Inform.*, 2002, 6: 350–351.
6. NCBI Resource Coordinators. Database resources of the National Center for Biotechnology Information. *Nucleic Acids Res.* 2015 43(Database issue): D6–D17.
7. Tateno, Y, Imanishi, T, Miyazaki, S, *et al.* DNA Data Bank of Japan (DDBJ) for genome scale research in life science. *Nucleic Acids Res.*, 2002, 30(1): 27–30.
8. Wilkinson, J. New sequencing technique produces high-resolution map of 5-hydroxymethylcytosine. *Epigenomics*, 2012 4(3): 249.
9. Kodama, Y, Kaminuma, E, Saruhashi, S, *et al.* Biological databases at DNA Data Bank of Japan in the era of next-generation sequencing technologies. *Adv. Exp. Med. Biol.* 2010, 680: 125–135.
10. Tatusova, T. Genomic databases and resources at the National Center for Biotechnology Information. *Methods Mol. Biol.*, 2010; 609: 17–44.
11. Khan, MI, Sheel, C. OPTSDNA: Performance evaluation of an efficient distributed bioinformatics system for DNA sequence analysis. *Bioinformation*, 2013 9(16): 842–846.
12. Posada, D. Bioinformatics for DNA sequence analysis. *Preface. Methods Mol. Biol.*, 2011; 537: 101–109.
13. Gardner, PP, Daub, J, Tate, JG, *et al.* Rfam: Updates to the RNA families database. *Nucleic Acids. Res.*, 2008, 37(Suppl 1): D136–D140.

14. Peter, S, Angela, NB, Todd, ML. The tRNAscan-SE, snoscan and snoGPS web servers for the detection of tRNAs and snoRNAs. *Nucleic Acids Res.*, 2007, 33(suppl 2): W686–W689.
15. Krishnamurthy, N, Sjölander, KV. Basic protein sequence analysis. *Curr. Protoc. Protein Sci.* 2005, 2(11): doi: 10.1002/0471140864.ps0211s41.
16. Xu, D. Computational methods for protein sequence comparison and search. *Curr. Protoc. Protein. Sci.* 2009 Chapter 2: Unit2.1.doi:10.1002/0471140864.ps0201s56.
17. Guex, N, Peitsch, MC, Schwede, T. Automated comparative protein structure modeling with SWISS-MODEL and Swiss-PdbViewer: A historical perspective. *Electrophoresis.*, 2009 (1): S162–S173.
18. He, X, Chang, S, Zhang, J, *et al.* MethyCancer: The database of human DNA methylation and cancer. *Nucleic Acids Res.*, 2008, 36(1): 89–95.
19. Pandey, R, Guru, RK, Mount, DW. Pathway Miner: Extracting gene association networks from molecular pathways for predicting the biological significance of gene expression microarray data. *Bioinformatics*, 2004, 20(13): 2156–2158.
20. Tamura, K, Peterson, D, Peterson, N, *et al.* MEGA5: Molecular evolutionary genetics analysis using maximum likelihood, evolutionary distance, and maximum parsimony methods. *Mol. Biol. Evol.*, 2011, 28(10): 2731–2739.
21. Frazier, TP, Zhang, B. Identification of plant microRNAs using expressed sequence tag analysis. *Methods Mol. Biol.*, 2011, 678: 13–25.
22. Kim, JE, Lee, YM, Lee, JH, *et al.* Development and validation of single nucleotide polymorphism (SNP) markers from an Expressed Sequence Tag (EST) database in Olive Flounder (Paralichthysolivaceus). *Dev. Reprod.*, 2014, 18(4): 275–286.
23. Nikitin, A, Egorov, S, Daraselia, N, MazoI. Pathway studio — the analysis and navigation of molecular networks. *Bioinformatics*, 2003, 19(16): 2155–2157.
24. Yu, H, Luscombe, NM, Qian, J, Gerstein, M. Genomic analysis of gene expression relationships in transcriptional regulatory networks. *Trends. Genet.* 2003, 19(8): 422–427.
25. Ku, CS, Naidoo, N, Wu, M, Soong, R. Studying the epigenome using next generation sequencing. *J. Med. Genet.*, 2011, 48(11): 721–730.
26. Oba, S, Sato, MA, Takemasa, I, Monden, M, Matsubara, K, Ishii, S. A Bayesian missing value estimation method for gene expression profile data. *Bioinformatics*, 2003 19(16): 2088–2096.
27. Yazhou, Wu, Ling Zhang, Ling Liu *et al.* Identification of differentially expressed genes using multi-resolution wavelet transformation analysis combined with SAM. *Gene*, 2012, 509(2): 302–308.
28. Dahlquist, KD, Nathan, S, Karen, V, *et al.* GenMAPP, a new tool for viewing and analyzing microarray data on biological pathways. *Nat. Genet.*, 2002, 31(1): 19–20.
29. Marcel, GS, Feike, JL, Martinus, TG. Rosetta: A computer program for estimating soil hydraulic parameters with hierarchical pedotransfer functions. *J. Hydrol.*, 2001, 251(3): 163–176.
30. Bock, C, Von Kuster, G, Halachev, K, *et al.* Web-based analysis of (Epi-) genome data using EpiGRAPH and Galaxy. *Methods Mol. Biol.*, 2010, 628: 275–296.
31. Barrett, JC. Haploview: Visualization and analysis of SNP genotype data. *Cold Spring HarbProtoc.*, 2009, (10): pdb.ip71.
32. Kumar, A, Rajendran, V, Sethumadhavan, R, *et al.* Computational SNP analysis: Current approaches and future prospects. *Cell. Biochem. Biophys.*, 2014, 68(2): 233–239.
33. Veneziano, D, Nigita, G, Ferro, A. Computational Approaches for the Analysis of ncRNA through Deep Sequencing Techniques. *Front. Bioeng. Biotechnol.*, 2015, 3: 77.
34. Wang, X. miRDB: A microRNA target prediction and functional annotation database with a wiki interface. *RNA*, 2008, 14(6): 1012–1017.

35. Bajorath, J. Improving data mining strategies for drug design. *Future. Med. Chem.*, 2014, 6(3): 255–257.
36. Giannoulatou, E, Park, SH, Humphreys, DT, Ho, JW. Verification and validation of bioinformatics software without a gold standard: A case study of BWA and Bowtie. *BMC Bioinformatics*, 2014, 15(Suppl 16): S15.
37. Le, TC, Winkler, DA. A Bright future for evolutionary methods in drug design. *Chem. Med.* 2015, 10(8): 1296–1300.
38. LeprevostFda, V, Barbosa, VC, Francisco, EL, *et al.* On best practices in the development of bioinformatics software. *Front. Genet.* 2014, 5: 199.
39. Chauhan, A, Liebal, UW, Vera, J, *et al.* Systems biology approaches in aging research. *Interdiscip. Top Gerontol.*, 2015, 40: 155–176.
40. Chuang, HY, Hofree, M, Ideker, T. A decade of systems biology. *Annu. Rev. Cell. Dev. Biol.*, 2010, 26: 721–744.
41. Manjasetty, BA, Shi, W, Zhan, C, *et al.* A high-throughput approach to protein structure analysis. *Genet. Eng.* (NY). 2007, 28: 105–128.

About the Author

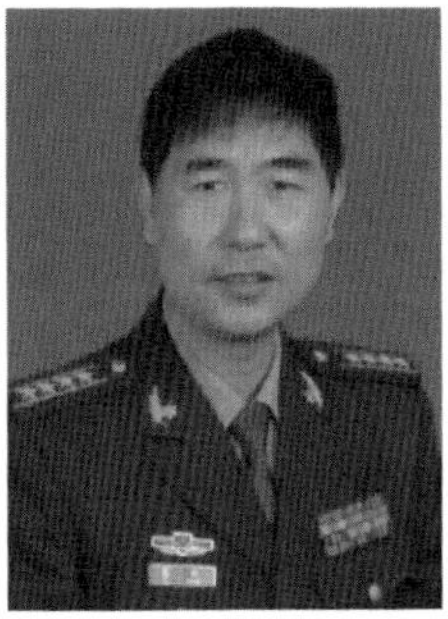

Dong Yi received a BSc in Mathematics in 1985, a MSc in Statistics in 1987, and a PhD in Computer Science in 1997 from Chongqing University. He finished a post-doc fellowship in Computer Science at Baptist University of Hong Kong in 1999 and joined the Division of Biostatistics in Third Military Medical University as Professor in 2002. His current teaching subjects are Medical Statistics/Health Statistics, Bioinformatics and Digital Image Processing and areas of research have primarily focused on the development of new statistical methods for health services research studies, for clinical trials with non-compliance, and for studies on the accuracy of diagnostic tests. In addition, he has been collaborating with other clinical researchers on research pertaining to health services, bioinformatics researches since 1999. He has been published a total of 31 peer-reviewed, SCI papers.

CHAPTER 24

MEDICAL SIGNAL AND IMAGE ANALYSIS

Qian Zhao*, Ying Lu and John Kornak

24.1. Random Signal[1,2]

Medical signal refers to the unary or multivariate function carrying the biological information, such as electrocardiogram signal, electroencephalograph signal and so on. Medical signals usually have randomness. For any $t \in T, X(t)$ is a random signal only if $X(t)$ is a random variable. When $T \subset R$ is a real set, $X(t)$ is called the continuous time signal or analog signal. When $T \subset Z$ is an integer set, $X(t)$ is called the discrete time signal or time series. A complex signal can be decomposed into some sinusoidal signals, where the sinusoidal is

$$X(t) = A\sin(2\pi ft + \varphi).$$

Here, A is amplitude, φ is initial phase and f is frequency, where amplitude and phase of random signal could vary over time. Random signal is also a stochastic process, which has the probability distribution and statistical characteristics such as mean, variance and covariance function, etc. (see Sec. 8.1 stochastic process). For the stationary of stochastic process, see Sec. 8.3 stationary process.

Non-stationary signal has the time-variant statistical characteristics, which is a function of time. This kind of signal often contains the information of tendency, seasonal or periodic characteristics. Cyclo-stationary signal is a special case of non-stationary signal, whose statistical characteristics is periodically stationary and can be expressed in the following forms: Mathematical expectation and correlation function of $X(t)$ are periodic functions

*Corresponding author: zhaoqian121@gmail.com

of time; Distribution function of $X(t)$ is a periodic function of time; The kth moment is a periodic function of time, where $k \leq n$, k and n are positive integers. The formulas for energy and power spectrum of random signal are

$$E\int_{-\infty}^{+\infty} X^2(t)dt = \int_{-\infty}^{+\infty} EX^2(t)dt$$

and

$$\lim_{T\to\infty}\frac{1}{2T}E\left|\int_{-T}^{+T} X(t)e^{-i\omega t}dt\right|^2$$
$$= \lim_{T\to\infty}\frac{1}{2T}\int_{-T}^{+T}\int_{-T}^{+T} E[X(t)\bar{X}(s)e^{-i\omega(t-s)}]dtds.$$

The inverse Fourier transform of power spectrum is the autocorrelation function of signal. Random signal system transforms between input and output signals. With the signal system T and input $X(t)$, the output $Y(t)$ is $T(X(t))$. Linear time invariant system satisfies linearity and time invariance at the same time. For any input signal $X_1(t)$ and $X_2(t)$, as well as constant a and b, linear system follows the linear rule as

$$T(aX_1(t) + bX_2(t)) = aT(X_1(t)) + bT(X_2(t)).$$

For any Δt, the time invariant system does not change the waveform of the output signal if the input is delayed. That is,

$$Y(t - \Delta t) = T(X(t - \Delta t)).$$

24.2. Signal Detection[3]

In medical signals, it usually requires to determine whether there exits a signal of interest. According to the number of detection assumptions, there are binary detection and multiple detections. The binary detection model is

$$H_0\colon x(t) = s_0(t) + n(t) \quad H_1\colon x(t) = s_1(t) + n(t).$$

where $x(t)$ is the observed signal and $n(t)$ is the additive noise. The question is to determine if source signal is $s_0(t)$ or $s_1(t)$.

The observation space D is divided into D_0 and D_1. If $x(t) \in D_0$, H_0 is determined to be true. Otherwise if $x(t) \in D_1$, H_1 is determined to be true. Under some criteria, the observation space D can be divided optimally.

(1) Bayesian Criterion: The cost factor C_{ij} indicates the cost to determine H_i is true when H_j is true. The mean cost is expressed as follows:

$$C = P(H_0)C(H_0) + P(H_1)C(H_1) = \sum_{j=0}^{1}\sum_{i=0}^{1} C_{ij}P(H_j)P(H_i|H_j),$$

$$C(H_j) = \sum_{i=0}^{1} C_{ij}P(H_i|H_j).$$

While minimizing the mean cost, we have

$$\frac{P(x|H_1)}{P(x|H_0)} \underset{H_0}{\overset{H_1}{\gtrless}} \frac{P(H_0)(C_{10} - C_{00})}{P(H_1)(C_{01} - C_{11})} = \eta,$$

where η is the test threshold for likelihood ratio.

(2) Minimum mean probability of error Criterion. When $C_{00} = C_{11} = 0$, $C_{10} = C_{10} = 1$, mean probability of error is

$$\bar{C} = P(H_0)P(H_1|H_0) + P(H_1)P(H_0|H_1).$$

While minimizing the mean probability of error, we have

$$\frac{p(x|H_1)}{p(x|H_0)} \underset{H_0}{\overset{H_1}{\gtrless}} \frac{P(H_0)}{P(H_1)}.$$

(3) Maximum likelihood Criterion: When $C_{00} = C_{11} = 0$, $C_{10} = C_{10} = 1$ and $P(H_0) = P(H_1) = 0.5$, we have

$$\frac{p(x|H_1)}{p(x|H_0)} \underset{H_0}{\overset{H_1}{\gtrless}} 1.$$

(4) Maximum a posteriori probability (MAP) Criterion: When $C_{10} - C_{00} = C_{01} - C_{11}$, we have

$$P(H_1|x) \underset{H_0}{\overset{H_1}{\gtrless}} P(H_0|x).$$

(5) Minimax Criterion: When cost factor C_{ij} is known and prior probability $P(H_0) = 1 - P(H_1)$ is unknown, the minimum mean cost $C_{\min}$ under Bayes Criterion is the function of $P(H_0)$. While maximizing $C_{\min}$, minimax equation is obtained to get the estimation of prior $P(H_0)$ and threshold η.

(6) Neyman–Pearson Criterion: When cost factor C_{ij} and prior probability $P(H_0)$ are both unknown, Neyman–Pearson criterion is to maximize $P(H_1|H_1)$ with the constraint $P(H_1|H_0) = \alpha$.

24.3. Signal Parameter Estimation[4,5]

Assuming the signal follows a known model and the model parameter θ is unknown, parameter estimation for medical signal is to get the optimum estimate $\hat{\theta}$ of θ with some criteria. There are some common parameter methods as follows:

(1) Bayesian estimation: The criterion is to construct the loss function $C(\hat{\theta}, \theta)$ and minimize risk function $E[C(\hat{\theta}, \theta)]$ to obtain Bayesian parameter estimation. The common loss functions include three forms: square type $|\hat{\theta} - \theta|^2$, absolute value type $|\hat{\theta} - \theta|$ and uniform type (given Δ, loss function is equal to 1 if $|\hat{\theta} - \theta| \geq \Delta$, else 0). The parameter estimate for square-type loss function is the estimation of mean squared error (MSE) as

$$\hat{\theta}_{\mathrm{MSE}} = E[\theta | x_1, \ldots, x_n].$$

The parameter estimate for absolute value type is $\hat{\theta}_{\mathrm{ABS}}$, which satisfies

$$\int_{-\infty}^{\hat{\theta}_{\mathrm{ABS}}} p(\theta | x_1, \ldots, x_n) dx_1 \cdots dx_n = \int_{\hat{\theta}_{\mathrm{ABS}}}^{+\infty} p(\theta | x_1, \ldots, x_n) dx_1 \cdots dx_n,$$

where $\hat{\theta}_{\mathrm{ABS}}$ is the median of posterior density function. The parameter estimate for uniform-type loss function is the estimation of MAP as $\hat{\theta}_{\mathrm{MAP}}$, which satisfies

$$\frac{\partial}{\partial \theta} p(\theta | x_1, \ldots, x_n)|_{\hat{\theta}_{\mathrm{MAP}}} = 0.$$

(2) Maximum likelihood estimation: Maximizing likelihood function, $\hat{\theta}_{\mathrm{ML}}$ satisfies

$$\frac{\partial}{\partial \theta} \ln p(x_1, \ldots, x_n | \theta)|_{\hat{\theta}_{\mathrm{ML}}} = 0.$$

The maximum likelihood estimate $\hat{\theta}_{\mathrm{ML}}$ is also uniform estimation. Give a large n, $\hat{\theta}_{\mathrm{ML}}$ approximately follows normal distribution with mean θ. When θ obeys uniform distribution, $\hat{\theta}_{\mathrm{ML}}$ is same as $\hat{\theta}_{\mathrm{MAP}}$.

(3) Linear MSE estimation: Assume the parameter θ is a linear function of the observations. To minimizing MSE, $\hat{\theta}_{\mathrm{LMS}}$ satisfies

$$\hat{\theta}_{\mathrm{LMS}} = \sum_{i=1}^{n} w_i x_i,$$

$$\sum_{i=1}^{n} w_i E[x_i x_j] = E[\theta x_j]|_{\hat{\theta}_{\mathrm{LMS}}},$$

where $w_i(i = 1, \ldots, n)$ is the coefficient of linear combination. The estimated error $(\hat{\theta} - \theta)$ is orthogonal to the observations. $\hat{\theta}_{\text{LMS}}$ is also Bayesian estimation $\hat{\theta}_{\text{MSE}}$ with square type loss function.

(4) Least square estimation: In the linear observation equation $X = A\theta + e$, where A is a known coefficient matrix and e is the observation error, $\hat{\theta}_{\text{LS}}$ is the estimate to minimize the square error $e^T e$. If $A^T A$ is invertible, $\hat{\theta}_{\text{LS}} = (A^T A)^{-1} A^T X$ is the unique solution and θ is called as parameter identifiability. If $A^T A$ is singular, same value of $A\theta$ may have different parameters θ. And now θ is called as parameter non-identifiability. If the components of error vector e are uncorrelated with the same variance, $\hat{\theta}_{\text{LS}}$ is also the optimum estimation with minimum variance. Considering the weight of error vector with weight matrix W, weighted least squares estimate of θ is $\hat{\theta}_{\text{WLS}} = (A^T W A)^{-1} A^T W X$ and the optimum weighted matrix is $[\text{Var}(N)]^{-1}$.

24.4. Signal Analysis of Time Domain[6]

Signal analysis of time domain, which studies the waveform of the signals changing over time, includes signal filter in time domain, calculation of statistical characteristics and correlation analysis, etc. Correlation analysis could measure the similarity between signals with auto-correlation function and cross-correlation function. Auto-correlation function studies synchrony and periodicity of signal itself as

$$R_{xx}(\tau) = E[x(t)x(t + \tau)].$$

And cross-correlation function discusses the degree of similarity between signals as

$$R_{xs}(\tau) = E[x(t)s(t + \tau)].$$

Signal filter in time domain, which makes a transform for input signal $x(t)$, extracts the useful information and obtains the output signal $y(t)$. For Linear time invariant system, the filter impulse response function is $h(t)$ and frequency response function is $H(\omega)$. The output signal $y(t)$ is shown as

$$y(t) = x(t) * h(t) = \int_{-\infty}^{\infty} h(\tau)x(t - \tau)d\tau,$$

$$Y(\omega) = X(\omega)H(\omega),$$

where $Y(\omega)$, $X(\omega)$ and $H(\omega)$ are the Fourier transforms of $y(t)$, $x(t)$ and $h(t)$, respectively. Consider signal model $x(t) = s(t) + n(t)$, where $n(t)$ is noise. There are three major types of discrete signal filter: matched filter, Wiener filter and Kalman filter.

(1) Matched filter: Matched filter is a linear optimal filter which seeks optimum $h(t)$ or $H(\omega)$ to maximize the signal noise ratio of output signal. When $n(t)$ is white noise with zero mean and unit variance, the frequency response function $H(\omega)$ satisfies the following formula:

$$|H_{\text{opt}}(\omega)| = |S(\omega)|,$$

where $S(\omega)$ is the Fourier transform of $s(t)$. When $n(t)$ is colored noise (non-white noise), the generalized matched filter is applied, which transforms the colored noise into white noise and then detects target signal with matched filter.

(2) Wiener filter: Wiener filter is a linear optimal filter which seeks optimum $h(t)$ or $H(\omega)$ to minimize MSE as

$$E[y(t) - s(y)]^2.$$

For causal filter, where $h(n) = 0$ if $n < 0$, cross-correlation function satisfies Wiener–Hopf function

$$R_{xs}(j) = \sum_{m=0}^{\infty} h_{\text{opt}}(m) R_{xx}(j - m) \quad j \geq 0.$$

(3) Kalman filter: Kalman filter is a linear optimal filter based on state space model which filters signal recursively to minimize MSE. With the estimate of previous signal $\hat{s}(n-1)$ and new observation $x(n)$, state equation and observation equation at time k of Kalman filter are established as follows:

$$S(k) = A(k)S(k-1) + w_1(k-1),$$
$$X(k) = C(k)S(k) + w_2(k),$$

where vector $S(k)$ and $X(k)$ are the system state and observation, $A(k)$ and $C(k)$ are the gain matrix, $w_1(k)$ and $w_2(k)$ are noise.

24.5. Signal Analysis of Frequency Domain[7]

With Fourier transform, signal is transformed into frequency domain to reveal the characteristic of signal frequency. Periodic signal can be expressed as the weighted sum of sine signals and non-periodic signal can be expressed as the weighted integral of sine signals.

Fourier transform: For continuous Fourier transform, the formulas of positive and inverse transform are as follows:

$$F(\omega) = \int_{-\infty}^{\infty} f(t)e^{-j\omega t}dt,$$

$$f(t) = \frac{1}{2\pi}\int_{-\infty}^{\infty} F(\omega)e^{j\omega t}d\omega.$$

$F(\omega)$ is called frequency spectrum and represented as

$$F(\omega) = |F(\omega)|e^{j\phi(\omega)},$$

which reflects the frequency distribution of each component of $f(t)$. $|F(\omega)|$ is the amplitude spectrum and $\phi(\omega)$ is the phase spectrum. For discrete Fourier transform, the formulas of positive and inverse transform are as follows:

$$F(k) = \sum_{n=0}^{N-1} f(n)e^{-j\frac{2\pi kn}{N}}, \quad 0 \le k \le N-1,$$

$$f(n) = \frac{1}{N}\sum_{k=0}^{N-1} F(k)e^{j\frac{2\pi kn}{N}}, \quad 0 \le n \le N-1.$$

Sampling theory: Sampling theory has two divisions in time domain and frequency domain.

Sampling theorem in time domain: assuming the frequency spectrum $F(\omega)$ ranges from $-\omega_m$ to ω_m and the sampling interval of time is $\boldsymbol{T}_s$, the sampled signal $f_s(t)$ could recover $f(t)$ if $1/T_s \ge 2\omega_m$.

Sampling theorem in frequency domain: assuming the signal $f(t)$ ranges from $-t_m$ to t_m and the sampling interval of frequency is ω_s, $f(t)$ could be uniquely represented by $F(n\omega_s)$, if $\omega_s/2\pi \ge 2t_m$.

There are some regular spectrums as follows:

(1) Amplitude spectrum

$$|F(\omega)| = \sqrt{[\mathrm{Re}(F(\omega))]|^2 + [\mathrm{Im}(F(\omega))]|^2},$$

which indicates the amplitude of each frequency component of $f(t)$.

(2) Phase spectrum

$$\phi(\omega) = \tan^{-1}(\mathrm{Im}(F(\omega))/\mathrm{Re}(F(\omega))),$$

which indicates the initial phase of each frequency component of $f(t)$. Those signals with same amplitude spectrum but different phase spectrum are completely different.

(3) Power spectrum: It is defined in Sec. 24.1. As is well known, there is Wiener–Khinchine theorem: for stationary signal $x(t)$ with zero mean, its auto-correlation function $R_{xx}(\tau)$ and power spectrum $P_{xx}(\omega)$ are Fourier transform pairs, which satisfy the following equation:

$$\int_{-\infty}^{\infty} P_{xx}(\omega)d\omega = E[|x(t)|^2] = R_{xx}(0).$$

Especially for the linear time-invariant system, the power spectrum of output signal $y(t)$ is

$$P_{yy}(\omega) = P_{xx}(\omega)|H(\omega)|^2,$$

where $H(\omega)$ is frequency response function of system and $x(t)$ is input signal.

24.6. Time-frequency Analysis[8]

Fourier transform is a kind of global transformation all in time domain or all in frequency domain, which can not figure out the local spectrum feature of signal over time. Time-frequency analysis can solve this problem. Time-frequency analysis comprises those techniques which can analyze signal in both time domain and frequency domain simultaneously such as linear time-frequency analysis and nonlinear time-frequency analysis.

Linear time-frequency analysis $T_s(t,\omega)$ is the time-frequency representation of signal $s(t)$. If $s(t)$ is the linear combination of some components: $s(t) = c_1 s_1(t) + c_2 s_2(t)$, $T_s(t,\omega)$ can be represented as

$$T_s(t,\omega) = c_1 T_{s1}(t,\omega) + c_2 T_{s2}(t,\omega),$$

$T_s(t,\omega)$ is called linear time-frequency representation.

(1) Short-time Fourier transform

$$\mathrm{STFT}_s(t,\omega) = \int_{-\infty}^{\infty} s(\tau)g^*(\tau - t)e^{-j2\pi\tau\omega}d\tau,$$

where $g(t)$ is window function of time and $*$ denotes complex conjugate. The time and frequency resolution are determined by T_p and $1/T_p$, respectively. T_p is the width of time window.

(2) Gabor transform

$$a_{mn} = \int_{-\infty}^{\infty} s(t)\gamma_{mn}^*(t)dt,$$

$$\gamma_{mn}(t) = \gamma(t - m\Delta t)e^{j2\pi n\Delta\omega t},$$

where Δt and $\Delta\omega$ are sampling intervals of time and frequency, respectively. $\gamma(t)$ is a window function which is biorthogonal with $g(t)$. Then, we have

$$s(t) = \sum_{m=-\infty}^{\infty} \sum_{n=-\infty}^{\infty} a_{mn} g_{mn}(t),$$

$$g_{mn}(t) = g(t - m\Delta t)e^{j2\pi n\Delta\omega t},$$

where a_{mn} is Gabor expansion coefficients and $g_{mn}(t)$ is Gabor basis function.

Nonlinear time-frequency analysis. Nonlinear time-frequency analysis often applies Wigner–Ville distribution, Cohen's class time-frequency distribution and wavelet transform. For the description of wavelet transform, see Sec. 24.7 wavelet analysis.

(1) Wigner–Ville distribution

$$W_s(t,\omega) = \int_{-\infty}^{\infty} s\left(t + \frac{\tau}{2}\right) s^*\left(t - \frac{\tau}{2}\right) e^{-j\tau\omega} d\tau.$$

When $s(t) = s_1(t) + s_2(t)$, we have

$$W_s(t,\omega) = W_{s_1}(t,\omega) + W_{s_2}(t,\omega) + 2\text{Re}[W_{s_1 s_2}(t,\omega)],$$

where

$$W_{s_1 s_2}(t,\omega) = \int_{-\infty}^{\infty} s_1\left(t + \frac{\tau}{2}\right) s_2^*\left(t - \frac{\tau}{2}\right) e^{-j\tau\omega} d\tau.$$

(2) Cohen's class time-frequency distribution

$$\begin{aligned} C_s(t,\omega) &= \int_{-\infty}^{\infty}\int_{-\infty}^{\infty} \phi_s(\tau,v) A_s(\tau,v) e^{-j(vt+\omega\tau)} d\tau dv A_s(\tau,v) \\ &= \int_{-\infty}^{\infty} s\left(t + \frac{\tau}{2}\right) s^*\left(t - \frac{\tau}{2}\right) e^{-jvt} dt, \end{aligned}$$

where $\phi_s(\tau,v)$ is weighted kernel function and $A_s(\tau,v)$ is the ambiguity function of $s(t)$. With the different kernel functions, Choi–Williams distribution (CWD), Born–Jordon distribution (BWD), Pseudo Wigner–Ville distribution (PWD) and Smoothed Pseudo Wigner–Ville distribution (SPWVD) could be derived.

24.7. Wavelet Analysis[9]

Wavelet analysis is a kind of analytical tool in time-frequency domain, which can adaptively adjust time and frequency windows based on the local feature of signal. It has characteristics of multi-resolution analysis and time-frequency localization, called as a mathematical microscope for analyzing signals.

(a) Wavelet function: If $\psi(t) \in L^2(R)$ and the Fourier transform $\hat{\psi}(\omega)$ satisfies the admissible condition as follows:

$$C_\psi = \int_{-\infty}^{\infty} \frac{|\hat{\psi}(\omega)|^2}{|\omega|} d\omega < \infty,$$

$\psi(t)$ is named as wavelet function or mother wavelet. $\psi(t)$ is often assumed as

$$\int_{-\infty}^{\infty} \psi(t) dt = 0.$$

Obviously, wavelet has the feature of volatility. Those common wavelets include Haar wavelet, Daubechies wavelet, Mexican hat wavelet, Morlet wavelet and Mayer wavelet, etc. Wavelet basis functions $\psi_{a,b}(t)$ are derived from the single wavelet function with dilation and translation.

$$\psi_{a,b}(t) = \frac{1}{\sqrt{a}} \psi\left(\frac{t-b}{a}\right), \quad (a, b \in R, a \neq 0),$$

where a and b are scale parameter and translation parameter.

(b) Continuous wavelet transform: $f(t)$ is a function of space $L^2(R)$. Continuous wavelet transform of $f(t)$ can be represented with wavelet basis functions as following:

$$(W_\psi f)(a, b) = \langle f(t), \psi_{a,b}(t) \rangle = \frac{1}{\sqrt{a}} \int_R f(t) \psi^* \left(\frac{t-b}{a}\right) dt$$

and* denotes the complex conjugate.

The inverse transformation is

$$f(t) = \frac{1}{C_\psi} \iint_{R^2} [(W_\psi f)(a, b)] \psi_{a,b}(t) \frac{1}{a^2} da db.$$

(c) Discrete wavelet transform: After discretization of wavelet function, the discrete scale and translation parameters are $a = a_0^j, a_0 > 0, j = 0, 1, \ldots$

and $b = ka_0^j, k \in Z$. The discrete wavelet basis functions are as follows:

$$\psi_{j,k}(t) \triangleq \psi_{a_0^j, ka_0^j}(t) = |a_0|^{-j/2}\psi(a_0^{-j}t - k)$$

Discrete wavelet transform and inverse wavelet transform are

$$(W_\psi f)(a_0^j, ka_0^j) = \langle f(t), \psi_{j,k}(t)\rangle,$$

$$f(t) = \sum_j \sum_k \langle f, \psi_{j,k}\rangle \psi^{j,k}(t),$$

where $\langle \psi_{j,k}, \psi^{l,m}\rangle = \delta_{j,l}\delta_{k,m}$.

(d) Multi-resolution analysis: W_j is the linear closure of $\{\psi_{j,k}(t)\}$ in space $L^2(R)$ and space $L^2(R)$ could be direct sum decomposed as $L^2(R) = \oplus_{j=-\infty}^{\infty} W_j$. Define closed subspace $V_j = \oplus_{k=-\infty}^{j-1} W_{j-1}$. If there exists $\phi(t) \in V_0$ and $\phi_{0,k}(t) \equiv \phi(t-k)$ is the basis of V_0, $\phi(t)$ is called wavelet scaling function. Space $\{V_j\}$ is the linear closure of $\{\phi_{j,k}(t)\}$ with $V_j \perp W_j$.

24.8. Independent Component Analysis (ICA)[10]

Under complex background, observed signal is often a mixture of multi-hannel signals. The process that the unknown source signals are separated from the mixed signals, is known as blind source separation (BSS). If the components of BSS are statistically independent, this process is called ICA, which first appeared in the cocktail party problem.

ICA model: Suppose that there are m observed signals and n independent source signals, the mixed model for observed signal is $X = AS$, where A is a mixing matrix of $m \times n$ and S is the vector of unknown source signals. The purpose of ICA is to calculate separation matrix W and obtain the estimation of source signals $Y = WX$, which allows the separated components of Y to be statistically independent but linearly mixed. There are some assumptions for traditional ICA model: The number of observed signal must be no less than that of original signals ($m \geq n$); when $m = n$, the optimal separation matrix is $Y = A^{-1}$; all components of source signal S are statistically independent; at most one of them could follow Gaussian distribution and the others obey non-Gaussian distribution; there are small noise or no noise in observed signals. Moreover, there are two uncertainties in the separated signals: the absolute amplitude and the sequence of signals.

Traditional methods for the solutions of ICA model are the following:

(1) Maximization of non-Gaussianity: Non-Gaussianity of estimate signal Y is measured.

Maximizing the non-Gaussianity, the independent signal components are extracted successfully. The classical measures of non-Gaussianity are kurtosis and negative entropy, which are shown in the following formulas, for a random variable y,

$$\text{kurt}(y) = E[y^4] - 3(E[y^2])^2,$$
$$J(y) = H(y_{\text{Gauss}}) - H(y),$$

where $H(y)$ is entropy. y_{Gauss} is a Gaussian variable with the same variance of y. The kurtosis and negative entropy of Gaussian variable is 0.

(2) Minimization of mutual information. The mutual information of vector Y is

$$I(Y) = \sum_{i=1}^{n} H(y_i) - H(Y),$$

$I(Y) \geq 0$. When all the components of $Y$are statistically independent, mutual information is 0.

(3) Maximization of likelihood estimation: In ICA model without noise, maximizing likelihood estimation is equivalent to minimizing mutual information. Then separation matrix W is obtained.

(4) Infomax ICA: For two independent source signals S_1 and S_2, we have

$$E\{f(S_1)g(S_2)\} = E\{f(S_1)\}E\{g(S_2)\},$$

where $f(g)$ and $\text{g}(g)$ are nonlinear functions. With the nonlinear function $\text{g}(g)$ in the output end, covariance matrix of the nonlinear output can be detected as a measure for independence. If all components of the output vector Y are independent, the covariance matrix of Y and $\text{g}(Y)$ are both diagonal matrices.

24.9. Higher-Order Statistics (HOS)[11]

HOS has higher order (≥ 3) than second-order statistics, such as higher-order moment, higher-order cumulant and higher-order spectrum. HOS is a powerful tool for non-Gaussian signal, non-stationary signal, nonlinear system and non-minimum phase system.

Characteristic function

$$\Phi(\omega) = E[e^{j\omega x}] = \int_{-\infty}^{\infty} e^{j\omega x} f(x)dx,$$

where $f(x)$ is the probability density function of the random variable x.

Second characteristic function

$$\Psi(\omega) = \ln \Phi(\omega).$$

***k*-order moment**

$$m_k = E[x^k] = (-j)^k \Phi^k(0).$$

***k*-order cumulant**

$$c_k = (-j)^k \left[\frac{d^k \Psi(\omega)}{d\omega^k}\right]\bigg|_{\omega=0} = (-j)^k \Psi^k(0).$$

***k*-order spectrum**

$$C_{kx}(\omega_1, \ldots, \omega_{k-1}) = \sum_{\tau_1=-\infty}^{\infty} \cdots \sum_{\tau_{k-1}=-\infty}^{\infty} c_{kx}(\tau_1, \ldots, \tau_{k-1}) e^{-j(\omega_1\tau_1 + \cdots \omega_{k-1}\tau_{k-1})}.$$

k-order moment and k-order cumulant are the coefficient of Taylor series for characteristic function and second characteristic function, respectively. They can transform into each other by C-M formula. k-order spectrum is the multidimensional Fourier transform of k-order cumulant. HOS has plenty of applications in signal detection, feature extraction and parametric estimation.

(1) System identification: For the parametric model such as AR, MA and ARMA model, k-order cumulants and auto-correlation function are used to build equations and estimate the model parameters and order. For non-parametric model with impulse response function $h(g)$ as follows:

$$y(k) = \sum_{i=0}^{q} h(i)x(k-i),$$

k-order cumulants are used to build equations and estimate the frequency response function and order q. That is,

$$H(\omega) = \sum_{i=0}^{q} h(i)e^{-j\omega_i}.$$

(2) Harmonic retrieval: Harmonic signal is expressed as

$$x(n) = \sum_{k=1}^{p} \alpha_k \exp[j(\omega_k n + \phi_k)],$$

where p is the number of harmonic signal. α_k, ω_k and ϕ_k are the amplitude, normalized frequency and initial phase for the kth harmonic component. If the observed signal is with noise as model $y(n) = x(n) + w(n)$, where the noise could be Gaussian or non-Gaussian, colored or white, symmetrical or asymmetric, k-order cumulants is powerful to estimate the parameters of harmonic signal.

HOS could restrain the influence of additive colored noise with unknown power spectrum, and extract the information from measuring non-Gaussianity. So it is applied widely in the field of signal processing to solve some problems such as signal reconstruction, adaptive-filtering, time delay estimation, blind de-convolution and blind equalization.

24.10. Image Digitization[12]

Image digitization is to convert an analog image signal into a digital image signal, which includes sampling and quantification. Analog image can be expressed with a 2D continuous function $I = F(x, y)$, whose spatial location and function value vary continuously. In spatial location, $I = F(x, y)$ is discretized into a matrix along the horizontal and vertical direction, where the points in the matrix are called pixel. The amplitude of every pixels is discretized into a integer value, which is called grayscale value. Each pixel has two attributes: spatial location and grayscale.

Sampling: It is the discretization of the image spatial coordinate, which describes image by pixels. The sampling frequency must be no less than twice the highest frequency of the original image.

Quantization: That is to convert the continuous gray value of pixel to a discrete integral value after sampling. Gray levels generally use binary digit such as $G = 2^g$, $G = 8, 64, 256$, etc., where g is the number of bits to store a pixel. If $G = 2$, the binary image is a black and white image, in which every pixel value is 0 or 1. If $G > 2$, the image is a grayscale image, which does not include color information. Color image consists of three components: red (R), green (G), blue (B). Each component is described with different gray levels.

In general, image digitization uses the uniform sampling and uniform quantization with the equal intervals. Non-uniform sampling can change the sampling interval according to the details of image. For the rich details, the sampling interval is small; otherwise the sampling interval is big. Non-uniform quantization can use a small G for the region with small changes in grayscale, while a big G for the region with rich grayscale. The quality of image digitization is decided by sampling interval and quantitative levels generally. If the sampling interval is large, it is of less pixels, low spatial resolution and poor image quality. Especially, checkerboard effect will appear with blocks when sample interval is larger. If quantitative levels are few, the image is degraded with low gray resolution and poor quality. False contour will appear. Therefore, with the smaller sampling interval and more quantitative levels, there is higher spatial and grayscale resolution with better quality image.

The digitalized image is a matrix with size $M \times N$ and gray level $G = 2^g$. The corresponding volume of image data is $M \times N \times$ g bits. Grayscale histogram can reflect the distribution of gray values in an image, which the abscissa is the gray value and the ordinate is the corresponding frequency (see also Chapter 2.3 histogram). Grayscale histogram can be used to evaluate the effect of image quantization, but not for the spatial location of each pixel. And there is no one-to-one relationship between image and its histogram. In other words, the different images could have the same histogram. For more details of local gray distribution, the image could be divided into multiple regions and the grayscale histogram could be produced accordingly. In addition, the sum of local histograms is still the histogram of original image.

24.11. Image Enhancement[13]

Image enhancement highlights the expected features and improves the visual effect of image with the transformation of original image. There are two kinds of enhancement: spatial domain and frequency domain.

For image enhancement in spatial domain, spatial transform operator $T(g)$ is used as

$$g(x, y) = T[f(x, y)],$$

where $f(x, y)$ is the original image. Spatial domain techniques operate directly on the pixels of an image. There are the following methods commonly used for enhancement.

(1) Grayscale transformation functions: This method is classified to linear and nonlinear representations according to the transform functions in the simplest way. The linear transformations include linear grayscale transformation, reverse transformation and piecewise linear grayscale transformation. The nonlinear methods involve logarithmic transformation, exponent transformation and power transformation.

(2) Histogram adjustment: Histogram adjustment involves histogram equalization and histogram matching. For histogram equalization, the transformation generates an image whose intensity appears approximately as uniform distribution, enhancing contrast of the image with good visual effect. For histogram matching, the transformation generates an image that has a specified histogram so that the gray range of interest is highlighted to improve the quality of image.
(3) Spatial filtering: Spatial filtering operators mainly contain the smoothing and sharpening filtering. Smoothing filtering can reduce the noise and remove some less important details, which includes mean, median, max and min filters. Sharpening filtering can enhance the details and contours of image with the first-order and the second-order differential operators, such as gradient operator and Laplacian operator.

Enhancement in frequency domain, which transform image from spatial domain into frequency domain via Fourier transform, lifts some frequency components of interest, reduces and even removes some other frequency components. Some traditional frequency domain filterings are shown as follows:

(1) Low-pass filtering: Low-pass filtering lets low frequency components pass through but blocks high frequency components, which reduces high frequency noise and image sharpness. Traditional low-pass filter involves ideal low-pass filter, Butterworth low-pass filter, Gaussian low-pass filter, exponential filter and ladder filter.
(2) High-pass filtering: High-pass filtering, by contrast, lets high frequency components pass through but blocks low frequency components, which weakens the low frequency information and sharpens image. Commonly, high-pass filtering covers ideal high-pass filter, Butterworth high-pass filter, Gaussian high-pass filter, exponential filter, ladder filter and Laplace operator.
(3) Homomorphic filtering: The image $f(x, y)$ is regarded as the product of the incident light $i(x, y)$ and reflected light $r(x, y)$. That is,

$$f(x, y) = i(x, y)r(x, y).$$

The incident light uniformly focuses on the low-frequency part, while the reflected light reflects the characteristics of surface targets and mainly focuses on the high-frequency part. Homomorphic filtering, which splits image into the incident light and reflected light, is a frequency domain operation to compress the image light area and enhance contrast.

(4) Wavelet transform filter: With wavelet transformation of image, wavelet coefficients of each level are filtered under a certain enhancement criterion such as soft-threshold algorithm. It is remarkable that the results of a filtered image are different if using different wavelet basis functions and decomposition levels. The details for wavelet transform can be found in Sec. 24.7.

24.12. Image Segmentation[14,15]

Image segmentation subdivides an image into its constituent regions or subsets, which focuses on obtaining the partition of image and extracting the regions of interest with a certain principle. Suppose that the partition of image R is $R_1, R_2, \cdots, R_n$, where R_i is a non-empty subset of R. Then we have

(1) $U_{i=1}^{n} R_i = R$;
(2) $R_i \cap R_j = \emptyset (i \neq j)$;
(3) For same subset, pixels in R_i are similar with each other.
(4) For different subsets, pixels in R_i and those in R_j have some difference.
(5) For each subsetR_i, R_i is a connected region.

So far there is no perfect method which can correctly segment all images, even no criterion to judge whether the segmentation is completely correct. So the quality of segmentation is based on the accuracy and efficiency, which guides the choice of suitable methods. The common segmentation approaches are as follows.

(1) Edge detection: Edge is the boundary of region with different gray value characteristics. There are two attributes for edge: direction and amplitude. Edge detection is by far the most common approach for detecting meaningful discontinuities. Such discontinuities are detected with the first- and second-order derivatives. Based on the first-order derivatives, there are Roberts, Sobel, Prewitt edge detectors. And based on the second-order derivatives, there are Laplacian of a Gaussian (LoG) and Canny edge detectors.

(2) Edge tracking: Edge tracking is a linking procedure to assemble edge pixels into meaningful edges. The traditional methods include edge linking, line detection with Hough transform and approaches based on the graph theory. Discontinuity points are connected with edge linking algorithm using the direction and amplitude of the gradient. Hough transform can be used to detect the parameters of boundary line and link a line segment in an image.

Edge tracing based on the graph theory is a global detection with graphic path and large time consumption.

(3) Thresholding: One obvious way to extract the image from the background is to set a threshold T that separates all pixels with $f(x, y) \geq T$ or $f(x, y) < T$. Then the image is divided into two parts: object and background. When T is a constant, this approach is called global thresholding, which is often histogram-based method based on the distribution of pixel properties. The optimal global thresholding could be obtained by maximizing the between-class variance or minimizing the probability of error. When T varies with locations, it is called local thresholding, which is particularly useful for image processing in non-uniform background. If there are some peaks and valleys in the histogram, multithreshold segmentation can be performed with locally varying threshold function.

(4) Region-based segmentation: Region growing is a typical segmentation based on finding regions directly. Starting with a set of seed pixels, region grows by appending to each seed those neighboring pixels which have predefined properties similar to the seed. Until no more pixels satisfy the criteria for inclusion in the region, region growing should stop and segmentation is completed.

(5) Watershed algorithm: A watershed is the ridge that divides areas drained by different river systems. The watershed transform considers a grayscale image as a topological surface, where the values of $f(x, y)$ are interpreted as heights. Then the catchment basins and ridge lines in image are found with distance transform or gradient magnitude to achieve segmentation.

24.13. Image Resampling[16]

Digital image $f(x, y)$ is represented with matrix and (x, y) is the spatial location for each pixel. If the coordinate (x_0, y_0) is not the sampling point of the original image, as the big black point shown in the Figure 24.13.1, the technique of interpolation for $f(x_0, y_0)$ will be performed as image resampling.

The common approaches for image resampling are as follows.

(1) Nearest neighbor interpolation: The interpolation kernel is a rectangle function. The value of $f(x_0, y_0)$ is the grayscale of the pixel which is the nearest to the point (x_0, y_0) in its neighborhood. This procedure does not generate the new value of $f(x, y)$ and has the advantages of high calculating

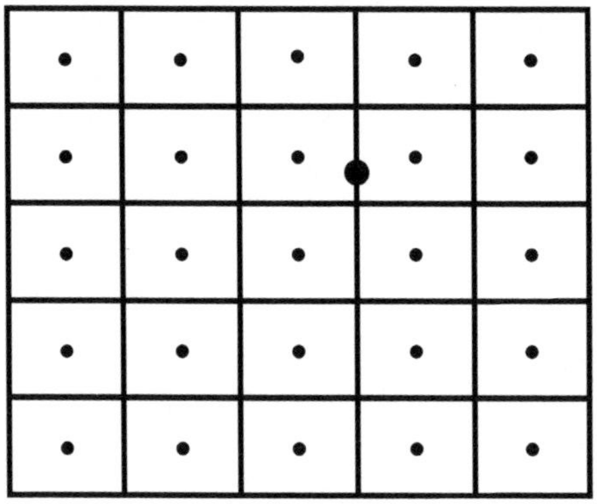

Fig. 24.13.1. Sampling points and resampling point.

speed. For image with rich details, this kind of interpolation may result in the location offset of pixels and cause mosaic.

(2) Bilinear interpolation: The interpolation kernel is a rectangle function in a triangle function. Setting (x_0, y_0) as the center, the nearest four points are searched in the neighborhood along the horizontal and vertical directions. Bilinear interpolation function is built with the distances between the four points and center. That is,

$$f(x_0, y_0) = W_{11}I_{11} + W_{12}I_{12} + W_{21}I_{21} + W_{22}I_{22},$$

where $W_{11} = (1 - \Delta x)(1 - \Delta y)$, $W_{22} = \Delta x \Delta y$, $W_{12} = (1 - \Delta x)\Delta y$ and $W_{21} = \Delta x(1 - \Delta y)$. I_{11}, I_{12}, I_{21} and I_{22} are the gray scales for the four points. Obviously, $f(x_0, y_0)$ is the weighted average of I_{11}, I_{12}, I_{21} and I_{22}, which is not good for edge detection. In addition, the new value $f(x_0, y_0)$ may be out of the range of original image grayscale.

(3) Cubic convolution: The interpolation kernel is a rectangle function in a cubic spline function. Setting (x_0, y_0) as the center, the nearest 16 points are searched in the neighborhood along the horizontal and vertical directions. The convolution function is the following formula:

$$f(x_0, y_0) = \sum_{i=1}^{4}\sum_{j=1}^{4} I(i, j)W(i, j),$$

where $W_{ij} = W(x_i)W(y_j)$ and $W(\mathrm{g})$ is weight coefficient. This kind of interpolation increases the number of neighboring pixels and improves the accuracy, but it is complex and has a large amount of calculation. Similarly, the new value $f(x_0, y_0)$ may be out of the range of original image grayscale.

Image resampling has a plenty of applications such as adjustment for different resolutions and scales. Another important application is digital image pyramid, which sets up hierarchical data structure with multiresolution and multidimension for multilevel image matching techniques.

24.14. Image Registration[17,18]

Searching the optimal transform, the floating image $I_1(x, y)$ and reference image $I_2(x, y)$ are matched in spatial locations. That is,

$$I_2(x, y) = g(I_1(f(x, y))),$$

where $f(g)$ is a two-dimensional space transform function and $g(\cdot)$ is a one-dimensional gray scale transform function.

In general, there are four steps for image registration: selecting feature space, constructing similarity criterion, defining searching space and developing search strategy.

(1) Feature space: Feature is extracted from the floating and reference images for registration. There are two types of features. One is grayscale of pixels in an image without segmentation. The gray-based registration is to search the optimal transform and maximize the similarity of intensity between the reference and floating images. The other type of image feature covers widely such as statistics, geometric characteristic, algebraic and frequency domain features and so on. For this case, the image needs to be segmented in advance and the features of the regions of interest are calculated. The feature-based registration is to search the optimal transform and maximize the similarity of features between the reference and floating images.

(2) Similarity criterion: Similarity is a measure to evaluate how well the floating image matches the reference image after each transformation. When the similarity approaches maximum, the two images are regarded as registered. Similarity always uses statistics such as mutual information, joint entropy, correlation and Euclidean distance.

(3) Searching space: A space of transformation, which covers the whole range of spatial transform for floating image, consists of global transformation, local transformation and optical flow-field transformation. Global transformation refers to the same transform for all pixels in image, such as shifting, rotating and scaling. Local transformation indicates the different regions with different spatial transforms. Optical flow-field transformation operates each pixel under the global constrain of offsets. In image registration, the commonly used transformation forms include rigid transformation,

affine transformation, projective transformation, perspective transformation, nonlinear transformation, etc.

(4) Search strategy: The good strategy to search the optimal transform in searching space has the merits of good estimate precision and high search speed. There are some algorithms to be chosen as follows: Powell algorithm, particle swarm optimization (PSO) algorithm, genetic algorithm and ant colony algorithm. Powell algorithm, optimizing the outcome of object function, obtains the optimal parameters of transform in the way of iteration with high search speed. PSO algorithm is an adaptive stochastic optimization algorithm based on group hunting strategy, which is an evolutionary algorithm with simple operations and few parameters.

To access the effect of registration, cost function is used to measure the error and loss of registered images in the aspects of accuracy, robustness, automaticity and adaptability.

24.15. Mathematical Morphology[19,20]

Mathematical morphology is a tool to extract image components that represents and describes the region shape such as boundaries, skeletons and the convex hull. Such operation is often defined in terms of set operations, which keep the properties of shape with the structuring elements. The common structuring element has a variety of shapes and size, such as disk-shape with radius r. A square structuring element with width three contains the nine neighbors: $B = \{(-1,-1), (-1,0), (-1,1), (0,-1), (0,0), (0,1), (1,-1), (1,0), (1,1)\}$. The fundamental morphological operations are erosion, dilation, opening and closing.

(1) Dilation: Dilation is an operation to grow or thicken objects in a binary image. The dilation of A by B is defined as

$$A \oplus B = \{z|(\widehat{B})_z \cap A \neq \emptyset\},$$

where $\emptyset$ is the empty set and B is the structuring element. $(\widehat{B})$ is the reflection of set B, $(\widehat{B})_z$ denotes the translation of set $(\widehat{B})$ by point z. The dilation of A by B is the set of $(\widehat{B})_z$ overlaps at least some part of A. So, dilation thickens objects, smoothes the contours and connects the narrow fractures.

(2) Erosion: Erosion shrinks and thins objects in a binary image. The erosion of A by B is defined as

$$A \ominus B = \{z|(B)_z \subseteq A\}.$$

$A \ominus B$ indicates the set of the translated B is a subset of A. Erosion shrinks objects, smoothes the contours and breaks thin connections. If we want to remove some small region and preserve the other structures, a structuring element with appropriate shape and size needs to be chosen.

(3) Opening: The opening of A by B is simply erosion of A by B, followed by dilation of the result by B, defined as

$$A \circ B = (A \ominus B) \oplus B.$$

Opening completely removes regions of an object which cannot contain the structuring element, particular for long thin gulfs and isolated regions.

(4) Closing: The closing of A by B is a dilation followed by an erosion, defined as

$$A \bullet B = (A \oplus B) \ominus B.$$

Unlike opening, it connects narrow breaks and fills holes smaller than the structuring element.

Morphological techniques are applied widely in image processing such as region filling, extraction of connected components and skeletons, thinning, thickening and pruning. More advanced progress contains fuzzy morphology, attribute morphology and morphological wavelet.

24.16. Image Classification[21,22]

In image processing, there is often no obvious edge between objects of interest such as the white matter and gray matter in magnetic resonance imaging. It is difficult to segment such objects. According to the properties and features, objects can be classified into different class. The procedure is called image classification or recognition. The common steps for image classification are: extracting features, selecting classification algorithm, setting discriminant rule and evaluating the outcome. With or without human intervention, approaches may be divided into two types: supervised and unsupervised classification.

(1) Supervised classification: Given the regions with known class as the training sample, the discriminant rule is obtained and used for the unknown regions. Supervised classification indicates learning pattern from training sample and assign test sample to their respective classes. The objects in a same class share a set of common properties of images. There are some supervised algorithms such as minimum distance algorithm, Mahalanobis distance algorithm, support vector machine, decision tree and so on. Grayscale and

texture feature are often used as image pattern descriptors. This type of image classification could select the categories of the training sample and remove some less important categories. So the classes for testing sample are limited in those in training sample, which seems somewhat subjective. In addition, supervised classifiers have the advantages of high precision and speed, while it needs a large amount of time and manpower to get training sample.

(2) Unsupervised classification: According to some image features and distribution rules, objects are clustered with a discriminant rule and without training sample as a prior. The similarity appears large for objects within the same cluster and small for objects between different clusters. The unsupervised classifiers divide an image into different clusters and can not specify the exact attributes of each cluster. Only after the classification, those attributes could be detected by other methods and the accuracy of classification will be tested in practice. There are some commonly used unsupervised classification algorithms such as K-means algorithm, fuzzy clustering, unsupervised neural network and iterative self-organization data analysis techniques. Unsupervised classification needs no prior information and reduces the artificial subjective error, especially for detecting the tiny clusters embodied in image, while it is hard to predict the attributes of classified clusters and computing speed is low.

The difference between supervised and unsupervised classifications lies in whether the prior information from training sample is used. In practice, the two kinds of classification are always combined together, clustering with unsupervised method and building classifiers with supervised method. This procedure could improve the speed and accuracy of classification algorithm. To access the quality of classification, classification accuracy, misclassification rate, confusion matrix and Kappa coefficient are commonly used. For evaluating the classification accuracy of medical image, it is always a problem. The typical solutions are phantom validation and visual inspection by specialist.

24.17. Image Compression[23]

Image compression addresses the problems of how to reduce the amount of data required. Removing redundancy is an efficient way to compress data for storage and transmission. Image compression consists of two distinct operators: encoding and decoding image.

Compression ratio: Let n_1 and n_2 denote the number of information carrying bits in the original and encoded images, compression ratio quantifies the degree of compression as

$$C_R = n_1/n_2$$

where n_1 refers to original image and n_2 refers to encoded image.

Data redundancy: The relative redundancy of original image is

$$R_D = 1 - 1/C_R.$$

There are three basic data redundancies as follows:

(1) Coding redundancy appears when the code words are less than the optimal. For example, the gray levels of an image are coded with a binary code.
(2) Inter-pixel redundancy results from correlations between the pixels. Since the values of pixels in image can be reasonably predicted from their neighbors, the information carried by the pixels is relatively small. The more pixels correlate, the more redundancy becomes.
Space redundancy in color spectrum, geometric redundancy in objects and inter frame redundancy in video belong to inter-pixel redundancy.
(3) Psycho-visual redundancy is due to data that is ignored by human visual system such as less important information for normal visual processing or color, luminance and spatial frequency out of the normal range received by human eyes. Elimination of psycho-visual redundancy is regarded as quantization and quantization is an irreversible operation without obviously degrading the quality of image.

In the procedure of encoding image, the input image is transformed into a format designed to reduce inter-pixel redundancy. With a predefined criterion, quantization attempts to eliminate the psycho-visual redundancy, and then the image is encoded which reduces the code redundancy. In the procedure of decoding image, the inverses operations of encoding without quantization are performed. There are lossless or loss compressions.

Lossless compression, which omits the operation of quantization in encoding, recovers the compressed image to the original one without any information loss. Lossless compression removes the code and inter-pixel redundancy, which preserves the high quality of image but has the low compression ratio. The commonly used coding methods for lossless compression are variable length coding, bit-plane coding, Lempel–Ziv–Welch coding and lossless predictive coding, which are used without any information loss such as satellite image and X-ray image.

Loss compression, which eliminates the psycho-visual redundancy in encoding steps, increases the compression ratio in cost of the accuracy of decoded image. The lost information comes from the psycho-visual redundancy and cannot be recovered. The common coding methods are loss predictive coding and transform coding, which are used in case tiny loss is acceptable such as the natural image.

For binary image, the compress standards widely used is G3 and G4 standard set by International Telephone and Telegraph Consultative Committee (CCITT). For static image (gray or color), one of the most popular compress standards is the Joint Photographic Experts Group (JPEG) standard, which is based on the discrete cosine transform. For dynamic image, Moving Picture Experts Group (MPEG) is a good standard to be chosen.

24.18. Three-dimensional (3D) Image Visualization[24,25]

With the modern imaging systems such as CT and MR, images of the object are always acquired with 2D display. 3D visualization generally refers to transformation and display of 3D objects so as to represent the 3D property of objects, especially for 3D structure information. For 3D data sets, various visualization methods are used in medical field, including image preprocessing and 3D display technique. Image preprocessing performs the operations such as enhancement, segmentation, registration and so on. 3D display techniques include surface rendering and volume rendering. Both techniques produce a visualization of selected structures.

(1) **Surface rendering:** This technique extracts the edges of image to define the surface of the structure and represents the surface by some connected polygons which join to form the complete surface. Surface tiling is performed at each contour point and then the surface is rendered visible with hidden surface removal and shading. The general procedure for surface rendering is as follows: acquiring 3D data of anatomy, segmenting objects of interest, identifying surface, extracting feature and adaptive tiling. The advantage of surface rendering is the fast rendering speed with small amount of contour data. Standard computer graphic hardware can support this technique. And the polygon-based surface is easy to be transformed to analytical description of structure. The disadvantage of this technique lies in the discrete contours defining the structure of surface to be visualized, which results in the information lost especially for slice generation or value measurement.

(2) Volume rendering: This technique is the most powerful tool for 3D image visualization, which is based on ray-casting algorithm with voxels. The algorithm for volume rendering may produce the optimal visualization of structure by changing the conditions of ray-casting. The different attributes of the voxels, such as voxel value and gradient, are used to produce on-the-fly surfaces cutting planes in the volume image. From the rendered image, any section of the actual image data is visualized and voxel values are measurable. Generally, there are two types of volume rendering algorithm: transmission and reflection. For the case of transmission such as X-ray radiograph, the rays transmit through the object and are recoded. The rendered voxel value is the integration of all voxels along the ray path. The common transmission algorithms include volumetric compositing, maximum intensity projection, minimum intensity projection and surface projection. For the case of refection such as photograph, the rays are reflected and then recorded. The rendered voxel value is a representation of each selected voxel which is the first one along the ray path that meets all the conditions of reflection model. Reflection algorithm defines surfaces within volume image with attributes of the voxel or specific object.

The technique of volume rendering preserves more details and context of the original volume image data, while high-performance computer hardware and highly optimal algorithm need to be met. Because of the huge amount of volume data, especially for high resolution image, rapid volume rendering seem to be the most important in a real time operation of medical field.

References

1. Oppenheim, AV, Schafer, RW. *Discrete-time Signal Processing.* (3rd edn.). New York: Prentice Hall, 2009.
2. Oppenheim, AV, Verghese, GC. *Signals, Systems and Inference.* (1st edn.). New York: Prentice Hall, 2015.
3. Schonhoff, T, Giordano, A. *Detection and Estimation Theory.* (1st edn.). New York: Prentice Hall, 2006.
4. Schonhoff, T, Giordano, A. *Detection and Estimation Theory and its Applications.* (1st edn.). New York: Prentice Hall, 2006.
5. Poor, HV. *An Introduction to Signal Detection and Estimation.* (2nd edn.). Berlin: Springer, 1998.
6. Haykin, SO. *Adaptive Filter Theory.* (5th edn.). New York: Prentice Hall, 2013.
7. Oppenheim, AV, Willsky, AS, Hamid, S. *Signals and Systems.* (2nd edn.). New York: Prentice Hall, 1996.
8. Cohen, L. *Time-frequency Analysis.* (1st edn.). New York: Prentice Hall, 1994.
9. Daubechies, I. *Ten Lectures on Wavelets.* (1st edn.). Philadelphia: SIAM: Society for Industrial and Applied Mathematics Press, 1992.
10. Hyvärinen, A, Karhunen, J, Oja, E. *Independent Component Analysis.* (1st edn.). Hoboken: John Wiley & Sons Inc., 2001.
11. Mendel, JM. Tutorial on higher-order statistics (spectra) in signal processing and system theory: Theoretical results and some applications. *Proceedings of the IEEE,* 1991, 79(3): 278–305.

12. Gonzalez, RC, Woods, RE. *Digital Image Processing.* (3rd edn.). New York: Prentice Hall, 2007.
13. Russ, JC, Neal, FB. *The Image Processing Handbook.* (7th edn.). Boca Raton: CRC Press, 2015.
14. Sonka, M, Hlavac, V, Boyle, R. Image Processing, Analysis and Machine Vision. (4th edn.). Boston: Cengage Learning Engineering, 2014.
15. Gonzalez, RC, Woods, RE. *Digital Image Processing.* (3rd edn.). New York: Prentice Hall, 2007.
16. Goshtasby, AA. *Image Registration: Principles, Tools and Methods.* London: Springer, 2012.
17. Goshtasby, AA. *Image Registration: Principles, Tools and Methods.* London: Springer, 2012.
18. Goshtasby, AA. *2-D and 3-D Image Registration for Medical, Remote Sensing, and Industrial Applications,* (1st edn.). Hoboken: Wiley Press, 2005.
19. Najman, L, Talbot, H. *Mathematical Morphology: From Theory to Applications.* (1st edn.). Hoboken: Wiley-ISTE, 2010.
20. Shih, FY. *Image Processing and Mathematical Morphology: Fundamentals and Applications.* (1st edn.). Boca Raton: CRC Press, 2009.
21. Theodoridis, S, Koutroumbas, K. *Pattern Recognition.* (4th edn.). Cambridge: Academic Press, 2008.
22. Bankman, I. *Handbook of Medical Image Processing and Analysis.* (2nd edn.). Cambridge: Academic Press, 2008.
23. Gonzalez, RC, Woods, RE. *Digital Image Processing.* (3rd edn.). UpperSaddle River: Prentice Hall, 2007.
24. Bankman, I. Handbook of Medical Image Processing and Analysis. (2nd edn.) Cambridge: Academic Press, 2008.
25. Haidekker, M. Advanced Biomedical Image Analysis. Hoboken: Wiley-IEEE Press, 2011.

About the Author

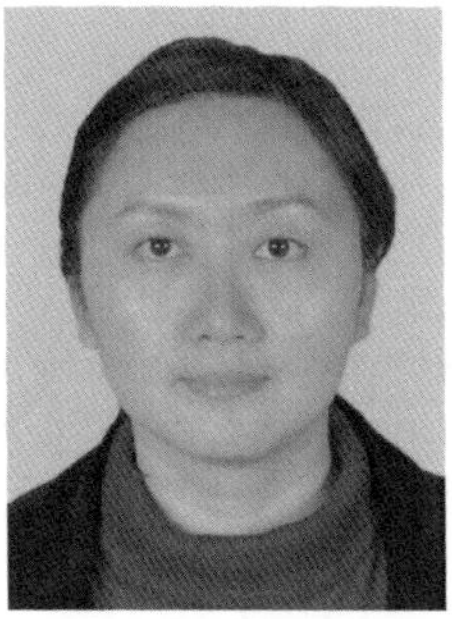

Zhao Qian has received a BSc in Mathematics in 2002, a MSc in Mathematics in 2005, and a PhD in Statistics in 2010 from Sun Yat-sen University. She was a scientific researcher in the Department of Radiology, University of California, San Francisco in 2007. Now she is an Associate Professor working in the Department of Statistics, School of Public Health, Guangzhou Medical University. She has some research projects supported by National Science Foundation. Her field of interest for research is Methodology in Biostatistics.

CHAPTER 25

STATISTICS IN ECONOMICS OF HEALTH

Yingchun Chen*, Yan Zhang, Tingjun Jin, Haomiao Li, Liqun Shi

25.1. Health Resources[1–3]

Broad health resources indicate the social resources (human, financial and material resources) that people use while launching healthcare activities. These resources include substances, materials, information and time which relate to geography, property, environment and social support system. Narrow health resources refer to the total sum of all kinds of factors of production occupied or consumed while society provides health services. Traditional accounting of health resources mainly contains health human resources, health material resources (health equipment), health financial resources (health expenditure), health information and technology. What health economics focuses on is the collection, distribution and use of health resources.

Health human resource, the most active resource among health resources, is the combination of quantity and quality of health manpower, which embodies laborers' intelligence, knowledge, experience, skill, physique, etc. in the field of health. The following are the common indicators reflecting health human resource: the amount of all kinds of health technical personnel, the number of health technical personnel based on population serviced such as the number of health technical personnel per thousand population, the number of doctors per thousand population, the number of health technical personnel based on institutions such as the number of doctors per township hospital, and indicators based on the structure of health human resource like the ratio of doctors and nurses or the constituent ratio of doctors and nurses in different levels.

*Corresponding author: chenyc2@qq.com

Health material resource refers to materials like basic constructions, medical equipment, medicines and health materials of health sectors. Common indicators include the number of regional medical institutions, beds and all kinds of special equipment.

Health financial resources is the financial resources used for medical health in the form of currency. It mainly means operating funds spent on medical and health service, and the money paid by residents while accepting health services.

Health information and technology refers to the information resources and technology used in the area of health. It is not only the main factor of health services provided, but also the basis of making plans, policies and decisions.

Health resources are counted according to their types or forms. In China, information of health resources are collected through the bottom-up straight quote system, and displayed on health statistics yearbook decreed by various levels of organizations.

As a kind of economic resource, health resources confront the contradiction of the limitation of resources, diversity of usage and indefiniteness of demands, so that health resources must be collected, distributed and validly used. The distribution of health resources should be based on and health services demand. We must take the service target method, demand method and health demand method into consideration when health resources are allocated. We use different methods to reckon the amount needed for different health resources. For instance, hospital beds can be reckoned by the demand approach:

$$\text{Hospital bed demand } = (P \times M \times L)/N,$$

in which P is the target population, M is the actual hospitalization rates per person per year, L is the average hospitalization days, and N refers to the days of open beds per bed.

$$\text{Demand of medical technicians } = (P \times C \times D \times T)/S$$

in which P is the target population, C is the annual average incidence per capita, D is the average service times per patient, T is the time consumed per service, annual work time per medical technician.

25.2. Total Health Expenditure, (THE)[3–5]

THE is the total monetary expense on the health services in a country or a region during a period of time (usually one year). THE, taking currency as a comprehensive measurement method, reflects the fundraising and distribution and effects brought by it from the perspective of the whole society. It is the key evidence of the national health management and health reform. The amount of THE, the percentage of THE in GDP and the average THE per capita represent its level of THE. According to the requirements of the World Health Organization (WHO), THE should not be under 5% in GDP, and it was 5.55% in China in 2014.

National Health Account adopts the bottom-up accounting mechanism. The National-level Accounts is also called National Health Account and each province also has its own THE. The accounting methods of THE include Financing Sources Method Expenditure by Provider Method and Function Using Method.

Financing Sources Method is to collect data and calculate expenses according to sources and ways of THE raising. According to the international rules, THE usually consists of the part supported by the government (which includes the pure government expenditure on health and the social health expenditure) and the part paid personally. These are the main sources of THE in China. Common indices used in the analysis of fundraising include the percentage of the part paid by the government and that paid personally and so on. Figure 25.2.1 indicates the components of THE in China.

Expenditure by Provider Method means that the sum of health fund distributed to different levels of health institutions reflects the distribution of the funds in different departments, areas and levels. Expenditure by Provider Method is to calculate the expenditure spent on different institutions including hospital expenditure, outpatient expenditure, expenditure of drugs, and other expenditure of retail institutions of medical supplier, public health agency, health administration and medical insurance management, and other expenditure on health.

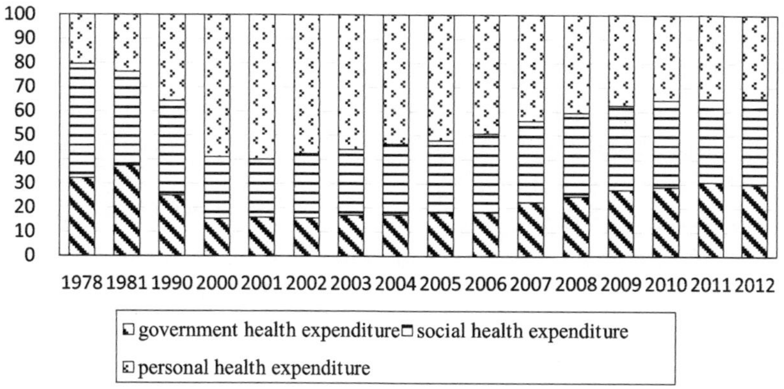

Fig. 25.2.1. The components of THE in China.

Function Using Method is to account the use of THE in all kinds of health service functions. In China, the functions are treatment, recovery, long-term care, supporting health services, outpatient medical supplies, prevention and public health services, health administration and medical insurance management services, etc. WHO presented *System of Health Accounts* in 2003 and provided the improved accounting framework of THE, System of Health Accounts (SHA) in 2011, which made the content and the arithmetic of the indicators much clearer.

25.3. Health Services Demand[2,3,6–9]

Health services demand refers to health services and its quantity that a consumer is willing to and able to purchase at a particular moment and a certain price that might be charged for that health services. Demand requires both willingness and ability to buy the service. The health services demand cannot exist if a consumer desires to purchase health services but cannot afford it or if a consumer may be able to afford to buy certain health services but he is unwilling to purchase.

Health services demand needs to follow its theorem that the price and quantity demanded for health services change in the opposite directions if other conditions remain unchanged. Health services demand drops when the price is up, on the contrary, the demand is up when the price drops.

Health services demand function can be taken to illustrate the relationship between quantity demanded for health services and its influencing factors. In the case that influencing factors are independent variables, the quantity demanded is the dependent variable, health services demand function may be as follows:

$$Q_d = f(T, I, P_x, E \ldots).$$

In this functional relationship, Qd is the quantity demanded of health services, T is preference, I refers to income; P is the price of health services, E refers to consumer expectations for the future and other factors.

Health services demand can be divided to individual demand and market demand from a standpoint of structure, and it can be separated into the demand transferred from needs and the demand without needs from a perspective of root. According to its urgency and importance, health services demand can be divided into three categories: (1) Health services demand for sustaining life, which refers to the demand for such diseases threatening patients' life; (2) General health services demand, which refers to that for some diseases that is not threatening life, as well as some discomfort in body;

(3) Healthcare demand for prevention, which refers to the demand for disease prevention and healthcare.

Health services demand is mainly affected by individual's health conditions, social economy, health services supply, social policies and so on. Questionnaire can be adopted to explore health services demands of residents, the willingness and ability to pay for health services and the actual utilization of health services. In China, many investigations, such as National Investigation of Health Services for all residents, National Investigation of Health of the Elderly Population, Health and Nutrition Survey, provide large sample data for the research of health services demand. In general, we use index of actual health service utilization and unmet health services, such as participation rate of health education, hospital visiting rate, unmet outpatient care ratio, hospitalization rate, unmet impatient care ratio and the rate of different health services utilization and so on, to reflect the status of health services demand. According to National Investigation of Health Services for all residents in 2013, 17.1% of the patients who need hospitalization were not hospitalized, 23.7% of these patients did not believe they needed inpatient treatment, and 43.2% of these patients did not come to hospital because of financial hardship.

25.4. Elasticity of Health Service Demand[2,6,7,10]

Elasticity illustrates the responsiveness of one variable to a change in another variable when there is a functional relationship between the two economic variables. In general, the elastic coefficient is used to represent the elasticity, and describe the sensitivity of the relative change of the dependent variable.

$$\text{Elastic cofficient } = \frac{\text{the percentage change of dependent variable}}{\text{the percentage change of independent variable}}.$$

The point elasticity and the arc elasticity can be used to measure elasticity: the point elasticity refers to the degree of change in the dependent variable when a delicate change in the independent variable occurs; the arc elasticity reflects the degree of change of the dependent variable which is caused by the change of the independent variable in a certain range.

1. Price elasticity of health services demand

The price elasticity of health services demand describes the percentage change in quantity demanded of health services resulting from a change in the price. It may be expressed in the following form:

$$\text{Edp} = \frac{\text{the percentage change in the quantity demanded of health service}}{\text{the percentage change in the price of health service that caused it}}.$$

2. Income elasticity of health services demand

The income elasticity of health services demand describes how great a change in quantity demanded results from a change in the income. Income elasticity may be positive (if a normal good) or negative (if an inferior good). In the case of the income elasticity of demand, it may be expressed in the following form:

$$\text{EdI} = \frac{\begin{array}{c}\text{the percentage change in the quantity}\\ \text{demanded of health service}\end{array}}{\begin{array}{c}\text{the percentage change in the}\\ \text{income level of consumer}\end{array}} = \frac{\Delta Q}{\Delta I} \cdot \frac{I}{Q}.$$

3. Cross-elasticity of health service demand

The quantity demanded of health services is influenced by its price. Cross-elasticity of demand relates to the percentage change in the quantity demanded for a product (service Y) to the percentage change in the price of another product (service X).

$$\text{Epxy} = \frac{\begin{array}{c}\text{the percentage change in the}\\ \text{quantity demanded of health service}\end{array}}{\begin{array}{c}\text{the percentage change in the price of}\\ \text{different health service that caused it}\end{array}} = \frac{\Delta Q_y}{\Delta P_x} \cdot \frac{P_x}{Q_y}$$

Epxy refers to cross-elasticity of service Y, and P_x describes the price of service X; Q_y refers to the demand of service Y.

The main factors affecting the elasticity of health services demand include the availability of substitute products, the urgency and intensity of demand, the percentage of price in consumer cost, the capacity of payment of third party and the duration of service or product and so on.

People often combine Power Model Method and Two-Part Model to estimate the price elasticity coefficient of demand. The main form of the function of the power function model is as follows:

$$D = \alpha P^{\beta} I^{\gamma} e^{\mu}.$$

Here, D is demand, and P refers to price, and I describes consumer income, and β, γ, μ are indexes of each variable in function, which are demand elasticities of variables.

25.5. Health Services Supply[2,6,7]

Health services supply refers to the amount of health services that a health services provider is willing to and able to provide at a particular moment and at each possible price. Health services supply requires both willingness and ability to provide health services. For example, health services providers need to master the technology of providing health services, have appropriate support personnel, basic facilities and conditions to provide health services.

Health services supply needs to follow the theorem of health service supply, namely the price and quantity of health service supply change in same directions in case were other conditions are unchanged. Health services supply increases with the rise of the price. Meanwhile, the supply will decline when the health services price falls.

The quantity supplied for health services is affected by many factors, mainly including the price of health services, motivation of health services provider, health resources allocation policies, technical level of health services staff and health equipment, as well as service pattern and management level and so on. In fact, the underlying determinants are the economy development level and productivity development level of a nation or region. Functions, curves and figures are often used to reflect quantity-dependent relationship among quantity supplied and influencing factors.

Health services supply function can be taken to illustrate the relationship between quantity supplied for health services and its influencing factors. In the case that the quantity supplied is the dependent variable reflected by Q_s, influencing factors are independent variables reflected by $a, b, \ldots, n$. Health services supply function may be describe as follows:

$$Q_s = (a, b, \ldots, n).$$

Assuming all other variables constant in the case and only taking price which is a major factor into consideration, we can simply show supply function as follows:

$$Q_s = f(P).$$

If there is a linear relationship between the quantity supplied for health services and its price, supply function will be a linear supply function. It may be described as follows:

$$Q_s = c + d \times P.$$

If there is a nonlinear relationship between the quantity supplied for health services and its price, supply function will be a nonlinear supply function. It

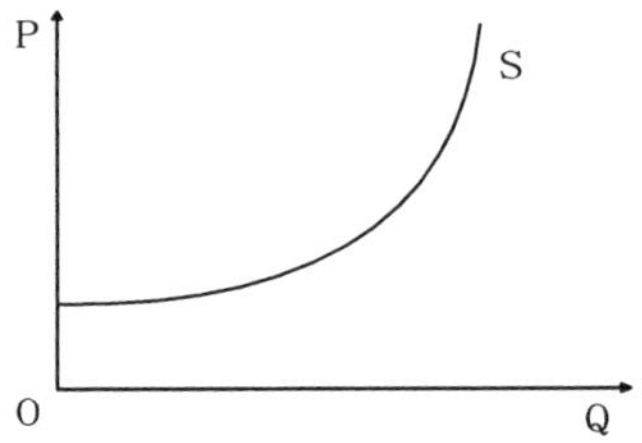

Fig. 25.5.1. The health services supply curve.

may be described as follows:

$$Q_s = \lambda P^{\beta}.$$

Here c, d, λ and β are all positive.

Usually, health services supply curve is used to graphically reflect health services supply function Q_S, which describes the relationship between quantity supplied for health services and its price (see Figure 25.5.1). Supply curve has a positive slope, which is a right upper left lower right curve.

25.6. Elasticity of Health Services Supply[2,3,7,11]

Elasticity of health service supply describes how great a change in quantity supplied resulting from a change in its price is. The elastic coefficient refers to the ratio of the percentage change in the quantity supplied and the percentage change in its price that caused it. E_S refers to the elastic coefficient of health services supply. Q and ΔQ reflect the quantity supplied and its change respectively, P and ΔP reflect the price and its change, respectively. The elasticity of health services supply would then appear as follows:

$$E_S = \frac{\Delta Q/Q}{\Delta P/P} = \frac{\Delta Q}{\Delta P} \times \frac{P}{Q}.$$

The elasticity of health services supply is used to describe the sensitivity of the relative change of supply caused by the change of price, namely percentage change in health services supply caused by 1% change in health services price. The elastic coefficient of health services supply reflects the relationship between the change in price and the quantity supplied. The relationship can be shown in formula form as follows:

$$\text{Esp} = \frac{\text{the percentage change in the quantity supplied of health service}}{\text{the percentage change in the price of health service that caused it}}.$$

Point elasticity and Arc elasticity can also be used to measure this elasticity.

Different from elastic coefficient of health services demand, the elastic coefficient of health services supply is positive, namely the quantity supplied and its price would change in the same direction. For example, if the elasticity coefficient of supply for a kind of health services is 2, it means the quantity supplied will increase by 2% if its price increases by 1%.

The main factors affecting the elasticity of health services supply include the feasibility of production adjustment, the feasibility of production scale and change, the quantity and similarity of substitute products, the cost variety and so on.

According to the numeric of elasticity of supply, elasticity of health services supply can be grouped into five categories: inelastic, elastic, unitary elastic, perfectly inelastic and infinitely elastic. Characteristics of all kinds of elasticity are shown in Table 25.6.1, and visualized in Figure 25.6.1.

Table 25.6.1. Elasticity of health services supply.

Elasticity Coefficient	Elasticity Category	Relationship Between Price and Quantity Supplied	Counterpart Diagram
$E_s = 0$	Perfectly inelastic	No change	(a)
$E_s = \infty$	Infinitely elastic	Raising infinity	(b)
$E_s = 1$	Unitary elastic	The rise is exactly equal to 1%	(c)
$E_s < 1$	Inelastic	The rise is smaller than 1%	(d)
$E_s > 1$	Elastic	The rise is greater than 1%	(e)

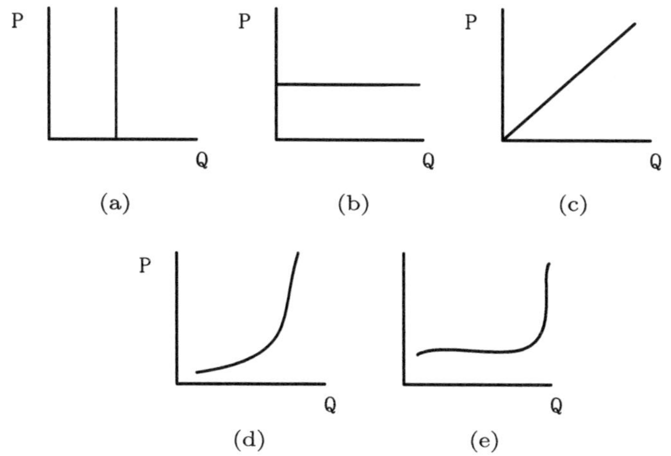

Fig. 25.6.1. Categories of elasticity of health services supply.

25.7. Cobb–Douglas Production Function[44,2,7]

It is proposed by American mathematician Charles Cobb and economist Paul Dougla which is based on U.S. industrial production statistics during 1899–1922 and widely used to represent the technological relationship between amounts of two or more inputs. Cobb–Douglas production function is one of the earliest application models in the production function model. It may be expressed as follows:

$$Q = AL^{\alpha}K^{\beta}.$$

In this function, Q is the output, A is the constant, L refers to the quantity of labor, K is the quantity of capital; α and β represents the elastic coefficient of labor and capital, respectively. Output elastic coefficient refers to the increase in percentage caused by 1% increase of input when other factors remain the same. Input elastic coefficient of labor refers to the sensitivity of the output change caused by labor change, which means the increase percentage of output caused by 1% increase of labor quantity. Similarly, input elastic coefficient of capital refers to the sensitivity of the output change caused by capital change.

The economic definitions of α and β are contributions made by all kinds of production factors. If $\alpha+\beta > 1, \alpha$ and β represent the relative importance of labor and capital, respectively, during production. In other words, α and β reflect proportions of labor and capital in gross production, respectively. In general, the contribution of labor is greater than that of capital. Cobb–Douglas production function was once used to calculate the contribution of labor and capital, of which the former was about 3/4 and the latter was about 1/4.

According to the output elastic coefficient in Cobb–Douglas production function, we can estimate the profits of input scale. There are three kinds of different conditions: (1) $\alpha+\beta > 1$, increasing returns to scale, which means that the percentage increased in the quantity of health services output would be greater than the percentage increased in input. In this case, the more the input of production factors of health services institutions, the higher the efficiency of resource utilization. (2) $\alpha+\beta = 1$, constant returns to scale, which means that the percentage increased in the quantity of health services output would be exactly equal to the percentage increased in input, and in this condition, the highest profit has been obtained in health services institutions. (3) $\alpha+\beta < 1$, decreasing returns to scale, which means that the percentage increased in the quantity of health services output would be smaller than the percentage increased in input. In this case, inputs of production factors should not be increased.

Assuming CT examination of a hospital conforms to Cobb–Douglas production function, and all kinds of production factors can be classified into two categories: Capital (K) and Labor (L). We could get production function of CT examination by analyzing input and output level for many times in the following equation:

$$Q = AL^{0.8}K^{0.2}.$$

According to output elastic coefficient of labor and capital (α and β), the analysis of the output changes caused by the changes of various production factors can be made to determine whether the input should be increased or decreased in health services.

Cobb–Douglas production function is mainly used to describe the relationship between the input and the output in production factors. In practical application, the difference of production, production scale and period leads to different elastic coefficients. The difficulty in the application of this function lies in the measure of coefficient. And we can use production coefficient of similar products or long-term production results to calculate elastic coefficient of a specific product.

25.8. Economic Burden of Disease[3,12,13,14]

The economic burden of disease which is also known as Cost of Illness (COI) refers to the sum of the economic consequence and resource consumption caused by disease, disability and premature deaths. Total economic burden of disease covers direct economic burden, indirect economic burden and intangible economic burden. Direct economic burden refers to the cost of resources used for the treatment of a particular disease, including direct medical costs (such as registration, examination, consultation, drugs) and non-medical direct costs (the cost for support activities during the treatment), such as costs for transportation, diet change or nursing fees. Indirect economic burden refers to the income lost that resulted from disability or premature deaths.

Direct economic burden can be estimated by the bottom-up approach or the top-down approach. The bottom-up approach estimates the costs by calculating the average cost of treatment of the illness and multiplying it by the prevalence of the illness. It is difficult to get the total cost for an illness in most circumstances. For specific types of health services consumed by patients, the average cost is multiplied by the number of actual use of the health services. Take the case of calculating direct medical costs as an example:

$$\mathrm{DMC}_i = [\mathrm{PH}_i \times \mathrm{QH}_i + \mathrm{PV}_i \times \mathrm{QV}_i \times 26 + \mathrm{PM}_i \times \mathrm{QM}_i \times 26] \times \mathrm{POP},$$

in which DMC is the direct medical cost, i is the one of the particular illness, PH is the average cost of hospitalization, QH is the number of hospitalizations per capital within 12 months, PV is the average cost of outpatient visit, QV is the number of outpatient visits per capital within 2 weeks, PM is the average cost of self-treatment, QM is the number of self-treatment per capital within 2 weeks and POP is the number of population for a particular year.

The top-down approach is mainly used to calculate the economic burden of a disease caused by exposure under risk. The approach often uses an epidemiological measure known as the population-attributable fraction (PAF). Following is the calculation formula:

$$\mathrm{PAF} = p(RR - 1)/[p(RR - 1) + 1],$$

in which p is the prevalence rate and RR is the relative risk. Then the economic burden of a disease is obtained by multiplying the direct economic burden by the PAF.

Indirect economic burden is often estimated in the following ways: the human capital method, the willingness-to-pay approach (25.16) and the friction-cost method. Human capital method is to calculate the indirect economic burden according to the fact that the patients' income reduce under the loss of time. By this method, the lost time is multiplied by the market salary rate. To calculate the indirect economic burden caused by premature death, the lost time can be represented by the potential years of life lost (PYLL); human capital approach and disability-adjusted life years (DALY) can be combined to calculate the indirect economic burden of disease. The friction cost method only estimates the social losses arising from the process lasting from the patient's leaving to the point a qualified player appears. This method is carried under the assumption that short-term job losses can be offset by a new employee and the cost of hiring new staff is only the expense generated during the process of hiring, training and enabling them to be skilled. We call the process train time.

25.9. Catastrophic Health Expenditure[15–17]

Catastrophic health expenditure exists when the total expenditure of a family's health services is equal to or greater than the family's purchasing power or is equal to or higher than 40% of the family's household expenditure. In 2002, WHO proposed that catastrophic health expenditure, being connected with the family's purchasing power, should be the main indicator of a family's financial burden caused by diseases. And health expenditure will be viewed as catastrophic when the family's has to cut down on necessities to pay for one or more family members' health services. Specifically, health expenditure will be viewed as catastrophic whenever it is greater than or equal to 40% of a household's disposable income.

Let us assume T as out-of-pocket health expenditure (OOP), x as total household expenditure, $f(x)$ as food expenditure, or more broadly non-discretionary expenditure. When T/x or $T/[x - f(x)]$ is over a certain standard (z), it means a family suffered catastrophic health expenditure. The general research proposed that catastrophic health expenditure appears if the denominator is total household spending (x) and z is 10%. WHO takes 40% as a standard when the family's purchasing power ($[x - f(x)]$) is viewed as the denominator.

(1) The frequency of catastrophic health expenditures is the sum of the families suffering from catastrophic health expenditures among the families surveyed.

$$H = \frac{1}{N}\sum_{i=1}^{N} E_i,$$

in which N is the number of families surveyed, and E means the family suffered from catastrophic health expenditure: $T_i/x_i > z, E = 1; T_i/x_i < z, E = 0$.

(2) The intensity of catastrophic health expenditures is the index of T/x or $T/[x - f(x)]$ minus the standard (z) divided by the number of families surveyed, which reflects the severity of catastrophic health expenditures, in which N is the number of families surveyed.

$$O_i = E_i\left(\frac{T_i}{x_i} - z\right),$$

$$O = \frac{1}{N}\sum_{i=1}^{N} O_i.$$

(3) The average gap of catastrophic health expenditure, reflecting the extent of household health expenditure over the defined standard, equals the difference between the percentage of OOP of the family suffering catastrophic health expenditure of the total household consumption

expenditure and the defined standard (z). Dividing all the average gaps of catastrophic health expenditure of the family summed up by the sample households, we could get the average gap of catastrophic health expenditure, which reflects the whole social severity of the catastrophic health expenditure.

The frequency of catastrophic health expenditures can be taken to make a comparison among different areas and to analyze the tendency of different periods of the same area. As time goes by, the whole influences of OOP towards the average household living conditions in the region are weakened, if the incidence and average gap of catastrophic health expenditure in a region are narrowing; otherwise, the influences are strengthened. At the same time, the research of catastrophic health expenditure can also detect the security capability of a nation's health insurance system.

25.10. Health Service Cost[1,2,18,19]

Health service cost refers to the monetary expression of resources consumed by health services provider during the process of providing some kinds of health services. The content of cost can be different according to the classification methods: (1) In accordance with the correlation and traceability of cost and health services scheme, cost can be divided into direct cost and indirect cost. Cost that can be directly reckoned into health services scheme or directly consumed by health services scheme is the direct cost of the scheme, such as drug and material expenses, diagnosis and treatment expenses, outpatient or hospitalization expenses and other expenses directly related to the therapeutic schedule of one disease. Indirect cost refers to the cost which is consumed but cannot be directly traced to a vested cost object. It could be reckoned into a health services scheme after being shared. (2) In accordance with the relationship between change of cost and output, cost can be divided into unfixed cost, fixed cost and mixed cost. Fixed cost is defined as the cost which will not change with health services amount under a certain period and a certain production. Unfixed cost is the cost which changes with the health services amount proportionately. Mixed cost refers to the cost changing with the quantity of output but not necessarily changing with a certain proportion and it contains both fixed and unfixed elements.

Health service cost usually consists of the following aspects: human cost, fixed asset depreciation, material cost, public affair cost, business cost, low value consumables cost and other costs.

One focus of counting Health service cost is to ascertain the objects being calculated and the scope of cost.The objects being calculated means that the cost should be categorized to a certain health services project, a certain health planning or a certain health services provider. The scope of cost refers to the category of resources consumed which should be categorized to the object of cost measurement, and it involves such problems as the correlation or traceability between the resources consumed and the object of cost measurement, the scalability of cost and so forth.

There are two elements in the measurement of direct cost: utilization quantity and price of the resources consumed. The utilization quantity can be obtained by retrospect of service processes such as hospital records, logbook, etc. For most service forms, the units cost of a service can be expressed by price, while the cost of all kinds of services units can be determined by the current market price. The resource consumption lacking market price, such as doctors' work time or patients' delayed admission time, can be replaced by the market wage rate. Thus, accounting is usually replaced by average wage rate. For the time patients and their families consume, we need to evaluate whether it should be paid as work time or spare time, etc. Accordingly, we can calculate their time cost.

To calculate indirect cost, like the service cost, hospital administration and logistics consume, we should allocate indirect costs of different participants to different service items. The common methods of allocation include direct allocation method, ladder allocation method and iteration step allocation method. In the process of allocation, different resource consumption has different ways to calculate parameters and coefficients of allocation. For instance, when a hospital needs to allocate its human cost of non-business departments to business departments, the consumption of human cost usually uses personnel number as allocation parameter, and allocates to departments using cost departments' personnel number/the total personnel number of the hospital.

25.11. Cost-effectiveness Analysis, (CEA)[2,3,20,21,22]

CEA refers to analysis or evaluation by combining health intervention projects or treatment protocols' input and output or cost and effectiveness, thereby choosing economic optimal method. It can be used in choosing project and analysis for disease diagnosis and treatment schemes, health planning, health policy, etc. Generalized effectiveness refers to all outcomes produced after the implementation of health services scheme. Specific effectiveness refers to the outcomes which meet people's needs. It is often reflected by the change of index of health improvement such as prevalence, death rates, life expectancy, etc. The basic idea of CEA is to get the maximum effect of output with the minimum cost of input. In the comparison and selection of different schemes, the scheme which has optimal effect with the same cost or has minimal cost with the same effect is the economic optimal scheme. The common indices for CEA are cost-effectiveness ratio and incremental cost-effectiveness ratio.

Cost-effectiveness ratio method is to choose a scheme according to the value of cost-effectiveness ratio, which is based on the idea regarding the scheme with the lowest ratio as optimal scheme. Cost-effectiveness ratio connects cost with effectiveness and is reflected by cost of unit effect such as the cost of each patient detected in tumor screening and the cost of keeping his life for a year. Calculation formula of cost-effectiveness ratio is

$$\text{Cost} - \text{effectiveness ratio} = C/E,$$

in which C means cost and E means effectiveness.

Incremental cost-effectiveness ratio method is used to choose optimal scheme when there is no budget constraint, both cost of input and effect of output are different, and when the maximum efficiency of the fund is considered. For instance, in the field of health, the progress of health services technology is to get better health outcomes and usually new technology with better effect costs more. At this point, we can use the incremental cost-effectiveness in the evaluation and selection of schemes.

The steps of incremental cost-effectiveness ratio method are: Firstly, calculate the increasing input and the increasing output after changing one scheme to the alternative one. Secondly, calculate the incremental cost-effectiveness ratio, which reflects the extra cost needed for an unit of additional effect. At last, combine budget constraints and policy makers' value judgment to make evaluation and selection of schemes. The calculation formula of incremental cost-effectiveness ratio is

$$\Delta C/\Delta E = (C_1 - C_2)/(E_1 - E_2),$$

in which ΔC is the incremental cost; ΔE is the incremental effect; C_1 is the cost of scheme 1; C_2 is the cost of scheme 2; E_1 is the effect of scheme 1; E_2 is the effect of scheme 2.

About CEA, there are several problems that should be paid attention to: (1) Determine effectiveness indexes of different alternatives for comparing, and the indexes should be the most essential output result or can exactly reflect the implementation effectiveness of the scheme. (2) Determine the category and calculation methods of all alternatives' cost and effectiveness.

(3) The cost needs to discount, so does the output result. (4) Only when the alternatives have the same kind of effectiveness can they be compared.

25.12. Cost-Benefit Analysis (CBA)[20,23,24]

CBA is a way to evaluate and choose by comparing the whole benefit and cost between two or among several schemes. The basic idea of evaluation and optimization is: choose the scheme with the maximum benefit when costs are the same; choose the scheme with the minimum cost when benefits are the same. Health services benefit is the health services effectiveness reflected by currency, and it contains direct benefit (like the reduced treating fee as a result of incidence' decline), indirect benefit (like reduced loss of income or growth brought to production) and intangible benefit (like the transformation of comfortable sensation brought by physical rehabilitation). The common indexes for CBA are net present value (NPV), cost-benefit ratio (C/B), net equivalent annual benefit and internal rate of return, etc. When the initial investment or planning period is the same, we can use NPV or cost-benefit ratio to make evaluation and optimization among multiple alternatives; otherwise, we can use net equivalent annual benefit and internal rate of return. As far as money's time value is considered, we should convert costs and benefits at different time points to the same time point when doing cost-benefit analysis.

1. Net present value (NPV)

NPV is defined as the difference between health service scheme's sum of benefit (present value) and cost (present value). NPV method is to evaluate and choose schemes by evaluating the difference between the whole benefit of health services and the sum of the cost of different schemes during the period. Calculation formula of NPV is

$$\mathrm{NPV} = \sum_{t=1}^{n} \frac{B_t - C_t}{1 - r},$$

in which NPV is the NPV (net benefit), B_t is the benefit occurring at the end of the t year, C_t is the cost occurring at the end of the t year, n is the age of the scheme, r is discount rate. If NPV is greater than 0, it means the scheme can improve benefit and the scheme of NPV is optimal.

2. Cost benefit ratio (C/B)

(C/B) is to evaluate and choose schemes by evaluating the ratio of schemes' benefit (present value) and cost (present value) through the evaluation period. Calculation formula of C/B is

$$\text{Cost Benefit ratio} = C/B,$$

$$C = \sum_{t=1}^{n} \frac{C_t}{(1+r)^t},$$

$$B = \sum_{t=1}^{n} \frac{B_t}{(1+r)^t},$$

in which B is the total benefit (present value), C is the total cost (present value), r is the known discount rate. If the C/B is smaller or B/C is greater, the scheme is more optimal.

CBA can be used to evaluate and select schemes with different output results. One of the difficulties is to ensure the currency value for health services output. At present, human capital method and willingness-to-pay (WTP) method are the most common ones to be used. Human capital method usually monetizes the loss value of health session or early death by using market wage rates or life insurance loss ratio.

25.13. Cost-Utility Analysis (CUA)[11,20,25,26]

CUA is an assessment method for health outcomes particularly of producing or abandoning health services project, plan or treatment options, and it is to evaluate and optimize alternatives by combining cost input and utility output. The utility of health services scheme means health services scheme satisfies people's expectation or satisfaction level in specific health condition, or means the ability to satisfy people's need and desire to get healthy. Common evaluation indexes are quality adjusted life years and disability adjusted life years, etc.

As the measurement of utility needs to consume biggish cost, CUA is mainly used for the following situations: (1) when quality of life is the most important output; (2) when alternatives affect both the quantity and quality of life while decision makers want to reflect these two outputs with only one index; (3) when the target is to compare a health intervention with other health interventions that has been assessed by CUA.

Cost utility ration method can be used to do CUA. The method can assess scheme's economic rationality by comparing different schemes' cost effectiveness ration.

For example, there are two treatment schemes for a disease named A and B. Scheme A can prolong lifespan for 4.5 years with ¥10000; Scheme B prolongs lifespan for 3.5 years with ¥5000. But quality of life (utility value) of two schemes is different as A's quality of life is 0.9 in every survival year while B is 0.5.

CEA result shows: For scheme A, cost is ¥2222.22 for every survival year while scheme B is ¥1428.57. Scheme B is superior to scheme A.

CUA result reveals: Scheme A's cost-utility ratio is 2469.14 while scheme B is 2857.14. Scheme A is superior to scheme B.

If the quality of life during survival was more concerned, CUA is better to assess and optimize schemes and scheme A is superior to scheme B.

At present, about the calculation of the utility of quality of life (QOL weight), mainly the following methods are used: Evaluation method, literature method and sampling method. (1) Evaluation method: Relevant experts make assessments according to their experience, estimate the value of health utility or its possible range, and then make sensitivity analysis to explore the reliability of the assessments. (2) Literature method: Utility indexes from existing literature can be directly used, but we should pay attention whether they match our own research, including the applicability of the health status it determines, assessment objects and assessment methods. (3) Sampling method: Obtain the utility value of quality of life through investigating and scoring patients' physiological or psychological function status, and this is the most accurate method. Specific methods are rating scale, standard gamble, time trade-off, etc. Currently, the most widely used measuring tool of utility are the WHOQOL scale and related various modules, happiness scale/quality of well-being index (QWB), health-utilities index (HUI), Euro QOL five-dimension questionnaire (EQ-5D), SF-6D scale (SF-6D) and Assessment of Quality of Life (AQOL).

25.14. Premium Rate[2,27,28]

The premium rate is the proportion of insurance fee the insured paid to the income. Premium is the fee the insured paid for a defined set of insurance coverage. The insurers establish insurance fund with the premium to compensate the loss they suffered from the accidents insured.

Premium rate is composed of pure premium rate and additional premium rate. The premium rate is determined by loss probability. The premium collected according to pure premium rate is called pure premium, and it is used for reimbursement when the insurance risks occur. The additional premium rate is calculated on the basis of the insurer's operating expenses, and the additional premium is used for business expenditures, handling charges and part of profits.

$$\text{Pure Premium Rate} = \text{Loss Ratio of Insuarance Amount} + \text{Stability Factor},$$

$$\text{Loss Ratio of Insurance Amount} = \frac{\text{Reparation Amount}}{\text{Insurance Amount}},$$

$$\text{Addition a Premium Rate} = \frac{\text{Operation Expenditures} + \text{Proper Profits}}{\text{Pure Premium}}.$$

At present, there are two ways, wage-scale system and flat-rate system, to calculate premium rate.

(1) In the wage-scale system, the premium is collected in a certain percentage of salary. It is the most common way of premium collection.

   (a) Equal Premium Rate: The premium rates paid by the insured and the employers are the same. For example, the premium rate paid by the old, the disabled and the dependent is 9.9% of the salary, and the insured and the employers have to pay 4.95% of the salary separate.
   (b) Differential Premium Rate: The premium rates paid by the insured and the employers are different. For example, for the basic medical insurance system for urban employees in China, the premium rate paid by the insured is 2% of the salary, while the employers have to pay 6% of the salary of the insured.
   (c) Incremental Premium Rate: The premium rate will increase if the salary of the insured increases. In other words, the premium rate is lower for the low-income insured, while higher for the high-income ones.
   (d) Regressive Premium Rate: A ceiling is fixed on salary, and the exceeding part of the salary is not levied. The French annuity system and the unemployment insurance are examples.

(2) In the flat-rate system, the premium rate is all the same for different insured irrespective of the salary or position.

The premium rates of social security system of different countries are shown in Figure 25.14.1.

Calculation of the premium rate is mainly influenced by the healthcare demand of residents, the effects of the security system and the government financial input. As the security system and the government financial input

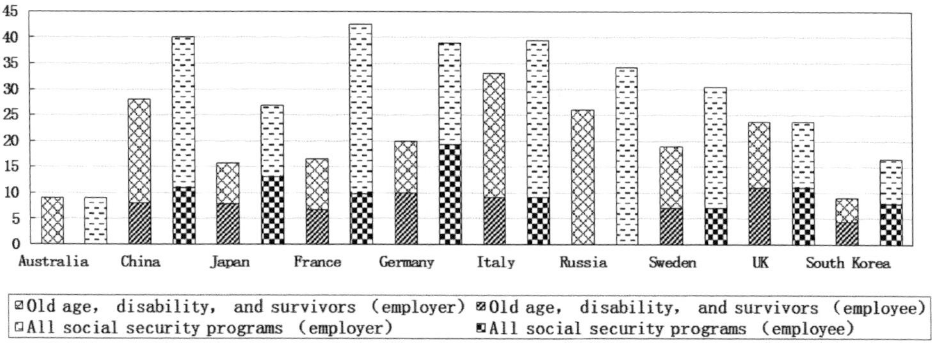

Fig. 25.14.1. The premium rates for social security programs of different countries, 2010 (in percent).
Source: Social Security Programs throughout the World in 2010

are usually fixed, the calculation of the premium rate is to ascertain the total financing mainly by estimating the assumption of residents. After the total financing is determined, individual premium can be ascertained, further, the premium rate is calculated according to the individual salary.

25.15. Equity in Health Financing[29–31]

The equity in health financing is the requirement that all people be treated equally in entire health financing system. It mainly focuses on the relationship between the health financing and the ability to pay. The equality of health financing determines not only the availability of health services, but also the quantity of families falling into poverty because of illness.

The equity in health financing mostly focuses on the household contributions to the health financing. No matter who pays the health expenditure, all of the health payment will eventually spread over each family of the whole society. The equity in health financing includes the vertical equity and the horizontal equity. The level of the residents' health expenditure should be corresponded to his ability to pay, which means that the residents with higher payoff capacity should raise more money than those with lower payoff capacity. Vertical equity means the family with the same capacity to pay should make a similar contribution for health financing, whereas vertical equity means that a family with a higher capacity to pay should have a higher ratio of health expenditure to household income. For vertical equity, health-financing system is progressive when the ratio of health expenditure to household income is higher, and is regressive when the ratio of health expenditure to household income is lower. When the ratio for each family is the same, the health-financing system can be seen proportional. Generally, the advanced health-financing system should be a progressive system.

There are many indexes to measure the fairness in health financing, such as Gini coefficient, concentration index (CI), Kakwani index, fairness of financing contribution (FFC), redistributive effect (RE), catastrophic health expenditure and so on.

The Kakwani index is a common measure to evaluate vertical equity or progressivity of a health-financing system. It is equal to the difference between the Gini index for the health financing and the Gini index for the capacity to pay, which is twice the area between the Lorenz curve and the concentration curve. Theoretically, the Kakwani index can vary from −2 to 1. The value is positive when the health-financing system is progressive; when the health-financing system is regressive, it is negative. When the Kakwani index is zero, the health-financing system is proportional.

FFC reflects the distribution of health-financing contribution, which is calculating the proportion of household health-expenditure to the household disposable income, known as household health financing contribution (HFC).The equation may be described as follows:

$$\mathrm{HFC}_h = \frac{\text{Household Health Expenditure}}{\text{Household Diaposable Income}}.$$

FFC is actually a distribution of HFC, and the equation follows as

$$\mathrm{FFC} = 1 - \sqrt[3]{\sum_{h=1}^{n} \frac{|\mathrm{HFC}_h - \mathrm{HFC}_0|^3}{n}},$$

In which HFC_h is the ratio of the healthcare expenditure to the disposable income. FFC can vary from 0 to 1. The larger the value, the more equity for the health financing. It indicates absolute fairness when the index is 1.

We need to study the family's capacity of payment in order to calculate the equity in health financing, and we usually get the statistics of the household consumption expenditure and household health expenditure through family investigation.

25.16. WTP[12,32,33]

WTP is the payment which an individual is willing to sacrifice in order to accept a certain amount of goods or services after valuing them by synthesizing individuals' cognitive value and the necessity of goods or services.

There are two methods, stated preference method and revealed preference method, to measure an individual's WTP. The stated preference method is a measure to predict the WTP for goods based on the consumers' responses under a hypothetical situation so as to get the value of the goods. The revealed preference method is used to measure the maximum amount during exchanging or developing their health after looking for an individual's action on the health risk factors in the actual market. The stated preference technique includes contingent valuation method (CVM), conjoint analysis (CA) method and choice experiments (CE) method. Among them, the CVM is the most common way to measure WTP.

1. Contingent Valuation Method (CVM)

CVM is one of the most popular and effective techniques to estimate the value of public goods. Consumers are induced to show their favors to public goods by providing a hypothetical market and a way of being questioned, so that they would like to spend maximum amount protecting and developing the goods. In a practical application of the CVM, the most crucial element is the guidance technology or questionnaire to elicit the maximum WTP. Nowadays, the guidance technology of CMV includes continuous WPT guidance technology and discrete WPT guidance technology.

2. Conjoint Analysis (CA)

CA, known as the comprehensive analysis, is commonly used in marketing studies to measure the preference that consumers make among two or more attributes of an analog product under a hypothetical market. According to the consumers' responses to these products, researchers can separately estimate the utility or relative values of the products or services with the method of mathematical statistics. Therefore, the best products could be found by studying the consumers' favor in purchasing and the potential measure of value about products and the consumers' favor of the products.

3. Choice Experiments (CE)

CEs is a technique of exploring consumer preference or WTP for the attributes of various goods in a hypothetical market on the basis of attribute value and random utility maximization. A CE presents consumers with a set of alternatives combination composed by different attributes and consumers are asked to choose their favorite alternative. Researchers can estimate separate values for each attribute or the relative value for attribute combination of any particular alternative according to consumer's responses. Multinomial Logit Model is a basic model in choosing experiment models.

25.17. Data Envelopment Analysis, (DEA)[34–36]

DEA is an efficiency calculating method for multiple decision-making units (DMU) with multi-input and output. For maximum efficiency, DEA model can compare the efficiency of a specific unit with several similar units providing same services. A unit is called relative efficiency is unit if the efficiency equal to 100%, while a unit is called inefficiency unit if the efficiency score is less than 100%. There are many DEA models, and the basic linear model can be set up as the following steps:

Step 1: Define variables

Assume that E_k is the efficiency ratio, uj is the coefficient of output j, which means the efficiency decrease is caused by a unit decrease in output. And v_I $(I = 1, 2, \ldots, n)$ is the coefficient of input I, which means the efficiency decrease is caused by a unit decrease in input. DMU_k consumes amount I_{jk} of input I, and produces amount O_{jk} of output j within a certain period.

Step 2: Establish the objective function

We need to find out a group of coefficient u and v to make sure the highest possible efficiency of the valuated unit.

$$\max E_e = \frac{u_1 O_{1e} + u_2 O_{2e} + \cdots + u_M O_{Me}}{v_1 I_{1e} + v_2 I_{2e} + \cdots + v_m I_{Me}},$$

in which e is the code of the valuated unit. This function satisfies a constraint that the efficiency of the comparative units will not be more than 100% when the same set of input and output coefficients (u_i and v_i) is fed into any other comparative units.

Step 3: Constraint conditions

$$\frac{u_1 O_{1k} + u_2 O_{2k} + \cdots + u_M O_{Mk}}{v_1 I_{1k} + v_2 I_{2k} + \cdots + v_M I_{Mk}} \leq 1.0.$$

Here, all coefficients are positive and non-zero.

If the optimal value of the model is equal to 1, and two slack variables are both equal to 0, the DMU is DEA-efficient. If two slack variables are not equal to 0, the DMU is weakly efficient. If the optimal value of the model is less than 1, the DMU is DEA-inefficient, which means the current production activity is inefficient neither in technique nor in scale. We can reduce input while keeping output constantly.

DEA is a non-parametric analysis method, which does not add any hypothesis on the potential distribution of inefficiency parameters, and assumes all the producers away from the efficient frontier are inefficient. As regards the result of DEA analysis, efficient is relative, while inefficient is absolute. The current study of DEA analysis focuses on the selection of input and output indicators. We can select indicators by literature study, Delphi method or in professional view. We should select suitable DEA analysis model, such as CCR, BCC, CRS, and so on for different problems. The most direct software used currently is DEAP2.1, which is developed by Australia University of New England, and SAS, SPSS, Excel can also be used to do the calculation.

25.18. Stochastic Frontier Analysis, (SFA)[37–39]

SFA is put forward and developed to overcome the limitations of data envelopment analysis (DEA, 25.17). In the SFA, error consists of two components. The first one is one-side error, which can be used to measure inefficiency and restrict the error term to be one side error, so as to guarantee the productive unit working above or under the estimated production frontier. The second error component, pure error, is intended to capture the effect of statistical noise.

The basic model of SFA is

$$y_i = \beta_i x_i + \mu_i + v_i.$$

Clearly, y_i is output, x_i is input, and β_i is constant; μ_i is the first error component, and v_i is the second error component.

It is difficult to integrate all outputs into a single indicator in estimating the production frontier in the research of health services. However, it is easy to integrate the cost into a single indicator when it is presented by currency. Thus, SFA is used to estimate the cost frontier instead of production frontier. What is more, stochastic frontier cost function is another production function, so it is an effective method to measure the productivity. The stochastic frontier cost function is

$$C_i = f(p_i, y_i, z_i) + \mu_i + v_i,$$

in which C_i is the cost of outputs, p_i is the price of all inputs, and z_i represents the characteristics of producers. In a research of hospital services, for example, we can put the hospital characteristics and cases mixed into the model, and discuss the relationship between these variables and productivity from the statistics. It is worth noting that we need logarithmic transformation in the stochastic frontier cost function, which can expand the test scope of cost function and maintain the original hypothesis.

When we encounter a small sample size in the research of hospital efficiency, we need aggregate inputs and outputs. When we estimate inefficiency and error, we can introduce a function equation less dependent of data, such as the Cobb–Douglas production function. However, we avoid taking any wrong hypothesis into the model.

SFA is a method of parametric analysis, whose conclusion of efficiency evaluation is stable. We need to make assumptions on the potential distribution of the inefficient parameter, and admit that inefficiency of some producers deviating from the boundaries may be due to the accidental factors. Its main advantage is the fact that this method takes the random error into consideration, and is easy to make statistical inference to the results of the analysis. However, disadvantages of SFA include complex calculation, large sample size, exacting requirements of statistical characteristics about inefficient indicators. Sometimes, SFA is not easy to deal with more outputs, and accuracy of results is affected seriously if the production function cannot be set up properly. Nowadays, the most direct analysis software is frontier Version 4.1 developed by University of New England in Australia, Stata, SAS, etc.

25.19. Gini Coefficient[2,40,41]

Gini coefficient is proposed by the famous Italian economist Corrado Gini on the basis of the Lorenz curve, which is the most common measure of inequality of income or of wealth. It is equal to the ratio of the area that lies between the line of perfect equality and the Lorenz curve over the total area under the diagonal in Figure 25.19.1.

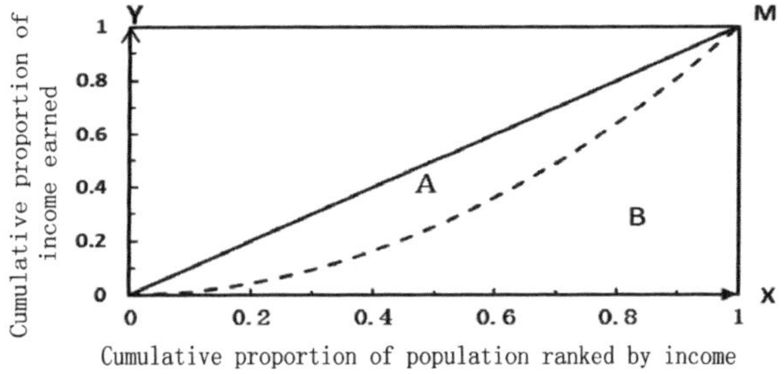

Fig. 25.19.1. Graphical representation of the Gini coefficient and the Lorenz curve.

Figure 25.19.1 depicts the cumulative portion of the population ranked by income (on the x-axis) graphed with the cumulative portion of earned income (on the y-axis). The diagonal line indicates the "perfect distribution", known as "the line of equality", which generally does not exist. Along this line, each income group is earning an equal portion of the income. The curve above the line of equality is the actual income curve known as Lorenz curve. The curvature degree of Lorenz curve represents the inequality of the income distribution of a nation's residents. The further the Lorenz curve is from the diagonal, the greater the degree of inequality.

The area of A is enclosed by the line of equality and the Lorenz curve, while the area of B is bounded by the Lorenz curve and the fold line OXM, then the equation of Gini coefficient follows as

$$G = \frac{A}{A+B}.$$

If Lorenz curve is represented by a function $Y = L(X)$, then

$$G = 1 - 2\int_0^1 L(X)dx.$$

According to the income of residents, the Gini coefficient is usually defined mathematically based on the Lorenz curve, which plots the proportion of the total income of the population that is cumulatively earned by the bottom X% of the population. Nowadays, there are three methods fitting the Lorenz curve,

(1) Geometric calculation: to calculate the partition approximately by geometric calculation based on grouped data. The more the number groups divided, the more accurate the result.
(2) Distribution function: to fit the Lorenz curve by the probability density function of the income distribution;
(3) Fitting of a curve: to select the appropriate curve to fit the Lorenz curve directly, such as quadratic curve, index curve, power function curve.

The Gini coefficient can theoretically range from 0 (complete equality) to 1 (complete inequality), but in practice, both extreme values are not quite reached. Generally, we always set the value of above 0.4 as the alert level of income distribution (see Table 25.19.1).

Table 25.19.1. The relationship between the Gini coefficient and income distribution.

Gini Coefficient	Income Distribution
Lower than 0.2	Absolute equality
0.2–0.3	Relative equality
0.3–0.4	Relative rationality
0.4–0.5	Larger income disparity
Above 0.5	Income disparity

25.20. Concentration Index (CI)[2,42,43]

CI is usually defined mathematically from the Concentration curve, which is equally twice the area between the curve and the 45-degree line, known as "the line of equality". This index provides a measure of the extent of inequalities in health that are systematically associated with socio-economic status. The value of CI ranges from −1 (all the population's illness is concentrated in the hands of the most disadvantaged persons) to +1 (all the population's illness is concentrated in the hands of the least disadvantaged persons). When the health equality is irrelevant to the socio-economic status, the value of CI can be zero. CI is defined as positive when there is nothing to do with the absolute level of health (or ill-health) and income.

The curve labelled L(s) in Figure 25.20.1 is a concentration curve for illness. It plots the cumulative proportions of the population ranked by socio-economic status against the cumulative proportions of illness. The further

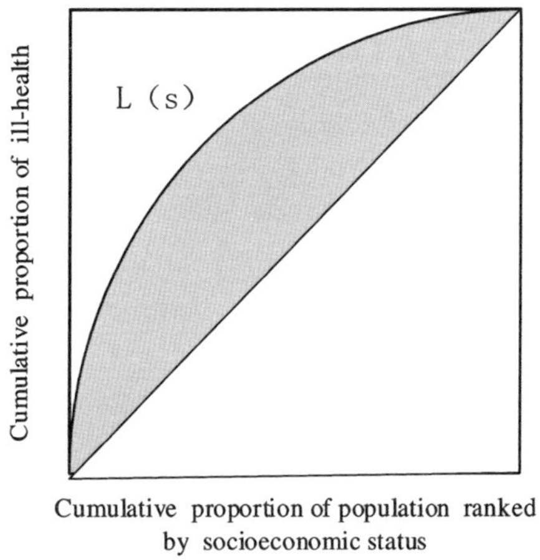

Fig. 25.20.1. Illness CI.

the L(s) is from the diagonal, the greater the degree of inequality. If the illness is equally distributed among socio-economic groups, the concentration curve will coincide with the diagonal. The CI is positive when L(s) lies below the diagonal (illness is concentrated amongst the higher socio-economic groups) and is negative when L(s) lies above the diagonal (illness is concentrated amongst the lower socio-economic groups).

The CI is stated as

$$\mathrm{CI} = \frac{2}{\overline{y}}\mathrm{cov}(y_i, R_i),$$

in which CI is the concentration index, y_i is the healthcare utilization of income group $i, \overline{y}$ is the mean healthcare use in the population, and R_i is the cumulative fraction of population in fraction income group i. The unweighted covariance of y_i and R_i is

$$\mathrm{cov}(y_i, R_i) = \sum_{i=1}^{i=n} \frac{(y_i - \overline{y})(R_i - \overline{R})}{n}.$$

Clearly, if richer than average, $(R_i - \overline{R}) > 0$, and more healthy than average at the same time, $(y_i - \overline{y}) > 0$, then CI will be positive. But if poorer and less healthy than average, the corresponding product will also be positive.

If the health level tends to the rich but not to the poor, the covariance will tend to be positive. Conversely, a bias to the poor will tend to result in a negative covariance. We understand that a positive value for CI suggests a bias to the rich and a negative value for CI suggests a bias to the poor.

The limitation of the CI is that it only reflects relative relationship between the health and the socio-economic status. While CI will give the same result among the different groups even the shapes of the concentration curve are in great difference. Then, we need to standardize the CI. Many methods, such as multiple linear regression, negative binomial regression and so on, can be used to achieve CI standardized. Keeping the factors that affect the health status at the same level, Health Inequity Index is created where it suggests the unfair health status caused by economic level under the same demands for health.

The Health Inequity Index is defined as

$$\mathrm{HI} = \mathrm{CI}_M - \mathrm{CI}_N,$$

in which CI_M is the non-standardized CI and CI_N is the standardized CI to affect health factors.

References

1. Cheng, XM, Luo, WJ. *Economics of Health.* Beijing: People's Medical Publishing House, 2003.
2. Folland, S, Goodman, AC, Stano, M. *Economics of Health and Health Care.* (6th edn.). San Antonio: Pearson Education, Inc, 2010.
3. Meng, QY, Jiang, QC, Liu, GX, *et al. Health Economics.* Beijing: People's Medical Publishing House, 2013.
4. OECD Health Policy Unit. *A System of Health Accounts for International Data Collection.* Paris: OECD, 2000, pp. 1–194.
5. World Health Organization. *System of Health Accounts.* Geneva: WHO, 2011, pp. 1–471.
6. Bronfenbrenner, M, Sichel, W, Gardner, W. *Microeconomics.* (2nd edn.), Boston: Houghton Mifflin Company, 1987.
7. Feldstein, PJ. *Health Care Economics* (5th edn.). New York: Delmar Publishers, 1999.
8. Grossman, M. On the concept of health capital and the demand for health. *J. Poli. Econ.*, 1972, 80(2): 223–255.
9. National Health and Family Planning Commission Statistical Information Center. *The Report of The Fifth Time National Health Service Survey Analysis in 2013.* Beijing: Xie-he Medical University Publishers, 2016, 65–79.
10. Manning, WG, Newhouse, JP, Duan, N, *et al.* Health Insurance and the Demand for Medical Care: Evidence from a Randomized Experiment. *Am. Eco. Rev.*, 1987, 77(3): 251–277.
11. Inadomi, JM, Sampliner, R, Lagergren, J. Screening and surveillance for Barrett esophagus in high-risk groups: A cost-utility analysis. *P Ann. Intern. Medi.*, 2003, 138(3): 176–186.
12. Hodgson, TA, Meiners, MR. Cost-of-illness methodology: A guide to current practices and procedures. *Milbank Mem. Fund Q.*, 1982, 60(3): 429–462.
13. Segel, JE. Cost-of-illness Studies: A Primer. RTI-UNC Center of Excellence in Health Promotion, 2006: pp. 1–39.
14. Tolbert, DV, Mccollister, KE, Leblanc, WG, *et al.* The economic burden of disease by industry: Differences in quality-adjusted life years and associated costs. *Am. J. Indust. Medi.*, 2014, 57(7): 757–763.
15. Berki, SE. A look at catastrophic medical expenses and the poor. *Health Aff.*, 1986, 5(4): 138–145.
16. Xu, K, Evans, DB, Carrin, G, *et al. Designing Health Financing Systems to Reduce Catastrophic Health Expenditure: Technical Briefs for Policy — Makers.* Geneva: WHO, 2005, pp. 1–5.
17. Xu, K, Evans, DB, Kawabata, K, *et al.* Household catastrophic health expenditure: A multicounty analysis. *The Lancet*, 2003, 362(9378): 111–117.
18. Drummond, MF, Jefferson, TO. Guidelines for authors and peer reviewers of economic submissions to the BMJ. The BMJ Economic Evaluation Working Party.[J]. *BMJ Clinical Research*, 1996, 313(7052): 275–283.
19. Wiktorowicz, ME, Goeree, R, Papaioannou, A, *et al.* Economic implications of hip fracture: Health service use, institutional care and cost in canada. *Osteoporos. Int.*, 2001, 12(4): 271–278.
20. Drummod, ME, Sculpher, MJ, Torrance, GW, *Methods for the Economic Evaluation of Health Care Programmes.* Translated by Shixue Li, Beijing: People's Medical Publishing House, 2008.

21. Edejer, TT, World Health Organization. Making choices in health: WHO guide to cost-effectiveness analysis. *Rev. Esp. Salud Pública*, 2003, 78(3): 217–219.
22. Muennig, P. *Cost-effectiveness Analyses in Health: A Practical Approach.* Jossey-Bass, 2008: 8–9.
23. Bleichrodt, H, Quiggin, J. Life-cycle preferences over consumption and health: When is cost-effectiveness analysis equivalent to cost-benefit analysis?. *J. Health Econ.*, 1999, 18(6): 681–708.
24. Špačková, O, Daniel, S. Cost-benefit analysis for optimization of risk protection under budget constraints. *Neurology*, 2012, 29(2): 261–267.
25. Dernovsek, MZ, Prevolnik-Rupel, V, Tavcar, R. *Cost-Utility Analysis: Quality of Life Impairment in Schizophrenia, Mood and Anxiety Disorders.* Netherlands: Springer 2006, pp. 373–384.
26. Mehrez, A, Gafni, A. Quality-adjusted life years, utility theory, and healthy-years equivalents. *Medi. Decis. Making*, 1989, 9(2): 142–149.
27. United States Social Security Administration (US SSA). Social Security Programs Throughout the World. Asia and the Pacific. 2010. Washington, DC: Social Security Administration, 2011, pp. 23–24.
28. United States Social Security Administration (US SSA). Social Security Programs Throughout the World: Europe. 2010. Washington, DC Social Security Administration, 2010, pp. 23–24.
29. Kawabata, K. Preventing impoverishment through protection against catastrophic health expenditure. *Bull. World Health Organ.*, 2002, 80(8): 612.
30. Murray Christopher, JL, Knaul, F, Musgrove, P, *et al. Defining and Measuring Fairness in Financial Contribution to the Health System.* Geneva: WHO, 2003, 1–38.
31. Wagstaff, A, Doorslaer, EV, Paci, P. Equity in the finance and delivery of health care: Some tentative cross-country comparisons. *Oxf. Rev. Econ. Pol.*, 1989, 5(1): 89–112.
32. Barnighausen, T, Liu, Y, Zhang, XP, *et al.* Willingness to pay for social health insurance among informal sector workers in Wuhan, China: A contingent valuation study. *BMC Health Serv. Res.*, 2007(7): 4.
33. Breidert, C, Hahsler, M, Reutterer, T. A review of methods for measuring willingness-to-pay. *Innovative Marketing*, 2006, 2(4): 1–32.
34. Cook, WD, Seifod, LM. Data envelopment analysis (DEA) — Thirty years on. *Euro. J. Oper. Res.*, 192(2009): 1–17.
35. Ma, ZX. *Data Envelopment Analysis Model and Method.* Beijing: Science Press, 2010: 20–49.
36. Nunamaker, TR. Measuring routine nursing service efficiency: A comparison of cost per patient day and data envelopment analysis models. *Health Serv. Res.*, 1983, 18(2 Pt 1): 183–208.
37. Bhattacharyya, A, Lovell, CAK, Sahay, P. The impact of liberalization on the productive efficiency of Indian commercial banks. *Euro. J. Oper. Res.*, 1997, 98(2): 332–345.
38. Kumbhakar, SC, Knox, Lovell, CA. *Stochastic Frontier Analysis.* United Kingdom: Cambridge University Press, 2003.
39. Sun, ZQ. *Comprehensive Evaluation Method and its Application of Medicine.* Beijing: Chemical Industry Press, 2006.
40. Robert, D. A formula for the Gini coefficient. *Rev. Eco. Stat.*, 1979, 1(61): 146–149.
41. Sen, PK. The gini coefficient and poverty indexes: Some reconciliations. *J. Amer. Stat. Asso.*, 2012, 81(396): 1050–1057.
42. Doorslaer, EK AV, Wagstaff, A, Paci, P. On the measurement of inequity in health. *Soc. Sci. Med.*, 1991, 33(5): 545–557.

43. Evans, T, Whitehead, M, Diderichsen, F, *et al. Challenging Inequities in Health: From Ethics to Action.* Oxford: Oxford University Press 2001: pp. 45–59.
44. Benchimol, J. Money in the production function: A new Keynesian DSGE perspective. *South. Econ.*, 2015, 82(1): 152–184.

About the Author

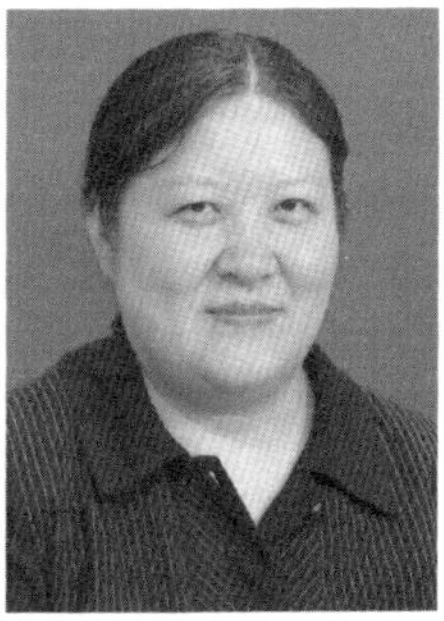

Dr Yingchun Chen is Professor of Medicine and Health Management School in Huazhong University of Science & Technology. She is also the Deputy Director of Rural Health Service Research Centre which is the key research institute of Human & Social Science in Hubei Province, as well as a member of the expert group of New Rural Cooperative Medical Care system of the Ministry of Health (since 2005). Engaged in teaching and researching in the field of health service management for more than 20 years, she mainly teaches Health Economics, and has published Excess Demand of Hospital Service in Rural Area — The Measure and Management of Irrational Hospitalization; what is more, she has been engaged in writing several teaching materials organized by the Ministry of Public Health, such as *Health Economics and Medical Insurance.* As a senior expert in the field of policy on health economy and rural health, she has been the principal investigator for more than 20 research programs at national and provincial levels and published more than 50 papers in domestic and foreign journals.

CHAPTER 26

HEALTH MANAGEMENT STATISTICS

Lei Shang*, Jiu Wang, Xia Wang, Yi Wan and Lingxia Zeng

26.1. United Nations Millennium Development Goals, MDGs[1]

In September 2000, a total of 189 nations, in the "United Nations Millennium Declaration" committed themselves to making the right to development a reality for everyone and to freeing the entire human race from want. The Declaration proposed eight MDGs, including 18 time-bound targets. To monitor progress towards the goals and targets, the United Nations system, including the World Bank and the International Monetary Fund, as well as the Development Assistance Committee (DAC) of the Organization for Economic Co-operation and Development (DECD), came together under the Office of the Secretary-General and agreed on 48 quantitative indicators, which are: proportion of population below $1 purchasing power parity (PPP) per day; poverty gap ratio (incidence multiplied by depth of poverty); share of poorest quintile in national consumption; prevalence of underweight children under 5 years of age; proportion of population below minimum level of dietary energy consumption; net enrolment ratio in primary education; proportion of pupils starting grade 1 who reach grade 5; literacy rate of 15–24 year-olds; ratio of girls to boys in primary, secondary and tertiary education; ratio of literate women to men, 15–24 years old; share of women in wage employment in the non-agricultural sector; proportion of seats held by women in national parliaments; under-five mortality rate; infant mortality rate; proportion of 1-year-old children immunized against measles; maternal mortality ratio; proportion of births attended by skilled health personnel; HIV prevalence among pregnant women aged 15–24 years; condom use rate

*Corresponding author: shanglei@fmmu.edu; 1615675852@qq.com

of the contraceptive prevalence rate; ratio of school attendance of orphans to school attendance of non-orphans aged 10–14 years; prevalence and death rates associated with malaria; proportion of population in malaria-risk areas using effective malaria prevention and treatment measures; prevalence and death rates associated with tuberculosis; proportion of tuberculosis cases detected and cured under directly observed treatment short course; proportion of land area covered by forest; ratio of area protected to maintain biological diversity to surface area; energy use (kilogram oil equivalent) per $1 gross domestic product (GDP); carbon dioxide emissions per capita and consumption of ozone-depleting chlorofluorocarbons; proportion of the population using solid fuels; proportion of population with sustainable access to an improved water source, urban and rural; proportion of population with access to improved sanitation, urban and rural; proportion of households with access to secure tenure; net official development assistance (ODA), total and to the least developed countries, as a percentage of OECD/DAC donors' gross national income; proportion of total bilateral, sector-allocable ODA of OECD/DAC donors to basic social services (basic education, primary healthcare, nutrition, safe water and sanitation); proportion of bilateral ODA of OECD/DAC donors that is untied; ODA received in landlocked countries as a proportion of their gross national incomes; ODA received in small island developing states as a proportion of their gross national incomes; proportion of total developed country imports (by value and excluding arms) from developing countries and from the least developed countries, admitted free of duty; average tariffs imposed by developed countries on agricultural products and clothing from developing countries; agricultural support estimate for OECD countries as a percentage of their gross domestic product; proportion of ODA provided to help build trade capacity; total number of countries that have reached their heavily indebted poor countries (HIPC) decision points and number that have reached their HIPC completion points (cumulative); debt relief committed under HIPC Initiative; debt service as a percentage of exports of goods and services; unemployment rate of young people aged 15–24 years, each sex and total; proportion of population with access to affordable essential drugs on a sustainable basis; telephone lines and cellular subscribers per 100 population; personal computers in use per 100 population and 90 Internet users per 100 population.

26.2. Health Survey System of China[2,3]

The Health Survey System of China consists of nine parts, which are the: Health Resources and Medical Service Survey System, Health Supervision

Survey System, Diseases Control Survey System, Maternal and Child Health Survey System, New Rural Cooperative Medical Survey System, Family Planning Statistical Reporting System, Health And Family Planning Petition Statistical Reporting System, Relevant Laws, Regulations and Documents, and other relevant information. The seven sets of survey system mentioned above include 102 questionnaires and their instructions, which are approved (or recorded) by the National Bureau of Statistics. The main contents include general characteristics of health institutions, implementation of healthcare reform measures, operations of medical institutions, basic information of health manpower, configurations of medical equipment, characteristics of discharged patients, information on blood collection and supply. The surveys aim to investigate health resource allocation and medical services utilization, efficiency and quality in China, and provide reference for monitoring and evaluation of the progress and effectiveness of healthcare system reform, for strengthening the supervision of medical services, and provide basic information for effective organization of public health emergency medical treatment.

The annual reports of health institutions (Tables 1-1–1-8 of Health Statistics Reports) cover all types of medical and health institutions at all levels. The monthly reports of health institutions (Tables 1-9,1-10 of Health Statistics Reports) investigate all types of medical institutions at all levels. The basic information survey of health manpower (Table 2 of Health Statistics Reports) investigates on-post staff and civil servants with health supervisor certification in various medical and health institutions at all levels (except for rural doctors and health workers). The medical equipment questionnaire (Table 3 of Health Statistics Reports) surveys hospitals, maternity and childcare service centers, hospitals for prevention and treatment of specialist diseases, township (street) hospitals, community health service centers and emergency centers (stations). The hospital discharged patients questionnaire (Table 4 of Health Statistics Reports) surveys level-two or above hospitals, government-run county or above hospitals with undetermined level. The blood collection and supply questionnaire (Table 5 of Health Statistics Reports) surveys blood collection agencies.

Tables 1-1–1-10, Tables 2 and 4 of the Health Statistics Reports are reported through the "National Health Statistics Direct Network Report system" by medical and health institutions (excluding clinics and village health rooms) and local health administrative departments at all levels, of which Table 1-3, and the manpower table of clinics and medical rooms are reported by county/district Health Bureaus, and Table 1-4 is reported by its township hospitals or county/district health bureau. The manpower table of civil servants with health supervisor certification is reported by their health administrative department. Provincial health administrative departments report Table 5 information to the Department of Medical Administration of the National Health and Family Planning Commission.

To ensure accurate and timely data reporting, the Health Statistics Information Center of the National Health and Family Planning Commission provides specific reporting timelines and completion demands for various types of tables, and asks relevant personnel and institutions to strictly enforce requirements. In accordance with practical needs, the National Health and Family Planning Commission also provides revision of the health survey system of China.

26.3. Health Indicators Conceptual Framework[4]

In April 2004, the International Standards Organization Technical Committee (ISO/TC) issued the Health Informatics — Health Indicators Conceptual Framework (HICF, ISO/TS 21667) (Table 26.3.1), which specifies the elements of a complete expression of health indicator, standardizes the selection and understanding of health indicators, determines the necessary information for expression of population health and health system performance and their influence factors, determines how information is organized together and its relationship to each other. It provides a comparable way for assessing health statistics indicators from different areas, different regions or countries. According to this conceptual framework, appropriate health statistics indicators can be established, and the relationship among different indicators can be defined. The framework is suitable for measuring the health of a population, health system performance and health-related factors. It has three characteristics: it defines necessary dimensions and subdimensions for

Table 26.3.1. Health indicators conceptual framework by international standards organization technical committee (ISO/TS 21667; 2010).

Health Status					↑
Well-being	Health Conditions		Human Function	Deaths	
Non-Medical Determinants of Health					
Health Behaviors	Socioeconomic Factors	Social and Community Factors	Environmental Factors	Genetic Factors	**Equity**
Health System Performance					
Acceptability	Accessibility		Appropriateness	Competence	
Continuity	Effectiveness		Efficiency	Safety	
Community and Health System Characteristics					
Resources	Population		Health System		↓

description of population health and health system performance; the framework is broad enough to adapt to changes in the health system; and, the framework has rich connotation, including population health, health system performance and related factors.

At present, other commonly used indicator frameworks include the OECD health system performance measurement framework and the World Health Organization (WHO) monitoring and evaluation framework. The OECD health indicators conceptual framework includes four dimensions, which are quality, responsiveness, efficiency and fairness, focusing on measuring health system performance. The WHO monitoring and evaluation framework includes four monitoring and evaluation sectors, which are inputs and processes, outputs, outcomes, and effect, aiming at better monitoring and evaluating system performance or specific projects. The framework will be different based on different description targets and the application scenarios of indicator systems, which can be chosen according to different purposes.

26.4. Hospital Statistics Indicators[5,6]

Hospital statistical indicators were generated with the advent of hospitals. In 1860, one of the topics of the Fourth International Statistical Conference was the "Miss Nightingale Hospital Statistics Standardization Program", and F Nightingale reported her paper on "hospital statistics". In 1862, Victoria Press published her book "Hospital Statistics and Hospital Planning", which was a sign of the formal establishment of the hospital statistics discipline. The first hospital statistical indicators primarily reflect the quantity of medical work, bed utilization and therapeutic effects. With the development of hospital management, statistical indicators gradually extended to reflect all aspects of overall hospital operation. Due to the different purposes of practical application, the statistical indicators of different countries, regions or organizations are diverse. The representative statistical indicators are:

The International Quality Indicator Project (IQIP) is the world's most widely used medical results monitoring indicator system, which is divided into four clinical areas: acute care, chronic care psychiatric rehabilitation, and home care with a total of 250 indicators. The user can choose indicators according to their needs.

The Healthcare Organizations Accreditation Standard by the Joint Accreditation Committee of U.S. Medical Institutions has two parts: the patient-centered standard and the medical institutions management standard, with a total of 11 chapters and 368 items. The patient-centered standard has five chapters: availability of continuous medical care, rights of patients and family members, patient's assessment, patient's medical care, and education for patients and families. The medical institutions management standard has six chapters: quality improvement and patient safety; prevention and control of infection; management departments, leadership and guidance; facilities management and security; staff qualification and education; information management. Each chapter has three entries, and each entry has core standards and non-core standards, of which the core standards are standards that medical institutions must achieve.

America's Best Hospitals Evaluation System emphasizes the equilibrium among structure, process, and results. Its specific structure indicators include medical technology projects undertaken (19 designated medical technologies, such as revascularization, cardiac catheter insertion surgery, and cardiac monitoring), number of discharges, proportion of full-time registered nurses and beds. The process indicator includes only the hospital's reputation scores. The outcome indicator includes only fatality. The calculated index value is called the "hospital quality index".

America's Top Hundred Hospitals Evaluation System has nine indicators: risk-adjusted mortality index; risk-adjusted complications index; diseases classification adjusted average length of stay; average medical cost; profitability; growth rate of community services; cash flow to total debt ratio; fixed asset value per capita; and rare diseases ratio.

In addition to the evaluation systems described above, international evaluation or accreditation standards with good effect and used by multiple countries include the international JCI standard, the international SQua standard, the Australia EQuIP standard and the Taiwan medical quality evaluation indicators.

26.5. Health Statistical Metadata[7–9]

Metadata is data which defines and describes other data. It provides the necessary information to understand and accurately interpret data, and it is the set of attributes used to illustrate data. Metadata is also data that can be stored in a database it can also be organized by data model. Health statistics metadata is the descriptive information on health statistics, including any information needed for human or systems on timely and proper use of health statistics during collection, reading, processing, expression, analysis, interpretation, exchange, searching, browsing and storage. In other words, health statistics metadata refers to any information that may influence and control people or software using health statistics. These include general definition, sample design, document description, database program, codebooks and classification structure, statistical processing details, data verification, conversion, statistical reporting, design and display of statistical tables. Health statistics metadata is found throughout the life cycle of health statistics, and includes a description of data at various stages from survey design to health statistics publication.

The purposes of health statistical metadata are (1) for the people: to support people to obtain the required data easily and quickly, and to have a proper understanding and interpretation; (2) for the computer: to have a well-structured and standardized form, to support machine processing data, and to facilitate information exchange between different systems.

The importance of health statistical metadata: (1) health statistics data sharing; (2) statistical data archiving: complete preservation of health statistical data and its metadata is the base for a secondary user to correctly use a health statistical data resource; (3) resource discovery: metadata can help users easily and quickly find the needed data, and determine the suitability of data; (4) accounting automation: health statistical metadata can provide the necessary parameters for the standardization of statistical processing, guiding statistical processes to achieve automation. Health statistical metadata sets up a semantic layer between health statistical resources and users (human or software agent), which plays an important role for accurate pinpointing of health statistical information, correct understanding and interpretation of data transmission exchange and integration.

Generation and management of statistical metadata occur throughout the entire life cycle of statistical data, and are very important for the long-term preservation and use of statistical data resources. If there is no accompanying metadata, the saved statistics cannot be secondarily analyzed and utilized. Therefore, during the process of statistical data analysis, much metadata should be captured, making statistical data and its metadata a complete information packet with long-term preservation, so as to achieve long-term access and secondary utilization.

26.6. World Health Statistics, WHS[10]

The World Health Statistics series is WHO's annual compilation of health-related data for its member states. These data are used internally by WHO for estimation, advocacy, policy development and evaluation. They are also widely disseminated in electronic and printed format. This publication focuses on a basic set of health indicators that were selected on the basis of current availability and quality of data and include the majority of health indicators that have been selected for monitoring progress towards the MDGs. Many health statistics have been computed by WHO to ensure comparability, using transparent methods and a clear audit trail.

The set of indicators is not intended to capture all relevant aspects of health but to provide a snapshot of the current health situation in countries. Importantly, the indicators in this set are not fixed — some will, over the years, be added or gain in importance while others may become less relevant. For example, the content is presented about both 2005 and 2015 in Table 26.6.1.

Table 26.6.1. The content about both 2005 and 2015.

2005
Part 1: World Health Statistics
Health Status Statistics: Mortality
Health Status Statistics: Morbidity
Health Services Coverage Statistics
Behavioral and Environmental Risk Factor Statistics
Health Systems Statistics
Demographic and Socio-economic Statistics
Part 2: World Health Indicators
Rationale for use
Definition
Associated terms
Data sources
Methods of estimation
Disaggregation
References
Database
Comments
2015
Part I. Health-related MDGs
Summary of status and trends
Summary of progress at country level
Part II. Global health indicators
General notes
Table 1. Life expectancy and mortality
Table 2. Cause-specific mortality and morbidity
Table 3. Selected infectious diseases
Table 4. Health service coverage
Table 5. Risk factors
Table 6. Health systems
Table 7. Health expenditure
Table 8. Health inequities
Table 9. Demographic and socio-economic statistics
Annex 1. Regional and income groupings

Several key indicators, including some health MDG indicators, are not included in this first edition of World Health Statistics, primarily because of data quality and comparability issues.

As the demand for timely, accurate and consistent information on health indicators continues to increase, users need to be well oriented on what exactly these numbers measure; their strengths and weaknesses; and, the assumptions under which they should be used. So, World Health Statistics cover these issues, presenting a standardized description of each health indicator, definition, data source, method of estimation, disaggregation, references to literature and databases.

26.7. Global Health Observatory, GHO[11]

GHO is WHO's gateway to health-related statistics from around the world. The aim of the GHO portal is to provide easy access to country specific data and statistics with a focus on comparable estimates, and WHO's analyses to monitor global, regional and country situation and trends.

The GHO country data include all country statistics and health profiles that are available within WHO. The GHO issues analytical reports on priority health issues, including the World Health Statistics annual publication, which compiles statistics for key health indicators. Analytical reports address cross-cutting topics such as women and health.

GHO theme pages cover global health priorities such as the health-related MDGs, mortality and burden of disease, health systems, environmental health, non-communicable diseases, infectious diseases, health equity and violence and injuries. The theme pages present

- highlights the global situation and trends, using regularly updated core indicators;
- data views customized for each theme, including country profiles and a map gallery;
- publications relevant to the theme; and
- links to relevant web pages within WHO and elsewhere.

The GHO database provides access to an interactive repository of health statistics. Users are able to display data for selected indicators, health topics, countries and regions, and download the customized tables in a Microsoft Excel format.

GHO theme pages provide interactive access to resources including data repository, reports, country statistics, map gallery and standards. The GHO data repository contains an extensive list of indicators, which can be selected by theme or through multidimension query functionality. It is the WHO's main health statistics repository. The GHO issues analytical reports on the current situation and trends for priority health issues. A key output of the GHO is the annual publication of World Health Statistics, which compiles statistics on key health indicators on an annual basis. World Health Statistics also include a brief report on annual progress towards the health-related MDGs. Lastly, the GHO provides links to specific disease or program reports with a strong analytical component. The country statistical pages bring together the main health data and statistics for each country, as compiled by WHO and partners in close consultation with Member States, and include descriptive and analytical summaries of health indicators for major health topics. The GHO map gallery includes an extensive list of maps on major health topics. Maps are classified by themes as below, and can be further searched by keyword. Themes include alcohol and health, child health, cholera, environmental health, global influenza virological surveillance, health systems financing, HIV/AIDS, malaria, maternal and reproductive health, meningococcal meningitis, mortality and Global Burden of Disease (GBD). The GHO standard is the WHO Indicator and Measurement Registry (IMR) which is a central source of metadata of health-related indicators used by WHO and other organizations. It includes indicator definitions, data sources, methods of estimation and other information that allows users to get a better understanding of their indicators of interest.

26.8. Healthy China 2020 Development Goals[12,13]

Healthy China 2020 is a Chinese national strategy directed by scientific development. The goals are maintenance and promotion of people's health, improving health equity, achieving coordinated development between socio-economic development and people's health based on public policy and major projects of China. The process is divided into three steps:

- The first, to 2010, establishes a basic healthcare framework covering urban and rural residents and achieving basic health care in China.
- The second step, to 2015, requires medical health services and healthcare levels to be in the lead of the developing countries.
- The third step, to 2020, aims to maintain China's position at the forefront of the developing world, and brings us close to or reaching the level of moderately developed countries in the Eastern area and part of the Midwest.

As one of the important measures in building a prosperous society, the goal of the Healthy China 2020 strategy is promoting the health of people. The emphasis is to resolve issues threatening urban and rural residents' health. The principle is to persist in combining both prevention and treatment, using appropriate technologies, mobilizing the whole society to participate, and strengthening interventions for the issues affecting people's health to ensure the achievement of the goal of all people enjoying basic health services.

The Healthy China 2020 strategy has built a comprehensive health development goal system reflecting the idea of scientific development. The goal is divided into 10 specific targets and 95 measurable detailed targets.

These objectives cover the health service system and its supporting conditions for protection and promotion of people's health. They are an important basis for monitoring and evaluating national health, and regulating health services. These specific objectives include:

(1) The major national health indicators will be improved further by 2020; the average life expectancy of 77 years, the mortality rate of children under five years of age dropping to 13%, the maternal mortality rate decreasing to 20/100,000, the differences in health decreasing among regional areas.
(2) Perfecting the health service system, improving healthcare accessibility and equity.
(3) Perfecting the medical security system and reducing residents' disease burden.
(4) Controlling of risk factors, decreasing the spread of chronic diseases and health hazards.
(5) Strengthening prevention and control of infectious and endemic diseases, reducing the hazards of infectious diseases.
(6) Strengthening of monitoring and supervision to ensure food and drug safety.
(7) Relying on scientific and technological progress, and adapting to the changing medical model, realizing the key forward, transforming integration strategy.
(8) Bringing traditional Chinese medicine into play in assuring peoples' health by inheritance and innovation of traditional Chinese medicine.
(9) Developing the health industry to meet the multilevel, diversified demand for health services.
(10) Performing government duties, increasing health investment, by 2020, total health expenditure-GDP ratio of 6.5–7%.

26.9. Chinese National Health Indicators System[14,15]

The National Health Indicators System is a set of indicators about the health status of a population, health system performance and health-related determinants. Each of the indicators set can reflect some characteristic of the target system. These indicators are closely related. They are complementary to each other or mutually restrained. This health indicator system is a comprehensive, complete and accurate indicators system for description of the target system.

In 2007, in order to meet the needs of health reform and development, the Health Ministry of the People's Republic of China developed a national health statistical indicators system. The indicators system included 215 indicators covering health status, prevention and healthcare, medical services, health supervision and health resources. Each of the indicators was described from the perspectives of investigation method, scope, frequency, reporting method, system of data collection and competent authorities.

National health indicator data for China come from the national health statistical survey system and some special surveys, such as the National Nutrition and Health Survey which takes place every 10 years, and the National Health Services Survey which takes place every 5 years.

In order to make better use of statistical indicators, and enhance comparability of statistical indicators at the regional, national and international level, standardization of statistical indicators is required. At present, Statistical Data and Metadata Exchange (SDMX, ISO/TS 17369: 2005) is the international standard accepted and used widely. For effective management and coordination of its Member States, according to SDMX, WHO has developed an IMR which provides a metadata schema for standardization and structural description of statistical indicators. IMR is able to coordinate and manage the definitions and code tables relating to indicators, and maintain consistent definitions across different statistical domains. The National Health and Family Planning Commission of China conducted research relating to Chinese national health statistical indicators metadata standards according to WHO IMR. The results will be released as a health industry standard.

The national health statistical indicators system and its metadata standards will be significant for data collection, analysis and use, publishing and management. The health statistical indicators system is not static. It must be revised and improved according to the requirements of national health reform and development in order to meet the information requirements of administrators, decision makers and the public, making it better in supporting management and decision making.

26.10. Civil Registration System[16,17]

The civil registration system is a government data repository providing information on important life events, a series of laws and regulations, statistics, and information systems. It includes all the legal and technical aspects when civil registration needs to be fulfilled based on a country's specific culture and social situations by the standard of coordination and reliability.

The United Nations defines civil registration as the continuous, permanent, compulsory and universal recording of the occurrence and characteristics of vital events pertaining to the population as provided through decree or regulation in accordance with the legal requirements of a country. Vital events include live birth, death, foetal death, marriage, divorce, annulment of marriage, judicial separation of marriage, adoption, legitimization and recognition. Civil registration is the registration of birth, death, marriage and other important issues. Its basic purpose is to provide the legal identity of the individual, ensuring people's civil rights and human rights. At the same time, these records are the best source of the statistics of life, which can be used to describe population changes, and the health conditions of a country or a region.

Individual civil registration includes legal documents such as birth certificate, marriage certificate, and death certificate. Family registration is a type of civil registration, which is more concerned with events within the family unit and very common in Continental Europe and Asian countries, such as Germany, France, Spain, Russia, China (Hukou), Japan (household registration), and South Korea (Hoju). In addition, in some countries, immigration, emigration, and any change of residence also need to be registered. Resident registration is a major concern for current residential civil registration.

Complete, accurate and timely civil registration is essential for quality vital statistics. The civil registration system is the most reliable source of birth, death and death cause. When a country's civil registration system is perfect, information relating to death reports and causes of death is accurate. Those countries which did not establish a perfect civil registration system often have only a few rough concepts relating to their population, life and health.

The Global Disease Study by the WHO divided death data rates around the world into 4 grades and 8 sections, and special death data quality into 4 grades and 6 sections. Sweden was the first nation to establish a nationwide register of its population in 1631. This register was organized and carried out by the Church of Sweden but on the demand of The Crown. The civil registration system, from the time it was carried out by the church to its development today, has experienced a history of more than 300 years. The United Nations agencies have set international standards and guidelines for the establishment of the civil registration system.

At present, China's civil registration system mainly includes the children's birth registration information system, the maternal and child healthcare information system based on the maternal and childcare service center, the cause of registration system from the Centers for Disease Control and Prevention, and the Residents' health records information system based in the provincial health department.

26.11. Vital Statistics[18]

Vital statistics are statistical activity for population life events. They contain information about live births, deaths, fetal deaths, marriages, divorces and civil status changes. Vital statistics activities can be summed up as the original registration of vital statistics events, data sorting, statistics and analysis.

The most common way of collecting information on vital events is through civil registration. So vital statistics will be closely related to the development of civil registration systems in countries. The United Nations Children's Fund (UNICEF) and a number of non-governmental organizations (Plan International, Save the Children Fund, World Vision, etc.) have particularly promoted registration from the aspect of human rights, while the United Nations Statistics Division (UNSD), the United Nations Population Fund (UNFPA) and the WHO have focused more on the statistical aspects of civil registration.

In western countries, early birth and death records are often stored in churches. English demographer and health statistician J Graunt firstly studied the survival probability of different ages based on death registration by using life tables, and then did some research on how to use statistical methods to estimate the population of London.

The government's birth and death records originated in the early 19th century. In England and Wales, both parliaments passed birth and death registration legislation and set up the General Register Office in 1836. The death registration system of the General Register Office played a key role in controlling the cholera epidemic in London in 1854. It opened government decision making and etiological study by using the statistical data of vital statistics. Vital statistics includes fertility, maternal and child health, death statistics and demography.

Fertility statistics describe and analyze fertility status from the perspective of quantity. Common statistical indicators for measuring fertility are crude birth rate, general fertility rate, age-specific rate, and total fertility rate. Indicators for measuring reproduction fertility are natural increasing gross reproduction rate, and net reproduction rate. Indicators for measuring birth control and abortion mainly include contraceptive prevalence rate, contraceptive failure rate, pearl pregnancy rate, cumulative failure rate and induced abortion rate.

Maternal and child health statistics mainly study the health of women and children, especially maternal and infant health issues. Common indicators for maternal and child health statistics are infant mortality rate, newborn mortality rate, post-neonatal mortality rate, perinatal mortality rate, mortality rate of children under 5-years, maternal mortality rate, antenatal examination rate, hospitalized deliver rate, postnatal Interview rate, rate of systematic management children under 3-years, and rate of systematic maternal management.

Death statistics mainly study death level, death cause and its changing rule. Common indicators for death statistics include crude death rate, age-specific death rate, infant mortality rate, newborn mortality rate, perinatal mortality rate, cause-specific death rate, fatality rate, and proportion of dying of a specific cause.

Medical demography describes and analyzes the change, distribution, structure, and regularity of population from the point of view of healthcare. Common indicators for medical demography are population size, demographic characteristics, and indictors on population structure, such as sex ratio, old population coefficient, children and adolescents coefficient, and dependency ratio.

26.12. Death Registry[19,20]

Death registration studies mortality, death causes and its changing rule of residents. It can reflect a country or a region's resident health status, and provide scientific basis for setting up health policy and evaluating the quality and effects of health work. Accurate and reliable death information is of great significance for a nation or a region to formulate population policies, and determine the allocation of resources and key intervention.

In order to meet the needs of communication and comparison among different countries and regions, and to meet the needs of the various statistical analyses in different periods, the WHO requires its members to code and classify the cause of death according to the international classification of diseases and use "underlying death cause", and have a unified format of the international medical death certificate. The definition of underlying death cause is (1) illness or injury, which directly leads to the death of the first in a series of pathological events, (2) Lethal damage accidents or violence.

Although different nations have different cause-and-death information report processes, different personnel responsibilities are clearly defined by the relevant laws and regulations in order to ensure the completeness and accuracy of cause-and-death information reports.

The developed countries, such as the United States and the United Kingdom, usually have higher economic levels, and more reliable laws and regulations. They collect information on vital events such as birth, death, marriage, and divorce through civil registration. In developing countries, owing to the lack of complete cause-and-death registration systems, death registration coverage is not high. Death registration is the basis of a death registry. According to China's death registration report system, all medical and health departments must fill out a medical death certificate as part of their medical procedures. As original credentials for cause of death statistics, the certificate has legal effect. Residents' disease, injury and cause of death information becomes part of legal statistical reports, jointly formulated by the National Health and Family Planning Commission and the Ministry of Public Security, and approved by the National Bureau of Statistics.

In China, all medical institutions at or above the county level must report the related information on deaths in the direct form of the network, and complete cause of death data by using the National Disease Prevention and Control Information System. Then the Center for Health Statistics and Information, and the National Health and Family Planning Commission will report, publishing the information in the annual report after sorting and analyzing the collected data.

Death investigations must be carried out when the following situations happen: the cause of death is not clear, or does not conform to the requirements of the unified classification of cause of death, or is difficult to classify according to the international classification of diseases; the basis of autopsy is not enough or not logical. Memory bias should be avoided in death investigation. In addition, cause of death data can be obtained by death review in the district without a perfect death registration report system, or can be collected by a special death investigation for a particular purpose. All measures above are necessary supplements to a death registration and report.

26.13. Health Service Survey[2,21]

A health service survey, carried out by health administrative departments at all levels, refers to a sampling survey of information about residents' health status, health service demand and utilization, and healthcare costs. A health service survey is essential for national health resource planning and health service management, and its fundamental purpose is to evaluate the health service, to ensure health services reach the expected standard, and provide the basis for improving health services. The findings of the health service survey are important for the government to formulate a health policy and health career development plan, to improve the level of health management, and to promote national health reform and development.

The health service survey is widespread, not only including all aspects of the health service accepted by residents, such as their experience of and feelings about health services, their demand for health services as well as the suitability of health services, efficiency, and the evaluation of medical and healthcare costs, the special needs of key groups in health services and the situation of meet, but also including the information of grass-roots health institutions and health service staff, such as medical staff work characteristics, work experience and practice environment.

The quality of survey data can be judged by internal logical relationships, or evaluated by the representation of the four indicators, the leaf index, the test of goodness fit, the Delta similarity coefficient and the Gini concentration.

In the 1950s, the United States and other western countries established health services research, the emphasis of which was on the continuity of health inquiry. In the 1970s, Britain, Canada, Japan and other developed countries gradually established health inquiry systems.

In recent years, some developing countries have conducted one-time or repetitive cross-sectional sample health service surveys. The National Health Service survey started relatively late in China, but development was fast and the scale was wide. Since 1993, there has been a national health services survey every 5 years.

The main contents of investigation include population and socio-economic characteristics of urban and rural residents, urban and rural residents health service needs, health service demands and utilization by urban and rural residents, urban and rural residents' medical security, residents satisfaction, key groups such as children under the age of five and childbearing women aged 15–49 in special need of health services, medical staff work characteristics, work experience, practice environment, county, township and village health institutions HR basic situation, personnel service capabilities, housing and main equipment, balance of payments, services, and quantity and quality. National Health Service survey methods can be divided into two categories, sampling surveys and project surveys.

Sampling surveys include family health inquiry, grassroots medical institutions, and a medical personnel questionnaire. The unified survey time is formulated by the nation. The project survey is a pointer to a special investigation and study, such as the ability of grassroots health human resources and services, grassroots health financing and incentive mechanism, doctor–patient relationships, and new rural cooperative medical research. The project survey is carried out in a different survey year according to the requirements.

26.14. Life Tables[22]

In 1662, John Graunt proposed the concept of life expectancy tables when he analyzed mortality data from London. In 1693, Edmund Halley published the first Breslaw city life table. After the mid-18th century, the U.S. and Europe had developed life tables.

A life table is a statistical table which is based on a population's age-specific death rates, indicating the human life or death processes of a specific population. Due to their different nature and purpose, life tables can be divided into current life tables and cohort life tables. From a cross-sectional study observing the dying process of a population, current life tables are one of the most common and important methods which can be used to evaluate the health status of a population. However, cohort life table longitudinally studies the life course of a population, which is mainly used in epidemiological, clinical and other studies. Current life tables can be divided into complete life tables and abridged life tables. In complete life tables, the age of 1-year-old is taken as a group, and in abridged life tables the age group is a group of teens, but the 0-year-old age group is taken as an independent group. With the popularization and application of the life table, in the medical field there is deriving a cause eliminated life table, an occupational life table, and a no disability life table.

Key in preparing a life table is to calculate death probability in different age groups by using an age-specific death rate. Popular methods include the Reed–Merrell method, the Greville method and the Chin Long Chiang method. In 1981, WHO recommended the method of Chin Long Chiang for all member countries. The main significance and calculation of the life table function are as follows:

(1) Death probability of age group: refers to the death probability of the generation born at the same time that died in a certain age group $x \sim (x+n)$, indicated as ${}_nq_x$, where x refers to age (years), n refers to the length of the age interval. The formula is

$$ {}_nq_x = \frac{2 \times n \times {}_nm_x}{2 + n \times {}_nm_x}. $$

${}_nm_x$ is the mortality of the age group $x \sim (x+n)$. Usually, the death probability at 0-year-old is estimated by infant mortality or adjusted infant mortality.

(2) Number of deaths: refers to the number of people who were alive at x, but died in the age interval $x \sim (x+n)$.

(3) Number of survivors: also called surviving number, it represents the number of people who survive at age x.

The relationship of number of survivors l_x, the number of deaths ${}_nd_x$, and the probability of death ${}_nq_x$ are as follows:

$$ {}_nd_x = l_x \cdot {}_nq_x, \quad l_{x+n} = l_x + {}_nd_x. $$

(4) Person-year of survival: it refers to the total person-years that the x-year-old survivors still survive in the next n years, denoted by ${}_nL_x$. For the Infant group, the person-year of survival is $L_0 = l_1 + a_0 \times d_0, a_0$ is a constant generated based on historical data. The formula for age group $x \sim (x+n)$, $x \neq 0$, is ${}_nL_x = n(l_x + l_{x+n})/2$.

(5) Total person-year of survival: it refers to the total person-years that x-year-old survivors still survive in the future, denoted by T_x. We have $T_x = {}_nL_x + {}_nL_{x+n} + \cdots = \sum_k {}_nL_{x+kn}$.

(6) Life expectancy: it refers to the expected years that an x-year-old survivor will still survive, denoted by e_x, we have $e_x = T_x/l_x$. Life expectancy is also called expectation of life. Life expectancy at birth, e_0, is an important indicator to comprehensively evaluate a country or region in terms of socio-economics, living standards and population health.

26.15. Healthy Life Expectancy (HALE)[23,24]

In 1964, Sanders first introduced the concept of disability into life expectancy and proposed effective life years. Sullivan first used disability-free life expectancy (DFLE) in 1971, and put forward the calculation of life expectancy through synthesizing mortality and morbidity. In 1983, Katz first proposed active life expectancy to represent the sustaining expected life for elderly people with activities of daily living that can be maintained in good condition. In the same year, Wilkins and Adams pointed out that the drawback of DFLE was using dichotomy weighted scores so that no matter what state, as long as there was a disability, it was given a zero score, causing sensitivity in distinguishing the degree of disability. They proposed to give the appropriate weight according to different disability levels, and converted the number of life-years in various states into equivalent number of years living in a completely healthy state, accumulated to form the disability-adjusted life expectancy (DALE). DALE comprehensively considers the impact of disability and death to health, so it can more accurately measure the health level of a population. The World Bank proposed the disability-adjusted life year (DALY) in 1992 and Hyder put forward healthy life years in 1998; both of these further improved HALE. The WHO applied more detailed weight classification to improve the calculation of DALE in 2001, and renamed it to HALE.

In a life table, the person-year of survival ${}_nL_x$ in age-specific group $x \sim (x+n)$ includes two states, H (healthy survival, disease-free and disability) and SD (survival, illness or disability). Assuming that the proportion of state SD is ${}_{SD}R_x$, and the person-years of survival with state H is ${}_nH_x = {}_nL_x(1 - {}_{SD}R_x)$. The life expectancy ${}_He_x$ is calculated according to the life table which is prepared by ${}_nH_x$ and mortality of each age group m_x, and ${}_He_x$ as the HALE for each age group, indicating that the life expectancy of a population has been maintained in state H.

The complexity of a healthy life is mainly in defining the status of SD and estimating the ${}_{SD}R_x$ which is stratified by gender. And the easiest way is that SD is dichotomy, ${}_{SD}R_x$ and is estimated by the prevalence of chronic disease that are stratified by sex, and age group. However, the healthy survival person-years needs to be weighted when the SD has multiple classifications. For example, when the ${}_{SD}R_x$ has no change in a given age group, according to the severity of disability classification and corresponding weights (W_j), the estimated value of ${}_nH_x$ is: ${}_nH_x = (1 - {}_{SD}R_x)\sum W_{in}L_i$.

HALE considers the non-complete healthy state caused by a disease and/or disability. It is able to integrate morbidity and mortality into a whole, and more effectively takes into account the quality of life. It is currently the most-used and representative evaluation and measurement indicator of disease burden.

26.16. Quality-adjusted Life Years (QALYs)[25,26]

With the progress of society and medicine, people not only require prolonged life expectancy, but also want to improve their quality of life. As early as 1968, Herbert and his colleagues had proposed the concept of quality-adjusted life year, and this was the first time of consolidation for survival time and quality of life. It was based on the descriptive indicators which integrated survival time and the physical ability that conducted by economists, operational researchers and psychologists in 1960s, and it had been used in "health state index study" in 1970s. In the 1980s, the definition of quality-adjusted life year was actually brought forward. Phillips and Thompson analyzed that it was a formula used to evaluate treatment, change quality of life and quantity brought by care. Malek defined the quality-adjusted life year as a method of measuring results, which considers both the quantity and quality of the life year prolonged by healthcare interventions; it is the mathematical product of life expectancy and quality of remaining life years. Fanshel and Bush noted that quality-adjusted life year was different from other health outcome indicators, which include not only the length of survival or life, but also disease, or quality of life. Since the 1990s, quality-adjusted life year has become the reference standard of cost-effectiveness analysis.

The calculation of quality-adjusted life year (1) describe the health status, (2) establish the score value of health status, that is, the weights of health-related quality of life w_i; (3) integrate the different health status score w_i and corresponding life y_i, then calculate QALYs $= \sum w_i y_i$.

So far, the measurement tools which are used to assess health status are the Good State Quality Scale, the Health Utilities Index, Health and Activity Limitation Indicators and the European Five Dimension Quality of Life Scale. Because different measurement tools describe various constituent elements of health, the overall evaluation of health status is different. At present, there is still a lack of a universally accepted gold standard for comparison of the results.

There are two categories of confirming weights of quality of life, the first is proposed by Williams. He thought the quality of life weights are decided by certain social and political groups or policy decision-makers, and there is no need to reflect individual preferences, which aims to maximize policy makers' preset targets. The second category was suggested by Torrance, and he thought that the weight measurements of quality of life should be based on preferences of health status, and his advocates include three specific calculation methods: the Grade Scale Method, the Standard Game Method and the Time Trade-off Method.

The advantages of quality-adjusted life year is that quality-adjusted life year alone can represent the gains which extend and improve the quality of life, and can explain why people have different value preferences of different results. It can confirm that patients get benefits of quantity and quality of prolonged life from health services, making sure of the utilization and the allocation of resources to achieve maximum benefit.

26.17. DALY[27,28]

To measure the combined effects of death and disability caused by disease to health, there must be a measurement unit which can be applicable for both death and disability. In the 1990s, with the support of the World Bank and the WHO, when the Harvard University research team conducted their GBD study, they presented the DALY. DALY consists of Years of Life Lost (YLL) which is caused by premature death and Years Lived with Disability (YLD) which is caused by disability. Single DALY is loss of healthy life year only. The biggest advantage of DALY includes not only considering the burden of disease caused by premature death. It also takes into account the burden of disease due to disability. The unit of DALY is in years, so that fatal and non-fatal health outcomes can be compared in terms of seriousness at the same scale. And it provides a comparison method to compare the burden of disease in different diseases, ages, genders and regions.

DALY is constituted of four aspects, the healthy life years that are lost by premature death, non-healthy life years under disease and disability state which are measured and converted in relation to the healthy life years lost by death, the relative importance of age and time of healthy life year (age weight, time discount), and it is calculated as: DALY $= \frac{KDCe^{-\beta a}}{(\beta+\gamma)^2}[(e^{-(\beta+\gamma)}(1+(\beta+\gamma)(l+a))-(1+(\beta+\gamma)a)]+\frac{D(1-K)}{\gamma}(1-e^{rl})$. Among which, D means disability weight (the value between 0 and 1, 0 represents health, 1 represents death), γ: discount rate, a: age of incidence or death, l: loss of life expectancy year due to disability duration or premature death; β: age weight coefficient, C: continuous adjustment coefficient, K: sensitivity analysis of age weights parameters (basic values is 1).

This formula calculates the DALY loss for an individual aged a sufferer of a particular disease, or death at age a due to a disease. In the study of disease burden and the DALY calculation formula, the parameters γ value is 0.03, β value is 0.04, K value is 1, C value is 0.1658. When $D = 1$, that is the formula of YLL; when D is between 0 and 1, that is the formula for YLD. For a disease in a crowd, its formula is DALY = YLL + YLD.

DALY considers death and disability, which more fully reflects the actual situation of the disease burden that can be used to compare the cost-effectiveness of different interventions. Using the cost of a relatively healthy saved life can not only help evaluate the technical efficiency of interventions, but also the efficiency of resource allocation.

26.18. Women's Health Indicator[11,29,30]

Reproductive health is a state of complete physical, mental and social well-being, and not merely the absence of disease or infirmity, in all matters relating to the reproductive system and to its function and processes.

Women's health, with reproductive health as a core and focus on disease prevention and healthcare, is carried out throughout the entire process of a woman's life (puberty — premarital period — perinatal period — perimenopause — old age) in order to maintain and promote women's physical and mental health, reduce prenatal and neonatal mortality and disability in pregnant women and newborn babies, to control the occurrence of disease and genetic disease, and halt the spread of sexually transmitted diseases.

Women's health statistics are used to evaluate the quality of women's health with statistical indicators based on comprehensive analysis on available information to provide evidence for work planning and scientific research development. Common indicators used to assess women's health in China are as follows:

(1) Screening and treatment of gynecological diseases: core indicators include the census rate of gynecological diseases, the prevalence of gynecological diseases, and the cure rate of gynecological diseases.
(2) Maternal healthcare coverage: core indicators include the rate of prenatal care coverage, prenatal care, postpartum visit and hospital delivery.
(3) Quality of maternal healthcare: core indicators include the incidence of high-risk pregnant women, hypertensive disorders in pregnancy, postpartum hemorrhage, puerperal infection, and perineum rupture.
(4) Performance of maternal healthcare: core indicators include the perinatal mortality, maternal mortality, neonatal mortality, and early neonatal mortality.

The WHO has developed a unified concept definition and calculation method of reproductive health and women's health indicators used commonly in order to facilitate comparison among different countries and regions. Besides the indicators mentioned above, it also includes: adolescent fertility rate (per 1,000 girls aged 15–19 years), unmet need for family planning (%), contraceptive prevalence, crude birth rate (per 1,000 population), crude death rate (per 1,000 population), annual population growth rate (%), antenatal care coverage — at least four visits (%), antenatal care coverage — at least one visit (%), births by caesarean section (%), births attended by skilled health personnel (%), stillbirth rate (per 1,000 total births), postnatal care visit within two days of childbirth (%), maternal mortality ratio (per 100,000 live births), and low birth weight (per 1,000 live births).

26.19. Growth Curve[30,32]

The most common format for the anthropometry-based gender-specific growth curve consists of a family of plotting curves with values which combine with mean ($\bar{x}$) and standard deviations (SD) or selected percentiles of given growth indicators, starting at $\bar{x} - 2SD$ (or 3rd percentile) as the lowest curve and with $\bar{x}$ + 2SD (or 97th percentile) as the highest. The curves with entire age range of interest scaled in the x-axis and growth indicators scaled in the y-axis are made up of common used intervals ($\bar{x}$ − 2SD, $\bar{x}$ − 1SD, $\bar{x}$, $\bar{x}$ + 1SD, $\bar{x}$ + 2SD) or consist of 3rd, 10th, 25th, 50th, 75th, 90th, 97th percentiles. Growth curves can be used to assess growth patterns in individuals or in a population compared with international, regional or country-level "growth reference", and help to detect growth-related health and/or nutrition problems earlier, such as growth faltering, malnutrition, overweightness and obesity.

For individual-based application, a growth curve based on continuous and dynamic anthropometry measurement including weight and height should be used as a screening and monitoring tool to assess child growth status, growth velocity and growth pattern by comparing it with a "Growth reference curve".

For population-based application, a growth curve based on age- and gender-specific mean or median curve can be used adequately for cross-comparison and monitoring time trend of growth by comparing it with the mean or median curve from the "Growth reference curve".

Growth curves provide a simple and convenient approach with graphic results to assess the growth of children, and can be used for ranking growth level, monitoring growth velocity and trends, and comparing growth patterns in individuals or in a population. Growth curves should be constructed based on different genders and different growth indicators separately. They cannot evaluate several indicators at the same time, nor can they evaluate the symmetry of growth.

Currently, WHO Child Growth Standards (length/height-for-age, weight-for-age, weight-for-height, body mass index-for-age), are the most commonly used growth reference and are constructed by combining a percentile method and a curve graph, providing a technically robust tool that represents the best description of physiological growth for children and adolescents, and can be used to assess children everywhere. For individual-based assessment, a growth curve can be used, ranking a child development level as "$< P_3$", "$P_3 \sim P_{25}$", "$P_{25} \sim P_{75}$", "$P_{75} \sim P_{97}$" or "$> P_{97}$" by comparing the actual anthropometry measurement of a child, such as weight and/or height, with cut-off values of 3rd, 25th, 50th, 75th, and 97th percentiles from the "reference curve". As a visually and intuitive method, a growth curve is suitable for accurate and dynamic assessment of growth development.

For population-based assessment, P_{50} an individual curve or a curve combined with other percentile curves including P_{10}, P_{25}, P_{75} and P_{90} can be used not only to compare the regional differences of child growth in the same time period but also to indicate the trend of child growth over a long time period.

26.20. Child Physical Development Evaluation[33,34]

The Child Physical Development Evaluation consists of four aspects of content which are the level of growth and development, velocity of growth, development evenness and physique synthetic evaluation. These are used not only for the individual but also for groups. Commonly used evaluation methods are as follows:

(1) Index method: Two or more indicators can be transformed into one index. There are three types of index commonly used: the habitus index (Livi index, Ratio of sitting height to height, Ratio of basin width to shoulder width, and the Erisman index and so on), the nutritional index (Quetelet index, BMI, Rohrer index) and the functional index (Ratio of grip strength to body weight, Ratio of back muscle strength to body weight, Ratio of vital capacity to height, and Ratio of vital capacity to body weight).
(2) Rank value method: The developmental level of an individual on a given reference distribution can be ranked according to the distance between standard deviation and mean of a given anthropometry indicator. The rank value of developmental of an individual is stated in terms of the rank of the individual in the reference distribution with the same age and gender.
(3) Curve method: The Curve method is a widely used model to display evolution of physical development over time. A set of gender and age-specific

reference values, such as mean, mean ±1 standard deviation, and mean ±2 standard deviation, can be plotted on a graph, and then a growth reference curve can be developed by connecting the reference values in the same rank position by a smoothed curve over age. Commonly, a growth reference curve should be drawn by difference gender. For individual evaluation, a growth curve can be produced by plotting and connecting the consecutive anthropometry measurements (weight or height) into a smooth curve. A growth curve can be used not only to evaluate physical developmental status, but also to analyze the velocity of growth and growth pattern.

(4) Percentile method: Child growth standards (for height, weight and BMI), which were developed by utilizing a percentile method and curve method combined, became the primary approach to child physical development evaluation by the WHO and most counties currently. For individual application, physical developmental status can be evaluated by the position which individual height or weight is located in the reference growth chart.

(5) Z standard deviation score: Z score can be calculated as the deviation of the value for an individual from the mean/median value of the reference population, divided by the standard deviation for the reference population: $Z = \frac{x-\bar{x}}{s}$, then a reference range can be developed by using ±1, ±2, ±3 as cutoff points. By means of these procedures, the development level can be ranked as follows: >2 top; $1 \sim 2$ above average; $-1 \sim 1$ average; $-1 \sim -2$ below average, and; < -2 low.

(6) Growth velocity method: Growth velocity is a very important indicator for growth and health status. Height, weight and head circumference are most commonly involved in growth velocity evaluation. The growth velocity method can be used for individual, population-based or growth development comparison among different groups. The most commonly used method for individual evaluation is growth monitor charts.

(7) Assessment of development age: Individual development status can be evaluated according to a series of standard developmental ages and their normal reference range which are constructed by using indicators of physical morphology, physiological function, and secondary sex characteristic development level. Development age includes morphological age, secondary sexual characteristic age, dental age, and skeletal age.

In addition, another technique including the correlation and regression method and assessment of nutritional status can be involved in evaluation of child growth and development.

References

1. Millennium Development Goals Indicators. The United Nations site for the MDG Indicators. 2007. http://millenniumindicators.un.org/unsd/mdg/Host.aspx?Content=Indicators/About.htm.
2. Bowling, A. Research Methods in Health: Investigating Health and Health Services. New York: McGraw-Hill International, 2009.
3. National Health and Family Planning Commission. *2013 National Health and Family Planning Survey System*. Beijing: China Union Medical University Press, 2013.
4. ISO/TC 215 Health informatics, 2010. http://www.iso.org/iso/standards_ development/technical_committees/list_of_iso_technical_committees/iso_technical_committee.htm?commid=54960.
5. AHA Hospital Statistics, 2015. Health Forum, 2015.
6. Ouircheartaigh, c, Burke, C, Murphy, W. The 2004 Index of Hospital Quality, U.S. News & World Report's "America's Best Hospitals" study, 2004.
7. Westlake, A. The MetNet Project. *Proceedings of the 1'st MetaNet Conference*, 2–4 April, 2001.
8. Appel, G. A Metadata driven statistical information system. In: EUROSTAT (ed.) *Proc. Statistical Meat-Information Systems*. Luxembourg: Office for Official Publications, 993; pp. 291–309.
9. Wang Xia. *Study on Conceptual Model of Health Survey Metadata*. Xi'an: Shaanxi: Fourth Military Medical University, 2006.
10. WHO, World Health Statistics. http://www.who.int/gho/publications/world_health_statistics/en/ (Accessed on September 8, 2015).
11. WHO, Global Health Observatory (GHO). http://www.who.int/gho/indicator_ registry/en/ (Accessed on September 8, 2015).
12. Chen Zhu. The implementation of Healthy China 2020 strategy. *China Health*; 2007, (12): 15–17.
13. Healthy China 2020 Strategy Research Report Editorial Board. *Healthy China 2020 Strategy Research Report*. Beijing: People's Medical Publishing House, 2012.
14. Statistics and Information Center of Ministry of Health of China. The National health statistical Indicators System. http://www.moh.gov.cn/mohbgt/pw10703/200804/18834.shtml. Accessed on Augest 25, 2015.
15. WHO Indicator and Measurement Registry. http://www.who.int/gho/indicatorregi stry (Accessed on September 8, 2015).
16. Handbook on Training in Civil Registration and Vital Statistics Systems. http://unstats.un.org/unsd/demographic/ standmeth/handbooks.
17. United Nations Statistics Division: Civil registration system. http://unstats.un.org/UNSD/demographic/sources/civilreg/default.htm.
18. Vital statistics (government records). https://en.wikipedia.org/wiki/Vital_ statistics _(government_records).
19. Dong, J. *International Statistical Classification of Diseases and Related Health Problems*. Beijing: People's Medical Publishing House, 2008.
20. International Classification of Diseases (ICD). http://www.who.int/classifications/icd/en/.
21. Shang, L. *Health Management Statistics*. Beijing: China Statistics Press, 2014.
22. Chiang, CL. The Life Table and Its Applications. Malabar, FL: Krieger, 1984: 193–218.
23. Han Shengxi, Ye Lu. The development and application of Healthy life expectation. *Health Econ. Res.*, 2013, 6: 29–31.

24. Murray, CLM, Lopez, AD. *The Global Burden of Disease*. Boston: Harvard School of Public Health, 1996.
25. Asim, O, Petrou, S. Valuing a QALY: Review of current controversies. *Expert Rev. Pharmacoecon Outcome Res.*, 2005, 5(6): 667–669.
26. Han Shengxi, Ye Lu. The introduction and commentary of Quality-adjusted life year. *Drug Econ.*, 2012, 6: 12–15.
27. Murray, CJM. Quantifying the burden of disease: The technical basis for disability-adjusted life years. *Bull. World Health Organ*, 1994, 72(3): 429–445.
28. Zhou Feng. Comparison of three health level indicators: Quality-adjusted life year, disablity-adjusted life year and healthy life expectancy. *Occup. Environ. Med.*, 2010, 27(2): 119–124.
29. *WHO. Countdown to 2015. Monitoring Maternal, Newborn and Child Health: Understanding Key Progress Indicators*. Geneva: World Health Organization, 2011. http://apps.who.int/iris/bitstream/10665/44770/1/9789241502818_eng.pdf, accessed 29 March 2015.
30. Chinese Students' Physical and Health Research Group. *Dynamic Analysis on Physical Condition of Han Chinese Students During the 20 Years Since the Reform and Opening Up. Chinese Students' Physical and Health Survey Report in 2000*. Beijing: Higher Education Press, 2002.
31. Xiao-xian Liu. *Maternal and Child Health Information Management Statistical Manual/Maternal and Child Health Physicians Books*. Beijing: Pecking Union Medical College Press, 2013.
32. WHO Multicentre Growth Reference Study Group. WHO Child Growth Standards: Length/Height-for-Age, Weight-for-Age, Eight-for-Length, Weight-for-Height and Body Mass Index-for-Age: Methods and development. Geneva: World Health Organization, [2007-06-01]. http://www.who.int/zh.
33. Hui, Li. Research progress of children physical development evaluation. *Chinese J. Child Health Care*, 2013, 21(8): 787–788.
34. WHO. *WHO Global Database on Child Growth and Malnutrition*. Geneva: WHO, 1997.

About the Author

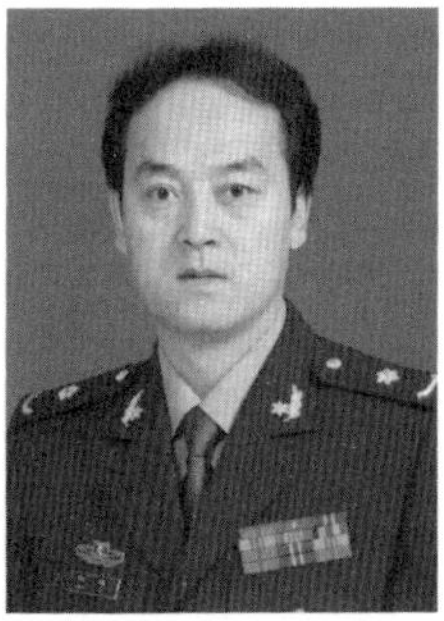

Lei Shang PhD, Professor, Deputy Director in, Department of Health Statistics, Fourth Military Medical University. Dr. Shang has worked on health statistics' teaching and research for 24 years. His main study interests are statistic method in child growth and development evaluation, statistic in health management, children's health-related behaviors evaluation, etc. He is a standing member of Hospital Statistics Branch Association, a member of Statistical Theory and Method Branch Association of Chinese Health Information Association, a member of Health Statistics Branch Association of Chinese Preventive

Medicine Association, a standing member of Biostatistics Branch Association of Chinese Statistics Education Association, a standing member of PLA Health Information Association. An editorial board member of *Chinese Journal of Health Statistics and Chinese Journal of Child Health.* In recent years, he has got 11 research projects, including in National Natural Science Foundation, etc. He has published 63 papers in national or international journals as the first or corresponding author, among these papers, 28 papers were published in international journals. As an editor-in-chief, he has published two professional books. As a key member, he got the first prize at National Science and Technology Progress Awards in 2010.

INDEX